FOURTH EDITION

INFORMATICS and NURSING: OPPORTUNITIES and CHALLENGES

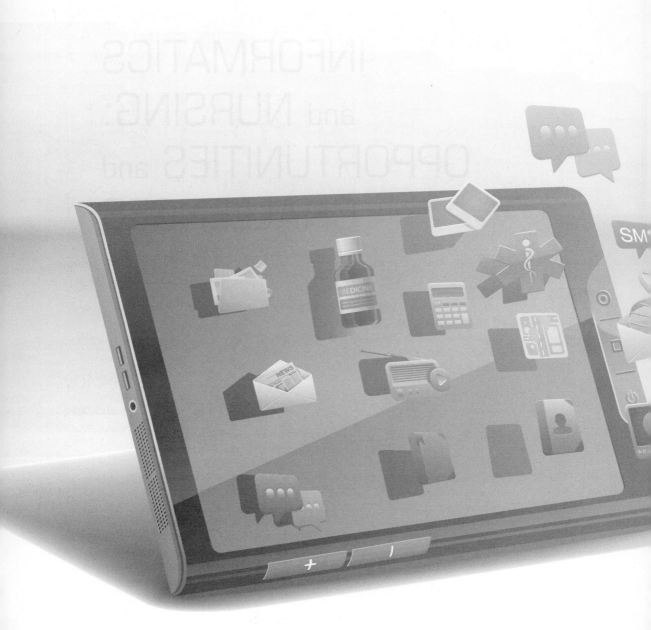

FOURTH EDITION

INFORMATICS and NURSING: OPPORTUNITIES and CHALLENGES

Jeanne Sewell, MSN, RN

Assistance Professor, School of Nursing
College of Health Sciences
Georgia College & State University, Milledgeville, GA

Linda Q. Thede, PhD, RN-BC

Editor, *CIN: Computers, Informatics, Nursing Plus*
Lippincott, Williams & Wilkins, Philadelphia, PA

Wolters Kluwer | Lippincott Williams & Wilkins
Health

Philadelphia • Baltimore • New York • London
Buenos Aires • Hong Kong • Sydney • Tokyo

Acquisitions Editor: Hilarie Surrena
Product Manager: Annette Ferran
Editorial Assistant: Jacalyn Clay
Design Coordinator: Holly McLaughlin
Illustration Coordinator: Brett MacNaughton
Manufacturing Coordinator: Karin Duffield
Prepress Vendor: SPi Global

4th edition

Library of Congress Cataloging-in-Publication Data
Sewell, Jeanne P.
  Informatics and nursing : opportunities and challenges / Jeanne P. Sewell, Linda Q. Thede. — 4th ed.
        p. ; cm.
  Rev. ed. of: Informatics and nursing / Linda Q. Thede, Jeanne P. Sewell. 3rd ed. c2010.
  Includes bibliographical references and index.
  ISBN 978-1-60913-695-6
  1. Nursing informatics. I. Thede, Linda Q. II. Thede, Linda Q. Informatics and nursing. III. Title.
  [DNLM: 1. Nursing Informatics. 2. Computers. 3. Internet. 4. Medical Records Systems, Computerized. WY 26.5]

  RT50.5.T483   2013
  610.73—dc23
                                    2011027051

Contributors

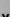

Deborah Ariosto, MSN, RN
Assistant Director of Clinical Informatics
Deborah Heart and Lung Center
Browns Mills, New Jersey

Pam Correll, RN, BSN
Nursing Informatics Consultant
Maine Center for Disease Control and Prevention
Public Health Nursing Program
Bangor, Maine

Karen H. Frith, PhD, RN, CNAA
Associate Professor
University of Alabama in Huntsville
College of Nursing
Huntsville, Alabama

Judy Hornbeck, MHSA, BSN, RN
Highland, Illinois

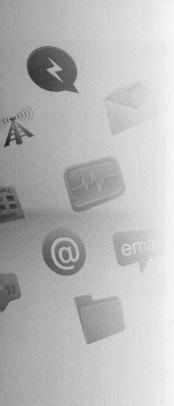

Reviewers

Barbara H. Baker, PhD, RN
Assistant Professor
University of Central Missouri
Warrensburg, Missouri

Kathleen R. Crane, MSN, RN-BC, CNE
Assistant Professor
Texas A&M University–Corpus Christi
Corpus Christi, Texas

Joan M. Krug, MSN, RN
Instructor of Nursing
Mount Alouysius College
Cresson, Pennsylvania

Carol Persoon Reid, MSN, RN
Assistant Professor
Metropolitan State University
St. Paul, Minnesota

Debra P. Shelton, EdD, APRN-CS, CNA, BC, OCN, CNE
Associate Professor
Northwestern State University
Shreveport, Louisiana

Bonnie Webster, MS, RN, BC
Assistant Professor
University of Texas Medical Branch School of Nursing
Galveston, Texas

Preface

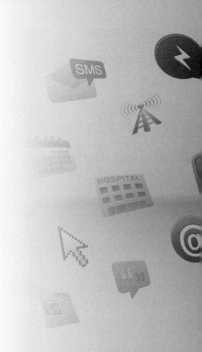

Writing a text in a field like informatics, in which today's news is easily outdated within months, continues to be a challenge. The first edition of this textbook was titled *Computers in Nursing* and published in 1999. It was one of the first textbooks to address core informatics competencies for all nurses. Each new addition of the textbook, including this fourth edition, was designed to capture the cutting edge advancement in nursing informatics core competencies and applications. In this fourth edition, we have tried to keep the best of the third edition, add topics that have entered the field since the last edition, and make it all interesting – and yes, thought provoking – to you, the reader. In just a little over a decade, the importance of informatics is now recognized not only in nursing, but also in the entire healthcare arena.

There are several significant updates in the fourth edition. In Unit I on "Informatics Basics," readers are introduced to information on the newest versions of office software, including Google cloud computing software, OpenOffice.org, and Microsoft Office 2010. A new feature in this edition is that the users can download digital versions of all of the examples used for the office software chapters. Units IV, V, and VI were updated to reflect changes coordinated by the United States Office of the National Coordinator for Health Information Technology (ONC). The implications of Health Information Technology for Economic and Clinical Health (HITECH) Act, "meaningful use," certification of the electronic health record (EHR), and Health Insurance Portability and Accountability Act (HIPAA) are threaded throughout chapters in the three units. Concepts related to business continuity planning and disaster recovery were added to Chapter 18 on electronic healthcare systems. Information on hardware is included in the textbook appendix.

Besides providing information for anyone who is just beginning to learn about nursing informatics, the book has been designed to be used either as a text for a course in nursing informatics or with a curriculum in which informatics is a vertical strand. The first two units, Informatics Basics and Computers and Your Professional Career, provide background information that would be useful in introductory courses, or as an introduction to computers and information management. The third unit, Information Competency, would be useful at any point in a curriculum. Units IV and V, The New Healthcare Paradigm and Healthcare Informatics, provides information that would be useful at more advanced levels, whereas the last unit, Computer Uses in Healthcare beyond Clinical Informatics, can either be used as a whole or its individual chapters matched with a course. The information in this textbook is what we believe every nurse should know.

Advancements in computer technology and the Internet have made the use of informatics pervasive in our society worldwide. Simply stated, informatics is the use of computers to discover, manipulate, and understand information. Information literacy and computer literacy skills provide foundational knowledge for informatics. Information literacy refers to the ability to identify pertinent information for retrieval and discovery of knowledge. Computer literacy is the ability to use computers. Nursing has been given direction to incorporate nursing informatics as a core competency into all levels of education programs by the two United States nursing accrediting bodies as well as the International Council of Nurses, and the Tiger Initiative. Furthermore, informatics is required to address nursing transformation addressed by the 2010 Institute of Medicine report, The Future of Nursing.

The major accrediting organizations for nursing, American Association of Colleges of Nursing (AACN) and the National League for Nursing Accrediting Commission (NLNAC) have identified informatics as an essential competency for all nurses, ranging from the beginning practitioner to the doctor of nursing practice (DNP), doctor of philosophy (PhD), and doctor of nursing science (DNSc) (American Association of Colleges of Nursing, 1996, 2006, 2008, 2010, 2011; National League for Nursing, 2008; National League for Nursing Accrediting Commission, 2008). It should be noted that although the term "informatics" was not commonly used in 1996, the 1996 *Essentials of Master's Education for Advanced Practice Nursing* (American Association of Colleges of Nursing, 1996) indicated that nurses should have the knowledge and skills "to use computer hardware and software to understand statistics and research methods" and "access current and relevant data needed to answer questions identified" in nursing practice (p. 6).

The importance of informatics is also recognized by the International Council of Nurses (ICN). The ICN website includes information about the importance of informatics to nurses. The ICN informatics fact sheet notes that informatics helps to make nursing visible in healthcare data sets. Informatics is identified as a "critical component of effective decision-making" and promotes nursing research (International Council of Nurses, 2010).

A call for nursing education to adopt informatics competencies for all levels of education came from the Tiger Initiative. The Tiger Initiative stemmed from a grant funded invitation of nursing education and other healthcare stakeholders to address use of informatics "in practice and education to provide safer, higher-quality patient care" (Technology Guiding Education Reform, 2007, 4).

In December 2010, the Institute of Medicine (IOM) published a report on the future of nursing (Institute of Medicine, 2010). Two of the IOM messages require informatics competencies (p. S-3):

- Nurses should be full partners, with physicians and other health professionals, in redesigning healthcare in the United States.
- Effective workforce planning and policy making require better data collection and an improved information infrastructure.

Evidence-based decision making using informatics tools should be used for healthcare redesign and improvements in data collection and information infrastructure. Clearly, there is agreement that informatics is an essential tool needed to address the need to provide evidence-based care with improved outcomes for individuals and populations. The informatics competencies and applications discussed in the fourth edition of this book are pertinent for all levels of nursing education ranging from undergraduate to all levels of graduate nursing programs.

This book comes with a set of instructor resources that can be accessed on thePoint, LWW's very popular Web-based content portal. With the materials you find on thePoint, you will be able to enhance your lectures with PowerPoint presentations, which provide an easy way for you to integrate the textbook with your students' classroom experience through either slide shows or handouts. In addition to the PowerPoint slides, the Test Generator lets you put together exclusive new tests from a bank containing over 250 questions, to help you in assessing your students' understanding of the material. These questions are formatted to match the NCLEX (National Council Licensure Examination), so that your students can have practice in preparing for this important examination. Additionally, the authors have provided a website that includes all Web addresses in the book, more information to supplement the text, and websites that are pertinent to each chapter. The Web page can be found at http://dlthede.net/Informatics/Informatics.html

Jeanne P. Sewell, MSN, RN
Linda Q. Thede, PhD, RN-BC

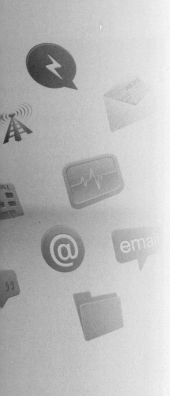

Acknowledgments

F ew writers, if any, know enough about a topic to write entirely from their own knowledge bank and what they can learn from the literature and the Web, even with two authors, as is the case with this edition of the text. We wish to thank Andy Salner, MD, for his help regarding the CHESS (Comprehensive Health Enhancement Support System) program. We also appreciate the help of both Kathy Lesh, RN, EdM, MS, technical manager of clinical informatics for the KEVRIC Company, and Susan Matney, MSN, RN, and Karen Martin, RN, MSN, FAAN. Thanks also to Barry Lung, MSN, RN, BC, informatics clinical consultant; Jill Williams, MSN, RN, CPHQ, MCSM, system analyst/program administrator; and Karen Childers, MSN, RN, systems analyst, for adding their expertise. In addition, we thank Karen Frith, PhD, RN, for writing Chapters 23 and 24. We would be remiss if we didn't acknowledge the personal feedback from the many students and faculty who have used the textbook.

In an effort to add a personal touch, there are three displays, whose authors freely gave of their time to write: Deborah Ariosto, MS, RN, tells of her experiences with an online support program, CHESS, in Chapter 14. In Chapter 16, Pam Correll, RN, BSN, writes about why she finds standardized terminologies helpful, and Judi Hornback, MHSA, BSN, RN, again contributes her typical day as an informatics nurse in Chapter 17. We hope you find these entertaining as well as informative. There were numerous others who assisted us in editing and rewriting, including Rebecca von Gillern, our Developmental Editor; we are truly indebted to you for all of your guidance and assistance.

Contents

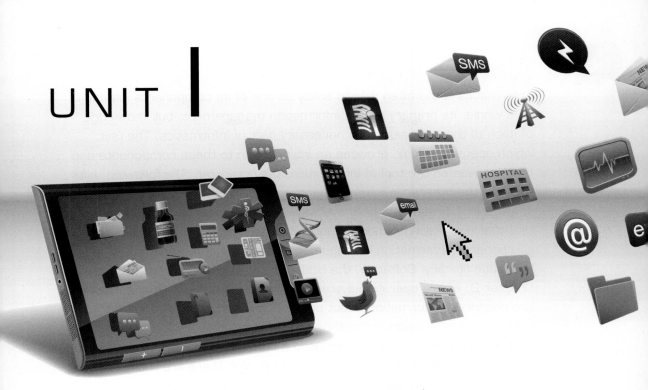

UNIT I

Informatics Basics

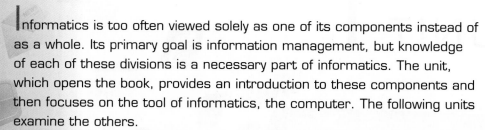

Informatics is too often viewed solely as one of its components instead of as a whole. Its primary goal is information management, but knowledge of each of these divisions is a necessary part of informatics. The unit, which opens the book, provides an introduction to these components and then focuses on the tool of informatics, the computer. The following units examine the others.

Chapter 1 presents a brief overview of informatics, what it is, the factors that are making it more important in healthcare, and a look at its components: information management, computer competency, and information literacy. Software, the brains of computers, is addressed in Chapter 2, where operating systems and general categories of software are described. Information about open source software, a concept that is finding some support in healthcare, and software copyright are also included. To those who have never used a computer, or whose experience is limited, facing one may seem intimidating. Yet, there are many features, which when learned can be applied across all genres of software. It is these topics that are explored in Chapter 3. The last chapter in this section, Chapter 4, examines the technology behind the scenes of computer networks.

CHAPTER 1

Introduction to Nursing Informatics: Managing Healthcare Information

Objectives

After studying this chapter you will be able to:

▶ Describe some of the forces inside and outside healthcare that are driving a move toward a greater use of informatics.

▶ Define nursing informatics.

▶ Distinguish between the computer and informatics.

▶ Explain the need for all nurses to have basic skills in informatics.

▶ Analyze the effects of informatics on healthcare.

▶ Interpret the need for nurses to be computer fluent and information literate to today's healthcare environment.

Key Terms

Aggregated Data
American Association of
    Colleges of Nursing (AACN)
American Nurses
    Association (ANA)
Computerized Provider
    Order Entry (CPOE)
Data
Decision Support Systems
Deidentified Data
Electronic Health Record (EHR)
Electronic Numerical Integrator
    and Computer (ENIAC)
Evidence-Based Care
Genomics
Healthcare Informatics
Health Information
    Technology (HIT)
Informatics
Information Literacy
Information Technology

Institute of Medicine (IOM)
Listserv
National League for Nursing
    (NLN)
Nursing Informatics
President's Information
    Technology Advisory
    Committee (PITAC)
Problem-Oriented Medical
    Information System
    (PROMIS)
Problem-Oriented Medical
    Record (POMR)
Protocols
Quality and Safety Education
    for Nurses (QSEN)
Secondary Data
Standardization
Technology Informatics
    Guiding Educational
    Reform (TIGER)

In attempting to arrive at the truth, I have applied everywhere for information, but in scarcely an instance have I been able to obtain hospital records fit for any purposes of comparison. If they could be obtained, they would enable us to decide many other questions besides the ones alluded to. They would show subscribers how their money was being spent, what amount of good was really being done with it, or whether the money was not doing mischief rather than good ..." (Nightingale, 1863, p. 176).

Informatics Introduction

What is informatics? Isn't it just about computers? Taking care of patients is nursing's primary concern, not thinking about computers! These are not unusual thoughts for nurses to have. Transitions are always difficult, and a transition to using more technology in managing information is no exception. The use of **information technology** (IT) in healthcare is known as **informatics**, and its focus is information management, not computers. Whether nursing uses informatics effectively or not will determine the quality of future patient care as well as the future of nursing.

Information management is an integral part of nursing. Think about your practice for a minute. When you are caring for patients, what besides the knowledge that nursing education and experience has provided do you depend on to provide care? You need to know the patient's history, medical conditions, medications, laboratory results, and more. Could you walk into a unit and care for a patient without this information? How this information is organized and presented to you affects the care that you can provide as well as the time you spend finding it.

The old way is to record and keep the information for a patient's current admission in a paper chart. Today, with several specialties, consults, medications, laboratory reports, and procedures, the paper chart is inadequate. A well-designed information system, developed with you and for you, can facilitate finding and using information that you need for patient care. Informatics skills enable you to participate in and benefit from this process. Informatics does not perform miracles; it requires an investment by you, the clinician, to assist those who design information systems so the systems are helpful and do not impede your workflow.

If healthcare is to improve, it is imperative that there be a workforce that can innovate and implement IT (American Health Information Management Association & American Medical Informatics Association, 2006). There are two roles in informatics: the informatics specialist and the clinician who must use **health information technology (HIT)**. This means that in essence every nurse has a role in informatics. Information, the subject of informatics, is the structure on which healthcare is built. Except for purely technical procedures (of which there are few, if any), a healthcare professional's work revolves around information. Is the laboratory report available? When is Mrs. X scheduled for surgery? What are the contraindications for the prescribed drug? What is Mr. Y's history? What orders did the physician leave for Ms. Z? Where is the latest x-ray report?

An important part of healthcare information is nursing documentation. When information systems are designed for nursing, this documentation can also be used to expand our knowledge of what constitutes quality healthcare. Have you ever wondered if the patient for whom you provided care had an outcome similar to others with the same condition? From nursing documentation, are you easily able to see the relationship between nursing diagnoses, interventions, and outcomes for your patients? Without knowledge of these chain events, you have only your intuition and old knowledge to use when making decisions about the best interventions in patient care. Because observations tend to be self-selective, this is often not the best information on which to base patient care. Informatics can furnish the information needed to see these relationships and to provide care based on actual patient **data**.

If Florence Nightingale were with us today, she would be a champion of the push toward more use of healthcare IT. Information in a paper chart essentially disappears into a black hole after a patient is discharged. Because we can't easily access it, we can't learn from it and use it in patient care. This realization is international. Many countries, especially those with a national health service, have long realized the need to be able to use information buried in charts. Tommy Thompson (2004), the then US Secretary of Health and Human Services, in a talk at the May 6, 2004, Health Information Technology Summit said that "the most remarkable feature of this 21st-century medicine is that we hold it together with 19th-century paperwork. This is just inexcusable. And it has to change."

Thompson's statement was backed up with the introduction of bills in the US Congress.

The **President's Information Technology Advisory Committee (PITAC)** was created to support for greater use of informatics. PITAC responsibilities were transferred to the President's Council of Advisors on Science and Technology in the Office of Science and Technology Policy in 2005 (Office of Science and Technology Policy, 2010).

In 2004, President Bush called for adoption of interoperable **electronic health records (EHRs)** for most Americans by 2014. He also established the position of National Coordinator for Health Information Technology. The 2008–2012 strategic plan (Department of Health & Human Services Office of the National Coordinator for Health Information Technology, 2008) was released to address "the federal activities necessary to achieve the nationwide implementation of this technology infrastructure throughout both the public and private sectors." The strategic plan formulated two goals that affect nurses and healthcare. They are as follows:

1. Patient-focused healthcare – provide higher quality, cost-efficient care using electronic information exchange among healthcare providers, patients, and their designees. The strategies for achieving this goal are as follows:
   a. Facilitate electronic exchange of the patient's health information while protecting privacy and security of the information.
   b. Make the information exchange interoperable so that it is available when and where it is needed.
   c. Promote nationwide adoption of EHRs and personal health records.
   d. Establish collaborative governance to guide the HIT infrastructure.
2. Population health – allow for access and "use of electronic health information to support public health, biomedical research, quality improvement, and emergency preparedness." The strategies for achieving this goal are as follows:
   a. Provide for information access and use of population health while protecting privacy and security of the information.
   b. Make the information exchange interoperable to support population-oriented uses.
   c. "Promote nationwide adoption of technologies and technical functions that will improve population and individual health."
   d. Establish collaborative governance to support the information use for population health.

To fulfill these goals, information, which is the structure on which healthcare is built, can no longer be managed with paper. If we are to provide **evidence-based care**, the mountains of data that are hidden in medical records must be made to reveal their secrets. Bakken (2001) proposed that five components are needed to provide evidence-based care:

1. **Standardization** of terminologies and structures used in documentation.
2. The use of digital information.
3. Standards to permit healthcare data exchange between heterogeneous entities.
4. The ability to capture data relevant to the actual care provided.
5. Competency among practitioners to use this data.

All of these components are parts of informatics.

The complexity of today's healthcare milieu, added to the explosion of knowledge, makes it impossible for any clinician to remember everything needed to provide high-quality patient care. Additionally, healthcare consumers today want their healthcare providers to integrate all known relevant scientific knowledge in providing their care. We have passed the time when the unaided human mind can perform this feat: Modern information management tools as well as a commitment by healthcare professionals are needed to change practices when more knowledge becomes available.

 Information Overload

Informatics at Your Service

Informatics is about managing information. The tendency to relate it to computers comes from the fact that the ability to manage large amounts of information was born with the computer and progressed as computers became more powerful and commonplace. However, human ingenuity is the crux of informatics. The term "informatics" originated from the Russian term "informatika" (Sackett & Erdley, 2002). A Russian publication, Oznovy Informatiki (Foundations of Informatics), published in 1968 is credited with the origins of the general discipline of informatics (Bansal, 2002). At that time, it was described within the context of computers. "Medical informatics" was the first term used to identify informatics in healthcare. It was defined as the information technologies that are concerned with patient care and the medical decision-making process. Another definition stated that medical informatics is complex data processing by the computer to create new information. As with many healthcare enterprises, there was debate about whether "medical" referred only to informatics focusing on physician concerns, or whether it refers to all healthcare disciplines. Increasingly, it is seen that other disciplines have a body of knowledge separate from medicine, but part of healthcare, and the term **healthcare informatics** is becoming more commonly used. In essence, informatics is the management of information, by using cognitive skills and the computer.

Healthcare Informatics

Healthcare informatics focuses on managing information in healthcare. It is an umbrella term that describes the capture, retrieval, storage, presenting, sharing, and use of biomedical information, data, and knowledge for providing care, problem solving, and decision making (Shortliffe & Blois, 2001). The purpose is to improve the use of healthcare data, information, and knowledge in supporting patient care, research, and education (Delaney, 2001). The focus is on the subject, information, rather than the tool, the computer. The distinction is not always obvious because of the need to master computer skills to enable one to manage this information. The computer is used in acquiring, organizing, manipulating, and presenting the information. It will not produce anything of value without human direction in how, when, and where the data is acquired and how it is treated, interpreted, manipulated, and presented. Informatics provides that human direction.

Nursing Informatics

Healthcare has many disciplines, and thus it is not surprising that healthcare informatics has many specialties of which nursing is one. The **American Nurses Association (ANA)** recognized **nursing informatics** as a subspecialty of nursing in 1992. The first informatics certification examination was given in the fall of 1995 (Newbold, 1996). Managing information pertaining to nursing is the focus of nursing informatics. Specialists in this area look at how nursing information is acquired, manipulated, stored, presented, and used. Informatics nurses work with practicing nurses to identify the needs of nurses for information and support, and with system developers in the development of systems that work to complement the practice needs of nurses. Nursing informatics specialists bring to system development and implementation a viewpoint that supports the needs of the clinical end user. The objective is an information system that is not only user friendly for data input, but presents the clinical nurse with needed information in a manner that is timely and useful. This is not to say that nursing informatics stands alone; it is an integral part of the interdisciplinary field of healthcare informatics, hence related to and responsible to all the healthcare disciplines.[1]

Definitions of Nursing Informatics

The term "nursing informatics" was probably first used and defined by Scholes and Barber in 1980 in their address that year to the MEDINFO conference in Tokyo. There is still no definitive agreement on exactly what this term means. As Simpson (1998) once said, defining nursing informatics is difficult because it is a moving target. The original definition said that nursing informatics was the use of computer technology in all nursing endeavors: nursing services, education, and research (Scholes & Barber, 1980). Hannah, Ball, and Edwards (1994) wrote another early definition that followed the broad definition by Scholes and Barber. Hannah et al. (1994) defined nursing informatics as any use of information technologies in carrying out nursing functions. Like the definition by Scholes and Barber, the

---

1 The nursing informatics subspecialty will be explored in more detail in Chapter 17.

one by Hannah et al. focused on the technology. They could be interpreted to mean any use of the computer, from word processing to the creation of artificial intelligence for nurses, as long as the computer use involved the practice of professional nursing.

The shift from a technology orientation in definitions to one that is more information oriented started in the mid-1980s with Schwirian (Staggers & Thompson, 2002). Schwirian (1986) created a model to be used as a framework for nursing informatics investigators. The model consisted of four elements arranged in a pyramid with a triangular base. The top of the pyramid was the desired goal of the nursing informatics activity and the base was composed of three elements: (1) users (nurses and students), (2) raw material or nursing information, and (3) the technology, which is computer hardware and software. They all interact in nursing informatics activity to achieve a goal. The model was intended as a stimulus for research.

The first widely circulated definition that moved away from technology to concepts was from Graves and Corcoran (Staggers & Thompson, 2002). They defined nursing informatics as "a combination of computer science, information science and nursing science designed to assist in the management and processing of nursing data, information and knowledge to support the practice of nursing and the delivery of nursing care" (Graves & Cocoran, 1989, p. 227). This definition secured the position of nursing informatics within the practice of nursing and placed the emphasis on data, information, and knowledge (Staggers & Thompson, 2002). Many consider it the seminal definition of nursing informatics.

Turley (1996), after analyzing previous definitions, added another discipline, cognitive science, to the base for nursing informatics. Cognitive science emphasizes the human factor in informatics. Its focus is the nature of knowledge, its components, development, and use. Goossen (1996), thinking along the same lines, used the definition by Graves and Corcoran as a basis and expanded the meaning of nursing informatics to include the thinking that is done by nurses to make knowledge-based decisions and inferences for patient care. By using this interpretation, he felt that nursing informatics should focus on analyzing and modeling the cognitive processing for all areas of nursing practice. Goossen (1996) also stated that nursing informatics should look at the effects of computerized systems on nursing care delivery.

In 1992, the first ANA definition added the role of the informatics nursing specialist to the definition by Graves and Corcoran. The 2001 ANA definition stated that nursing informatics combines nursing, information, and computer sciences for the purpose of managing and communicating data, information, and knowledge to support nurses and healthcare providers in decision making (American Nurses Association, 2001). Information structures, processes, and technology are used to provide this support. In the latest ANA Scope and Standards of Practice, the definition was reiterated, albeit in slightly different wording (American Nurses Association, 2008), with the addition of wisdom to the data, information, and knowledge conceptual framework. The most recent definition emphasized again, that the goal of nursing informatics is to optimize information management and communication to improve the health of individuals, families, populations, and communities.

Staggers and Thompson (2002), who believe that the evolution of definitions will continue, pointed out that in all of the current definitions, the role of the patient is underemphasized. Some early definitions included the patient, but as a passive recipient of care. With the advent of the Internet, more and more patients are taking an active role in their healthcare. This factor not only changes the dynamics of healthcare but also permits a definition of nursing informatics that recognizes that patients as well as healthcare professionals are consumers of healthcare information. Patients may participate in keeping their medical records current. Staggers and Thompson (2002) also pointed out that the role of the nurse as an integrator of information has been overlooked and should be considered in future definitions.

Despite these definitions, the focus of much of today's practice informatics is still on capturing data at the point of care and presenting it in a manner that facilitates the care of an individual patient. Although this is a vital first step, thought needs to be given to **secondary data** analysis, or analysis of data for purposes other than for which it was originally collected in the system design process. You can make decisions based on actual patient care data by using **aggregated data**, or the same piece(s) of data. For example, you can analyze outcomes of a given intervention for many patients. Understanding how informatics can serve you as an individual nurse, as well as the profession, puts you in a position to work with informatics specialists to retrieve data needed to improve patient care.

Forces Driving Toward More Use of Informatics in Healthcare

The ultimate goal of healthcare informatics is a lifetime EHR with **decision support systems**. These records will include standardized data, permit consumers to access their records, and provide for secondary use of healthcare data. President Bush set a goal of 2014 for every American to have an EHR; however, many issues must be addressed before this becomes a reality.

National Forces

Federal efforts behind a move to EHRs include not only the creation of PITAC but also efforts to standardize data. The **Institute of Medicine (IOM)**, an independent body that acts as an adviser to the US[2] government to improve healthcare, has completed several reports aimed at improving healthcare, all of which foresee a large role for IT. The IOM report *Health Professions Education: A Bridge to Quality* (Greiner & Knebel, 2003) includes informatics as a core competency required of all healthcare professionals. In the report *Crossing the Quality Chasm: A New Health System for the 21st Century* (Committee on Quality of Health Care in America & Institute of Medicine, 2001), IT is seen as an important force in improving healthcare. Some of the IT themes in this report are a national information infrastructure, computerized clinical data, the use of the Internet, clinical decision support, and evidence-based practice integration (Staggers, 2004).[2]

Nursing Forces

Nursing has recognized the need for informatics. In 1962, Dr. Harriet Werley recognized the value of nursing data and insisted that the ANA make research about nursing information a priority before the term informatics was coined. There many articles were written about informatics in the intervening years. In addition, the journal *Computers in Nursing*[3] was started as a mimeograph sheet in 1982. However, few nurses realized the value of and need for informatics.

In 1993, the National Center for Nursing Research released the report *Nursing Informatics: Enhancing Patient Care* (Pillar & Golumbic, 1993), which set the following six program goals for nursing informatics research:

1. Establish a nursing language (useful in computerized documentation).
2. Develop methods to build clinical information databases.
3. Determine how nurses give patient care using data, information, and knowledge.
4. Develop and test patient care decision support systems.
5. Develop workstations that provide nurses with needed information.
6. Develop appropriate methods to evaluate nursing information systems.

In 1997, the Division of Nursing of the Health Resources and Services Administration convened the National Advisory Council on Nurse Education and Practice. The council produced the *National Informatics Agenda for Education and Practice*, which made the following five recommendations (National Advisory Council on Nurse Education and Practice, 1997, p. 8):

1. Educate nursing students and practicing nurses in core informatics content.
2. Prepare nurses with specialized skills in informatics.
3. Enhance nursing practice and education through informatics projects.
4. Prepare nursing faculty in informatics.

---

2 See Chapter 15 for more information on US government efforts.

3 Now named *CIN: Computer Informatics Nursing*, and since 1984, a fuel-fledged journal.

5. Increase collaborative efforts in nursing informatics.

In 2008, the **National League for Nursing (NLN)** published a position paper outlining recommendations for preparing nurses to work in an environment that uses technology (National League for Nursing, 2008). The paper outlined recommendations for nursing faculty, deans/directors/chairs, and the NLN. Examples of recommendations included the need for faculty to achieve informatics competencies and incorporation of informatics into the nursing curriculum.

The **American Association of Colleges of Nursing's (AACN's)** list of core competencies includes many recommendations in the area of information and healthcare technologies, such as the use of information and communication technologies, the use of ethics in the application of technology, and the enhancement of one's knowledge using information technologies (AACN, 2006, 2008, 2011).

The ANA has been another force moving nursing toward effectively using informatics. Starting in 1994 with two documents, Standards of Practice for Nursing Informatics and The Scope of Practice for Nursing Informatics, the association has since combined these documents. The third edition, which is greatly expanded, was released in 2008. The Committee for Nursing Practice Information Infrastructure and the National Information and Data Set Evaluation Center are two ANA committees whose work concerns informatics.

The current shortage of nurses in many countries, including the United States and Canada, is another driving force. A report from the Maryland Statewide Commission on the Crisis in Nursing (Womack, Newbold, Staugaitis, & Cunningham, 2004) examines technology's role in addressing the nursing shortage and makes many recommendations. A study conducted by the Robert Wood Johnson Foundation (2010) revealed that nurses believe technology can improve workflow, communication, and documentation; however, many technologies are still not "user-friendly." Although technology has the potential to improve nursing, there is still work that must be done. The bedside clinician has an integral role in that work. The clinical nurse with essential nursing competencies can and must assist in designing user-friendly technologies that improve care delivery and care outcomes.

The **Technology Informatics Guiding Educational Reform (TIGER)** initiative originated after several years of planning, with a 2-day invitation-only conference starting October 30, 2006. TIGER's objective is to make nursing informatics competencies part of every nurse's skill set, with the aim of making informatics the stethoscope of the 21st century (Technology Guiding Educational Reform, 2007). TIGER is working to ensure that nursing can be fully engaged in the digital era of healthcare by ensuring that all nurses are educated in using informatics, empowering them to deliver safer, high-quality, evidence-based care.

Other Driving Forces

Healthcare is an information-intensive industry, yet most healthcare providers often consider the management of their information as an onerous, unappreciated task (Korpman, 1990). Poorly organized and implemented documentation systems tend to hinder the process of finding and using the information one needs to provide high-quality care. Add to that time requirements for documentation, the frequent need to enter data in duplicate or even triplicate, time spent trying to locate patient records, and missing reports, and the reasons for dissatisfaction become clear.

Patient Safety

Patient safety is a primary concern and the one that drives many informatics initiatives. At least 10 patient safety databases use aggregated healthcare data to identify safety issues. Most, such as the National Nosocomial Infections Surveillance System from the Centers for Disease Control and Prevention (CDC) and the National Database of Nursing Quality Indicators from ANA, are voluntary, but two, the vaccine adverse event report system from the CDC and the U.S. Food and Drug Administration (FDA), are mandatory (Bakken, 2006).[4]

---

4 Providing the data for these reports is not possible without standardization of data, a topic that will be further investigated in Chapters 15 and 16.

The **Quality and Safety Education for Nurses (QSEN)** is a three-phase initiative funded by the Robert Wood Johnson Foundation (Quality and Safety Education for Nurses, 2010). The goals for phase I address IOM's five competencies – patient-centered care, teamwork and collaboration, evidence-based practice, quality improvement, and informatics – plus safety, for a total of six goals. Phase II integrates the competencies in pilot nursing programs. Phase III continues to promote the implementation and evaluation of knowledge, skills, and attitudes associated with the six competencies.

Some other informatics implementations that focus on safety include bar coding for medication administration and **computerized provider order entry (CPOE)**. A well-designed CPOE system can not only prevent transcription errors but, when combined with a patient's record, can also flag any condition that might present a hazard or would need additional assessment. Clinical decision support systems that provide clinicians with suggested care information or remind busy clinicians of items easy to forget or overlook are also being pushed to improve patient safety.[5]

Costs

Healthcare costs are also driving the move to informatics. One example is the Leapfrog Group. Upset by the rising cost of healthcare, a group of chief executives of leading corporations in the United States met in 1998 to discuss how they could have an influence on its quality and affordability (Leapfrog Group, 2009a). The executives were spending billions of dollars on healthcare for their employees, but they lacked a way of assessing its quality or comparing healthcare providers. The Business Roundtable provided the initial funding, and this group took the name "Leapfrog Group" in November 2000. This move was given further impetus by the 1999 IOM report *To Err Is Human*, which reported up to 98,000 preventable hospital deaths and recommended that large employers use their purchasing power to improve the quality and safety of healthcare.

Today, the Robert Wood Johnson Foundation, Leapfrog members, and others also support the Leapfrog Group. Their mission is to improve the safety, quality, and affordability of healthcare by encouraging the availability of the information necessary for consumers to make informed healthcare decisions and the use of incentives and rewards to promote high-value healthcare (Leapfrog Group, 2009b). The Leapfrog Group mission goals are as follows:

1. Promoting the use of CPOE systems to reduce medication errors
2. Encouraging consumers and healthcare purchasers to select hospitals with extensive experience and good outcomes for certain high-risk surgeries
3. Promoting the staffing of intensive care units (ICUs) with intensivists or doctors with special training in the care of ICU patients
4. Assessing hospitals' progress on the National Quality Forum – endorsed safe practices.

Efforts toward this last goal are met by collecting data voluntarily submitted by hospitals and posting this information on a website (http://www.leapfroggroup.org/cp) where consumers can check the outcomes of hospitals in their areas for selected procedures. Members of the Leapfrog Group also educate their employees about patient safety and the importance of comparing healthcare providers. They will offer financial incentives to their covered employees for selecting care from hospitals that meet their standards. Healthcare providers without information systems will have a difficult time in providing the information that these healthcare buyers demand and could see themselves losing patients.

As healthcare informatics moves to solve these problems, the need for interdisciplinary, enterprise-wide, information management becomes clearer. The advances of IT coupled with the evolution of the EHR will create a steady progression to this end. Integration, however, is not without its perils. Any discipline that is not ready for this integration may find itself lost in the process. For nursing to be a part of healthcare informatics, all nurses must become familiar with the value of

---

5 CPOE will be further discussed in Chapter 20 and decision support systems in Chapter 20.

nursing data, how it can be captured, the terminology needed to capture it, and methods for analyzing and manipulating it. True integration of data from all healthcare disciplines will improve patient care and the patient experience, as well as enabling economic gains.

The Information Management Tool: Computers

In 1850, all the medical knowledge known to the Western world could be collected into two large volumes, making it possible for one person to read and assimilate all this information. The situation today is dramatically different. The number of journals available in healthcare and the research that fills them have increased many times over. Even in the early 1990s, if physicians read two journal articles a day, by the end of a year, they would be 800 years behind in their reading (McDonald, 1994). In the early 2000s, healthcare clinician could be expected to know something about 10,000 different diseases and syndromes, 3,000 medications, 1,100 laboratory tests, and the information in the more than 400,000 articles added to the biomedical information each year (Davenport & Glaser, 2002). The number of journals, books, blogs, and news articles is growing exponentially on a daily basis. Additionally, current knowledge is constantly changing: one can expect much of one's knowledge to be obsolete in 5 years or less.

In healthcare, the increase in knowledge has led to the development of many specialties, such as respiratory therapy, neonatology, and gerontology, and subspecialties within each of these. As these specialties have proliferated and spawned the development of many miraculous treatments, healthcare has too often become fractionalized, resulting in difficulty in gaining an overview of the entire patient. The pressure of accomplishing the tasks necessary for a patient's physical recovery usually leaves little time for perusing a patient's record and putting together the bits and pieces so carefully charted by each discipline. Even if time is available, there is simply so much data, in so many places, that it is difficult to merge the data with the

knowledge that a healthcare provider has learned, as well as with new knowledge needed to provide the best patient care. We are drowning in data but lack the time and skills to transform it to useful information or knowledge.

The development of the computer as a tool to manage information can be seen in its history. The first information management task "computerized" was numeric manipulation. Although not technically a computer by today's terminology, the first successful computerization tool was the abacus, which was developed about 3000 BC. Although when one developed skill, real speed in these tasks was possible, but the operator of the abacus still had to manipulate data mentally (Dilson, 1968). All the abacus did was store the results step-by-step. Slide rules came next, in 1622 (The Oughtred Society, 2007), but like the abacus, they required a great deal of skill on the part of the operator. The first machine to add and subtract by itself was Blaise Pascal's "arithmetic machine," built between 1640 and 1642 AD (Freiberger & Swaine, n.d.). The first "computer" to be a commercial success was Jacquard's weaving machine built in 1803 ("Jacquard, Joseph Marie (1752–1834)," 2009). Its efficiency so frightened workers at the mill where it was built that they rioted, broke apart the machine, and sold the parts. Despite this setback, the machine proved a success because it introduced a cost-effective way of producing goods.

The difference and analytical engines, early computers designed by Charles Babbage in the mid-19th century, although never built, laid the foundation for modern computers (Millar, Millar, Millar, & Millar, 2002). The first time that an automatic calculating machine was successfully used was in the 1900 census. Herman Hollerith (who later started IBM) used the Jacquard loom concept of punch cards to create a machine that enabled the 1900 census takers to compile the results in 1 year instead of the 10 required for the 1890 census (Bellis, n.d.). The first computer by today's perception was the **Electronic Numerical Integrator and Computer (ENIAC)** built by people at the Moore School of Engineering at the University of Pennsylvania in partnership with the US government. When completed in 1946, it consisted of 18,000 vacuum tubes, 70,000 resistors, and 5 million soldered joints. It consumed enough energy to dim the lights in an entire section of Philadelphia (Moye, 1996). The progress in hardware since then is phenomenal; today's "palmtop" computers have more processing power than ENIAC did.

Computers and Healthcare

Computers in healthcare use originated in the late-1950s and early-1960s, as a way to manage financial information. This was followed in the late-1960s by the development of a few computerized patient care applications (Saba & Erdeley, 2006). Some of these hospital information systems included patient diagnoses and other patient information as well as care plans based on physician and nursing orders. Because of the lack of processing power then available, these systems were unable to deliver what was needed and never became widely used.

Early Healthcare Informatics Systems

One of the interesting early uses of the computer in patient care was the **Problem-Oriented Medical Information System (PROMIS)** begun by Dr. Lawrence Weed in 1968 at the University Medical Center in Burlington, Vermont (McNeill, 1979). The importance of this system is that it was the first attempt at providing a total, integrated system that covered all aspects of healthcare, including patient treatment. It was patient oriented and used as its framework the **problem-oriented medical record (POMR)**. The unit featured an interactive touch screen and was known for fast responsiveness (Schultz, 1988). At its height, it consisted of more than 60,000 frames of knowledge.

PROMIS was designed to overcome four problems that are still with us today: lack of care coordination, reliance on memory, lack of recorded logic of delivered care, and lack of an effective feedback loop (Jacobs, 2009). The system provided a wide array of information to all healthcare providers. All disciplines recorded their observations and plans and related them to a specific problem. This broke down barriers between disciplines, making it possible to see the relationship between conditions, treatments, costs, and outcomes. Unfortunately,

this system did not have wide acceptance. To embrace it meant a change in the structure of healthcare, something that did not begin to happen until the 1990s, when managed care in all its variations reinvigorated a push toward more patient-centered information systems, a push that continues even today.

Another early system that became functional in 1967 and still functioning is the Help Evaluation through Logical Processing (HELP) system developed by the Informatics Department at the University of Utah School of Medicine. It was first implemented in a heart catheterization laboratory and a post–open-heart ICU. It is now operational in many hospitals in the Intermountain Healthcare system (Gardner, Pryor, & Warner, 1999). This is not only a hospital information system but also integrates a sophisticated clinical decision support system that provides information to clinical areas. It was the first hospital information system that collected data for clinical decision making and integrated it with a medical knowledge base. Clinicians accepted the system. The HELP system demonstrated that a clinical support system is feasible and can reduce healthcare costs without sacrificing quality.

Progression of Information Systems

As the science of informatics has progressed, there have been changes in information systems. Originally, computerized clinical information systems were process oriented. That is, they were implemented to computerize a specific process, for example, billing, order entry, or laboratory reports. This led to the creation of different software systems for different departments, which unfortunately could not share data, creating a need for clinicians to enter data more than once. An attempt to share data by integrating data from disparate systems is a difficult and sometimes impossible task. Even when possible, the results are often disappointing and can leave negative impressions of computerization in users' minds. These barriers are being overcome slowly with the introduction of data standards, both in terminology and in **protocols** for passing data from one system to another.

Newer systems, however, are organized by data and are designed to use the same piece of data many times, thus requiring that the entry be made only once. The primary design is based on how data is gathered, stored, and used in an entire institution rather than on a specific process such as pharmacy or laboratory. For example, when a medication order is placed, the system can have access to all the information about a patient including his or her diagnosis, age, weight, allergies, and eventually **genomics**, as well as the medications that he or she is currently taking. The order and patient information can also be matched against knowledge, such as what drugs are incompatible with the prescribed drug, the dosage of the drug, and the appropriateness of the drug for this patient. If there are difficulties, the system can deliver warnings at the time the medication is ordered instead of requiring clinician intervention either in the pharmacy or at the time of administration. Another feature in a data-driven system is the ability to make the same information available to the dietician planning the patient's diet and the nurse providing patient care and doing discharge planning, thus enabling a more complete picture of a patient than one that would be available when separate systems handle dietetics and nursing.

Evidence-based practice will result not only from research and practice guidelines but also from unidentifiable (data minus any patient identification) **aggregated data** from actual patients. It will also be possible to see how patients with a given genomics react to a drug, thus helping the clinician in prescribing drugs. This same aggregated data will help clinicians make decisions by providing information about treatments that are most effective for given conditions, replacing the current system, which is too often based on "what we have always done" rather than empirical information. These systems will use computers that are powerful enough to process data so that information is created "on the fly," or immediately when requested. Systems that incorporate these features will require a new way of thinking. Instead of having all one's knowledge in memory, one must be comfortable both with needing to access information and with changing one's practice to accommodate the new knowledge.

Computerization will affect healthcare professionals in other ways. Some jobs will change focus. As nurses, we may find that our job as a patient care coordinator has shifted from transcribing and checking orders to accessing this information on the computer. To preserve our ability to provide full care for our patients, and as an information integrator for other disciplines, we will need to make our information needs known to those who design the systems. To accomplish this, we all need to be aware of the value of both our data and our experience. We need to be able to identify the data we need to perform our job, as well as to appreciate the value of the data that others add to the healthcare system.

Benefits of Informatics

The information systems described earlier will bring many benefits to healthcare. These benefits can be seen in the ability to create and use aggregated data, prevent errors, ease working conditions, and provide better healthcare records.

For Healthcare in General

One of the primary benefits of informatics is that data that were previously buried in inaccessible records become usable. Informatics is not only about collecting data but also about making it useful. When data are captured electronically in a structured manner, they can be retrieved and used in different ways, both to assimilate easily information about one patient and as aggregated data. Aggregated data are the same piece or pieces of data for many patients. **Table 1-1** shows some aggregated data for postsurgical infections sorted by physician and then by the organism. Because infections for some patients are caused by two different pathogens as presented in **Table 1-1**, you see two entries for some patients; however, this is all produced from only one entry of the data. With just a few clicks of a mouse, these same data could be organized by unit to show the number of infections on each unit. This is possible because data that are structured as in **Table 1-1** and standardized can be presented in many different views.

When aggregated data are examined, patterns can be seen that might otherwise take several weeks or months to become evident or might never become evident. When patterns, such as the prevalence of infections for Dr. Smith emerge (**Table 1-1**), it is possible to investigate what the patients

Table 1-1 Aggregated Data

First Name	Last Name	Unit	Surgery	Physician	Pathogen
Charles	Babbage	3 West	Cholecystectomy	Black	E. coli
Jack	Of All Trades	4 West	Appendectomy	Black	Strep
George	Washington	4 West	Tonsillectomy	Black	Strep
John	Wayne	2 East	Herniorrhaphy	Greene	E. coli
Gloria	Swanson	2 East	Cholecystectomy	Greene	E. coli
Gloria	Swanson	2 East	Cholecystectomy	Greene	Strep
Susan	Anthony	3 West	Tubal ligation	Jones	Strep
Alexander	Hamilton	2 East	Cholecystectomy	Smith	E. coli
Florence	Dayingale	4 West	Hysterectomy	Smith	E. coli
Abigail	Adams	2 East	Herniorrhaphy	Smith	Staph
Johnny	Appleseed	3 West	Open reduction, left femur	Smith	Staph
Davey	Jones	3 West	Transurethral resection	Smith	Staph
Alexander	Hamilton	2 East	Cholecystectomy	Smith	Strep
Florence	Dayingale	4 West	Hysterectomy	Smith	Strep

Note: Fictitious patient names are used here to help in understanding the concept; real secondary data should be unidentifiable.
E. coli, Escherichia coli; Staph, Staphylococcus; Strep, Streptococcus.

have in common. However, caution should be observed. The aggregated data in **Table 1-1** are insufficient to draw conclusions; the data serve only as an indication of a problem and clues to where to start investigating. Aggregated data are a type of information or even knowledge, but wisdom says that they are incomplete[6]. If these data were shared outside of an agency or with those who don't need to have personal information about a patient, it would be **deidentified**; that is, there would be no patient names and probably no physician names. Deciding who can see what data is one of the current issues in informatics.

Informatics through information systems can improve communication between all healthcare providers, which will improve patient care and reduce stress. Additional benefits for healthcare include making the storage and retrieval of healthcare records much easier, quicker retrieval of test results, printouts of needed information organized to meet the needs of the user, and fewer lost charges because of easier methods of recording charges. The computerization of administrative tasks such as staffing and scheduling saves time and money.

Benefits to the Nursing Profession

Each healthcare discipline will benefit from its investment in informatics. In nursing, informatics will not only enhance practice but also add to the development of nursing science. Informatics will improve documentation and, when properly implemented, can reduce the time spent in documentation. Nurses spend more than 15%–25% of their time documenting patient care (Gugerty et al., 2007). Entering vital signs both in nursing notes and on a flow sheet, wastes time and invites errors. In a well-designed clinical documentation system, these data will be entered once, retrieved, and presented in many different forms to meet the needs of the user.

Paper documentation methods create other problems such as inconsistency and irregularity in charting as well as the lack of data for evaluation and research as mentioned above. An electronic clinical information system can remind users of the need to provide data in areas apt to be forgotten and can provide a list of terms that can be clicked to enter data. The ability to use patient data for both quality control and research is improved vastly when documentation is complete and electronic.

---

6 Aggregated data will be further discussed in Chapter 9.

Despite Florence Nightingale's emphasis on data, for much of nursing's history, nursing data have not been valued. They are either buried in paper patient records that make retrieving it economically infeasible, or worse, discarded when a patient is discharged, hence unavailable for building nursing science. With the advent of electronic clinical documentation, nursing data can be made a part of the EHR and become available to researchers for building evidence-based nursing knowledge. The Maryland report on the use of technology to address the nursing shortage demonstrated that informatics could be used to improve staff morale and patient care (Gugerty et al., 2007). For example, paper request forms can be eliminated, work announcements can be more easily communicated, the time for in-services can be reduced, and empty shifts can be filled by using Internet software.

In understanding the role and value that informatics adds to nursing, it is necessary to recognize that the profession is not confined to tasks but that it is cognitive. Providing data to support this is a joint function of nursing informatics and clinicians. Identifying and determining how to facilitate data collection is an informatics skill that all nurses need.

Nursing Informatics Competencies and Information Literacy

The need to manage complex amounts of data in patient care demands that all nurses, regardless of specialty area, have informatics skills (Gaumer, Koeniger-Donohue, Friel, & Sudbay, 2007; Nelson, 2007). Informatics skills for all nurses require basic computer skills as one component (American Nurses Association, 2008). Another skill needed for proficiency in informatics is **information literacy**. The ANA, NLN, and AACN have identified both computer and information literacy skills as necessary for evidence-based practice.

Computer Fluency

The 20th century was described as the information age; the present century will be the information-processing age, that is, the use of data and information to create more information and knowledge. The term "computer literacy" is used broadly to mean the ability to perform various tasks with a computer. Given the rapid changes in technology and in nursing, perhaps a better perspective on computer use can be gained by thinking in terms of computer fluency rather than literacy. The term "fluency" implies that an individual has a lifelong commitment to acquiring new skills for being more effective in work and personal life (National Research Council [U.S.] Committee on Information Technology Literacy, 1999). This necessitates a goal of gaining sufficient foundational skills and knowledge to enable one to acquire new skills independently. Thus, computer literacy is a temporary state, whereas computer fluency involves being able to increase one's ability to effectively use a computer when needed.

A perusal of **Listserv**[7] archives in informatics reveals periodic requests for instruments to measure the computer competency of staff. Unfortunately, there is little agreement on specific competencies needed, let alone an instrument to measure this, but there is consensus that it involves knowledge, attitude, and competencies in the use of computers, computer technology, and hardware and software. Nurses must be able to visualize the overall benefits to nursing practice and patient care outcomes. More than a decade ago, Simpson (1998) pointed out the need for nurses to master computers to avoid extinction. A computer is a mind tool that frees us from the mental drudgery of data processing, just as the bulldozer frees us from the drudgery of digging and moving dirt. Similar to the bulldozer, however, the computer must be used intelligently or damage can result.

Given the forces moving healthcare toward more use of informatics, it is important for nurses to learn the skills associated with using a computer for managing information. Additionally, knowing how to use graphical interfaces and application programs such as word processing, spreadsheets, databases, and presentation programs is as an important an element in a professional career as mastering technology skills (McCannon & O'Neal, 2003).

---

7 A Listserv is an e-mail discussion list that has participants who discuss various aspects of a topic such as informatics.

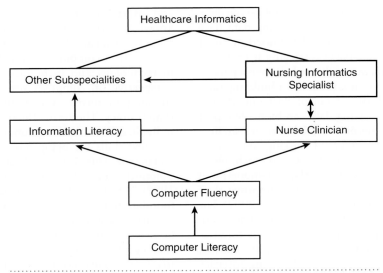

Figure 1-1 Skill set in nursing informatics.

Just as anatomy and physiology provide a background for learning about disease processes and treatments, computer fluency skills are necessary to appreciate more complex informatics concepts (McNeil & Odom, 2000) and for learning clinical applications (Nagelkerk, Ritolo, & Vandort, 1998).

Ronald and Skiba (1987) were the first to look at computer competencies required for nurses. In the late-1990s and early part of this century, this issue was revisited, but the focus became the use of computer skills as part of informatics skills (McCannon & O'Neal, 2003; McNeil et al., 2003; Utley-Smith, 2004). Staggers, Gassert, and Curran (2001, 2002) defined four levels of informatics competencies for practicing nurses. The first two pertain to all nurses, and the last two pertain to informatics nurses:

1. The beginning nurse should possess basic information management and computer technology skills. Accomplishments should include the ability to access data, use a computer for communication, use basic desktop software, and use decision support systems.
2. Experienced nurses should be highly skilled in using information management and computer technology to support their major area of practice. Additional skills for the experienced nurse include being able to make judgments on the basis of trends and patterns within data elements and to collaborate with nursing informatics nurses to suggest improvements in nursing systems.
3. The informatics nurse specialist should be able to meet the information needs of practicing nurses by integrating and applying information, computer, and nursing sciences.
4. The informatics innovator will conduct informatics research and generate informatics theory.[8]

Information Literacy

Information literacy, or the ability to know when one needs information and how to locate, evaluate, and effectively use it (National Forum on Information Literacy, 2011), is an informatics skill. Although it involves computer skills, similar to informatics, it requires critical thinking

---

8 A Word document containing the complete list of the levels and competencies is available at http:// www.nurs.utah.edu/ informatics/competencies.htm (or from the book web page at http://dlthede.net/Informatics/Competencies2008.doc).

and problem solving. Information literacy is part of the foundation for evidence-based practice and provides nurses with the ability to be intelligent information consumers in today's electronic environment[9] (Jacobs, Rosenfeld, & Haber, 2003).

The level of computer fluency needed by nurses to be both information literate and informatics capable in their practice is what is expected of any educated nurse (see **Figure 1-1**). In this book, the chapters addressing basic computer skills will emphasize concepts that promote the ability to learn new applications. These chapters provide information underlying the use of informatics in professional life. In future chapters, these principles will be built upon to allow the reader to start to gain new informatics skills, including the ability to find and evaluate information from electronic sources. Additional chapters will allow the reader to develop skills necessary to work with nursing informatics specialists in providing effective information systems and the use of nursing data.

Summary

Healthcare is in transition and nursing is being affected by these changes. Part of these changes involves informatics. Whether the change will be positive or negative for patient care and nursing depends on nurses. For the change to be positive, nurses need to develop skills in information management, known in healthcare as informatics. To gain these skills, a background in both computer and information literacy skills is necessary.

As knowledge continues to expand logarithmically, data and information can no longer be managed solely by the human mind. The use of technology tools to aid the human mind has become mandatory. Healthcare has been behind most industries in using technology to manage its data. However, government- and private-level forces are working to change this. With these pressures, healthcare informatics is rapidly expanding. Nursing is one of many subspecialties in healthcare informatics. Embracing informatics will allow

nurses to assess and evaluate practice just as a stethoscope allows the evaluation and assessment of a patient.

The use of computers in healthcare started in the 1960s, mostly in financial areas, but with the advance in computing power and the demand for clinical data, computers are being used more and more in clinical areas. With this growth has come a change in focus for information systems from providing solutions for just one process, to an enterprise-wide patient-centered system that focuses on data. This new focus provides the functionality that allows one piece of data to be used in multiple ways. To understand and work with clinical systems, as well as to fulfill other professional responsibilities, nurses need to be computer fluent, information literate, and informatics knowledgeable.

APPLICATIONS AND COMPETENCIES

1. Investigate one of the forces outside healthcare that are driving a move toward the greater use of informatics, and briefly discuss some pros and cons for this force.

2. Using the definitions of nursing informatics in this chapter or from other resources, create your own nursing informatics definition that would apply to your clinical practice.

3. Support the statement: "The computer is a tool of informatics, but not the focus."

4. Take one instance of informatics used in healthcare and analyze its effect on nurses and patient care.

5. List reasons why every nurse needs to have informatics skills.

6. The results of the Delphi study by Staggers et al. (2002) are available at http://www.nurs.utah.edu/informatics/competencies.htm (or from the book web page at http://dlthede.net/Informatics/Competencies2008.doc) as a Word document. Download the list and rate yourself for each of the competencies. Select one for which you need to improve your skills and design a plan for reaching competency.

7. Analyze all the information beyond your immediate knowledge that you need and use in caring for one of your patients on just one shift.

---

9 Information Competency will be discussed in Unit III.

Where does this information originate? When do you need it for care? How do your obtain it? How do you use it?

8. Write one or two paragraphs on how you now think a practicing nurse can use computer fluency and information literacy to advance in a career. Save this and at the end of this book, compare it with how you then see these two skills affecting a nursing career.

REFERENCES

American Health Information Management Association, & American Medical Informatics Association. (2006). *Building the workforce for health information transformation.* Retrieved June 9, 2010, from http://library.ahima.org/xpedio/groups/public/documents/ahima/bok1_030746.pdf

American Association of Colleges of Nursing. (2006, October). *The essentials of doctoral education for advanced nursing practice.* Retrieved July 28, 2011, from http://www.aacn.nche.edu/DNP/pdf/Essentials.pdf

American Association of Colleges of Nursing. (2008, October 20). *The essentials of baccalaureate education for professional nursing practice.* Retrieved June 10, 2010, from http://www.aacn.nche.edu/education/pdf/baccessentials08.pdf

American Association of Colleges of Nursing. (2011, March 21). *The essentials of master's education in nursing.* Retrieved July 28, 2011, from http://www.aacn.nche.edu/Education/pdf/Master'sEssentials11.pdf

American Nurses Association. (2001). *Scope and standards of nursing informatics practice.* Washington, DC: American Nurses Publishing.

American Nurses Association. (2008). *Nursing informatics: Scope and standards of practice.* Washington, DC: American Nurses Publishing.

Bakken, S. (2001). An informatics infrastructure is essential for evidence-based practice. *Journal of the American Medical Informatics Association, 8*(3), 199–201.

Bakken, S. (2006). Informatics for patient safety: A nursing research perspective. *Annual Review of Nursing Research, 24,* 219–254.

Bansal, M. (2002). *Medical informatics: A primer.* Cincinnati, OH: McGraw-Hill.

Bellis, M. (n.d.). *Herman Hollerith – Punch cards.* Retrieved June 10, 2010, from http://inventors.about.com/library/inventors/blhollerith.htm

Committee on Quality of Health Care in America, & Institute of Medicine. (2001). *Crossing the quality chasm: A new health system for the 21st century.* Retrieved from http://books.nap.edu/catalog.php?record_id=10027#toc

Davenport, T. H., & Glaser, J. (2002). Just-in-time delivery comes to knowledge management. *Harvard Business Review, 80*(7), 107–111. Retrieved from http://hbswk.hbs.edu/archive/3049.html

Delaney, C. (2001). Health informatics and oncology nursing. *Seminars in Oncology Nursing, 17*(1), 2–6.

Department of Health & Human Services Office of the National Coordinator for Health Information Technology. (2008, June 3). *The ONC-coordinated federal health IT strategic plan: 2008–2012.* Retrieved June 9, 2010, from http://healthit.hhs.gov/portal/server.pt/gateway/PTARGS_0_10741_848083_0_0_18/HITStrategicPlan508.pdf

Dilson, J. (1968). *The abacus: A pocket computer.* New York, NY: St. Martin's Press.

Freiberger, P. A., & Swaine, M. R. (n.d.). *Arithmetic machine – Encyclopedia Britannica.* Retrieved June 10, 2010, from http://www.britannica.com/EBchecked/topic/725527/Pascaline

Gardner, R. M., Pryor, T. A., & Warner, H. R. (1999). The HELP hospital information system: Update 1998. *International Journal of Medical Informatics, 54*(3), 169–182. doi: S1386505699000131.

Gaumer, G. L., Koeniger-Donohue, R., Friel, C., & Sudbay, M. B. (2007). Use of information technology by advanced practice nurses. *CIN: Computers Informatics Nursing, 25*(6), 344–352. doi: 10.1097/01.NCN.0000299656.59519.06.

Goossen, W. T. (1996). Nursing information management and processing: A framework and definition for systems analysis, design and evaluation. *International Journal of Biomedical Computing, 40*(3), 187–195.

Graves, J. R., & Cocoran, S. (1989). The study of nursing informatics. *Image: Journal of Nursing Scholarship, 21,* 227–231.

Greiner, A. C., & Knebel, E. (Eds.). (2003). *Health professions education: A bridge to quality.* Washington, DC: National Academy Press.

Gugerty, B., Maranda, M. J., Beachley, M., Navarro, V. B., Newbold, S., Hawk, W., et al. (2007, May). *Challenges and opportunities in documentation of the nursing care of patients.* Retrieved May 24, 2007, from http://www.mbon.org/commission2/documenation_challenges.pdf

Hannah, K. J., Ball, M. J., & Edwards, M. J. A. (1994). *Introduction to nursing informatics.* New York, NY: Springer-Verlag.

Jacobs, L. (2009). Interview with Lawrence Weed, MD – The father of the problem-oriented medical record looks ahead. *The Permanent Journal, 13*(3). Retrieved from http://xnet.kp.org/permanentejournal/sum09/Lawrence_Weed.pdf

Jacobs, S. K., Rosenfeld, P., & Haber, J. (2003). Information literacy as the foundation for evidence-based practice in graduate nursing education: A curriculum-integrated approach. *Journal Professional Nursing, 19*(5), 320–328.

Jacquard, Joseph Marie (1752–1834). (2009). *The Hutchinson dictionary of scientific biography.* Abingdon, UK: Helicon Publishing.

Korpman, R. A. (1990). Patient care automation the future is now: Introduction and historical perspective, part 1. *Nursing Economics, 8*(3), 191–193.

Leapfrog Group. (2009a). *About us.* Retrieved June 10, 2010, from http://www.leapfroggroup.org/about_us

Leapfrog Group. (2009b). *The Leapfrog Group fact sheet.* Retrieved June 10, 2010, from http://www.leapfroggroup.org/about_us/leapfrog-factsheet

McCannon, M., & O'Neal, P. V. (2003). Results of a national survey indicating information technology skills needed by nurses at time of entry into the work force. *Journal of Nursing Education, 42*(8), 327–340.

McDonald, M. D. (1994). Telecognition for improving health. *Healthcare Forum Journal, 37*(2), 18–21.

McNeil, B. J., & Odom, S. K. (2000). Nursing informatics education in the United States: Proposed undergraduate curriculum. *Health Informatics Journal, 6*(1), 32–38.

McNeil, B. J., Elfrink, V. L., Bickford, C. J., Pierce, S. T., Beyea, S. C., Averill, C., et al. (2003). Nursing information technology knowledge, skills, and preparation of student nurses, nursing faculty, and clinicians: A U.S. survey. *Journal Nursing Education, 42*(8), 341–349.

McNeill, D. G. (1979). Developing the complete computer-based information system. *Journal of Nursing Administration, 9*(11), 34–46.

Millar, D., Millar, I., Millar, J., & Millar, M. (2002). Babbage, Charles (1791–1871). In *The Cambridge dictionary of scientists* (2nd ed., pp. xii, 428). Cambridge, UK: Cambridge University Press.

Moye, W. T. (1996, January). *ENIAC: The army-sponsored revolution*. Retrieved June 10, 2010, from http://ftp.arl.army.mil/~mike/comphist/96summary/

Nagelkerk, J., Ritolo, P. M., & Vandort, P. J. (1998). Nursing informatics: The trend of the future. *Journal of Continuing Education in Nursing, 29*(1), 17–21.

National Advisory Council on Nurse Education and Practice. (1997, December). *A national informatics agenda for nursing education and practice.* Retrieved June 10, 2010, from ftp://ftp.hrsa.gov//bhpr/nursing/nireport/NIFull.pdf

National Forum on Information Literacy. (2011). *National forum on information literacy: 21st century skills.* Retrieved July 27, 2011, from http://infolit.org/

National League for Nursing. (2008). *Position statement: Preparing the next generation of nurses to practice in a technology-rich environment: An informatics agenda.* Retrieved June 10, 2010, from http://www.nln.org/aboutnln/PositionStatements/informatics_052808.pdf

National Research Council (U.S.) Committee on Information Technology Literacy. (1999). *Being fluent with information technology.* Washington, DC: National Academy Press.

Nelson, R. (2007). U.S. hospitals need staffing makeover. *American Journal of Nursing, 107*(12), 19. doi: 10.1097/01.NAJ.0000301004.88450.83.

Newbold, S. K. (1996). The informatics nurse and the certification process. *Computers in Nursing, 14*(2), 84–85, 88.

Nightingale, F. (1863). *Notes on hospitals* (3rd ed.). London, England: Longman, Green, Longman, Roberts, and Green.

Office of Science and Technology Policy. (2010, June 9). *Science, technology and innovation.* Retrieved June 9, 2010, from http://www.whitehouse.gov/administration/eop/ostp

Pillar, B., & Golumbic, N. (1993). *Nursing informatics: Enhancing patient care.* Bethesda, MD: National Center for Nursing Research, U.S. Department of Health and Human Services.

Quality and Safety Education for Nurses. (2010). *Project overview: QSEN – Quality & safety education for nurses.* Retrieved May 17, 2010, from http://www.qsen.org/overview.php

Robert Wood Johnson Foundation. (2010, May 6). *Improving the nurse work environment on medical-surgical units through technology.* Retrieved June 10, 2010, from http://www.rwjf.org/pr/product.jsp?id=62869

Ronald, J., & Skiba, D. (1987). *Guidelines for basic computer education in nursing.* New York, NY: National League for Nursing.

Saba, V. K., & Erdeley, W. S. (2006). Historical perspectives of nursing and the computer. In V. K. Saba & K. A. McCormick (Eds.), *Essentials of nursing informatics* (4th ed., pp. 9–27). New York, NY: McGraw-Hill.

Sackett, K. M., & Erdley, W. S. (2002). The history of health care informatics. In S. Englebardt & R. Nelson (Eds.), *Healthcare informatics from an interdisciplinary approach* (pp. 453–477). St. Louis, MO: Mosby.

Scholes, M., & Barber, B. (1980). Towards nursing informatics. In D. A. D. Lindberg & S. Kaihara (Eds.), *MEDINFO: 1980* (pp. 7–73). Amsterdam, the Netherlands: North Holland.

Schultz, J. R. (1988). A history of the PROMIS technology: An effective human interface. In A. Goldberg (Ed.), *A history of personal workstations* (pp. 1–46). Reading, MA: Addison-Wesley.

Schwirian, P. (1986). The NI pyramid – A model for research in nursing informatics. *CIN: Computers in Nursing, 4*(3), 134–136.

Shortliffe, E. H., & Blois, M. S. (2001). The computer meets medicine: Emergence of a discipline. In E. H. Shortliffe & L. E. Perrault (Eds.), *Medical informatics: Computer applications in healthca*re (pp. 3–40). New York, NY: Springer-Verlag.

Simpson, R. (1998). The technologic imperative: A new agenda for nursing education and practice, part 1. *Nursing Management, 29*(9), 22–24.

Staggers, N. (2004). Assessing recommendations from the IOMs quality chasm report. *Journal of Healthcare Information Management, 18*(1), 30–35.

Staggers, N., Gassert, C. A., & Curran, C. (2001). Informatics competencies for nurses at four levels of practice. *Journal of Nursing Education, 40*(7), 303–316.

Staggers, N., Gassert, C. A., & Curran, C. (2002). *Results of a Delphi study to determine informatics competencies for nurses at four levels of practice.* Retrieved July 28, 2011, from http://nursing.utah.edu/programs/masters/specialty/informatics/competencies.doc

Staggers, N., & Thompson, C. B. (2002). The evolution of definitions for nursing informatics: A critical analysis and revised definition. *Journal of the American Medical Association, 9*(3), 255–261.

Technology Guiding Educational Reform. (2007). *The TIGER initiative: Evidence and informatics transforming nursing: 3-year action steps toward a 10-year vision.* Retrieved May 17, 2010, from http://www.aacn.nche.edu/Education/pdf/TIGER.pdf

The Oughtred Society. (2007, September 16). *Slide rule history.* Retrieved June 10, 2010, from http://www.oughtred.org/history.shtml

Thompson, T. G. (2004, May 6). *Health Information Technology Summit.* Retrieved June 9, 2010, from http://www.hhs.gov/news/speech/2004/040506.html

Turley, J. (1996). Toward a model for nursing informatics. *Image: Journal of Nursing Scholarship, 28*(4), 309–313.

Utley-Smith, Q. (2004). 5 competencies needed by new baccalaureate graduates. *Nursing Education Perspectives, 25*(4), 166–170.

Womack, D., Newbold, S. K., Staugaitis, H., & Cunningham, B. (2004). *Technology's role in addressing Maryland's nursing shortage: Innovations & examples.* Baltimore, MD: Technology Workgroup, Maryland Statewide Commission on the Crisis in Nursing.

CHAPTER 2
Software: Information Management

Objectives

After studying this chapter you will be able to:

▶ *Describe features of operating systems.*

▶ *Apply basic features of operating systems.*

▶ *Differentiate application software.*

▶ *Define a computer algorithm.*

▶ *Explain the importance of user groups.*

▶ *Differentiate the various types of software copyright.*

Key Terms

Active Window	Mouse
Algorithm	Office Suites
Application Program	Open Source
Cloud Computing	Operating System
Code	Point and Click
Crash	Quick Launch Bar
Desktop	Shareware
Disk Operating System (DOS)	Software
Flowchart	Software Piracy
Freeware	Speech Recognition
Graphical User Interface (GUI)	Task Bar
Groupware	Title Bar

The computer, despite all its parts, will do nothing but act as an expensive paperweight unless it is told what to do. These instructions, which allow us to manage data and information, come in the form of **software**, or computer programs. Many kinds of software exist. Basically, software manages either the computer system itself or information. Software that manages the computer system includes two overall items: those programs and utilities that reside in read-only memory (ROM), which enable the computer to boot, and system software. This latter category includes the **operating system** that controls the computer and the utilities that allow the user some control over that operating system. Software that manages user information is known as **application programs**. Application programs include information systems in healthcare agencies and off-the-shelf generic applications that can perform a variety of tasks. Examples of the latter include the many **office suites** such as Microsoft Office®, OpenOffice.org, Corel WordPerfect Office®, and Lotus Symphony®. **Speech recognition** software that can convert spoken words to text is another type of application program. There are also software packages that allow users to organize and edit photos, create graphics including animation, create learning packages, and many other tasks.

Operating Systems

Hands down, the most important program on your computer is the operating system. It coordinates input from the keyboard with output on the screen, responds to **mouse** clicks, heeds commands to save a file, retrieves files, and transmits commands to printers and other peripheral devices. It is the software platform on top of which all application programs run. Application programs are written to work with a specific operating system. Thus, the operating system that you select determines which applications you can run. Personal computers (PCs) today and most notebooks use a version of Microsoft Windows®. The Apple Macintosh® uses a different operating system, as do larger computers. The operating system on mobile Internet devices and personal digital assistants varies.

The operating systems for large servers, such as those that control hospital information systems, have large responsibilities and powers (Webopedia, 2011a). They must act like a traffic cop – making sure that different programs and users do not interfere with one another, as well as accept, store, and retrieve data. They are also responsible for ensuring that unauthorized users cannot access the system. In this chapter, we will concern ourselves only with operating systems and software that one is likely to encounter on a PC.

DOS

Early PCs used the DOS operating system, which is an acronym for **disk operating system**. Although it could refer to any operating system, the term "DOS" came to mean the operating system developed by Microsoft® for PCs. DOS was text based, and it required users to remember a set of commands such as Delete, Run, Copy, and Rename. Unlike today's operating systems, DOS allowed only one program at a time to be operational. Transferring information between programs was difficult and time-consuming, as was creating anything that was not text.

Graphical User Interfaces

In a **graphical user interface** (GUI – pronounced "gooey"), users no longer had to remember esoteric commands. Instead, commands are entered by "pointing and clicking." Pointing and clicking refers to moving a mouse,[1] which moves the screen mouse pointer in the direction that the mouse is moved. When the mouse pointer is in the desired location, the user taps (clicks) the left mouse button. GUIs are oriented to this **point and click** method of giving commands and to icons or small pictures instead of words.

GUIs were designed by the Xerox Corporation's Palo Alto Research Center in the 1970s (Webopedia, 2011a, 2011b, 2011c). Because they required more central processing unit (CPU) power and a high-quality monitor, which were then prohibitively expensive, they were slow to be accepted. It was the Apple Macintosh that first employed them, followed in the late 1980s by PCs. Most healthcare agencies use PCs with Windows; thus, this book concentrates on that computer and operating system. Many home computers are Macintoshes; although the exact implementation of commands will not translate, most of the principles and features that are discussed in this chapter and others that address PCs will be useful.

Microsoft Windows® Operating System

Because GUIs are easy to use, most healthcare information systems use a GUI operating system, usually a version of Microsoft Windows®. For this reason, as well as the computer fluency demanded of healthcare professionals, it is appropriate to review some basics of using Windows. When a PC is turned on and finishes booting (often a 3- to 5-minute process), the **desktop** screen appears. The desktop has icons representing many of the application programs that are installed on the computer. Below these icons is the name of the application that the icon

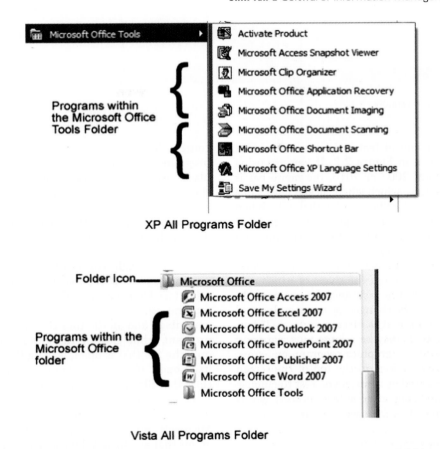

XP All Programs Folder

Vista All Programs Folder

Figure 2-1 All programs folders.

represents. When "clicked" (putting the mouse pointer on the icon and left-clicking), the program the icon represents will open.

Opening a Program in a PC

As with all things with Microsoft Windows®, there are several ways to start a program when using a PC. Clicking the icon on the desktop, mentioned earlier, is often used when the computer is first turned on. If an icon for the desired program is not on the desktop, the user should click the Start button, then click All Programs, and click the name of the program on that list. The Start button, so called because it "starts" processes, is located in the lower left corner of the screen. In Windows Vista®, the start button is the Windows logo surrounded by a blue circle.

Some programs that are together in a suite such as OpenOffice.org, Corel Office®, Lotus Symphony™, or Microsoft Office® may require that the folder containing all of them be opened and then the program selected from the secondary menu contained in the folder. In XP, this will be indicated by a black triangle mark pointing to the right. In Vista, a container for more programs will be the folder icon as seen in **Figure 2-1**. In either case, clicking the container will show the programs with that folder, and you can make your selection from there.

Working With a Program in a PC

Once a program is opened, you will see the work screen, which may look like any of those in **Figure 2-2**. The choices on the menu bar can be

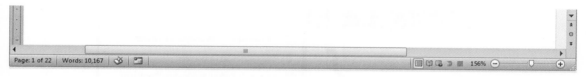

Figure 2-2 Program window.

clicked for a menu of features classified by that choice as shown in **Figure 2-3**. If you are using Microsoft Word® 2007 or 2010, the menu bar is replaced with tabs, which when clicked have icons for the features classified under that tab. When first starting to use a new application program, or a major update, using Help to find the feature you want is often necessary.

All programs will have a symbol, which represents the mouse pointer, the shape of which may vary according to the task and the program. In some cases, it can be changed by the user. In word processing software, it is often a vertical "I" bar; in spreadsheets, it may be a large plus sign; and in a presentation or graphics program, an arrow. Although many choices on the top of the screen may be represented by icons, if you rest the mouse pointer on an icon, after a few seconds words describing what the icon is will appear.

Multiple Windows

One of the advantages of GUIs is the ability to have multiple programs open at the same time and to easily move data between them. This makes it possible to copy a graph from a spreadsheet into a word processing document, or a graphic from PowerPoint into a spreadsheet or word processing document.

Closing Files and Programs

In the context of a PC, the term "windows" may refer to the operating system or to the various content boxes that appear on the screen. Each program that is open creates its own window and places a tab on the **task bar** on the bottom of the screen. If a word processor and a spreadsheet program are open simultaneously, two program windows are open; both may or may not be visible on the screen at the same time. Closing the window in any program involves clicking on an X in the upper right corner of the screen. In some programs, you will see two Xs, one on top of the other (see **Figure 2-4**). In these cases, clicking the top one, which is usually red, will close the program itself and all the files that are open in that program, while clicking the lower one will close only the file that is open, leaving the application itself open. If there is only one X, clicking it will close that file and instance of the program.

Looking at the task bar at the bottom of the screen tells you how many instances of each Microsoft® program are open, and any other programs that are open. When so many programs are open that there is no room on the task bar, multiple instances of the same program will be grouped under one icon, meaning that you will have to click that tab and select which file you wish to use for that program.

Navigating Between Programs and Files

GUIs provide the ability to have many different windows open at one time and aid in productivity. As mentioned earlier, when you have more than one program or file open, the program name will be

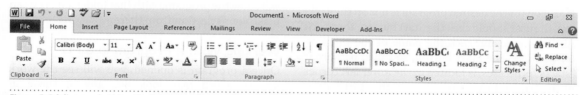

Figure 2-3 Microsoft Word® ribbon toolbar.

Two X's in the upper right corner

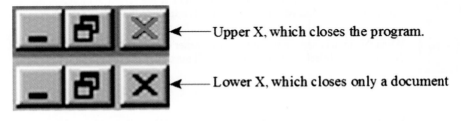

—————Upper X, which closes the program.

—————Lower X, which closes only a document

One X in the upper right corner

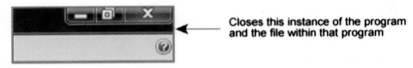

Closes this instance of the program
and the file within that program

Figure 2-4 Closing files and programs.

on the task bar, which is at the bottom of the screen. If this line is not visible, place your mouse pointer on the bottom of the screen, and it will appear.

Part of the left side of the task bar is the **Quick Launch bar** to which you can drag icons either from the desktop or the program list for programs that you frequently use. Then instead of using the desktop or All Programs from the Start button to open a program, you can click the icon in the Quick Launch bar that represents the program you wish to open. If you can't remember what the icons represent, rest your mouse pointer a second or two on it and the name of the program will appear.

Maximizing and Minimizing a Window

Not only does Windows allow you to have more than one window open at a time, it lets you see multiple windows at the same time. Often, when you open a program, you will see that it does not take up the entire screen. You may even see another program or the desktop behind it. In this format, the window is said to be "minimized." This holds true whether it takes up almost the entire screen or is reduced to just the **title bar** (see **Figure 2-5**). You can maximize it by clicking the square in the upper right corner of the screen and minimize it by clicking the three-dimensional square that replaces the original square when the window is maximized.

In a minimized format, you can place your mouse pointer on the sides of the window until it becomes a double-edged arrow ($\leftrightarrow$), and then drag the side to change the size of the window. To move a window, place the mouse pointer in the title bar, or the top line of the window that has the name of the program and often of the file itself, and drag the window wherever you want it. If the windows overlap, the window that is the **active window**, or the window in which you are working, will be on top. Clicking in a window makes it the active window. If the windows are side by side, the active window is the one where the mouse pointer is, although sometimes the title bar will be a little darker in color in the active window. Placing windows side by side or one on top of the other can be very useful when working on two files in the same program, or needing to synchronize files from different programs.

Accessories and Utilities

Operating systems usually come with some utilities and built-in software. Certain utilities are helpful with disk maintenance, such as the disk utilities ScanDisk and Disk Defragmenter discussed in Appendix A. Additional accessories such as Paint, a simple drawing program, allow a user to create drawings or various shapes, such as circles, squares, or triangles, in any of the colors available

When this icon is seen in the upper right corner of the screen, it indicates that the document is **maximized**. Clicking on it will minimize the document.

 When this icon is seen in the upper right corner of the screen, it indicates that the document is **minimized**. Clicking on it will maximize the document.

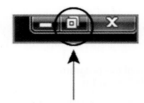

Click this button to make Window smaller or minimize the Window

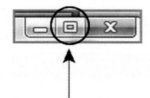

Click this button to make Window fill entire screen or maximize the Window

Figure 2-5 Maximizing and minimizing a window.

in the program. Also available are writing accessories such as Notepad, a product that is useful in creating files in ASCII (American Standard Code for Information Interchange), which is a format that can be read by many different programs.

Ease of Access

Given the prevalence of computers in today's society, and the increasing use that is being made of the web for patient empowerment, nurses need to be aware of the various options available for helping those with disabilities to use computers. Both Apple® Computers and Microsoft® maintain pages that provide information about the various options to assist those whose disabilities present problems with using computers. Some examples of the adjustments that can be made with both Windows XP® and Vista® are changing how items on the screen are displayed, a screen magnifier, and an option to provide visual warnings for system sounds. There are also many options for changing how the keys on a keyboard work as well as the way the mouse behaves. In Windows XP, information about making these changes is available from the Accessibility Wizard; Windows Vista has an Ease of Access choice on the classic view of the Control Panel (accessible from the Start button). There is even a narrator that will read each character

that is entered when using Microsoft Office® products. Microsoft's website at http://www.microsoft .com/enable/ provides links to information about using these utilities in addition to tutorials and guides to accessibility options for many disabilities including dexterity problems. Apple Computer maintains a similar site for Macintosh users at http://www.apple.com/accessibility/

Exiting the Operating System

In the earlier sections, we discussed how to close a file on which you are working and how to close a program. Before shutting down a computer, it is necessary to exit the operating system. Although invisible to users, Microsoft Windows®, like all operating systems, actually works very hard behind the scenes to provide its many functions, as do many of the application programs. To do this, application programs and Microsoft Windows® have to have easy access to specific information. Often, this is accomplished by creating files on the hard disk of the information that the application needs to use. These files are temporary and unknown to the users. They are created, changed, and deleted as users change what they are doing. Before quitting Windows, the application programs need to be able to shut these files down. If users do not exit all programs and close the operating system properly, these temporary files are left on the disk and can cause problems as well as fill up your hard disk. To exit Windows and shut down your computer, click the Start button in the lower left corner of the screen, select Shut Down from the menu, and let the computer go through the shutdown process, which may take a minute or more. If, during the time you have used the computer, a program or the operating system has downloaded some updates, you may see a message saying, "Files are being updated. Please don't turn off the computer." This message may or may not add that the computer will be turned off by the program, when the installation is complete, but in most cases this will occur.

Handling Minor Problems

As robust as today's computers are, they sometimes get themselves tangled up and, through no fault of the user, refuse to respond to commands. This is most apt to happen to an individual program, not the entire computer. If you are working in a computer laboratory, or on an agency computer, leave the computer alone and notify the laboratory or network manager. If, however, you are home, there are some things you can do. If you get a message saying, "This program is not responding" and are asked if you want to shut it down, you have no choice except to say yes. It may or may not shut down. If it does not, this is the time to use what is affectionately referred to as the "three-finger salute," because it requires three fingers to execute. To carry it out, you press down and hold the Ctrl, Alt, and Delete keys until you get a menu on which one of the choices is to open the task manager (Microsoft Vista®) or the task manager itself (Microsoft XP®). From there you can locate the offending program and click the End Task button (see **Figure 2-6**). You may then get still another window telling you that the program is not responding and asking you if you want to end it. You may need to tell it yes more than once! But eventually it will close the program.

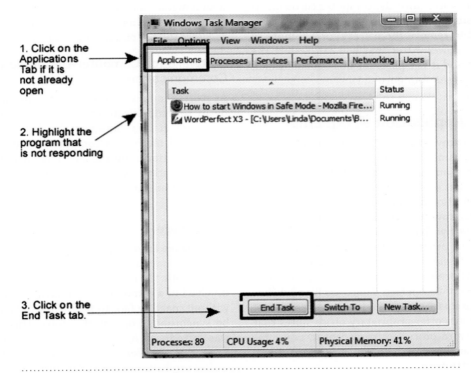

Figure 2-6 Closing a nonresponding program.

After letting it rest for a few minutes, you can then restart that program if you wish.

The biggest drawback is that when a program **crashes**, you will lose whatever you have not saved, which is a reason to save continually as you work! However, most of today's programs will do a backup save every 10 or 15 minutes, a time that you can set in the preferences. After a program crash, when you reopen the program, you will be told that it did not close properly last time and be asked about files that were open and not saved. The best approach is to look at each one and match with what you have on disk to see which is the latest version, the backup or the one you can retrieve from the disk.

On rare occasions, the above approach does not work, and the computer seems bent on doing its own thing with absolutely no regard for what you want. No matter what you do, you can't seem to get its attention. Those who program operating systems, knowing that despite all their efforts occasionally this can happen, have provided an out. To turn off a nonresponding computer, press the power button (yes, the power button on the CPU) and hold it down until the computer turns off! If you are using a laptop or other mobile device, you may need to remove the battery for a minute to cut off its power. After that you can restart the computer, and it will probably be back to normal! Beyond this, see your guru!

Application Programs

There are many different types of software application programs. You are probably familiar with a hospital information system, and possibly even programs that access the web, or browsers, which are all application programs. There are many others that can improve your productivity professionally and personally. Word processors, spreadsheets, presentation programs, and databases form the bulk of professional use, whereas displaying, organizing, and printing photos are one of the main leisure uses of computers. There are many different software packages for any of these functions. Three vendors offer proprietary office suites that contain a word processor, spreadsheet, presentation program, and, in their professional version, a relational database.

Word processors have grown beyond simple text creation and editing to being able to include graphics in a document and produce pamphlets. Spreadsheets have many uses for tasks that focus on numbers. They even have limited statistical features, although a full-featured statistical package will serve this function far better. They are sometimes used as databases (Sewell, 2006), but unless the user needs only a simple database, a relational database works far better. Relational databases allow users to track, summarize, manipulate, and gain knowledge from data. Presentation programs allow users to create computer slide shows, although care must be taken to produce something that is truly useful to an audience. Productive use of each of these types of software will be examined in a separate chapter. There is also a free office suite called Open Office.org (http://www.openoffice.org/) that is compatible with the Microsoft Office™ products. The two other proprietary office suites, Corel™ and Lotus™, will also create files that are compatible with Microsoft Office® products. There are several photo editing and printing packages; some come with a digital camera, others are proprietary, such as Adobe Photoshop™, and some are even free, such as Picasa (http://picasa.google.com/).

Software for Computer-to-Computer Communication

As soon as computers could store information, the desire to share this information between computers arose. It was, however, the development of a standard method of computer communication and production of inexpensive modems that made this interaction available to the general public. This software includes e-mail and networking packages.

Groupware

Groupware is software that permits two or more persons to have a meeting, work on a file together, or do both. It is designed to facilitate people involved in a common task to achieve their goals without meeting face to face. These meetings can be synchronous or asynchronous. This category was introduced in 1989 when Lotus introduced Lotus Notes™ (Woolley, 1996), an outgrowth of an earlier product used on the mainframe. The term as currently used refers to software that promotes not only group discussion, but an array of activities such as scheduling and document sharing.

One can find a wide range in the features in groupware, as well as the definitions. Wikis, which are user-created information sites, are one type of groupware as is text messaging. Generally, however, the term refers to a more sophisticated product in which users share the work on a document or presentation. Both Google™ and Yahoo™ allow users to create private groups for this purpose without charge. There are also many proprietary products. Some of these products allow the meeting coordinator to show a screen that all see; some also allow the use of cameras. A quick search with a web search engine will find many such programs.

Speech Recognition

Speech, or voice, recognition in the context of computer input is the ability of a computer to recognize spoken words and translate them into printed text. This must not to be confused with understanding what is said; that is a function of a field called natural language processing (Webopedia, 2011a, 2011b, 2011c). With the increased power of computers and improved microphones, voice recognition systems have greatly improved since the early days when using one could be an exercise in frustration. The two types of voice recognition are discrete and continuous speech processing. Discrete speech processing, which is not used much today, requires the speaker to say one word at a time, pausing briefly after each word. In continuous speech processing, the user can speak at a normal rate, although speaking distinctly is necessary.

In the past, systems required the user to train the program extensively to understand the spoken word. The training consisted of the user repeating those words the computer would be required to understand, until the word was recognized as spoken by that person. Some systems today are capable of recognizing the spoken word from different people without this special training, but for optimal use of more than a few phrases, all require some training (Jackson, 2010). The accuracy of voice software is also affected by the quality of the microphone used for voice input.

Speech recognition has received a welcome reception in the field of medical transcription. To meet this need, and because the vocabulary used is quite different from everyday use, several companies have introduced systems that have a large built-in vocabulary that focus on a specific field, such as radiology. No matter how good a speech recognition program is, proofing the result is very necessary.

Microsoft® made speech recognition software available as an accessory that could be downloaded with Service Pack 1 for Windows XP™. With Windows Vista® and Windows 7®, speech recognition is an integral part of the operating system and is an accessory. A quick way to locate the feature is to use the Windows Start menu icon and type *speech recognition* in the Search Programs and Files box, although you may have to use the Help and Support options to find it. With training, it can provide good speech recognition.

Cloud Computing

Cloud computing refers to the ability to access software and file storage on remote computers using the Internet. Many of the cloud computing office application and file storage resources provide the ability to share files and folders with others. The user simply enters the e-mail name(s) for shared files. Examples of cloud computing software include Microsoft Office® Live (Word, Excel, and PowerPoint) and Google Docs (Document, Presentation, Spreadsheet, Form, Drawing). Microsoft Office® Live also provides off-site file storage capabilities. Many of the cloud computing resources provide 2–25 GB of free file storage (**Table 2-1**).

 Installing Software

Installing a legal copy of software, after the computer hard drive is set up for use, is usually quite easy. A good rule of thumb to follow is to first close all other applications before installing something new. After that, insert the disk that the program is on and follow the screen directions. At one point you will have to check a box, indicating that you accept the licensing agreement. Unless you are very versed in file and disk anatomy, it is best to

Table 2-1 Cloud Computing Resource Examples

Cloud Computing Application	URL	Office Applications	File Storage
Office Live	http://www.officelive.com/en-us/	X	X
Google Docs	http://docs.google.com	X	X
Zoho	http://www.zoho.com/	X	X
Dropbox	https://www.dropbox.com/		X
Box	http://www.box.net/		X
iDrive	http://www.idrive.com/		X
aDrive	http://www.adrive.com/		X

Remote data backup is a common cloud computing feature for antivirus software such as Norton and Symantec. Remote backup is used to restore a computer system configuration in the event of a problem created by an unsuspected virus or malware. For additional information on how cloud computing storage works, go to http://communication.howstuffworks.com/cloud-storage.htm

let the program decide into what folder (named container on a disk) it will install itself, and select the usual installation process. In Windows Vista, you must have administrator privileges to do the installation, a process that can prevent programs that would harm the computer from installing themselves without user knowledge. On laboratory or agency computers, you will probably not be allowed to install any program on the computer. This protects the agency against illegal software and software that could interfere with the network system.

Creating Software

Software is created using a programming language, of which there are many. There are also different levels of languages. These levels depend on the degree to which the language approaches "natural language" – the higher the level, the closer to regular language. The drawback is that as the level of the language increases the flexibility of the language decreases. The lowest level, machine language, communicates directly with the zeros and ones that represent bits. The next level, assembly language, uses cryptic names instead of numbers to translate commands to the machine language. Level three, or the so-called high-level languages, includes such well-known languages as COBOL, FORTRAN, and Basic. Fourth-level languages are designed for a specific purpose. Structured query language is a fourth-level language designed specifically to query relational databases. Ultimately,

no matter which level language is used or which language a program is written in, it must be translated to machine language in a process called compiling.

Computer software works by taking a user's commands and quickly providing the computer with a detailed step-by-step set of instructions in such a manner that the computer can understand and comply. These instructions are called **code**. Before a single line of code is written, it is necessary to define the problem the computer is to solve and develop a **flowchart** of instructions. From this flowchart, a detailed set of instructions can be developed and turned into code. These instructions are known as an **algorithm**. A flowchart in computer programming is like a flowchart used to model any process. It is a pictorial representation of the process or project being planned with decision points. Flowcharts provide people with a common understanding of the process. **Figure 2-7** shows an example of a flowchart.

As a healthcare professional, a nurse may be called on to assist in defining a problem or testing the proposed solution. Defining a problem with enough accuracy and detail so that the computer can be used to solve it is a difficult task. A simple problem such as asking the computer to flag vital signs that require nursing attention requires attention to many details. First, the nurse needs to determine the limits of normal. This may sound easy until the nurse remembers that in some cases, a temperature elevated by 2.25°F may not be of any concern. In the same way, the nurse also must

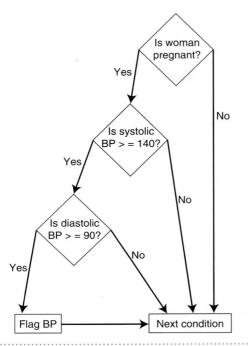

Figure 2-7 A flowchart that is the basis for an algorithm.

define "normal" pulse and respiration rates and blood pressures. To do this, the nurse must come up with a set of rules or algorithms stating what readings need flagging under which conditions.

This information is then programmed using "if-then-else" statements that tell the computer what to do if a certain condition exists. In the situation in **Figure 2-7**, an if/then statement would be part of the code for each of the decisions depicted. When one considers the many variables that impinge on clinical decisions, it becomes easy to see why humans must always evaluate computer output. Evaluation is helped if the nurse knows what limits were placed on each variable. In this example, the user would want to know that the computer flags the blood pressure for a pregnant woman only when the systolic exceeds 140 mm Hg and diastolic 90 mm Hg. Because it is highly unlikely that every condition can be programmed, it is imperative that computer users not rely solely on computer output for determining anomalies. There is no substitute

for critical thinking by a perceptive healthcare professional. Common sense and expert intuition will never be replaced by a computer.

Open Source Software

Open source software is software that is copyrighted, but whose source code is available to anyone who wants it. The idea behind this is that when the source code is available, many programmers, who are not concerned with financial gain, will make improvements to the code and produce a more useful, bug-free product (Beal, 2005). This concept is based on using peer review to find and eliminate bugs, a process that is unfortunately absent in many proprietary programs. Open source grew in the technological community as a response to proprietary software owned by corporations.

User Groups

When learning to use any software, sources of help can be extremely useful. Whether using a book, teacher, or other source of instruction, questions arise for which answers are not readily available. One excellent source of help is a user group, which is a gathering of people who meet regularly for the purpose of sharing information about a given topic. There are user groups for PC application programs and hospital information systems. User group members range from novices to those who make a living as consultants for the program. The level of formal organization varies with the size and purpose of the group. Most user group meetings have an agenda that includes both a question-and-answer session and a presentation by a member or invited guest on some aspect of the group's focus.

There are few geographic areas today in the United States that do not have a computer user group for PCs or Macintoshes. In large cities, there may be one umbrella group with smaller significant interest groups that meet independently to learn more about a specific program. For more information about user groups and how to find a group, see the website for the Association of Personal

Computer User Groups at http://www.apcug.org, or call a local computer store. Computer stores usually have information on the groups in the area. In fact, they may even be the sites for meetings.

Information system user groups for health information systems are of two types: internal and external. An internal group consists of users of a system within a given institution, whereas an external group has members from healthcare institutions all over the country (or even the world). Like other software user groups, they share experiences both positive and negative. If a nurse from each unit is not a member of a user group for the information system in his or her institution, nurses are missing opportunities to improve the program so that it serves nursing better, be a powerful advocate for nursing, and learn shortcuts for using the information system that can be shared with colleagues.

Software Program Copyright

When selling software, many vendors believe that the users are not buying the software, but instead buying a license to use it. In this thinking, breaking the shrink-wrap means the user agrees to the conditions of the license. These licenses generally state that the software cannot be sold or given away without the permission of the vendor and that the vendor cannot be held responsible for any problems the software might cause the computer. Depending on the vendor, users may be told that they can install the software on only one computer or, in some cases, on more than one computer if only one copy will be used at a time.

Today, installing most proprietary software such as Microsoft Office Suite™ requires the user to register the software – a process that generally requires the user to be connected to the Internet (online). During installation, one must enter a number that may be called the serial number, product key, or some other designation, which can be found on either the installation disks or the envelope in which the software disk came. The program then checks to see if the program has been registered before, and if not, it allows the installation to go forward. Some products that allow trial

periods will give the user a chance to register either after a given number of days or when it is installed if the product is already purchased. In any case, keep a record of these numbers in case they are needed at a later date. Product numbers may be matched to a number in the BIOS. Should the hard disk crash, the software can be easily reinstalled on a new disk on that computer if the user still has the registration information.

Today, given the ease with which programs can be checked to see if they are legitimate, pirated software is more a problem than illegal installations of legitimate software. Most problems are from countries outside the Western world. The Fourth Annual Business Software Report found that for every $2 spent on legitimate software, $1 was lost to pirated software, but that this ratio was reversed in some countries (Business Software Alliance, 2007). In 1992, Congress passed the Software Copyright Protection Bill, which raised **software piracy** from a misdemeanor to a felony (Nicoll, 1994). Penalties of up to $100,000 for statutory damages and fines of up to $250,000 can be levied for this crime, plus the people responsible can be sentenced to a jail term of up to 5 years.

Healthcare and educational organizations are not immune from prosecution. One western university paid $130,000 to the Software Publishers Association when it was found to have illegal software in a laboratory. A hospital in Illinois was fined about $161,000 when they were found engaging in unauthorized software duplication (Chicago hospital caught pirating, 1997). Organizations without an enforced software oversight policy are possible candidates for investigation. To want to spend less for software is always tempting, but beware of pirated copies. Besides opening the owners up to lawsuits, jail terms, and economic losses, they can carry viruses that can affect the computer. The Business Software Alliance is so serious about pirated software that they provide an online method of reporting software piracy (https://reporting.bsa.org/usa/home.aspx).

Some software is distributed as **shareware**. Software of this type is often found on the Internet. The publishers of shareware encourage users to give copies to friends and colleagues to try out. They request that anyone who uses the program after a trial period pay them a fee.

Registration information is included in the program. Continuing to use shareware without paying the registration fee is considered software piracy. In many cases, access to the program may be denied after a given period of time, which will be stated when the program is installed.

Freeware is an application the programmer has decided to make freely available to anyone who wishes to use it. Although it may be used without paying a fee, the author usually maintains the copyright, which, unless the program is open source, generally means a user cannot do anything with the program other than what the author intended. Some freeware programs available on the Internet are in the public domain and for which the author states that they can be used any way the user desires, including making changes. When users accept software through any channel but a reputable reseller, they should be certain that they know whether the software is proprietary, shareware, freeware, or in the public domain. And, unless the vendor is very well known, download the program file, save it, and use a virus checker to see if the file is carrying a virus before installing it.

Summary

There are many different types of software that are useful in managing information. Yet, it can be said that software is generally of two overall types: software that manages systems and software that allows people to manage information. Systems software consists of utilities and operating systems.

An operating system determines what application software you can use. This software includes not only the operating systems but also accessories that help you to manage the computer and some other programs such as those that create ASCII text or graphics. There are also programs such as a calendar and a calculator.

Software that allows users to manage information includes many different varieties including computer-to-computer communication and other special niche programs such as photo editing and speech recognition. There are different vendors for application programs, each of which approaches the task of implementing functions a little differently, but, essentially, all produce the same finished product. Several vendors offer office suites, which consist of a word processor, spreadsheet, presentation package, and database. Office suites from one vendor are designed for the programs they contain to integrate well with each other.

Programming languages can be classified as machine language, assembly, high-level, or fourth-level languages. Machine language consists solely of zeros and ones, whereas assembly language, which is one level higher, uses some word-like characters in its code. Fourth-level languages come the closest to natural language. Writing applications involves defining the problem to be solved and translating that to code.

Although there is some open source and free software, most of the software used is proprietary and copyrighted. Using a copy of a proprietary program for which a user does not hold a license is software piracy. Shareware is software that can be tried for free, but a registration fee should be paid if it is regularly used. Only freeware can be used without cost.

APPLICATIONS AND COMPETENCIES

1. Identify the current operating system on the computer you are using.

2. Identify the application software that is available on that computer.

3. Practice maximizing, minimizing, and dragging a window.

4. Open two or three application programs and navigate between them.

5. Write down as many rules as you can think of that define when deviations, either more or less than the normal temperature of 98.6°F (37°C), are cause for action by a nurse.

6. Create a flowchart of the steps for giving a PRN medication. Use a diamond shape for a decision, a rectangle for a process, and a parallelogram for data.

7. A friend gives you a CD-ROM with a program on it for you to install. What things should you consider before doing so?

8. You wish to install a program that you have at home on your computer at work. What things need to be considered?

REFERENCES

Beal, V. (2005, September 26, 2008). *All about open source*. Retrieved November 15, 2008, from http://www. webopedia.com/DidYouKnow/Computer_Science/2005/ open_source.asp

Business Software Alliance. (2007). *2006 piracy study*. Retrieved November 15, 2008, from http://portal.bsa.org/ idcglobalstudy2007/studies/2006globalpiracystudy-en.pdf

Chicago hospital caught pirating. (1997, January). *Healthcare Informatics, 20*.

Jackson, J. (2010, August 5). Speech recognition systems must get smarter, professor says. *PC World*. Retrieved January 30, 2011, from http://www.pcworld.com/ businesscenter/article/202692/speech_recognition_ systems_must_get_smarter_professor_says.html

Nicoll, L. H. (1994). Modern day pirates: Software users and abusers. *Journal of Nursing Administration, 24*(1), 18–20.

Sewell, J. P. (2006). Getting the most from your software: Using excel as the poor man's database. *Computers, Informatics, Nursing, 24*(1), 13–17.

Webopedia. (2011a). *Operating system*. Retrieved July 27, 2011, from http://www.webopedia.com/TERM/o/operating_ system.html

Webopedia. (2011b). *Graphical user interface*. Retrieved January 30, 2011, 2010, from http://www.webopedia .com/TERM/G/Graphical_User_Interface_GUI.html

Webopedia. (2011c). *Voice recognition*. Retrieved January 30, 2011, from http://www.webopedia.com/TERM/v/voice_ recognition.html

Woolley, D. (1996). *Choosing conferencing software*. Retrieved January 30, 2011, from http://thinkofit.com/webconf/ wcchoice.htm

CHAPTER 3

Understanding Computer Concepts: Common Features

Objectives

After studying this chapter, you will be able to:

▶ Use the right mouse button effectively.

▶ Apply computer conventions appropriately.

▶ Use the "Help" option to learn to use software features.

▶ Select, copy, and move an object on a computer.

▶ Use "Save" and "Save As" functions appropriately.

▶ Employ file organizational principles.

▶ Differentiate between "Sleep" and "Hibernate" options.

Key Terms

Backwardly Compatible	Multitask
Clipboard	Object
Context-Sensitive Help	Overtype
Default	Point and Click
Dialog Box	Print Screen Key
Drop-Down Menu	Rtf File
Embed	Scroll Bar
Function Keys	Sleep
Hard Return	Status Line
Hibernate	System Tray
Icon	Tag
Insertion Point	Task Bar
Link	Toolbar
Logical	Vertical Bar
Menu Tab	Wizard
Mouse	Word Wrap

Remember the first time you cared for a patient? Everything took a long time and required absolute concentration while you moved through each procedure step by step. After you gained comfort and experience, you were able to adapt procedures to meet individual patient needs because you had developed baseline knowledge that was adaptable to new situations. For example, the first time you measured someone's blood pressure, the procedures involved in wrapping the cuff, pumping up the manometer, placing the stethoscope properly, and slowly releasing the pressure took your total concentration. After some experience, the tasks involved in taking a blood pressure became second nature and you were able to view it as a whole and concentrate on the patient instead of the task. Eventually, you developed the judgment needed to independently decide to take a blood pressure beyond routine assessment. You were now an expert in your approach to blood pressures. When required to learn a new procedure that is related to blood pressures, such as applying an automated blood pressure machine, you easily applied your knowledge to the new task, which shortened the learning curve.

Expanding Your Computer Horizons

This same progression from novice to competent to expert applies to computers. At first, a user may be very concerned about the keystrokes needed to perform each function. As more experience is gained, the tasks are automated and they are used appropriately. When it is necessary to learn a new program or information system, the command of the features that are common to all programs, such as editing text, scrolling the screen, and using the help menu and **mouse**, makes learning the new program much easier. Without realizing so, users internalize concepts that are transformed into quicker understanding and mastery of other computer tasks. This chapter will explore some of the basic concepts that are needed to get a start on this lifelong journey.

Keyboard Keys

Computer keyboards have keys other than letters and numbers that invoke actions, such as Ctrl (pronounced control) and Alt. The top line on the computer has **function keys**, such as F1 and F5, which are used to invoke features in software. How they are used varies among application programs, but a universal use for a function key is the help key, F1, which in all Microsoft Windows®–compatible applications accesses help for the active program. The "Ctrl" and "Alt" keys are often used together with other keys to implement a feature. When you see directions that read Ctrl + C, it means that you are to hold down the Ctrl key and while it is down, tap the C, and then release both keys. The Alt key works the same way. Sometimes you will see a command such as "Ctrl + Shift + D"

(double-underline function in Microsoft Word®). Then you hold down both the Ctrl and Shift keys while tapping the "D" key. When you see a plus (+) sign, it means that you are to hold the preceding key(s) down until you have finished the sequence.

Laptops also have a key near the left bottom of the keyboard labeled "FN." This key is used together with a function key to accomplish a task. Which function keys to use in conjunction with the FN key is generally vendor specific, but almost all use FN + F4 or F8 to cycle where the screen output is going from the laptop screen to a projector, or to both.

Default

Default is a word you often see in conjunction with computers. Defaults are properties or attributes that may be changed but are how something will be done unless otherwise specified. For example, when using a word processor, there is a default font and size of the font. Unless these are changed, any text entered will use this font and size. If the default font is Calibri and the font size is 11, but a user needs to use Times New Roman with a font size of 12 and makes those changes, they become the default font for only that document. If something different from the default is used frequently, most programs provide a way to change the default so that it will be the default for all documents. They also provide a way to return all settings to the default.

Mice

The basics of **pointing and clicking** and the information on varieties of mice is available in Appendix A. There is another item connected with mice. Those for personal computers (PCs) have at least two buttons: the left button that selects **objects** and the right button that shows features that can be applied to the selected object. Some mice now come with either a scrolling feature that allows you to scroll up and down the screen; others offer the ability to program buttons to perform any feature that you use frequently. If you are left handed, you can change the mouse configuration so that it can be operated by the left hand. From the Control Panel, in Windows XP®, select Mouse from Printers and Other Hardware; in Windows Vista® and Windows 7®, type mouse in the Control Panel search window. If you changed the mouse button configuration for use with the left hand, you would read a click as meaning the right mouse button and a right click as meaning a left mouse button click.

When interpreting the directions on a help screen, or anywhere else, when you see "click the mouse," it means that you should click the left mouse button. Although there are exceptions, generally one left mouse click selects an object, whereas a double click is required to implement a feature or open a program. If the right button is to be clicked, the instructions will specify that. Learning to use a mouse can be trying. There are several excellent resources available to assist users to gain skills using the mouse. Go to http://www.youtube.com or search the Internet by using the search term "using the mouse." To gain practice using the mouse and have some fun, play solitaire, which is one of the games that come with Microsoft Windows®. Open it by selecting Games from the All Programs menu.

Scroll Bars

When using most application programs, and even in healthcare information systems, the information

that you need may exceed the size of the screen. Most often you will need to scroll down the screen, but in some applications such as spreadsheets or databases, you also need to scroll to the right. This is easily accomplished by using either a scroll box (also called a bar) or the arrowhead on the right side or bottom of the screen. In **Figure 3-1**, you can see these tools. If you want to scroll down quickly, place your mouse pointer on the vertical **scroll bar**, hold down the left mouse button, and move the mouse in the direction that you wish to scroll. To scroll one line at a time, point to one of the arrowheads and click once. Holding down the left mouse button while pointing at the arrowhead will also scroll, but more slowly than using the scroll bar. Whether you see a scroll bar or a box is dependent on the amount of information, not on the screen. If you see a scroll bar, you will know that there is information that you cannot see. The size of the box varies with the amount of information that is not visible; the smaller the box, the larger the document, hence the less information visible on one screen. When you are reading a document, where the scroll bar or box is located on the

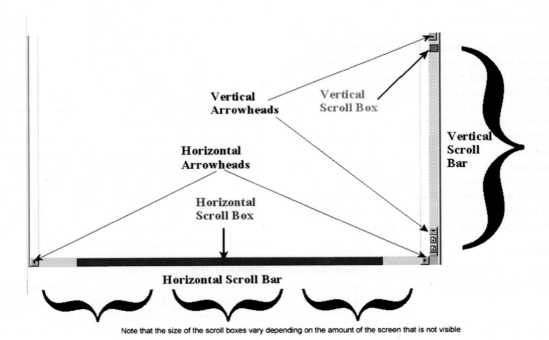

Vertical Arrowheads

Vertical Scroll Box

Horizontal Arrowheads

Vertical Scroll Bar

Horizontal Scroll Box

Horizontal Scroll Bar

Note that the size of the scroll boxes vary depending on the amount of the screen that is not visible

Figure 3-1 Horizontal and vertical scroll bars.

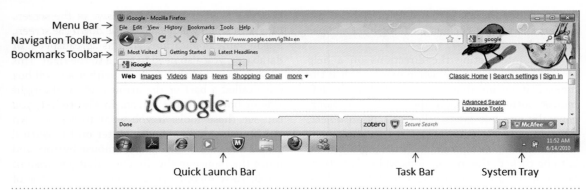

Menu Bar →
Navigation Toolbar →
Bookmarks Toolbar →

Quick Launch Bar   Task Bar   System Tray

Figure 3-2 Status bar, menu, and toolbars.

vertical bar tells you about how much more of the document is either above or below the screen view. If a screen does not have any scroll bars, it means that what you see on the screen is all there is.

Status Bar

In many application programs, a horizontal bar near the bottom of the screen is the status bar or the **status line**. In some programs, it may be called the application bar. The status line provides information about the file or document currently in the active window. This information varies among programs and vendors. In many word processors, this line indicates the page of a document, the line of text on that page, or how far from the left margin the **insertion point**[1] is located. The status bar may also indicate whether the Caps Lock is on or whether the user is in Insert mode (any characters entered will make room for themselves) or **Overtype** mode (a strikeover or typeover status in which entered characters will type over the characters already on the screen). The **task bar** on the bottom of the screen shows an **icon** for all the programs open at that time. Clicking any of these icons opens the associated window. **Figure 3-2** shows the status bar, menu, and **toolbars** when viewing the Firefox web browser on a PC.

Toolbars

All desktop applications, and even some health-care information system screens, have toolbars.

A toolbar is, as the name suggests, a line or bar of tools. The default is to have toolbars at the top of the screen, although provision is usually made to move them for users who would like to have one or all their toolbars on the sides or bottom of the screen. A "ribbon" in Microsoft Word® 2007 is really a toolbar, just a new name for an old feature (see **Figure 2-3** in Chapter 2). Although there are toolbars that are open by default, in programs other than Microsoft Office® 2007, users may choose to have others open or the defaults closed by clicking View on the menu line, then Toolbars, and checking or unchecking the desired toolbar. Sometimes toolbars are context sensitive, that is, when a feature such as the Outline feature is implemented, a special toolbar is added to those that are visible.

Many users are not happy with the default toolbars, colors of the screen, or other items. These can all be changed. The terminology used to provide this opportunity varies as does the option on the toolbar where it can be found, but when the word "preferences," "options," "settings," or "customize" is seen, selecting this option will allow making some changes. In XP programs, the most common place to find these options is under Tools. In Microsoft Office® 2007, select Options from the choices displayed when the Office logo button is clicked.

System Tray

In **Figure 3-2**, you will also notice the **system tray** in the status bar. The system tray has objects that generally represent changes that you can make to the system, such as the volume of the speakers or your antivirus program. If you place your mouse pointer

---

1 The insertion point used to be called a cursor. With either terminology, it means the place where the next object (remember, a character is an object) entered will be placed.

over an icon in the system tray, a **tag** will appear telling you what it represents. To access the features in the system tray, you often need to right-click the icon.

Drop-Down Menus, Dialog Boxes, and Menu Tabs

Windows is a very interactive system. Menus, **dialog boxes**, and **menu tabs** offer the ability to easily invoke features. When most off-the-shelf application programs open, you will see a line of menus across the top of the screen. In most application programs from any vendor prior to 2007 versions, when the mouse pointer is placed over a menu choice and the left mouse button clicked, a **drop-down menu** offering a choice of features appears. In the Microsoft Office® 2007 and 2010 programs, clicking any of those choices, instead of offering a drop-down box of features, causes a new "ribbon" of icons to appear that represent features that can be implemented. In application programs, including most healthcare information systems, items that are not available in the current context are grayed out, that is, appear faded or in gray type. When you see a triangle on a menu item, or on the right bottom of a ribbon group in Microsoft Office® 2007 programs, this indicates that clicking this icon or text menu choice will produce another menu of choices, usually in a drop-down box. In many programs, an ellipsis (...) will indicate that a pop-up dialog box, or a small window into which you give the computer more information about what you want to do, will appear. Sometimes a dialog box will have menu tabs near the top, as you see in **Figure 3-3**. The tab that is a different color than the rest is the one that is active. Clicking any of the other tabs will cause a new interactive window to appear. In **Figure 3-3**, the "Buttons" tab is active.

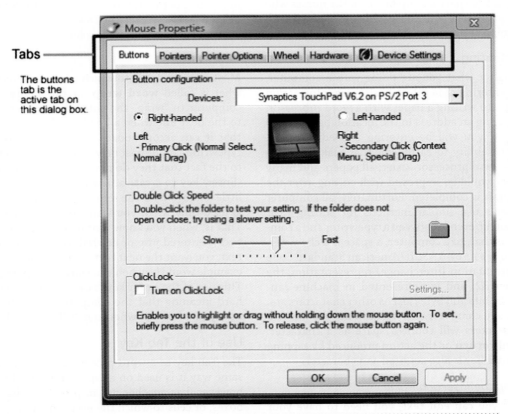

Figure 3-3 Tabs on a dialog box (Microsoft™ product screen shot reprinted with permission from Microsoft Corporation).

Many of these conventions are used in healthcare information systems. Making choices from one screen with drop-down menus, tabs, or dialog boxes is easier than going to a new screen. Drop-down boxes can also be used to facilitate data entry by presenting a menu of the usual choices for that entry. For example, a drop-down box is often used when there are fixed choices, such as smoking status or gender, that need to be entered into the system. A drop-down menu using the triangle option may also be used. To illustrate, in an intensive care unit, when users click the black triangle under "tubes" in the electronic medical record, a drop-down list appears, listing all the possible tubes or types of tubes that might be used. Clicking another black triangle, one that indicates drainage, produces a list of possible drainage tubes. The content of these lists is determined by nurses who work in these areas. Good information systems result from a partnership between the nurses who work in an area with those who are involved with designing and implementing the system.

Text Editing

No matter what you are doing with a computer, from entering data into a healthcare information system, to writing a paper with a word processor, to entering an address in the location bar of a web browser, you will be entering and editing text. It is the ability to easily edit that makes writing with a word processor easier; all papers and many memos would be improved with editing after the first draft is completed. Fortunately, all computer programs use similar methods for editing text. A major difference between a typewriter and a computer is that, to a computer, a space is a character. It even has its own ASCII (American Standard Code for Information Interchange) representation, the number 32, and is represented in machine language by bits and bytes just as other characters are. Thus, any computer entry that limits the number of characters will count a space as a character. A **hard return** or the action produced by tapping the Enter key is also counted as a character.

Moving the Insertion Point

Before you can edit text, you need to have your insertion point at the place where you want to edit. There are two ways to do this: using the arrow keys or the mouse. Using either method leaves the underlying text unchanged. Tapping an arrow key will move the insertion point, either line by line with the up and down arrows or character by character with the left and right arrows. To use the mouse, move the mouse pointer to the desired location, left click, and make the needed changes.

Erasing Text

Another universal feature is the use of the Delete and Backspace keys. When pressed, the Backspace key always erases the character to the insertion point's left, and the Delete key erases the character (a hard return is a character) to the insertion point's right. If you need to erase a large portion of text, it may be easier to select the text and then tap the Delete key. To select the text, place the mouse pointer at one end of the text to be deleted and then hold down the Shift key and use the arrow keys or mouse to move to the other end. When the text to be deleted is selected, tap the Delete key. Selected text will always be in a different color than other text.

Word Wrap

Most applications into which text is entered have what is called **word wrap**, or the ability of the computer to "wrap" the entered characters down to the next line when a line has all the characters that it can accommodate. Those who have used typewriters in the past may take a while to get used to the fact that they do not have to tap the return (Enter) key to create a new line. The Enter key, a little analogous to the return key on a typewriter, is used only when you want to force a new line. That is, when you know that no matter how much text is entered into or deleted from the preceding text, you want the next text to be on a new line. An example would be when you start a new paragraph. This use of the Enter key is called a "hard return," hard meaning that the computer is not to trifle with your choice of where a new line should go.

Use of the Tab Key

The Tab key in a word processor can be used the same way it is used on a typewriter. The Tab key, however, has another use in programs that have boxes, or cells to which the user must navigate. In a table, or a cell in a spreadsheet, tapping the Tab key moves the insertion point from the current cell to the next one. **Shift + Tab** moves the insertion point back one cell. This feature also works when filling out boxes on a web page. In short, almost anyplace where you are entering information into a box or cell, the Tab key can be used to navigate from one cell (box) to either the next or previous one.

Undo (Ctrl + Z) Redo (Ctrl + Y)

There will come a time when after you have completed an action you will realize that it was not what you wanted to do. Two commands that many application programs have, especially word processors, spreadsheets, and graphics programs, are "Undo" and "Redo." To undo something, click the icon that looks like a mirror image of a "C" but has an arrow at the top left (or tap Ctrl + Z). To redo something, click the icon resembling a "C" with an arrow at the top right (or tap Ctrl + Y). Undoing or redoing can be repeated more than once in many programs. The number of changes or types of changes that can be undone depends on the program being used. If you use "Redo," you need to know that this puts changes back in the order in which they were removed.

Icons

Computer application programs are more and more using icons, or small graphical pictures, rather than text. This can be seen in the use of icons for things that were once text. Fortunately, placing the mouse pointer over an icon for a few seconds causes a pop-up label to appear, telling you what the icon represents. There are also some fairly universal icons that are used in most programs. They can be seen in **Figure 3-4**.

Help

Feeling comfortable using a computer is often a matter of getting help when it is needed. Classes may provide some beginning skills, but when a user tries to use the functions learned or experiment with new functions, questions often arise. There are many sources of help available; some are on your computer, and others will require access to the web.

Printed manuals are not available for most applications. Instead, users are expected to use the application's help feature. Although help for basic features is available from information placed on your hard drive when a program is installed, more help is available online. Many programs have a menu option of Help; some use a question mark (?) instead of the word "help." Tapping F1 will access help in any program that works with the Microsoft Windows® operating system.

The appearance of the help screen varies from vendor to vendor. Some programs open up a screen and ask you to enter a search term. Others give you choices through tabs such as contents (generally like a table of contents), index (an index to the contents), and search. The most difficult thing may be deciphering what term to enter into the search box to indicate the topic of your search. For some programs, after you select the terms you want, you need to click the button on the bottom of that window that says "Display." For others, you can just click the item.

Using help works only if you know what features the application offers and can ask for help. Books about the software in use are helpful to acquaint you with an application's features. Many texts

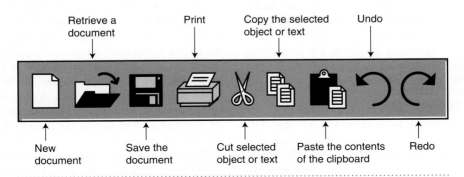

Figure 3-4 Universal icons.

about popular software products are available; however, there are so many that making a decision about which book to use is a personal decision. Some are written for beginners, whereas others are complete references for a program. Keep in mind that the beginning books are very limited in their coverage of a program's functions. They are helpful when one is first starting to use a program, but it might be more cost-effective in the long run to buy a more complete book. Look at several at a bookstore before making a decision to buy.

Books can be overwhelming in the material presented. If you are learning a program from a book, one suggestion is to work your way through the book until you feel reasonably comfortable with the program. Then using some of the features, create something, referring either to online help or the book when necessary. After becoming a little more comfortable with the program, take the time to peruse the rest of the book, noting what features are available. By knowing what is available, you can plan a document by using this information and learn how to implement the feature when you will use it.

Context-Sensitive Help

Many applications today, and this includes healthcare information systems, have what is called **context-sensitive help**. For example, if you are entering vital signs and need help, when you click the Help icon (which may be a question mark in the upper right corner of the screen), the Help screen appears with options for just that feature. This feature can save much time and frustration.

Wizards

Some application programs feature **Wizards**, which take you step by step through executing a task. Wizards can be helpful, but they cover only basic tasks. Depending on them for everything that you need to do with an application will limit what you can do with the program.

Read the Screen

Often the best help is to "read the screen." It sounds obvious, but most of us, when we are coping with learning a new feature, develop tunnel vision and will not see all the choices on the open window. Keep in mind that features are often nested, that

is, you need to go through a few options to get to the feature you want. Remember that any rectangle with text or an icon and a triangle pointing down will provide other choices when that triangle is clicked. Many of these drop-down boxes have scroll bars, so scroll up and down before concluding that the feature you want is not available. If you still don't see what you need, look on both the bottom and top of a window; sometimes the needed feature is there, sometimes, especially on web pages, in very small print.

Other Help

Some healthcare information systems will have printed help attached to the computer. Most also have help desks, which you can call. Application programs for PCs often have a local user group where you can learn more about the program. Whether learning to use an application program or a healthcare organization's information system, it is important that you locate the sources of help available and take advantage of them. Asking for help is a sign that the user is serious about learning to fully use a program, not just get by. Give yourself permission to learn, and ask for help when needed. It is an axiom that most people only use a small percentage of the features that any program has, thus making their job harder.

Selecting, Copying, and Moving Objects

Choices on a menu, as well as objects, are selected by moving the mouse pointer over them and clicking, that is, point-and-click. The principle of selecting and clicking is used in all computer applications, not only in menus but also as they apply to other features. The objects that can be selected vary from application program to application program. Note that the word "object" is applied to anything that is selected. This can be a letter, word, paragraph, page, entire document, cell or cells in a table or spreadsheet, an image, or pieces of that image. Text is selected as described above, and graphical objects are selected by clicking them. When graphical objects are selected, the selected object may show a border with either eight circles on the border, or dots at the corners and a square

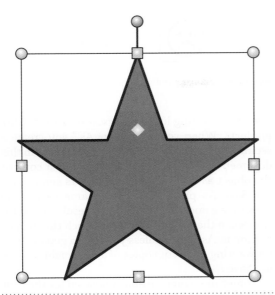

Figure 3-5 Selected graphical object.

on each side as seen in **Figure** 3-5. A selected object may be cut, copied, moved, pasted, or dragged.

When an object is cut, it is removed from where it was and placed in random access memory (RAM) in a space called the **clipboard**. When the object is copied, the object remains where it is, but a copy is placed on the clipboard. From the clipboard, objects are then pasted anywhere the user desires. To paste an object that is on the clipboard, move the mouse pointer or insertion point to the desired location and paste it. There are several ways to paste. A quick method is to hold down the Ctrl (pronounced Control) key and tap the letter "V," or use the Shift + Insert key method. Paste can also be invoked by selecting it from the edit menu or in Microsoft Office® 2007 programs from the Home tab. In all programs, objects on the clipboard can be pasted many times because they remain on the clipboard until replaced with another object. In Microsoft Office® programs since 2002, it is possible to place more than one object on the clipboard if the clipboard is open and then select the desired one when ready to paste. Objects on the clipboard can often be pasted into another application program, even one that is not from the same vendor, or open at the time the object is placed on the clipboard. Objects on the clipboard disappear when the computer is turned off.

When any text is highlighted, indicating that it is selected, one can simply type the replacement without deleting the original. For example, if a sentence is selected and the Enter key is tapped, the sentence will disappear and a new line will be entered. (Use the "undo" option to get it back!) This principle holds true in any computerized form or in a web browser on the address or location bar.

Graphics, or nontext items, such as pictures or photos that can be inserted into word processing programs, spreadsheets, and databases, as well as presentation or graphics programs, can also be copied or moved even in nongraphical–oriented programs such as word processors and databases. When a graphical object is selected and the right mouse button clicked, the options presented will be different than those for text. Some of the techniques for working with graphical objects in a presentation program will be addressed in Chapter 8. Tapping the **Print Screen key**, sometimes abbreviated "Prt Sc," will place a copy of the screen on the clipboard. Once on the clipboard, it can be pasted into any program.

Working With Objects That You Create

Remember that an object can be anything, such as a full document, parts of text, or pictures. When you are working on objects, they are only electronic bits in RAM. If the power goes off for some reason or the program crashes and the object has not been converted to a file by saving, it will be lost. This holds true for all computer programs. The only exception may be when entering data into a database. Desktop application databases save data as soon as the user leaves the field in which data were entered. The only thing you need to save in a database is an object such as a form or query that you create.[2]

The physical form onto which you save the document will vary depending on what you have available. It may be a flash drive, a CD, or a hard drive. To save time, this chapter will refer to all these physical locations as a disk. The location of the file on the disk is dependent on how the disk is organized and will be explained later in this chapter.

---

2 See Chapter 9 for more discussion of saving in a database.

Saving

Saving a document in any program involves invoking the Save command in one of three ways:

1. Clicking File on the menu line (the logo in the upper left corner in Microsoft Office® 2007) and then Save on the menu.
2. Clicking the disk icon on the toolbar for all applications except Microsoft Office® 2007 and 2010.
3. Tapping Ctrl + S.

When an object that you have created is saved, a copy of the object as it currently exists in RAM is saved to a disk. When additional changes are made to the object in RAM, these are not recorded on the file on the disk until the document is again saved. Thus, frequent saving keeps users from losing a document in its updated version (see **Figure 3-6**). More than one person has shed tears because he or she did not follow this rule. A good idea is to get into the habit of tapping Ctrl + S every few minutes.

The first time that an object is saved, the user is asked to name the file into which it will be placed. To make it easier to find the file the next time it is needed, the name chosen should reflect its contents. Names in Microsoft Windows® operating systems since 2002 can have up to 256 characters and include spaces.[3] Some characters may not be used in a file name (e.g., the hyphen and either slash). Letters and numbers are always safe to use in file names. After the file has been saved the first time, each time it is saved again is a repeat save, that is, the new version of the document replaces the one put on the disk by the previous save. The procedure to do a resave is identical to the first save except you do not need to give the name of the file.

There may be times when you want to preserve the original document but want to use it as a basis for a new document (**Figure 3-7**). In this case, you should select Save As. When using Save As, you should give the new file a different name. This choice can be found on the File menu on the menu

Prevent sad faces!
Save frequently.

Figure 3-6 Save frequently!

line or by clicking logo in Microsoft Office® 2007 products. When you do a "Save As," you create a separate file. Thus, you now have two files from this document: a copy of the last save plus a copy of the object as it now exists. Beginners sometimes use Save As providing a new name each time they save a document. This often results in confusion when they try to determine which the current version is. As a rule, unless you have a good reason for wanting different copies of a document, do not use Save As.

Sometimes when an object is saved for the first time, after you enter a name for the file, you will receive a message stating that a file by that name already exists. The program also asks whether the existing file by that name should be replaced. If you say "Yes," the file by that name will be overwritten. Retrieving a file by that name will then retrieve what was saved in the last save. The original file by that name will be forever gone. Thus, unless you know what is in the file on the disk that has that name and do not mind losing that file, you should click "No" and select a different name.

Automatic Backups

Many programs have a provision for an automatic backup. That is, after a given number of minutes, the computer will back up one's work without a command being given. Although this can be a lifesaver, there are some difficulties associated with it. Automatic backups work best when you are on your own computer, assuming that you have activated the feature to perform automatic backups. One difficulty with depending on this feature is that you may have spent the last 10 minutes creating something that required a lot of work. If the automatic backup time is every 15 minutes and a problem occurs before the next save, you will lose at least some of the work. Although this feature is available in word processing programs, it is not available in all programs. If you are on a computer

---

3 Although files with long file names can exist on most drives, some older CD creation programs will not tolerate a file with a name longer than eight characters, thus creating difficulties if you try to copy to a CD.

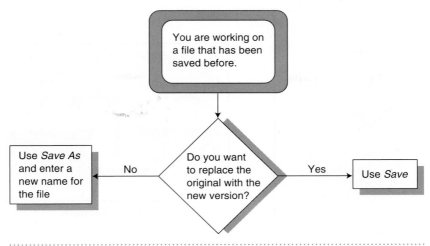

Figure 3-7 Decision tree for using Save or Save As.

in a lab, the ability to recover lost files is often not available. There is no substitute for regular saves and resaves!

Purposeful Backups of Objects

Remember that a file that is saved is only 0s and 1s on the storage medium. Files on all types of storage material can become corrupted. Smart people save important objects in more than one place. If the object is really important, such as a thesis or dissertation, copies of all the needed objects should be saved not only on more than one physical item, but some of these items should also be placed in different geographical locations in case of fire, tornado, or other disasters. This is why backups of healthcare information systems are placed in different geographical locations.

Print

Printing is another function that is available for objects that you create with computer programs, as well as items from the web. Printing a document from a word processor, or for some web pages, is fairly straightforward because these documents are oriented toward a printed page. However, when printing things such as spreadsheets or databases, or some web pages, it is easy to forget that a piece of paper has a finite size. It is common with either

of those program types to design a document that is wider than any paper a printer can use. When an attempt is made to print the document, the part that is too wide to fit on one sheet of paper may be completely omitted or it may print on another sheet.

If the document to be printed is not too large, there are two possible ways to solve this problem. One is to change the paper orientation from the default portrait to landscape (**Figure 3-8**). To do this, select Page Setup from the File menu or Orientation from the Page Layout tab in Microsoft Office® 2007 and 2010 products. In landscape orientation, the longer side is horizontal instead of the shorter side. Although this approach can take care of some width problems, it still cannot accommodate all cases. More room can be created by using a font of a smaller point size, but this solution has its limitations in readability. The best solution is to remember paper size when designing any item that will be printed.

Files

Once an object is saved to disk, it is a file. The file format, or the type of file created, is determined by the program that was used to create the document and save it. Applications from different vendors create files that are often incompatible with other programs, the same applications

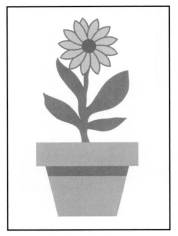

Portrait orientation

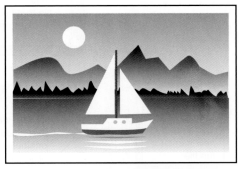

Landscape orientation

Figure 3-8 Page orientation.

from other vendors, and even different versions of the same program. Thus, a file created in Corel WordPerfect® may not open in Microsoft Works®.

File Extensions

The type of file is usually indicated by an icon before the file name and a file extension. When you see a list of files, such as when you use the "open file" option, or when using Microsoft Windows Explorer®, the file extension letters may or may not be visible but the icon always will be. Unless you are very familiar with these icons, you may wish to change the default file listings so that these extensions are shown. To learn how to do this, use Help after clicking the Start menu or the Microsoft® logo in Microsoft Vista® or Windows 7®. Enter "Show file name extension" into the search box and then follow the directions. Knowing the type of file is always important when you receive a file in an e-mail. If a file extension is unknown to you, go to http://www.sharpened. net/helpcenter/extensions.php and enter the letters into the search box.

Backward Compatibility

Generally, software is **backwardly compatible**; that is, a newer version will open files created by an older version, but in many cases, the reverse is not true. For example, the file

type created by default with Microsoft Office® 2007 applications cannot be opened by Microsoft Office® 2003 products without the use of special software (you can download this software at http://www.microsoft.com/downloads/details. aspx?familyid=941B3470-3AE9-4AEE-8F43-C6BB74CD1466&displaylang=en). Lack of backward compatibility, or using software of the same type from different vendors or different versions, is often the cause when recipients of file attachments are unable to open the attached files.

When using a later version of the same vendor's product, there is almost always a way to save the file in the format used by the older version. When this is done, any features in the new file that are not supported by the older program will be lost, but this is often not a problem. For example, a database created by Microsoft Word® 2007 and saved in the Microsoft Word® 2003 format loses any features that are new in Microsoft Word® 2007.

Saving in a Different File Format

To save a file in a different file format with the Save As window open, change the type of file by clicking the triangle at the end of the box on the bottom of the Save window labeled "Save as Type" and select the format you wish (see **Figure 3-9**). If you are working in Microsoft Word® 2007 or 2010 and want to enable someone to open the file by using Microsoft Word®

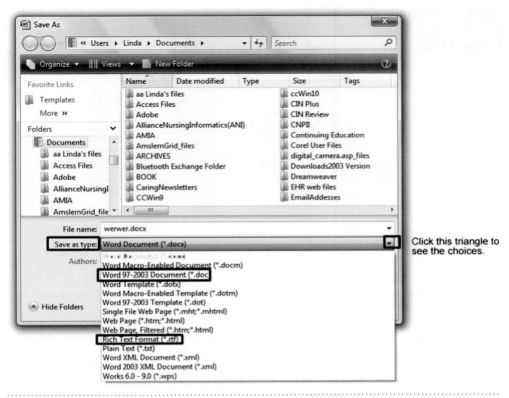

Figure 3-9 Saving a file as a different type (Microsoft™ product screen shot reprinted with permission from Microsoft Corporation).

2003, you would select "Word 97-2003 Document (*.doc)." Then you would click Save.

For word processing files, there is also a universal format that can be opened by any Microsoft Windows®–compatible word processor. This format is abbreviated **"rtf"** and is known as a rich text format. Thus, one can save a Microsoft Word® 2007 file in this format, and it can be opened by Corel WordPerfect®. Many programs can also save a file in the format of a file from an application by a different vendor.

Disk Organization

When the files are saved, they go to a **logical** (i.e., one visible to the user but which may have no relationship to the actual physical placement of the file) location on the disk. All internal hard disks are organized into folders that are similar to files in a filing cabinet except that the "folders" may have other folders nested within as well as files. Other disks can also be organized into folders. The ease with which one can find a file is directly proportional to the organization of the folders on the disk.

On the internal hard drive in a PC, the base folder where you store files may be called "My Documents" or, in Microsoft Vista® and Windows 7®, "Documents." In an attempt to keep pictures separated from documents, another folder called "My Pictures" is seen in PCs ("Pictures" in Microsoft Vista®). Folders are organized in what looks like a hierarchical organizational chart with the top of the chart, or what could be called "the boss," being the base of the hard drive or the base of the external disk.

Personal style is reflected in how a filing cabinet is organized and how users name their files and folders. In some organizations, protocols for both file naming and folder organization are used

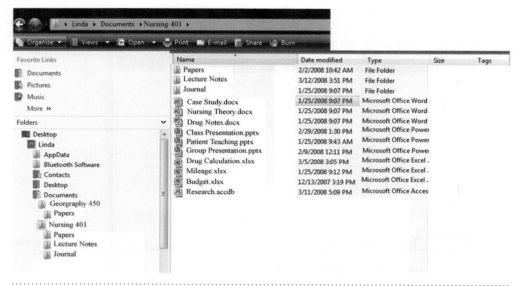

Figure 3-10 Folders and files (Microsoft™ product screen shot reprinted with permission from Microsoft Corporation).

by everyone to facilitate finding files that more than one person will use. Creating and using some type of organization will make backing up files to smaller disks a much easier process.

Figure 3-10 shows a view of folders and files in Microsoft Vista®.[4] On the left are the folders, and on the right, the contents of the open folder. On the top of the screen, you see "▸ Linda▸ Documents▸ Nursing 401 ▸." This information tells you that this account belongs to Linda and that the folder Nursing 401, the open folder, is a folder in her Documents folder. The names on the right-hand side of the screen are the folders and files in her folder Nursing 401. Notice that the Nursing 401 folder includes both subfolders and files. For hard drives, consider the base folder, in this case Documents, to be the top of the organizational chart for files. There is no limit to the number of nested folders one can have, just be sure that there is some organizational principle behind the nesting.

Windows 7® introduced the concept of "libraries" to organize files and folders (**Figure 3-11**). Libraries allow the user to organize and access files that may be located in a variety of locations, for example, an external hard drive or another computer. To learn more about working with libraries, enter the search terms "files and folders" or "libraries" in the Windows Help and Support search menu.

In both **Figures 3-10 and 3-11**, the account holders had changed the default so that file extensions show. The extensions belong to files created or used by Microsoft Office® 2007 and Firefox. The file extensions, docx, xlsx, and accdb are used by Microsoft Office® 2007 and 2010. The mht extension is a Multipurpose Internet Mail Extension document by Microsoft. Although disk organization exploring views for Microsoft Windows® vary with the different operating systems, the principles are identical, just as they are on other storage items such as flash drives.

Viewing a File List

There are several options for viewing file lists with Microsoft Windows®. The main choices for viewing the file names are lists, details, tiles, and different sizes of icons. Unless you are viewing pictures (pictures are often viewed by thumbnail), the two most important views are the list and details views. Details view provides information about the file such as its size and the date on which

---

4 To explore Windows, right click on either the Start button (XP) or the Microsoft Logo (Windows Vista and Windows 7) in the lower left corner of the screen.

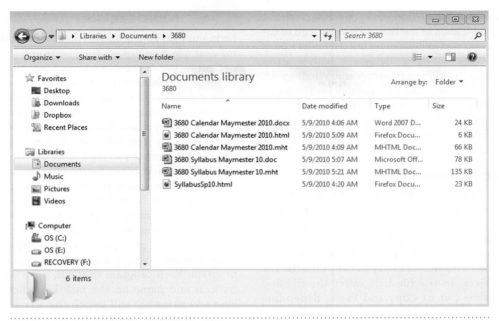

Figure 3-11 Folders and files in Windows 7®.

it was created. The default listing of files in either view is alphabetical. You can reorder the files by the data in any of these columns by clicking the name of the column. For example, clicking Date Modified will order the files starting with the one that was modified first. Clicking Date Modified a second time will reverse the file order in the list, that is, placing the one modified last first. The list view shows only the file name with the icon of the program that created it and the extension if this is enabled. **Figure 3-9** is a detailed view.[5] The order in which the files will appear in list view is determined by the last reordering of the files in the details view. The files in **Figure 3-10** are organized by file type. The files in **Figure 3-11** are organized by file name.

Tags

Although we organize our files in folders, some times making a distinction as to what folder a file belongs in is muddied because it may be useful in more than one circumstance. To permit this type of file management, Microsoft Office® 2007

added the ability to label a file by using what is called a tag. For example, you are writing a paper for a course and want to file it under the course folder. However, you realize that next time you want information about this topic, you may not remember for which course you wrote it, so you tag it with a label that tells the topic of the paper. This feature, however, is available only for files created with Microsoft Word®, Microsoft Excel®, and pictures that have an extension of "jpg."

Saving to a Specific Location

Understanding how files are organized on a disk makes it possible to save a file to the desired folder. When you click the Save icon or the Logo button in Microsoft Office® 2007 applications and select "Save," the file list will look a lot like as shown in **Figures 3-10 and 3-11**. If there are many files and folders, there will be scroll bars, either horizontal or vertical, depending on how the files are viewed. Except for navigating to a folder lower in the hierarchy, which is done by clicking on the folder name, navigating to the desired folder is done a little differently, depending on which version of the operating system you are using and the vendor of the program. In versions of the Microsoft Windows® prior to the

---

5 In Windows Vista and Windows 7, if the data that you wish to see are not items under details, right click on a blank portion of that bar, click on More ..., and select an item from that list.

Microsoft Vista® and Windows 7® operating systems, to move up folders in the hierarchy at the end of the box with the open folder name, click the folder icon of an open folder that has a sideways "L" with an arrow pointing up. In Microsoft Vista® and Windows 7®, you can move up a folder by clicking on the folder name on the folder name bar of the folder that you wish to open or the folder name on the left side. To create a folder, use the Help function and search for "create folder."

Copying or Moving Files

Copying or moving files or folders is a relatively simple procedure. It can be done by using the Cut or Copy options together with the Paste option from any Edit menu or by dragging the file in a Microsoft Windows Explorer® window. Cut, Copy, and Paste work exactly as they do with any other object. In the file list, select the file and apply either Cut or Copy and Paste, depending on your need. To drag a file or folder, select it on the right panel, and holding down the left mouse button, drag it to its new location in the left panel. There is a basic principle that you need to understand when using the dragging feature. When a file is dragged to a new location, if the new location is a different folder on the same disk, the file will be moved (analogous to cut) so that it is only in one location on the disk. If the new location is a different disk, the file will be copied.

Universal Key Presses

When there are mouse-activated features that you use frequently, you may want to learn to use the alternate key presses for those features. With all programs, with the exception of Microsoft Office® 2007 applications, when a menu is opened by clicking, the key presses that will activate that feature are listed on the right side of the menu, as can be seen in **Figure 3-12**. The ones in this figure are universal to all versions of Microsoft Windows®–compatible applications. There are many others including Ctrl + Home, which moves the insertion point to the beginning of a document, and Ctrl + End to move it to the end. An excellent resource to discover universal key presses for both PCs and Macs is at http://www.computerhope.com/shortcut.htm.

Multitasking

Living in today's world, you no doubt **multitask**; for example, you talk on the phone and look for a patient record at the same time. Since the advent of the graphical user interface, you can multitask with your computer. In computer terminology, this means having more than one program open at the same time and being able to quickly move between them. You can have as many programs open at one time as you wish, however, depending on the RAM and other facets of your computer; if you open too many at one time, the computer may slow down. Most computers today will allow at least four or more programs to be open at the same time without losing efficiency. Thus, you can have your word processor and spreadsheet open while you are creating a presentation in another program. Each program that you open will leave its icon and name on the task bar; clicking the icon and name bar will switch the active window to that program. By using the clipboard, you can easily copy objects from one program to another.

Having Different Files Open in One Program

With most programs today, you can also have more than one file open at the same time in a program. There is a difference in how one accesses open files in the same program, depending on the application. In all Microsoft Office® applications, every open file in a program opens another item on the task bar. In most other programs, open files within the same program are accessed by clicking "Windows" in the menu bar of the application.

Embedding and Linking

Any program that supports object **linking** and **embedding**, which includes all of the office applications, allows you to either embed a file from one program into another program or link to that file. For example, you may wish to have data from a spreadsheet in your word processing document. There is, however, a big difference in these processes. If you embed the file, you place a copy of the worksheet as it is when you embed the file in your document. It is termed static because the document will not reflect further changes to the worksheet. If you click the

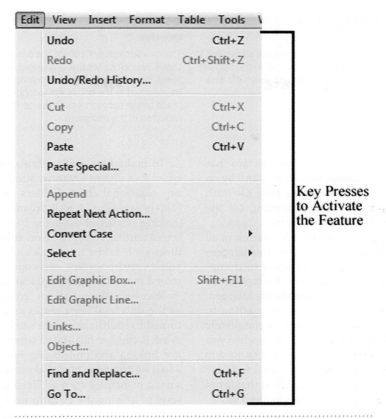

Figure 3-12 Key presses (Edit menu from Corel's WordPerfect® x3).

embedded file, changes you make are only in that document, they do not affect the spreadsheet. When a spreadsheet is linked to a document, what is seen in the document will change if the linked spreadsheet changes. Clicking the linked object will open the spreadsheet, and changes you make will be reflected in the word processing document after the spreadsheet is saved with the new changes.

For example, let's say that you keep a record of the monthly expenses for supplies for a unit on a spreadsheet. You need to report these expenses every month along with a narrative explaining some of the expenses. Because each document reflects that month, you want the document to reflect the spreadsheet as it looks when you create the document. Then you embed the file and save the document for that month. If, instead, you

need to do a report that is identical each time you report it, except for the data, you would link to the spreadsheet instead. Keep in mind that if you link, you will not have a record of any past documents. To learn how to do either, use the program's help feature (**Table 3-1**).

Sleep (Stand by) or Hibernate

Chapter 2 discussed closing programs and shutting down Microsoft Windows®, but not the options available to you when you close Windows. If you are using Microsoft Vista®, you will see a list of these options when you activate the Close option by clicking the Start logo and clicking the tiny triangle on the lower right side of that window. In other versions of Microsoft Windows®, once you click the Start button and select Shut Down, it is necessary to open the drop-down box to see these options.

Table 3-1 Linked and Embedded Files

Linked	Embedded
Changes made to either the spreadsheet while embedded in the document or the spreadsheet when open in the spreadsheet program will be reflected in both the document and the spreadsheet.	The spreadsheet will reflect the document at the time that it was embedded. Any changes made to the spreadsheet from within the word processing program will not be reflected in the actual spreadsheet, nor will changes made to the spreadsheet in the spreadsheet program be reflected in the document.

Most of these options are fairly clear; the two that may be confusing are **Sleep**, known as Stand by on many computers, and **Hibernate**. They are both power-saving features, although turning off the monitor in PCs is also a big power saver.

The Sleep option saves all the information in all your open files plus information about which programs are open to RAM. This cuts power consumption to a minimum because the monitor is powered down and the disk drives are completely stopped. Hibernate, however, saves all this information to the hard drive and shuts the computer completely down, thus requiring no power. Of course when you again use the computer, it will recover very quickly from Sleep mode because RAM retrieval is faster than hard disk retrieval. The downside is that if the power goes off while the computer is in Sleep mode, all the information that was not saved is lost.

 ## Summary

Computers are tools used to manage information. The task of learning to use a computer to manage information is facilitated when a user understands some of the computer conventions such as how to use a mouse, edit text, find files, and use the "Help" function. Help is useful to both beginners, who need direction on many things, and more experienced users, who need to learn a new feature or who infrequently use a feature. Many functions such as opening or saving a file, entering text, or printing follow the same principles in all application programs. Similarities also occur in the methods a computer uses with graphical objects, whether they are clip art, a drawing, an object that has been scanned, or the result of a screen capture. Understanding these principles makes transferring knowledge from one situation to another easier.

To make files easily retrievable, files are organized on a disk in a manner similar to a hierarchical organizational chart. Folders can contain nested folders and files. A well-organized disk facilitates making copies of files for backup purposes. All important files should be on at least two different disks such as the hard disk and a floppy diskette, and if very important, one copy, at least, should be stored in another geographical location.

Knowing shortcuts for computer tasks such as the universal key presses and becoming accustomed to multitasking are work- and time-savers. Work is further facilitated when you know how to use linking and embedding features. In this age when we are aware of global warming, using power-saving principles such as Sleep and Hibernate are ways of helping the environment.

When learning to use a computer, remember to give yourself permission to make mistakes – the computer could care less. It is you who becomes upset. Even experienced users make mistakes – there are very few from which it is not relatively easy to recover. Remember Ctrl + Z to undo!

APPLICATIONS AND COMPETENCIES

1. Examine a healthcare information system to see how many of the common features in this chapter are used. For example,
   a. Are there drop-down menus, dialog boxes, scroll bars, or tabs?
   b. Does F1 get help, or is there a question mark icon available?
   c. How is text edited?
   d. If text is selected and you type another character, does it replace that text?
   e. Is there context-sensitive help?

f. Is there a taskbar and system tray on the screen?

g. Will Ctrl + C copy an object? If it does, when should this not be used?

h. Select something and tap the right mouse button. What happens? (Try this in an Microsoft Office® suite program.)

2. You have selected a sentence and wish to move it to a new location in the paragraph. Which option would you use after selecting the sentence: Cut or Copy? Why?

3. Files, Folders, and Multitasking

a. Open Microsoft Windows Explorer® and navigate to the disk that you will use for backup copies (or originals if working in a lab).

b. By using Help, create two new folders.

c. Keeping Explore open, open a word processing program, create a simple file, and save it to one of the new folders by using the word processing program.

d. By using the task bar, switch to Explore and move this file to the other folder by

dragging it. Move it back to its original location by using the universal key presses, Ctrl + C (Copy) and Ctrl + V (Paste).

4. You are working on an important paper that will take several sessions at the computer to complete. How will you preserve this?

5. Draw an organizational file chart with Documents as the "boss" or master folder.

6. Every month, you need to do a report of the infections on your unit, which is kept in a spreadsheet along with a narrative that is in the word processor. This narrative will vary each month, but you wish to preserve each month's report. Will you embed the spreadsheet or link it? Why?

7. Make a chart of about 8–10 key presses that substitute for mouse actions for features that you use frequently.

8. You need to leave your computer for about 30 minutes. Which feature will you use, Sleep (Stand by) or Hibernate, and why?

CHAPTER 4
Computer Networking

Objectives

After studying this chapter, you will be able to:

▶ Discuss the overall technology of computer networking.

▶ Analyze the different methods of connecting to the Internet.

▶ Differentiate between the Internet and the World Wide Web.

▶ Identify uses of WWW technology for networking within an organization.

▶ Protect a computer against computer malware.

Key Terms

Active Server Pages (ASPs)
Active X
Adware
Bandwidth
Bookmarks
Botnet
Broadband
Case Sensitive
Client/Server Architecture
Computer Malware
Computer Virus
Distributed Denial of Service (DDoS)
Digital Subscriber Line (DSL)
Domain Name System
Download
Dynamic IP Address
Extensible Markup Language (XML)
Extranet
Favorites
Fiber Optic Cable
File Transfer Protocol (FTP)
Firewall
Graphical User Interface (GUI)
Hard Wired
Hoax
Home Page
Hypertext Markup Language (HTML)
Internet
Internet Protocol (IP)
Intranet
IP Address
Java

JavaScript
Local Area Network (LAN)
Markup Language
Megabits per Second
Modem
Net Neutrality
Network
Nodes
Peer-to-Peer Network
Pharming
Phishing
Plain Old Telephone Service (POTS)
Plug-In
Rich Internet Application
Spyware
Static IP Address
Streaming
Telephony
Transmission Control Protocol (TCP)
Trojan Horse
Universal Resource Locator (URL)
Upload
Urban Legend
Virtual Private Network (VPN)
Web Browser
Web Cookies
Wide Area Network (WAN)
Wired Equivalent Privacy (WEP)
Wireless
World Wide Web (WWW/W3)
Worm

Anurse encounters a patient with an unfamiliar disease. From an e-mail message, the nurse learns that a document on a computer in another country has information about caring for patients with this disease. Within 60 seconds of logging on to the **Internet**, the nurse prints out the document. This ability to exchange information on a global scale is changing the world. No longer do healthcare professionals have to wait for information to become available in a journal in the country in which they live. Nurses and other healthcare professionals can and do use computers to **network** with colleagues all over the world.

Healthcare depends on communication: communication between the nurse and the patient, communication between healthcare professionals, communication about organizational issues, and communication with the general public. As you can see, the methods used to communicate in healthcare are today being augmented with computer networking. Since the first computers talked to each other in the late-1960s, networking has progressed to the point where not only computers in an organization are connected to each other but also institutions are connected to a worldwide network known as the Internet.

Networks

A network can range in size from a connection between a smartphone and a personal computer (PC) to the worldwide, multiuser computer connection – the Internet. Variation in network size or the number and location of connected computers is often seen in the name used to denote the network, such as a **local area network (LAN)** or a **wide area network (WAN)**. A LAN is a network in which the connected computers are physically close to one another, such as in your home, hospital workplace, or college campus. A WAN is a network in which the connections are farther apart; a network of many LANs. WANs are sometimes referred to as enterprise networks because they connect all the computer networks throughout the entire organization or enterprise. The Internet, a network of LANs, is an example of a WAN. Healthcare organizations that span across several states or a nation, such as Kaiser Permanente and Mayo Clinics, network by using WANs.

Network Architecture

There are many different variations in how networks are constructed, or what is referred to as their architecture, often depending on the purpose of the network. For a home network, a **peer-to-peer network** in which each connected computer is a workstation is a normal approach. In this scheme, each computer can have a shared folder that is accessible by other computers. Often, the network is primarily for connecting to the Internet or for sharing hardware such as a printer.

Another type of architecture, often seen in healthcare agencies, is **client/server architecture**. The principles behind this model vary, but for most healthcare applications, they are similar to the "dumb terminal" model. A client computer has software that allows it to request and receive information from the server. The server has software that can accept these requests, find the appropriate information, and transmit it back to the client (**Figure 4-1**). The client views the information, enters data, and sends it back to the server for processing. Under this model, the client computer does no processing. Beyond making the initial request, rarely is any of this process visible to the user. Users sometimes have the misperception that the software and data reside on the computer/terminal that they are using, instead of the server.

There are other variations for networks. A computer in a healthcare facility may function as a client for the patient care information system but may have application software that allows users to do things such as word processing, in which case it acts like a regular computer. This computer may also be networked to another server that stores the files created by the networked computer, or the files may be stored on the computer that was used to create them. This computer may even be connected to the Internet through another server. Printers and scanners are usually connected to a network so that more than one computer/client can use them. Managing networks is an ongoing maintenance task performed by the network administrator.

Connections

Networks are connected physically with a variety of materials such as twisted-wire cables, phone lines, fiber optic lines, or radio waves. Computers

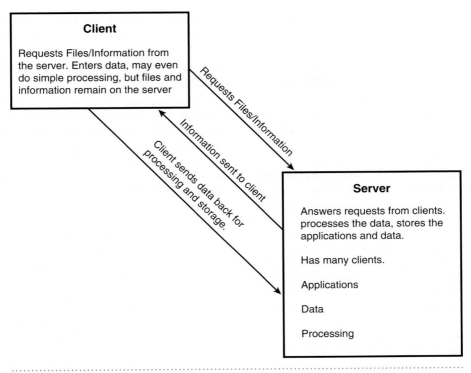

Figure 4-1 Client/server architecture.

that are wired together are said to be **hard wired**. When you see the term "hard" with another item, this means that the item is permanent, or that it physically exists. Most healthcare agency networks, even those that use **wireless**, are hard wired to some extent.

Wireless (Wi-Fi) transmissions are limited in distance, so they do not compete with other radio traffic. When a wireless system is installed, **nodes** are placed at strategic locations throughout the institution, locations that are determined after a thorough assessment of the building. A node in a wireless connection is a single point on the network that consists of a tiny router with a few wireless cards and antennas. These nodes pick up the signals sent by a user and transmit them to the central server, or even to another node for rebroadcast, and transmit signals back to the user's computer. Successful wireless communication depends on an adequate number of nodes or hardware that sends or rebroadcast the signal and on their placement. The distance of a device from

the node will affect both the speed of transmission and whether one can use the network.

Wireless transmission is less secure than hardwired transmission because the signal is available for use for anyone in range (Joan, 2009a). Security depends on the network administrators who follow procedures to secure the transmission. Many wireless networks, including those at home, use **wired equivalent privacy (WEP)**, the goal of which is to prevent disclosure or modifications of messages in transit. When this is employed, to connect to a network, a user must have the WEP key to enter before being allowed to use the network. In many cases, once a WEP key is entered on a computer, the computer remembers it and will automatically find it any time a user is in range of that network. Wi-Fi protected access (WPA) was designed with improved data encryption and user authentication to be more secure than WEP; however, hackers are able to use advanced tools to gain access to the network. WPA2 is the most secure measure to protect wireless networks (Joan, 2009b). The downside of

WPA2 is the required computing processing power and resulting slowed network speed.

Setting Up a Home Wireless Network

Home wireless systems are very popular. Besides allowing for shared printers and scanners, it also provides wireless access for use with mobile Internet devices (MIDs) and gaming devices, such as the Wii, Xbox 360, and PlayStation 3. To set up a home system, you will need to have a **broadband** connection with a **digital subscriber line (DSL)** or cable **modem**, a wireless router, and a computer with wireless network capabilities (Microsoft, 2009). If you have a home wireless system, you may want to upgrade the wireless router to one of the newer networking standards, which are 802.11g and 802.11n (CNET, 2009). The access range for 802.11g is 150 feet and 802.11n is 250 feet. The networking standard will be listed on the box of the wireless router.

Of course, you will want to read the instructions before beginning but the process is easy. First, connect the DSL/cable modem (it should be turned off) to the wireless router with Ethernet cable (should come with the wireless router). Second, connect the wireless router to your computer network adapter with an Ethernet cable. Turn on the DSL/cable modem first and then the wireless router. The last step is to configure the router with a unique name and a security code. There are several resources to assist in setting up the wireless system. Your DSL/cable provider is the primary resource. Others include Microsoft® (http://www.microsoft.com/athome/organization/wirelesssetup.aspx) and CNET (http://www.cnet.com/1990-7390_1-6213817-3.html).

Protocols

For networks to function correctly, it is necessary that there be agreements known as protocols, which prescribe how data will be exchanged between participating computers. These protocols include standards for tasks such as how the system will check for transmission errors, whether to use data compression, and, if so, how the sending machine will indicate that the message it has sent is complete and how the receiving machine will indicate that it has received the message.

Internet Protocol and Transmission Control Protocol

To ensure interoperable data transmission on the Internet, the **Internet protocol (IP)** and the **transmission control protocol (TCP)**, sometimes referred to as TCP/IP, were introduced in 1974 and are still in use, although consideration is being given to moving beyond the capabilities of these two protocols. The IP enables computers to find each other, and the TCP controls the tasks associated with data transmission.

Although invisible to the user, messages sent on the Internet are not sent as a whole. Instead they are broken up into what are called packets. Each packet may even take a different route to its destination. For each packet, a device called a router scans the routes available to the final destination, selects what is the shortest and the least congested route at that moment, and then sends the packet to another router that again makes a decision about the best route at that moment. This process continues for each packet until all the packets in a message reach their final destination. Under this process, it is not uncommon for packets in a message to take different routes to their destination.

File Transfer Protocol

Another process used on the Internet is the **file transfer protocol (FTP)**. This is the method used to exchange files (as opposed to retrieving a page from the web) with another computer. Until the early-1990s, this was a manual process and users had to learn commands to do it. Today, **web browsers** have automated this process for files that are retrieved from the **World Wide Web (WWW/W3)**. People who create pages for the WWW on their own computers use an FTP program to place their files on the server. There are several free FTP software applications available, for example, FileZilla (http://download.cnet.com/FileZilla/3000-2160_4-10308966.html?tag=mncol) and Ipswitch WS_FTP Home (http://download.cnet.com/Ipswitch-WS-FTP-Home/3000-2160_4-10018456.html?tag=mncol).

Internet: A Network of Networks

The Internet is, as its last three letters indicate, a network. Granted, it is a worldwide, amorphous network of interconnected computers, but it still is a network. Nothing in the world before has become so quickly assimilated into daily use. In the early-1990s, the Internet was relatively unknown by all but a few academics. By the summer of 1994, the popular culture took note of this phenomenon, as evidenced by a cartoon in the New Yorker showing two dogs at a computer, with one remarking to the other, "On the Internet no one knows you are a dog." Since then, the Internet has started to change how and with whom we communicate. It crosses national boundaries disregarding long-established international protocols and has created a situation in which laws designed for national entities are inadequate.

The Beginnings of the Internet

One of the positive legacies of the Cold War, the Internet was devised as a means of communication that would survive a nuclear war and provide the most economical use from then scarce, large computer resources. The journey from ARPANET (Advanced Research Projects Agency NETwork), which was established in 1969 to connect four nodes – the University of California, Los Angeles; Stanford Research Institute; the University of California, Santa Barbara; and the University of Utah (Howe, 2010) to today's Internet has been amazing. It is "one of the most successful examples of the benefits of sustained investment and commitment to research and development of information infrastructure" (Internet Society, 2010).

The underlying technical feature of the Internet is open architecture networking (Internet Society, 2010). That is, the choice of how connected networks were set up, or their network architecture, was immaterial as long as they could work with other networks using a metalevel "internetworking architecture." The government, industry, and academia have been, and continue to be, partners in evolving and implementing the Internet. The free and open access to basic documents, especially protocol specifications, has been a key to the rapid growth of the Internet.

Internet Service Provider

An Internet service provider (ISP) is any organization that provides access to the Internet. It can be an educational institution, an employer, a hotel, or a coffee shop. For home or business use, a private ISP provides this service. If you are using a dial-up Internet connection, the ISP can be any service; however, common sense says that the dial-up number should be a local number. For broadband connections, you are limited in your selection of ISPs to whoever provides telephone DSL or cable service to your location. A typical ISP offers e-mail with one or more addresses per account. The cost varies; for dial-up, it can range from free (10 hours/month) to $10 a month, whereas for broadband, it may be bundled with either phone or cable service.

Your choice of ISPs is often limited to where you live. Rural areas may be restricted to **plain old telephone service (POTS)**. Like all investments, it is worth exploring the returns before making a decision. Take time to conduct an Internet search for help. ISPcompared.com provides a directory and customer reviews of ISPs (ISPcompared.com, 2010).

Connections to the Internet

The last mile of connection to the Internet is determined by the user. When institutional networked computers are connected to the Internet, the connection is generally provided at the network level and is invisible to the user. For home computers, the user has several choices.

Types of Connection

There are different ways to connect to the Internet, many of which are determined by your ISP. They fall generally into two broad categories: POTS and broadband. These choices, somewhat limited by geographical location and available ISPs, determine the speed of the connection; that is, how quickly information will be transmitted. This speed is referred to as **bandwidth**; the higher the bandwidth, the faster the speed. Bandwidth varies throughout the Internet.

Telephone Modems

The original method of connecting computers to the Internet was through telephone lines. This system, still used especially in rural areas, requires a modem, or a device that will translate computer output (digital format) to electronic impulses that can be transmitted over telephone lines (analog format). Telephone modems are connected to the computer through a serial port and to the Internet through a telephone line. The speed with which information can be sent over a telephone line has increased dramatically from the original 25 characters per second (which was measured in baud) to 56,600 kilobits per second. Data transmission, however, often does not live up to its full capacity. To attain full speed, the phone line must be clear of noise or interference. More noise on the line, which is common in older lines, slows the connection. Picking up a phone extension while the line is being used for a computer connection and call waiting produce enough noise to interrupt a regular telephone connection to the Internet. Dial-up connection has probably reached its top speed.

Broadband Connections

Broadband refers to telecommunication in which one wire transmits a wide band of frequencies. This allows more information to be transmitted, just as a six-lane highway will permit more cars to travel at the same time. POTS allows only a single frequency to be transmitted at one time; hence, a broadband connection offers more speed. There are different broadband connections available for using the Internet, such as DSLs, cable, satellite, and **fiber optic cable** (see Table 4-1).

Digital Subscriber Lines

DSL, one form of broadband, offers much faster speeds than POTS, although it still uses a basic copper phone line (Franklin, 2000). Various types of DSL are available, and you will sometimes see it referred to as xDSL, meaning all the varieties. Asymmetric digital subscriber lines (ADSLs), which provide a faster connection than the original DSL, are an improvement to DSL; most DSL connections today in North America are of the ADSL type. Another type of DSL, symmetric digital subscriber line (SDSL), is more common in

Table 4-1 Pros and Cons of Broadband Connection Types

Connection Type	Pros	Cons
Fiber optic cable	Supports high-speed data transfer	More fragile than wire
	Excellent signal reliability	More expensive than DSL
Digital subscriber lines (DSL)	Faster than dial-up	Available only where there is phone service
	Uses a regular phone line (can use the phone and Internet connection at the same time)	
	Easy to install	Connection speed slowed by longer distances from the provider
Television cable	Faster than dial-up and DSL	Available only where there is cable television service
	Uses a television cable connection (can use Internet and television at the same time)	
	Supports high-speed data transfer	
Satellite	Faster than dial-up and DSL	Affected by weather (heavy cloud cover and storms)
	Available worldwide	More expensive than DSL and cable
	Can be powered by generator or battery power	
		Requires use of a satellite dish

Europe (Beal, 2005). The name symmetric is used because the data transmission rate is identical for upstream and downstream.

All types of DSL are able to use regular phone lines by employing a sophisticated scheme that packs digital data onto the existing phone lines, avoiding the translation of data to the analog format. A special modem is required for DSL service, along with what is called a splitter, on all the phone lines with the same number. Because DSL transmission uses parts of the telephone line not used in voice communication, unlike POTS service, DSL users can talk on the phone at the same time they are accessing the Internet.

With ADSL, **download** speed (receipt of information from the Internet) is usually set to be faster than the **upload** speed in the belief that most users download much more than they upload (Beal, 2005). Although ADSL is faster than POTS, the distance from the central office of the telephone company is still a factor. As you get farther away, the signal becomes weaker and the connection speed slows. The limit for ADSL service is now about 20,000 feet (6,096 m). Speeds also vary with the type of DSL, but it is always at least 100 times faster than POTS.

Cable

The last mile can also be provided by the cable used to transmit television. Like DSL, which uses unused portions of the telephone line, cable connections use unused bandwidth on a cable television network. A cable connection can attain speeds from 1 **megabits per second** (Mbps) and 30 Mbps bandwidth for downloads; however most service providers limit the download speed to 6 Mbps. The cable upload speed varies between 128 and 768 Mbsp (Mitchell, 2011). Subscriber needs can be met by configuring the upstream and downstream rates. The transmission of television signals is not interrupted by the use of the Internet. Cable connections, like the varieties of DSL, can make use of **telephony**, that is, the use of the Internet as a telephone by subscribing to a third party such as Skype® (Wikipedia, 2008).

Cable or DSL?

Whether cable or DSL is faster has been debated since the move from POTS, and as of yet, there is no clear winner. Although cable modem download speeds are typically two times faster than DSL, because this technology is based on shared bandwidth, many factors influence this speed (Wikipedia Contributors, 2011). With the varieties of DSL, the connection is only yours; with cable, it is shared with other users. Hence the speed varies with the number of users on the network. Cable providers seldom publish the speed of the connection. For uploading information, the speed is usually about the same. There are many websites that you can access to test the speed of your connection; search by using the type of connection and speed.

Fiber Optic Cable

Fiber optic cable is a popular connection for LANs. This cable consists of very thin, pure glass, which allows more fibers to be bundled in the size of a copper wire (What is fiber optic cable and why would I want it for my business?). Data travel over this cable in the form of light and is capable of speeds up to 100 gigabits per second (Hitchcock, 2007); however, the technology to use all this speed is still in development. The light signal in one fiber does not interfere with signals in other fibers, so it provides both faster data transfers and clearer phone conversations. Besides these advantages, the fiber does not corrode and has no known distance limitations. Its main disadvantage is that it is more fragile than wire, difficult to splice, and more expensive.

Satellite

Satellite Internet connections offer broadband connections to rural areas that cannot receive either DSL or cable. The download speed is approximately 768 kilobits per second to 5.0 megabits per second (Web Exordium, 2010). The cost is higher than DSL or cable for the setup, but the monthly cost is not much higher than other broadband services. The connection requires an antenna, transmit-and-receive electronics, and a satellite dish. Because the satellite dish needs a clear view of the skies, heavy rainstorms or other severe weather is likely to cause outages. Also, because of the distance that the Internet signal has to travel, there is a built-in delay of about a quarter of a second (Kawamoto, 2005). Like cable connections, subscribers compete with one another for bandwidth. A satellite connection may, however, be an answer for underdeveloped countries because it can be powered by a generator or battery power that is able to support a desktop computer system (Gardena, 2008).

IP Addresses

To make it possible for each computer on the Internet to be electronically located, each has an **IP address**, even the one you use to connect to the Internet at home. Because numbers are difficult for most people to remember, and because they may change, each computer is also assigned a name. Each time a message is sent, the Internet **Domain Name System** translates the computer name into its IP address. Using this system, only the domain name system must be updated when an IP numerical address change is required.

IP addresses can be static or dynamic. A **static IP address** will be the same each time the computer is logged on to the Internet. A **dynamic IP address** changes each time a user connects to the Internet. To facilitate each online computer having its own IP address, each ISP is assigned a given number of IP addresses, which they then assign to online computers, in either a static or a dynamic format.

Internet Domains

As part of the domain name system, it was decided to assign a suffix to a computer name to indicate the domain to which the computer belonged. When the Internet was first established, six domain suffixes, as shown in **Table 4-2**, were set up. As the web grew, the need for more domain names also grew. The Internet Corporation for Assigned Names and Numbers (ICANN) was established in 1998 (International Corporation for Assigned Names and Numbers (ICANN), 2010). The role of the agency is to coordinate the Internet's naming system. In 2000, ICANN approved seven new

top-level domains (TLDs). In 2004, six additional domains were added.

Originally, one could tell the type of organization sponsoring the web page by the domain suffix. This practice is still followed, but the number of domain suffixes continues to grow. In 2010, ICANN began accepting applications for new generic top-level-domains (gTLDs) (Marsan, 2009). The primary purpose of the change was to support non-English domains. The new suffixes can have 3–63 characters. One should pay attention to the domain suffix in a web address (URL) because people intent on deceiving others will take the name of the computer of a respected organization and obtain an Internet address with that name but with a different domain suffix. If you wonder whether this has been done, in the address bar of a browser, enter the same computer name, but use a different domain suffix.

Network Neutrality

Today, with the use of the Internet for everything, from its original purpose of open access for academic information to downloading full movies, the traffic on the Internet has grown to the point where there are traffic jams. This has raised several questions. Should payment for the privilege of being on the Internet be a flat fee for everyone, or should it be based on the amount of usage, much like cell phone service is billed? Another question involves the right of those who provide Internet service to prevent users from accessing some sites or prevent them from using any device from a nonsponsored vendor to connect to the Internet.

These have all become an object of concern in what has been named **net neutrality**. The definitions of this term vary, but the main meaning is that the Internet be free of restrictions on use or equipment used to access the Internet, or the type of use, regardless of the service that is providing connectivity to the Internet (PC Magazine, 2011) Several bills concerning net neutrality were introduced into the first session of the 110th Congress, none of which advanced beyond the committee stage. The Internet Freedom Preservation Act of 2008 (HR5353), a bill addressing network neutrality, was introduced n the second session of the 110th Congress. However, the bill died in committee. The bill "proposed adding a new section to the Communications Act of

Table 4-2 Original Domain Suffixes

Characters	Type of Organization
edu	Educational institution
mil	Military computer
gov	Government source
org	Nonprofit organization
com	Commercial enterprise

1934, which regulates the telecommunications and media industries and which was amended with the Telecom Act of 1996, to regulate broadband Internet communications" (Morgan, 2008).

Some ISPs are already altering service in an attempt to control bandwidth usage. In 2008, the Federal Communications Commission (FCC) upheld a complaint against Comcast for inhibiting users from using the high-speed file transfer software BitTorrent. Although Comcast admitted no wrongdoing, it settled the class-action lawsuit for $16 million (Bode, 2010). The lawsuit may make others pause before taking similar actions. Other ISPs are experimenting with a tiered pricing that raises prices for those who have a high-bandwidth usage. Where and how this will end is still up in the air; expect strong lobbying by both sides. The underlying fact is that the infrastructure required to keep the Internet working has to be paid for, and with the increase in traffic, it will need updating.

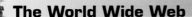

The World Wide Web

The WWW or W3, although the term is often used interchangeably with the term Internet, is a part of the Internet, but it is far from being the entire Internet. It began as a networked information project in 1989 at the European Organization for Nuclear Research (CERN). Its originator, Tim Berners-Lee, devised the system to enable the sharing of research materials and collaboration between physicists at many different locations (Howe, 2010). It first became operational in 1990. In less than 20 years, it became a large factor in the economy and lives of many in the world. Since Gutenberg's invention of movable type, there has not been an innovation that has so changed the speed with which new information could be made available and how we access this information.

The WWW can be regarded as a huge, worldwide library. By using it, one can find valuable information, such as the latest in cancer treatments, the full wording of bills pending before Congress, and any information that someone who has a point to make and access to a website wants to publish. Like its container, the Internet, the WWW is based on a set of protocols and conventions. Although the web is a wonderful contribution to the spread of knowledge, the fact that anyone can obtain a website and

post anything on it means that users must carefully evaluate the information they find on the web, a topic addressed in Chapters 11 and 14.

Web Browsers

The tool that enables users to retrieve and display files from the web is called a web browser, or just a browser. Using the client/server model of networking to retrieve a web document, the browser on the client computer requests a file by using a transmission protocol known as the hypertext transfer protocol (HTTP). With this same protocol, the server, by using special server software, receives that message, finds the file, and sends it off to the requesting computer. The web browser concept and popular web browsers are discussed in Chapter 2. Although you have probably used one or more browsers, you still may not have a clear understanding about how they work or the different **markup languages** used to display information.

Markup Languages

One of the protocols used by the web is a markup language. Markup languages are computer files that combine data and extra information that provides more information about the data. It was derived from the term used in publishing, to mark up the margins of a manuscript with symbols for the printer (Webopedia, 2011). Today, there are several markup languages; the first standardized of these was the standardized generalized markup language (SGML). By using syntax from SGML, Sir Time Berners-Lee developed the markup language most used on the web, Hypertext Markup Language (HTML). The **extensible markup language (XML)** finds a user in healthcare to extract information from electronic messages and documents.

Hypertext Markup Language

HTML is, as the term "markup" implies, a system of marking up a document. HTML adds tags to objects such as text or images that define the manner in which they should be displayed. The tags provide a browser with information about the color, font, attributes, and size to be used to display the text. The tags also provide instructions for hypertext links to other web pages and instructions for displaying any image files that the

```
<!DOCTYPE html PUBLIC "-//W3C//DTD XHTML 1.0 Transitional//EN"
"http://www.w3.org/TR/xhtml1/DTD/xhtml1-transitional.dtd">
<html xmlns="http://www.w3.org/1999/xhtml">
<head>
<meta http-equiv="Content-Type" content="text/html; charset=utf-8" />
<title>HTML</title>
</head>

<body>
<p align="center">Hypertext Markup Language</p>
<p>Hypertext markup language (HTML) is as the term in the name "mark-up" implies really a system
 of marking up a document by adding tags to objects such as text or images to define the manner
 in which they should be displayed. The tags provide a browser with information about what color
 to use for a piece of text as well as the font, attributes, and size to use to display the text.
 The tags also provide instructions for hypertext links to other web pages and instructions for
 displaying any image files that the document contains. Figure 5-3 shows some of the tags that
 are used to markup a Web document and how it is displayed by the browser.
</p>
</body>
</html>
```

Document retrieved by the Web browser

Hypertext Markup Language

Hypertext markup language (HTML) is as the term in the name "mark-up" implies really a system of marking up a document by adding tags to objects such as text or images to define the manner in which they should be displayed. The tags provide a browser with information about what color to use for a piece of text as well as the font, attributes, and size to use to display the text. The tags also provide instructions for hypertext links to other web pages and instructions for displaying any image files that the document contains. Figure 5-3 shows some of the tags that are used to markup a Web document and how it is displayed by the browser.

Document displayed in the Web browser

Figure 4-2 Web documents and HTML formatting tags.

document contains. **Figure 4-2** shows some of the tags that are used to markup a web document and how it is displayed by the browser. The name that would be displayed at the very top of the browser is located between the two title tags. The body tag starts the document and the p tag tells the browser to display all the text within this tag as a paragraph. Notice that tags exist in pairs. What symbol is used to tell the browser that this is the end of that type of formatting?[1] To see some live examples of html, on your browser's View tab click "Page Source" or simply "Source."

Extensible Markup Language

Another markup language, XML, is used in healthcare to improve data exchange (Schroeter, n.d.). It is also a system of tags, but the purpose of these tags is to define the meaning of the data, thereby making it easier to find information within a document, database, or website. Much healthcare information is in a free text or narrative format that lacks any

structure. Important information may be omitted if it is reduced to a computerized format without structure. XML enables tags to be used to identify items such as diagnosis, patient name, gender, and birth date in free text. XML is useful for both exchanging data between incompatible systems and extracting information from free text. Like information in a database, information tagged with XML tags can be displayed in many different ways, including on the web (J. Quiggle, personal communication, 2008).

Web Navigation

Navigating within a web document is identical to most applications in a **graphical user interface (GUI)** operating system. The four arrow keys will move in the document just as they will in any computer document, and the action of the vertical and horizontal scroll bars is also identical. Navigating from document to document (called pages) on the web is done using hyperlinks. Clicking a hyperlink, which is also known as a hot area, will retrieve the document whose web address is specified by that link. On most pages, hyperlinks are identified in

---

1 The backslash in the tag, for example.

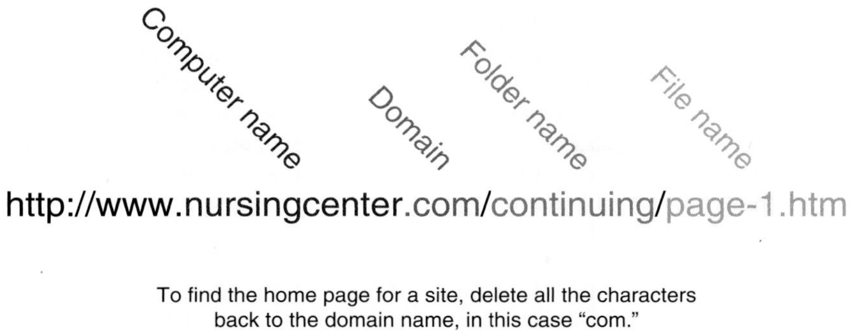

Computer name Domain Folder name File name

http://www.nursingcenter.com/continuing/page-1.htm

To find the home page for a site, delete all the characters
back to the domain name, in this case "com."

Figure 4-3 Anatomy of a URL.

text by the color blue and an underline.[2] Images can also be a hot area. A sure indicator that you are over a hot area is that the mouse pointer changes to a hand with the index finger pointing up.

Although the screens vary among the various browsers, they all have some things in common. For each open window, they keep a record of files that you access in that window, making it possible to move forward or backward in each browser window. The backward and forward arrows near the top of the screen on the left-hand side enable this movement. Hence, if in one window you have opened five documents, you will need to click the back arrow five times to return to the original document.

Not only is this history available for each window but also every web page that you access from any window is kept in an overall history. How long this history is kept depends either on the default duration or on a duration you set in preferences. This history is very helpful if you want to return to a document you left five clicks ago, or even 5 days ago. To see the history you can tap Ctrl + H. To return to a specific document, click the name of the desired document on the menu that appears. This feature is very helpful if you accidentally close a tab or window and want to open it again.

Sometimes when a link is clicked, a document opens in a new window, often smaller than the original, instead of in the current browser window. In this case, the back arrow on the menu line is grayed out. To return to your original document, you must close this window. Although sometimes opening another window is beyond your choice, you can always choose to have a link open in either a new window or, in most browsers today, a tab in that window. To see these choices, right-click a hot area. Two of these choices will be "Open link in new window" and "Open link in new tab." By using either of these, it is easy to switch back and forth between various documents without having to wait for each to be displayed again.

Universal Resource Locators

All documents on the WWW have an address, or a **universal resource locator (URL)**. These addresses are seen in commercials on television or in print advertising. Most URLs start with "http" (the acronym for hypertext transfer protocol), a colon, and two forward slashes (//), or you may see "https" at the beginning of the URL, indicating a secure website. After the introductory letters, some URLs then have the letters "www." The rest of the address varies. URLs may look like a conglomeration of characters when they are first encountered, but there is a pattern to them (see **Figure 4-3**). The name of the computer that hosts the document follows either the double forward slash or the dot after "www." The computer name includes the domain suffix, which is the letters following the last dot in the name before the leftmost single forward slash (/). The letters after the name of the computer are the name of the folder or folders on the host computer where the document is stored.

Some URLs have more than one directory name in them. For example, in the URL http://dlthede.net/Informatics/Chap05ComputerCommunications/

---

2 Some web designers whose desire to demonstrate that their design capabilities exceed their desire to make a site user-friendly will use different attributes to designate a hyperlink.

Chap05.html, there are two directory names between the name of the computer (dlthede.net), "Informatics" and "Chap05ComputerCommunications" and the file name. Just as on a storage disk, directories are organized hierarchically. A forward slash separates each folder from the one above it. The last part of the URL may or may not end with a file name. File names end in a dot and usually the letters "htm," "html," "pdf," or "asp."

Given the myriad features now offered on the web, marked by some very complicated disk organization, it is not surprising that many URLs are very long and have many characters in them, such as some cited in this book. These elements are all integral parts of an address and must not be omitted. One thing that all web addresses have in common, however, is that they contain no spaces and all slashes are forward slashes. Additionally, the characters in a URL after the domain name are often **case sensitive**; that is, if the letter in an URL is uppercase, it needs to be entered in uppercase; if in lowercase, it must be entered in lowercase. Because URLs can become very complicated, whenever you need to enter a complex URL, which is not a hyperlink, but is in an electronic document, select it, copy it to the clipboard, and paste it in the address bar of the browser. Use copy/paste also if you need to include the URL in a word processing, spreadsheet or database document. For this reason, all the URLs in this book will be on the web page for the book, so you can just click to access them (see http://dlthede.net/Informatics/Informatics.html).

Home Page

A concept that came with the WWW is the idea of a **home page**. On a browser, this refers to the page that opens when the browser is first opened. On websites, however, the home page is the primary point of the site, or the top page from which all others are linked. If you are accessing a page and want to know more about the originator of that page, in the address bar, delete the names of all the folders back to the domain suffix and tap the Enter key.

Other Web Page Tools

Active Server Page

You may have noticed that not all web addresses end in "htm" or "html." The web has grown to where it needs interactive pages. One of the most popular ways to create these is to combine HTML for the text part, and use **active server pages (ASPs)** to create interaction (Web Wiz Guide, 2010). ASP is server based, so independent of which browser a user has. It allows web pages to dynamically access databases to present real-time data.

Java and JavaScript

Java and **JavaScript**, both useful on the web, are two different items. Java is a programming language developed by Sun Microsystems® that is used to create small applications called applets that can be downloaded from the web. JavaScript is a scripting language written by Brendan Eich (Wilton-Jones, n.d.) that allows web designers to create interactive pages. A scripting language is enabled when it is run while a programming language such as Java is precompiled (already converted into machine language, thus starts quickly). JavaScript is an open language that can be used without purchasing a license.

Active X and Active X Control

Active X is a set of programming technologies and tools for the web, created by Microsoft®, used to create a self-sufficient program that can be run in Windows® and Macintosh® operating systems. An Active X control is a program similar to a Java applet. However, unlike Java applets, Active X controls have full access to the operating system, and they work only with Internet Explorer (IE). To protect you from unauthorized access to your operating system, when Active X is working on a website, the newer versions of IE will place an Information Bar near the top of your screen and warn you that a program wants to install something on your computer. Be certain of the legitimacy of a site before you agree to this.

Rich Internet Applications

A **rich Internet application** (RIA) is a built-in web browser application that has the features and functionality of a regular desktop application, with the processing done on the user's computer, but the data and program stored on the application server (Deb, 2010). It is called "rich" because it offers more user-interface functions than traditional

Internet offerings. The technologies for RIAs are Ajax (a combination of asynchronous JavaScript and XML), Microsoft Silverlight, Adobe Flash, and Java (Deb, 2010; TechTarget, 2011). Some of the benefits are improved performance, improved security, and less consumption of bandwidth.

Favorites (Bookmarks)

Entering URLs from a keyboard can become very tiresome as well as prone to transcription error. For this reason, browsers provide a way for users to easily record the URLs of sites that are frequently accessed. To access a site that has been recorded, click **Favorites** (IE) or **Bookmarks** (Netscape® and Firefox®), and click the site name on the list. To add a site to these lists, with the document displayed, click Favorites (Bookmarks) and select Add. These Bookmarks (Favorites) can be organized into folders.

Secure Web Pages

Many web users shop online, giving out their credit card numbers. A level of security is provided by web browsers by placing a locked lock icon on the screen when the site is a secure site. The placement of the lock varies; it is generally near one of the four corners of the screen. Some browsers will also change the color of the address bar; for example, in IE, the line becomes gray.

Web Cookies

A great deal of fear and misinformation are linked to **web cookies**. Web cookies are a collection of data that are sent to your computer by some websites and generally make the use of the web more convenient. The browser stores the information in a cookie file on your computer. They may be used when users fill out forms with their name, address, and phone number, on the web. You may have noticed being prompted by a web browser to "remember" a login and password. If you said "yes," you gave permission to create a cookie with that information. Some cookies, known as session cookies, expire when the user leaves the site. Persistent cookies exist for a given time (Beal, 2008).

Cookies do not normally act maliciously on computer systems. However, a trend toward using cookies that store and track your activity online exists. This information is used to build a profile that is sold to advertisers who use the information to target you for specific advertising. Cookies cannot be used to spread viruses, and they cannot access or read your hard drive. Cookies stored on your computer can be read by users, but the information is gibberish to most of us. Protections are, however, available against cookies.

Today's browsers allow you to set a default to delete any cookies when you exit the browser. Additionally, many malware and antivirus programs should flag suspicious **spyware** or **adware** cookies when scanning your system for viruses. To learn more about managing cookies, check the Help section of your browser. You can also search the Internet using the terms "how to delete cookies."

Plug-Ins/Helpers

A **plug-in** is a helper program for a browser. Browsers alone are capable only of interpreting html. The Internet, however, is capable of transmitting other types of files, such as those created by multimedia-authoring languages. Before one can use these files, his or her computer must have a program that can interpret the file and show it either in the browser or on a separate screen. Plug-ins perform this function.

One of the most common plug-ins is the Adobe Acrobat Reader®, which is used to read files that are in the portable document format (PDF). Unlike regular web pages that print according to the dictates of the printer used to output them, PDF files are designed to print in a specified way. This type of file is useful for things such as forms that are intended for printing. PDF files, however, are difficult to read online and take longer to download. Most plug-ins intended to display files from the web, such as Adobe Acrobat Reader®, Real Player®, Apple QuickTime®, or Shockwave®, can be downloaded for free.

Streaming

Streaming is a method of delivering information, usually either audio or video on the Internet. It allows the user to start seeing or hearing the file before the entire file has downloaded. This technique is becoming important because of the increase in the number of large files, such as multimedia applications, that users want to download. Its ability to work depends on the receiving computer's ability to collect the data and deliver it in a steady stream, despite the unsteady rate at which data are transmitted on the Internet. Audio files and video clips are sometimes sent in this manner.

Other Uses of WWW Technology

Intranet

An **intranet**[3] is a private network, usually within a corporation that uses html-formatted documents and the TCP/IP. They provide a cost-effective way to share information within agencies. Anyone in an organization who has struggled either to find the latest version of a procedure or to see that all who need updated information have it in their possession can appreciate an intranet. Intranets can be extremely useful for storing documents that need frequent updating, such as procedures, clinical pathways, policies, and drug information. Because there is only one official copy of these items, all that is required to make current information accessible is to update the one document on the intranet.

An intranet may or may not be connected to the Internet. If it is connected, the contents of the intranet will be protected from the outside world. Those within the institution can access both the intranet and the Internet, but outsiders cannot access the information on the intranet. Intranets can also provide some of the same kinds of features provided on the Internet, such as e-mail, mailing lists, or news groups, although unless they are connected to the Internet, these features will be limited only to those on the intranet.

Like information on the Internet, information on an intranet is also not limited to text. Graphics and multimedia files can also be made available through the intranet. Digital video cameras can be used to record a procedure and the file placed on the intranet, giving users the ability to play it in slow motion or to stop and start as necessary. This makes the intranet an ideal way to offer in-service continuing education programs and access to

procedures. Preparing these documents does not need to be difficult. Although they often comprise a very large file, or one not really suited to the full Internet, all the major application programs (word processors, databases, spreadsheets, and presentation programs) convert documents to web documents with a few mouse clicks. When preparing material for the intranet, thought should be given to adapting the material to take full advantage of browser capabilities, especially hyperlinking.

Extranet

An **extranet** is an extension of an intranet with added security features. Like an intranet, it uses HTTP and TCP/IP. It provides accessibility to the intranet to a specific group of outsiders, often business partners. To access the extranet, a valid username and password are needed. An extranet can be viewed as part of a company's intranet that is extended to users outside the company.

Virtual Private Network

A **virtual private network (VPN)** is a private network that uses a public network, usually the Internet, to connect the nodes (Beal, 2009). The information that the VPN transmits uses an encrypted tunnel and cannot be read by anyone else. It can be described as an extranet with an added layer of security. It can be used to provide access to current patient data from patient monitors to authorized healthcare professionals who are not physically present in the hospital. web-based patient portal software in use by many healthcare agencies and doctors' offices allows patients to communicate with their healthcare provider. With the VPN software, patients can send messages, make appointments, and request medication refills.

Online Security

One does not have to be web familiar to have heard about web security problems. Most of these can be prevented by a savvy user. Before becoming overly paranoid about this, know that most of the problems occur if one is lax about Internet security. Anyone connecting to the Internet with any type of broadband connection needs to protect their computer systems against invaders or viruses. POTS users, although less vulnerable, also need to take precautions.

---

3 Internet, because it is a formal name, is always capitalized; intranet is not a formal name, thus should not be capitalized.

Computer Malware

Computer malware is a term given to all forms of computer software designed by criminals specifically to damage or disrupt a computer system for a profit. Several types of such programs exist, all of which operate differently, but they all damage a computer. Malware is malicious; it can be hidden in advertisements on reputable websites such as Google, Yahoo, and Fox (Mills, 2010).

Although all computer users are vulnerable for a malware infection, there are preventative measures that we can employ. Like healthcare diseases, it is important to understand the problems and vulnerabilities. The language of the "dark world" sounds like child play, but make no mistake, it is a serious lucrative business for cyber criminals.

Botnets

Botnets are the newest fastest-growing malware threat. Botnets are networks of computers that have been hijacked by a malware virus or **worm** (Vaughn-Nichols, 2009). The botnet owner is termed a "herder," the infected computer is a "drone" or "zombie," and computer resources used to trap malware are termed "honeypots" (Shadowserver, 2007a, 2007b). The number of command and control botnet servers doubled to 6,000 between 2008 and 2010. They may lurk on popular websites such as social networking, financial institutions, online advertisements, online auction sites, and online stores.

Botnets are used for click fraud, **distributed denial of service (DDoS),** keylogging, warez, and spam. When the botnet "clicks" on a click fraud advertisement, the cyber crook absconds the award from visiting the site. DDoS is when the botnet prevents access to a website for a long time. The cyber crooks have even demanded ransom money to release the hijacked website. Botnets use keylogging to steal passwords and bank account numbers. They can also gain access to illegal and pirated software (warez). Finally, botnets are used to spread spam.

Phishing and Pharming

Phishing and **pharming** are older forms of web scams, and both try to get an individual to reveal personal information such as a bank account number or a social security number. Phishing and pharming are easy to detect. In phishing, the victim is sent an e-mail message with a web address hyperlink in it, with instructions to go to this website to confirm an account or perform some other task that will involve revealing personal information. Although the hyperlink text in the message looks authentic, clicking it will take a user to a website that is not the one seen in the URL in the message, although it may be a mirror image of the real one.

One can protect oneself against this type of fraud by placing the mouse pointer over the hyperlinked web address and looking at the lower left corner of the screen. In that area, you will see the real address to which you will be taken if you click this link (see **Figure 4-4**). Pharming, on the contrary, results when an attacker infiltrates a domain name server and changes the routing for addresses. Thus, when users of that domain name server enter an URL for a pharmed site, they are pharmed to the evil site. It results from inadequate security for the domain name server. Protection against this type of attack rests with those who maintain the domain name server servers.

Computer Viruses

A type of malware that you hear about most often is a **computer virus**. These are small software programs that are designed to execute and replicate themselves without your knowledge. Before the widespread use of the Internet, they usually were introduced by a disk inserted into the computer's drive. Today, they usually arrive from the Internet, with an e-mail attachment, a greeting card, or an audio or video file. They can corrupt or delete data on your computer or use your e-mail program to send themselves to everyone in your address book or even erase your hard drive.

Like the human variety, computer viruses cause varying degrees of harm. Some can damage hardware, others only cause annoying effects. Although a virus may exist on a computer, it cannot infect the computer until the program to which it is attached is run. After their initial introduction, viruses are usually spread unknowingly by sharing infected files or sending e-mails with an infected attachment.

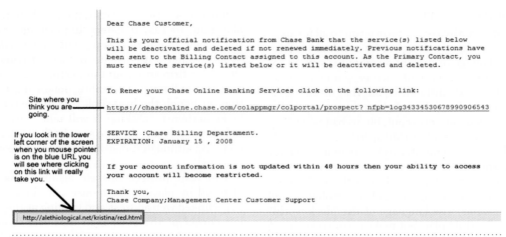

Dear Chase Customer,

This is your official notification from Chase Bank that the service(s) listed below will be deactivated and deleted if not renewed immediately. Previous notifications have been sent to the Billing Contact assigned to this account. As the Primary Contact, you must renew the service(s) listed below or it will be deactivated and deleted.

To Renew your Chase Online Banking Services click on the following link:

Site where you think you are going. → https://chaseonline.chase.com/colappmgr/colportal/prospect? nfpb=log34334530678990906543

SERVICE :Chase Billing Departament.
EXPIRATION: January 15 , 2008

If you look in the lower left corner of the screen when you mouse pointer is on the blue URL you will see where clicking on this link will really take you. → If your account information is not updated within 48 hours then your ability to access your account will become restricted.

Thank you,
Chase Company;Management Center Customer Support

http://alethiological.net/kristina/red.html

Figure 4-4 E-mail scam.

E-mail Virus. This type of virus can be attached to an e-mail message. One type, not too common anymore because of increased security, replicates itself by accessing the victim's address book and mailing itself to those in the list. More common is a virus that is attached to a file created by a legitimate program such as a word processor or a spreadsheet. To prevent this type of virus, most antivirus programs thoroughly vet each e-mail message.

Worm. A worm is a small piece of malware that uses security holes and computer networks to replicate itself. It is not completely a virus in that it does not require a human to run a program to become active; rather, it is considered a subclass of virus because it replicates itself. To accomplish replication, the worm scans the network for another machine with the same security hole and, using this, copies itself to the new machine, which in turn repeats this action creating an ever-growing mass of infection. Unlike a plain virus, worms do not need to attach themselves to an existing program. They always cause harm to a network, even if only by consuming bandwidth.

Koobface (Facebook anagram) is a fast-growing worm spread by social networking sites such as MySpace. It tricks users by appearing to be an invitation from a friend. The invitation will ask them to view a video but will mention the need to update the version of video player. The link to update the software update unleashes a Trojan code (Leydon,

2009; Olechoswski & Taylor, 2010). A video with an explanation of the malware is online http://edition.cnn.com/video/#/video/us/2009/03/02/barnett.facebook.worm.cnn?iref=videosearch (Barnett, 2009; Ferguson, 2010).

Trojan Horse. A **Trojan horse** is not technically a virus because it does not replicate itself. Like the historical Trojan horse, it masquerades as something it is not. For example, a Trojan horse may appear to be a program that performs a useful action or is fun, such as a game; but in reality, when the program is run, it damages your computer. Trojan horses may also create what is called a backdoor to the computer, which provides malicious users access to the computer. Trojan horses do not infect other files or self-replicate.

A keylogger trojan is malicious software that monitors keystrokes, placing them in a file and sending it to the remote attacker (Landesman, 2010b). Some keyloggers record all keystrokes; others are sophisticated enough to log keys only when you open a specific site such as a bank account. This type of software is also used by parents to monitor their children's online activities. Some sites prevent keylogging by having a user use the mouse to point to a visual cue instead of using the keyboard.

Adware and Spyware

Adware and spyware are neither a virus nor spam. Most adwares are legitimate, but some software that function as adware are actually spywares, which at the very least is a nuisance, or it may actually invade your privacy by tracking your Internet travels or installing malicious code (Beal, 2004).

Adware. Adware is a software that is often a legitimate revenue source for companies that offer free software. Software programs, games, or utilities that are designed and distributed as freeware, such as the e-mail program Eudora, often provide their software in what is called a sponsored mode (Beal, 2004). In this mode, depending on the vendor, most or all of the features will be enabled, but pop-up advertisements will be seen when you use the program. Paying to register the software will remove the advertisements. This software is not malicious but just paid advertisements that are randomly displayed when the program is used. It does not track your habits or provide personal information to a third party but is a legitimate source of income to those who provide free software.

Spyware. Spyware, in contrast to adware, tracks your web surfing to tailor advertisements for you. Some adwares unfortunately are spywares (Beal, 2004). This has given legitimate adware a bad name. Spyware can be compared to a Trojan horse because it comes aboard masquerading as what it is not. Downloading and installing peer-to-peer file swapping products, such as those allowing users to swap music files, is a common way to become infected. Although spyware appears to operate like legitimate adware, it is usually a separate program that can monitor keystrokes, including passwords and credit card numbers, and transmit this information to a third party. It can also scan your hard drive, read cookies, and change default home pages on web browsers. Sometimes, a licensing agreement, which few of us read before clicking Accept, informs users that spyware will be installed with the program, although this information is usually in obtuse, hard-to-read legalese, or misleading double-edged statements.

Protection Against Malware

Whether malware is a type of virus, spyware, or Trojan horse is not important. What is important is that a computer be protected against them, or that if a computer is infected, they be promptly removed. The first line of protection is to be careful of sites whose reputation is unknown. Downloading a file that you find in an open web search is always problematic. If you really must download it, scan the file with your antivirus program before installing or executing it. In fact, this is a good standard procedure with any file that is downloaded, no matter what the source.

Olechoswski (Olechoswski & Taylor, 2010), a security expert with Cisco advises us to take the following steps as protection against malware:

- Avoid password reuse.
- Use strong passwords.
- Avoid getting "too personal" on social networking sites.
- Always keep your antimalware software updated.
- Always download the latest software updates. Many of the updates fix security holes.
- Avoid the "it won't happen to me" syndrome.

Firewalls

A **firewall** for computers is like a firewall in a building; it acts to block destructive forces. On a computer, it is a program or hardware device that works closely with a router program to filter the traffic both coming into and, for many firewalls, going out of a network or a private computer. The difficulty comes with deciding what should be let through, that is, what level of security to set. For networks such as those in healthcare agencies, the network administrator sets the limits.

For a private computer, the best method is to accept the defaults. Windows® software includes a firewall. Reputable antivirus software will manage the Windows® firewall and alert you of a security risk if the firewall is turned off. Given that new methods of attack as well as new viruses come on the scene almost daily, make sure that the firewall is turned on. In addition to the Windows® firewall, most wireless routers for home use include a built-in hardware firewall.

Antivirus Software

Although you have antivirus software on your computer, the first step toward protecting one's data is to keep a backup of important files and store in another geographical location. There are many different vendors of antivirus software, including free versions, some of which are of high quality (Landesman, 2010a).

Details may differ between vendors, but antivirus software operates by scanning files or your computer's memory or both, looking for patterns based on the signatures or definitions of known viruses that may indicate an infection. Because virus authors are continually creating new viruses, antivirus software must be continually updated. In fact, once installed on your computer, most antivirus software immediately go to the Internet and download updates. Most antivirus software allows you to make continual updating automatic, for example, every Tuesday at noon. If the computer is not online at that time, or if you do not set automatic updates, you need to access the software and manually update it.

Once antivirus software is fully installed and updated, you should run a complete scan of the entire computer. After that, depending on the software and your choice, you may be able to configure the software to automatically scan specific files or folders at intervals that you set (McDowell & Householder, 2009a). Scanning the entire computer is often a lengthy process; it may even take 2–4 hours. This process uses much of the processing ability and usually slows down any work that you may wish to do. Therefore, you may want to set the scan for times when you are normally not using the computer, but it is on. Antivirus software can also scan individual files, which is usually a quick process. Scanning any e-mail attachments of web downloads is an excellent way to protect your system from malware.

The response when an antivirus program finds a virus varies with the software and whether the virus is found during an automatic or a manual scan. Some software packages will present you with a dialog box asking you if you would like the virus removed, and others will remove the virus without asking you.

Today, most antivirus software is combined with software to detect and remove both viruses and spyware as well as to have firewall-type protection. However, consider downloading a separate antimalware application in addition to the antivirus software (Nelson, 2009). You can run both antimalware and antivirus at the same time. You must never run your computer with more than one antivirus software application.

Once installed, this software operates in the background and checks all the incoming and outgoing data for malicious operations. However, if it is not regularly updated, it cannot offer much protection.

Hoaxes

The world has never known a shortage of practical jokers or those who enjoy sending sensational news to friends. Unfortunately, e-mail lends itself beautifully to these misguided individuals.

Virus Hoaxes

E-mails that warn of viruses are a **hoax** 99% of the time. Although, with few exceptions, these hoaxes are not harmful; they are a waste of time and clutter up the Internet and internal networks with useless messages. Hoaxes sound very credible, frequently citing sources such as an official from Microsoft® or Symantec®. The message contains the information that this virus will destroy a hard drive or perform other dire computer damage. They always tell the recipient to forward this message to anyone she or he knows. Despite containing the statement "This is not a hoax," such messages are a hoax. Discard these messages and do not forward them. When there is a real virus, you are most likely to hear about it in the regular mass media, especially if the virus is new and your antivirus program does not have any protection against it. There are several websites where a virus warning can be checked to see whether it is a hoax. One such site is http://www.trendmicro.com/vinfo/hoaxes/default.asp. About.com at http://urbanlegends.about.com/cs/nethoaxes/ht/emailhoax.htm provides excellent information on how to spot an e-mail hoax.

Urban Legends

Urban legends often are stories thought to be factual by those who pass them on. They may be cautionary or moralistic tales passed on by those who believe them. They are not necessarily untrue but are generally sensationalist, distorted, or exaggerated. They can even be found in a news story, but today, these are mostly passed via e-mail. The sender alleges that the incident happened to someone they or their friends know. Before passing on such information, check with a site that reports on urban legends, such as Snopes (http://www.snopes.com/).

Damaging Hoaxes

There is another type of hoax that is not exactly a hoax but a malicious practical joke that is also spread by e-mail. A user receives a message saying that if a file named "such and such" is on the recipient's computer, the recipient should delete it immediately because it is a logical virus that will execute in so many days and damage the computer, files, and so on. Included are elaborate instructions for how to determine whether the file is on the computer and equally elaborate instructions for deleting it. When a user searches for this file, it is found on the computer. Believing the message, the user deletes it. Unfortunately, it is often a file that is part of the operating system or other application program on the computer. Deleting the file causes a problem when the system or application program needs that file. Repairing the damage is often a lengthy chore.

If a recipient has any doubt that a message such as the one discussed in the previous paragraph is a malicious practical joke, after finding the file, he or she should maximize the Find Screen and look at the date that the file was created (use the details view). The recipient will probably find that the date the file was created shows that the duration mentioned in the warning has exceeded long ago, and hence, the file is not malicious. If the file is part of the operating system, the date will be the date that Windows® was installed on that computer or that a patch was applied. As a rule of thumb, except for deleting files that were user created with an application program, proceed very cautiously in deleting any file. Know exactly what the file that is to be deleted does, and be 100% certain that it is not an important file. A good way to discover what a file does is to enter the name into a web search tool.

Characteristics of This Type of Joke

E-mail warnings should arise suspicions if any of the following characteristics are present (McDowell & Householder, 2009b):

- The message says that tragic consequences will occur if you do not perform a given action.

- It is mentioned that you will receive money or a gift certificate for performing an action.
- Instructions or attachments claim to protect you from a virus that is undetectable by antivirus software.
- The e-mail says that it is not a hoax.
- The logic is contradictory.
- There are multiple spelling or grammatical errors.
- You are asked to forward the message.
- The message has already been forwarded multiple times, which is evidenced by a trail of e-mail headers in the body of the message.

Security Pitfalls

Believing that antivirus software and firewalls once installed are 100% effective is a guaranteed step toward problems. Although combining these technologies with good security habits reduces risk, if protective software is not updated frequently, you are at risk (McDowell, 2008). If you do not protect your computer, believing that there is nothing important on it, it becomes a fertile field for use by attackers who, unbeknownst to you, plant software that is used to attack other people in denial of service attacks. Some operating systems will not install a program without informing you, but it is only a matter of time until attackers learn to bypass this. Slowing down of your computer may be a sign that there are other processes or programs running in the background without your permission, usually to yours or the Internet's detriment. Ignoring patches for either the operating system or the software is another risk situation.

Summary

The time since the first two computers "talked" to each other to today's Internet has been short, but it has been a long journey. Never before in history have the methods of communication been as rapidly changed. The worldwide reach of the Internet and its features, such as the WWW and e-mail, provides the tools that are creating a truly international community.

Ways of connecting to the Internet have speeded up connections from the original 300 baud (slow enough to read the text as it was sent to your computer) to 56 kilobytes per second for POTS and up to 1,000 megabits per second for fiber, with the potential to keep increasing. Building on the use of protocols that join the Internet, the WWW has introduced a new level of knowledge dissemination. From the original HTML language have come variations such as Java and ASP, which have added new features to the web.

Organizations, understanding the benefits of Internet connections, have created network connections such as LANs and WANs. Unfortunately, people intent on doing damage to others have also been active in creating botnets, viruses, Trojan horses, and other methods of spying on web users. Fortunately, methods of protecting against these threats have kept up, and with common sense, it is possible to protect oneself against damages. Computer networking is here to stay and will continue to expand the ways that it can be used, limited not by technology, but by imagination and the willingness to adopt new methods.

APPLICATIONS AND COMPETENCIES

1. How do you see the rapid communication and availability of knowledge via the Internet affecting society in general? Healthcare?

2. Visit a website with many directory names. Parse the URL by working your way backwards until you read the domain name. What did you learn about the sponsor of the site?

3. Add two sites to Favorites (if using IE) or Bookmarks (if using Netscape® or Firefox®).

4. Learn how your browser manages cookies. Does it erase them when you close the browser, when you leave the site, or are they kept for a given number of days?

5. View the page source for a web page. Identify a tag for a paragraph.

6. Compare and contrast two Internet security products using a site that reviews these products. Which one would you select and why?

REFERENCES

Barnett, E. (2009, March 10). *New Facebook worm threat.* Retrieved March 28, 2010, from http://edition.cnn.com/video/#/video/us/2009/03/02/barnett.facebook.worm.cnn?iref=videosearch'

Beal, V. (2004, November 11). *The difference between adware & spyware.* Retrieved March 26, 2010, from http://www.webopedia.com/DidYouKnow/Internet/2004/spyware.asp

Beal, V. (2005, June 3). *Cable vs. DSL.* Retrieved March 26, 2010, from http://webopedia.com/DidYouKnow/Internet/2005/cable_vs_dsl.asp

Beal, V. (2008, September 4). *What are cookies and what do cookies do?* Retrieved March 26, 2010, from http://www.webopedia.com/DidYouKnow/Internet/2007/all_about_cookies.asp

Beal, V. (2009, September 18). *What is a virtual private network (VPN)?* Retrieved March 26, 2010, from http://www.webopedia.com/DidYouKnow/Internet/2007/virtual_private_network_VPN.asp

Bode, K. (2010, February 23). *Comcast P2P throttling settlement nets users "up to" $16.* Retrieved March 27, 2010, from http://www.dslreports.com/shownews/Comcast-P2P-Throttling-Settlement-Nets-Users-Up-To-16-107031

CNET. (2009, November 3). *Wireless network buying guide.* Retrieved March 26, 2010, from http://reviews.cnet.com/2719-7605_7-277-1.html?tag=page;page

Deb, B. (2010). *Rich Internet applications: A look into available technology choices.* Retrieved March 27, 2010, from http://www.jaxmag.com/itr/online_artikel/psecom,id,828,nodeid,147.html

Ferguson, R. (2010, March 1). *A variant of Koobface worm spreading on Facebook.* Retrieved March 28, 2010, from http://blog.trendmicro.com/new-variant-of-koobface-worm-spreading-on-facebook/

Franklin, C. (2000, August 7). *How DSL works.* Retrieved January 22, 2011 from http://www.howstuffworks.com/dsl.htm

Gardena, E. (2008, January 23). *Satellite Internet.* Retrieved March 26, 2010, from http://ezinearticles.com/?Satellite-Internet&id=944996

Hitchcock, R. (2007, May 8). *Copper and glass: A guide to network cables.* Retrieved March 27, 2010, from http://www.windowsnetworking.com/articles_tutorials/Copper-Glass-Guide-Network-Cables.html

Howe, W. (2010, March 24). *A brief history of the Internet.* Retrieved March 26, 2010, from http://www.walthowe.com/navnet/history.html

International Corporation for Assigned Names and Numbers. (2010, January 5). *What does ICANN do?* Retrieved March 28, 2010, from http://www.icann.org/en/participate/what-icann-do.html

Internet Society. (2010). *A brief history of the Internet and related networks.* Retrieved March 26, 2010, from http://www.isoc.org/internet/history/cerf.shtml

ISPcompared.com. (2010). *Internet providers directory – find an ISP – compare Internet service providers.* Retrieved March 27, 2010, from http://www.ispcompared.com/

Joan, B. (2009a, November 9). *Difference between WEP and WPA.* Retrieved March 26, 2010, from http://www.differencebetween.net/technology/difference-between-wep-and-wpa/

Joan, B. (2009b, October 26). *Difference between WPA and WPA2.* Retrieved March 26, 2010, from http://www.differencebetween.net/technology/difference-between-wpa-and-wpa2/

Kawamoto, W. (2005, February 1). *Satellite equals broadband lite.* Retrieved March 27, 2010, from http://www.small-businesscomputing.com/webmaster/article.php/3466881

Landesman, M. (2010a). *Review: Free antivirus software.* Retrieved March 26, 2010, from http://antivirus.about .com/od/antivirussoftwarereviews/a/freeav.htm

Landesman, M. (2010b). *What is a keylogger trojan?* Retrieved from http://antivirus.about.com/od/whatisavirus/a/key-logger.htm

Leydon, J. (2009, March 2). *Koobface variant worms across social networking sites.* Retrieved March 28, 2010, from http://www.theregister.co.uk/2009/03/02/ koobface_worm_returns/

Marsan, C. D. (2009). *ICANN: New domains coming in 2010.* Retrieved March 26, 2010, from http://www.network-world.com/news/2009/062409-icann-new-domains.html

McDowell, M. (2008, October 15). *Cyber security tip ST06-002: Debunking some common myths.* Retrieved March 26, 2010, from http://www.us-cert.gov/cas/tips/ST06-002.html

McDowell, M., & Householder, A. (2009a, June 30). *Cyber security tip ST04-005: Understanding anti-virus software.* Retrieved March 26, 2010, from http://www.us-cert.gov/ cas/tips/ST04-005.html

McDowell, M., & Householder, A. (2009b, June 25). *Cyber security tip ST04-009: Identifying hoaxes and urban legends.* Retrieved March 26, 2010, from http://www.us-cert.gov/ cas/tips/ST04-009.html

Microsoft. (2009). *4 steps to set up your home wireless network.* Retrieved March 27, 2010, from http://www.microsoft .com/athome/organization/wirelesssetup.aspx

Mills, E. (2010, March 22). *Malware delivered by Yahoo, Fox, Google ads.* Retrieved March 27, 2010, from http://news. cnet.com/8301-27080_3-20000898-245 .html?tag=rtcol;pop

Mitchell, B. (2011). *Cable speed – How fast is cable model Internet? About.com.* Retrieved July 28, 2011, from http:// compnetworking.about.com/od/internetaccessbestuses/f/ cablespeed.htm

Morgan, T. P. (2008, February 19). *Net neutrality comes around on the ferris wheel again.* Retrieved March 26, 2010, from http://www.itjungle.com/tlb/tlb021908-story06.html

Nelson, D. J. (2009, June 5). *Malware prevention with Spotbot, Defender, and Malwarebytes.* Retrieved March 27, 2010, from http://security-antivirus-software.suite101.com/ article.cfm/malware_prevention

Olechoswski, S., & Taylor, A. (2010, January 12). *Web 2.0, social media and the dark web – A web criminal's paradise?* Retrieved July 28, 2011, from http://www.experts123. com/q/web-2.0-social-media-and-the-dark-web-a-web-criminals-paradise.html

PC Magazine. (2011). *Net neutrality.* Retrieved January 22, 2011, from http://www.pcmag.com/encyclopedia_term/0, 2542,t=Net+neutrality&i=55962,00.asp

Schroeter, G. (n.d.). *How XML is improving data exchange in healthcare.* Retrieved March 27, 2010, from http://www .softwareag.com/xml/library/schroeter_healthcare.htm

Shadowserver. (2007a, November 12). *Botnets.* Retrieved March 28, 2010, from http://www.shadowserver.org/wiki/ pmwiki.php/Information/Botnets

Shadowserver. (2007b, November 12). *Honeypots.* Retrieved March 28, 2010, from http://www.shadowserver.org/wiki/ pmwiki.php/Information/Honeypots

TechTarget. (2011). *What is rich Internet application?* Retrieved January 22, 2011, from http://searchsoa.techtarget.com/ definition/Rich-Internet-Application-RIA

Vaughn-Nichols, S. J. (2009, August 14). *What is a botnet any-way?* Retrieved March 28, 2010, from http://www.itworld .com/security/74656/what-botnet-anyway

Web Exordium. (2010). *Satellite Internet service providers – High speed satellite Internet for rural areas.* Retrieved July 28, 2011, from http://www.high-speed-internet-access-guide.com/satellite/

Webopedia. (2011). *Markup language.* Retrieved January 22, 2011, from http://www.webopedia.com/TERM/M/ markup_language.html

Web Wiz Guide. (2010). *What are active server pages (classic ASP).* Retrieved March 26, 2010, from http://www.web-wizguide.com/kb/asp_tutorials/what_is_asp.asp

Wikipedia. (2008). *Digital Subscriber Line.* Retrieved November 20, 2011, from http://en.wikipedia.org/wiki/ Digital_subscriber_line

Wikipedia Contributors. (2011, July 28). *Digital subscriber line.* Retrieved July 28, 2011, from http://en.wikipedia. org/wiki/Digital_Subscriber_Line

Wilton-Jones, M. (n.d.). *The early Internet and the first genera-tion browsers.* Retrieved March 26, 2010, from http://www .howtocreate.co.uk/jshistory.html

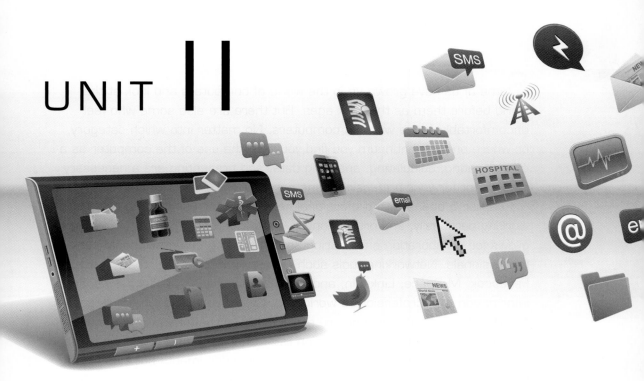

UNIT II

Computers and Your Professional Career

Some of us have grown up in the world of computers and look at the world before them as the dark ages. But there are also some who feel uncomfortable in the world of computers. No matter into which category, or where on the continuum you find yourself, the use of the computer as a tool in writing, calculating, analyzing data, and presenting are a necessary instrument for your professional and personal life.

Chapter 5 opens with professional networking, or using computer networking personally, and professionally. Web 2.0 tools, the interactive web, allows for collaboration and sharing among nursing and other healthcare professionals. Networking tools such as instant messaging, chat, Twitter, Facebook, MySpace, LinkedIn, and Plaxo allow nurses to collectively share information with professionals worldwide. Collective intelligence tools such as wikis, blogs, and mashups are explained as is the full world of e-mail including the use of e-mail discussion lists. Chapter 6 addresses word processing skills not only from writing professional documents but also using Cloud Computing word processor applications and features that allow for file sharing. The features discussed focus on improving productivity.

Chapters 7, 8, and 9 also address office computing skills that improve productivity and allow sharing of documents. You will examine Cloud Computing office applications and compare it with office suite software that resides on your computer. Chapter 8 on presentations are looks at both the pluses and minuses of using slide presentation programs and offers help to make their usage truly informational. Chapter 9 examines spreadsheets, software that can assist in managing numbers. The mathematical priority in formulas, tips to better spreadsheets, the use of graphs, and other spreadsheet features such as protecting data are investigated. Chapter 10, the last chapter in this unit, introduces databases, which are the key ingredient of all information systems. Starting with searching databases, the chapter examines other uses in nursing, such as for analyzing data pertinent to a unit, database structures, and the "one piece of data, many views" concept, and concludes with the use of data mining.

CHAPTER 5
Professional Networking

Objectives

After studying this chapter you will be able to:

▶ *Discuss Web 2.0 features.*

▶ *Discuss the advantages and disadvantages for use of social networking sites.*

▶ *Use e-mail effectively.*

▶ *Manage e-mail accounts.*

▶ *Be a responsible member of a discussion list.*

Key Terms

Backwardly Compatible
Bcc
Blog
Cc
Collective Intelligence
E-mail
Emoticon
Flame
Flame War
Folksonomy
Grass Roots Media
Hypertext Markup Language (HTML)
Instant Messaging
Internet Mail Access Protocol (IMAP)
Internet Service Provider (ISP)
Listserv
Login Name
Mashup
Pharming
Phishing
Podcast

Post Office Protocol 3 (POP3)
Rich Text File (RTF)
Real Simple Syndication and Rich Site Summary Feed
Semantic Web
Simple Mail Transfer Protocol (SMTP)
Spam
Telephony
Threaded Messages
User ID
Vodcast
Voice over the Internet Protocol (VoIP)
Web 3.0
Web Conferencing
Web 2.0
Webcast
Webinar
Wiki
Wikipedia®
Zipped File

Christina is a nurse in the quality improvement department of a rural county hospital. Kerrie is a nurse in a critical care step-down unit. Both Christina and Kerrie (not their real names) are working on nursing degrees and have become dependent on electronic communication, but both have had to devise "work-arounds" to get access to the Internet. Christina has access to **e-mail** and the Internet from her hospital but not at home. In the evenings and on weekends, she takes her laptop and textbooks and drives to the local library or coffee or sandwich shop to check e-mail and complete online course assignments. Kerrie doesn't have e-mail or Internet access at work, so to stay in touch with her instructors and fellow students during breaks, she checks e-mail by using her smartphone.

Like the two nurses mentioned earlier, online communication has become so important to daily life that when it is not easily available, people go out of their way to become connected. Free Wi-Fi™ (wireless fidelity)[1] connections to the Internet have become a selling point for coffee shops and hotels. Never before in history have new communication methods like those provided by the Internet and its by-products made such quick inroads into society. The Internet has given us inexpensive asynchronous discussions, synchronous instant communication, e-mail, electronic mailing lists, and the library known as the World Wide Web (WWW). Creative users, not content to have the WWW as just a repository of information, have given us social networking, interactive sites, instant news, and personal opinions not regulated by traditional media.

The networking thus provided allows us to communicate with colleagues worldwide and to stay abreast of standards of care and practice. History has taught us through recent devastating disasters that electronic networking can provide a means for organizing and delivering healthcare provider volunteer assistance, pharmaceuticals and medical supplies, and a way to provide care to those in need. Nurses trapped within the disasters have been able to connect to the Internet and chronicle events by using **instant messaging** (IM), e-mail, and online **blogs**.

Web 2.0

In the quest to make the web function in a more personal manner, a concept called **Web 2.0** was born. It does not have strict boundaries from the original web but is about people interacting, sharing, and collaborating. The term "Web 2.0" was first coined by O'Reilly and others to describe what online companies/services that survived the dot.com bubble burst in 2000 had in common (O'Reilly, 2005). Web 2.0 has emerged as a social technology that allows us to communicate and share information. Web 2.0 provides a rich medium to nurses and other healthcare professionals for interactive networking. A professional networking website is like a visit to one's colleague's office or home where one can see personal pictures and other decor that reflect his or her ideas and personality.

Before the concept of Web 2.0 existed, we used the web to read; now we use it to read, interact, and write. Information sharing can be video, data, text, or metadata. The provider determines the format, with the basic idea being that information is created and shared among many users. The result maximizes the **collective intelligence**. The outcomes can be commonly accepted content or opinion. This type of intelligence requires some type of regulation, often from users of the site. Examples include user recommendations on eBay or Amazon and reviews of various travel facilities by those who have used them.

Instant Messaging, Chat, and Twitter

IM, chat, and Twitter are very popular text-based communication worldwide. They all are classified as social networking and microblogging applications. Microblogging refers to very brief web journaling. A microblog could be simply a sentence fragment.

The immediacy of text-based communication resulted in the development of a new language system called "text speak" that uses letter, numbers, and symbols instead of spelling out words. For example, instead of "I have a question for you" the text-based representation would be "?4U." There is no standard that invokes the meaning of words used in IM; however, in English, the alphabet letter, number, or symbol that invokes meaning of a word is commonly used. For example, the letter r is used for the word "are" the number 2 is used instead of "to," and number 4 used instead of "for." Webopedia has an extensive listing of abbreviations used for

---

1 The Wi-Fi Alliance is a trade group that owns Wi-Fi™, which is the trademark to Wi-Fi.

quick messaging at http://www.webopedia.com/quick_ref/textmessageabbreviations.asp. Abbreviated language works well for information quick communication, but it should never be used in a professional setting such as school or workplace communication.

The prevalent use of smartphones and other mobile Internet devices (MIDs) has allowed IM to become the preferred method (over e-mail) for many to communicate (**Figure 5-1**). It is relatively unobtrusive and provides the ability for instant communication. IM is a feature in online services such as Google Chat®, Yahoo! Messenger®, and Windows Live Messenger®. Text messaging (short message service [SMS]) and multimedia messaging (multimedia message service [MMS]) are similar features that are standard on mobile phones.

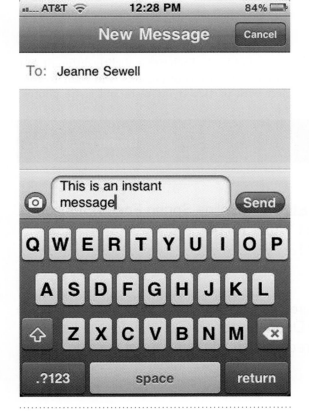

Figure 5-1 Instant messaging.

IM use continues to be a controversial topic. In school classrooms, students IM each other in class similar to the days some of us passed paper notes. Teachers voice concern that the students are inattentive to classroom lessons. Should there be laws against drivers using IM while operating vehicles? It is against the law in some states and still under debate in others (Governors Highway Safety Association, 2010).

Chat is interactive e-mail that has been around for a long time, but it has morphed into newer types of instant types. The main difference between IM and chat is that IM is messaging between two individuals, whereas chat can involve two or more individuals. Chat is an optional feature that is available in course Learning Management Systems (LMSs). In this milieu, the computer screen shows a list of the participants as they enter the chat room. Some chat software allows users use their real names or a "handle or alias." Chat users type their conversation, and tap the Enter key to send the message. Others in the chat room respond with their replies (**Figure 5-2**).

Twitter (http://twitter.com/) users send short (140 characters or less) message known as "tweets" to the Twitter website by using a computer or a mobile device. Twitter does require users to register, create login and password, but the service is free. The difference between Twitter and IM is that tweets are shared with collective others and IM is shared with just two individuals. Twitter uses the concept of "followers," meaning that you identify the organizations or persons that you want to glean information from their postings and others can follow your postings. Twitter is about tiny information bites that anyone wants to share (**Figure 5-3**).

Twitter allows us to keep up with breaking news from professional organizations such as the American Academy of Ambulatory Care Nursing, Interdisciplinary Nursing Quality Research Initiative, Healthcare Information Management Systems and Society, and the Centers for Disease Control and Prevention. Click on the "Follow People" and enter a topic or a person's name. The tweets for the organizations or people you are following will show up on your Twitter home page. The tweets are a great way to keep up with your particular interests.

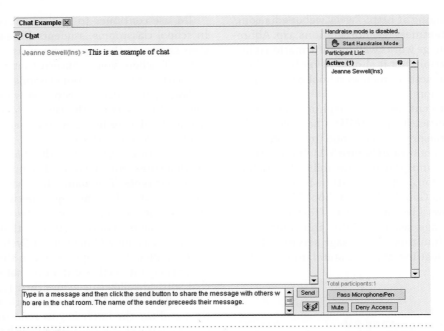

Figure 5-2 Chat.

Social Networking Service Trends

While microblogging serves the purpose of instant communication, it also has its limitations. Social networking sites such as Facebook, MySpace, Plaxo, and LinkedIn serve to connect millions of users worldwide. Each site is slightly different, but all meet the needs of persons who want to connect with particular interests and share photos,

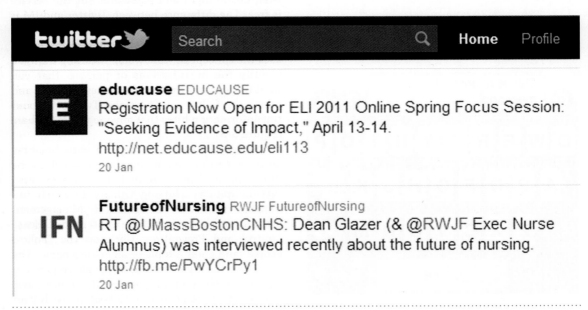

Figure 5-3 Twitter.

Table 5-1 Examples of Professional Associations Using Social Networking Sites

Look for the following groups in Facebook, LinkedIn, and Twitter:

- American Nurses Association
- Nursing Informatics Working Group (NIWG) of AMIA (American Medical Informatics Association)
- PubMed
- HIMSS (Healthcare Information and Management Systems Society)
- MERLOT (Multimedia Educational Resources for Learning and Online Teaching)

videos, stories, and experiences. The trend of social networking is still emerging, but there is a blur between the actual social networking site and the ability to use associated applications, such as games and office suite software.

Academia and corporate businesses initially shunned use of social networking. Today, many hospitals still block the use of social networking sites. However, many academic and healthcare settings have embraced the use of the sites to connect with groups of users on a more personal level with a sense of community. Examples of use at colleges and universities include connecting with enrolled students and alumni. Examples in nursing include professional associations and association group chapters (**Table 5-1**).

Social networking services have a short history beginning with Friendster (http://www.friendster.com/) in 2002 (Buckley, 2010). MySpace (http://www.friendster.com/) began in 2003 and became most popular until 2008, when Facebook took over. Facebook (http://www.facebook.com/) began in February 2004 when Mark Zuckerberg and three of his college friends decided to connect with other students by using a website from a Harvard University dorm (Facebook, 2011). One month later, the social networking site was in use by students at Columbia, Yale, and Stanford universities. Six years later, the site had more than 400 million active users. In 2010, 25% of the users accessed the site from mobile devices. According to Facebook, 25 billion pieces of content are shared monthly.

Plaxo (http://www.plaxo.com/) is a social networking online address book. It can also be classified as a cloud computing address book. Plaxo can be used to track feeds from other social networking sites such as Facebook and Twitter. As with other online services, you must create a login and password before accessing the site.

LinkedIn (https://www.linkedin.com) is a professional rather than a social networking site. Like Facebook, the users can choose individuals and groups with whom they want to connect. LinkedIn provides a way to connect with other business professionals, share information, or look for new career opportunities.

The popularity of Facebook and LinkedIn has gained the attention of nurses, professional nursing organizations, libraries, and corporate America. Marla Weston, American Nurses Association (ANA) chief executive noted, "ANA is now offering multiple ways for nurses to connect with each other and stay informed, as well as enhance a personal sense of community" ("American Nurses Association now on Facebook, LinkedIn groups," 2009). The trend of connecting with people where they tend to gather electronically is expected to continue.

Privacy is an issue with the Internet in general and the use of social networking services is no exception, privacy related to both the clinical setting and the social networking site user. Nurses have been fired for breaching patient privacy (AHC Media, 2009a). As an example, a nurse posted a photo that she took with her cell phone of an x-ray and then posted it on her Facebook page along with a discussion posting. A second nurse also photographed the same x-ray. An anonymous caller reported the incident to the local sheriff's department. The incident was referred to the Federal Bureau of Investigation. The nurses were subsequently fired for breaching the hospital's privacy policy. A potential misunderstanding about privacy is that it addresses only the patient's name or medical record number. Sharing information about a particularly unique case or condition might easily identify a particular patient. A breach of confidentiality is in violation of the Health Insurance Portability and Accountability Act. First, nurses should never take personal photographs of patients, patients' family members, or anything related to the patient care setting or the patient's record. Second, it is inappropriate to have any clinical discussion or blog related to patients or patient care in the public domain.

Personal privacy is also a very important consideration. Each social networking site should have privacy help information available. For example, Facebook maintains a site at http://www.facebook.com/#!/privacy/explanation.php. When logging into a social networking site for the first time, you should expect to have to input your birth date to ensure that you are not a child. However, you can hide that information and more. There are other choices. You do not need to accept invitations from others to befriend you. You can choose to ignore the invites. You also can "block" users from your site.

On a final note, it is important that we understand how others are using social networking sites. For example, the campus police use them to identify when and where large parties are occurring in preparation for roadblocks to detect driving under the influence of alcohol or other substances. Employers may use them to check on job applicants before making employment decisions or to monitor postings by current employees (AHC Media, 2009b). Teachers may use them to monitor the status of students or as a communication tool to connect with students. The benefits for use of social networking sites can outweigh the risks if prudent judgment is used.

Internet Telephone

Internet telephone or **telephony** refers to computer software and hardware that can perform functions usually associated with a telephone. Telephony products are often referred to as **voice over the Internet protocol (VoIP)**. VoIP provides a means to make a telephone call anywhere in the world with voice and video by using the Internet, thereby bypassing the phone company.

The free versions provide phone communication from computer to computer. Skype (http://www.skype.com) is an example of VoIP software. Skype allows free Skype-to-Skype calls, video calls, IM, and chat. For an Internet call, all you need is a microphone, speakers, and a sound card. If you have a video camera, you can have video calls. The connection, computer processor, and software determine the number of people and quality of the connection. For a small fee, you can choose to call telephone numbers on mobile phones and landlines by using the Internet. You can also download the software for your mobile phone or even purchase a Skype phone that allows you to make phone calls using Wi-Fi. Vonage (http://www.vonage.com/) and Evaphone (http://evaphone.com/) are examples of two other VoIP products. The choice of services is changing, so you may want to do your own search, using the search terms "Internet telephone." For additional information on how the Internet telephone works, go to CNET Reviews – Internet Phones at http://reviews.cnet.com/4520-9140_7-5131535-1.html.

Teleconferencing via the Internet

Conference calls by using the telephone have become a way of life for those belonging to committees whose members live in different geographical locations. In **web conferencing**, videos such as slideshows and other visuals can be added to the meeting. Some web conferencing software feature the ability of participants to mark up documents or images, as well as "chat" by using a keyboard. Web conferencing is similar to an open telephone call, but with the added element of video.

A **webcast** is a one-way presentation, usually with video, to an audience who may be present either in a room or in a different geographical location. Methods for the distant audience to ask questions are usually provided. Webcasts can be viewed "live" or recorded for distribution later as a link on a webpage or as an e-mail file attachment.

A **webinar**, on the other hand, is more like a live seminar. Users are directed to login to a website address. Although there is a speaker, the audience can ask questions, and the speaker can ask for feedback as the information is delivered. Most webcast and webinar software allow the sessions to be recorded, saved as a file, and shared with others. Participants can choose to participate by using a computer or a telephone connection. Like webcasts, webinar sessions can be recorded and distributed as a webpage link or an e-mail attachment.

Webinar software is available for enterprise and individual use. Faculty who teach courses online may use webinar software for office hours. Healthcare organizations use the software to conduct meetings and save employee inconvenience and travel costs. webinar software can be used alone or embedded with an LMS. Webinar software usually provides a means for video, audio, and chat. Free trial versions of webinar software are available for individual use. For more information, search the Internet by using the term "webinar."

Collective Intelligence Tools

Collective intelligence is defined as knowledge and understanding that emerges from large groups of people (Johnson, Levine, Smith, & Stone, 2010). Analysis of data that are collected over time will allow new patterns to emerge and in turn will result in new knowledge. The notion of collective intelligence has implications for changes in the educational process and the nursing profession. Use of collective intelligence applications in nursing education provides opportunities for grassroots problem solving and knowledge construction by students worldwide.

 ## Wikis

A **wiki** is one example of a collective intelligence application. A "wiki" is a piece of server software that allows users to freely create and edit a web page's content using any web browser. The work "wiki" is Hawaiian for "quick" (Wikipedia Contributors, 2010a). Wikis include a file manager, the ability to upload and download files, a text editor, and support for hyperlinks. Some wiki sites are available for private use without advertising; others charge a fee. The person who creates the wiki, the "owner," hosts a wiki site. The "owner" can then invite others into the site. Editing authority may be public, as in **Wikipedia®**, or by those invited to participate in the wiki.

Wikipedia® is a popular, free, publically edited, online encyclopedia, which began in 2001. Within the first 6 months of development, users had contributed 6,000 articles (Neus, 2001); as of March 2010, there were more than 14 million articles (Wikipedia Contributors, 2010b). Wikipedia® articles are collaboratively created and improved by users. To make any changes to Wikipedia® articles, users do not need to log into the site, although their computer Internet protocol address will be publically available in the edit history. Tabs at the top of the article provide a means for collaborative discussion on the topic, editing the topic, or viewing the history of changes (an audit trail). All changes are recorded and can always be undone. The strength of Wikipedia® is that it provides information on an ever-expanding number of topics. Critics are quick to point out that the quality of articles is inconsistent. For technical information, it is often one of the most up-to-date and the best sources of information.

Wikis are websites designed for sharing and collaborative work on documents. They are used for research endeavors, committee work, clubs, classrooms, and knowledge management. Wiki sites can be private or public, for example, a wiki designed for committee work or nursing research would be private. The wiki administrator identifies the membership using e-mail addresses, and the wiki automatically e-mails members with information on how to register for the wiki website.

There are numerous free wiki sites available. When selecting a wiki site, consider the purpose of the site, restrictions for numbers of users, and file sizes. Also, consider having to pay special fees to make the site free of advertisements and private. Examples (in alphabetical order) include the following:

- DooWiki (http://www.doowikis.com/)
- Google Sites (http://sites.google.com/)
- Wikidot (http://www.wikidot.com/)
- Wikispaces (http://www.wikispaces.com/)
- Wet Paint (http://www.wetpaint.com/)
- XWiki (http://www.xwiki.com)
- Zoho® wiki (http://wiki.zoho.com/)

The culture of the group is a factor that affects the effectiveness of collaboration (Harper & Watson, 2008). Users must be willing to share knowledge and exchange ideas. They must be open-minded and willing to seek new knowledge. When wikis are used as an updatable knowledge management repository, users must have the technical skills to upload and edit documents.

Acrobat.com

Acrobat.com is an Adobe shared workspace like a wiki; however, it has a few unique features. By default, the shared workplace is free, is private, and does not have advertisements. You can access the feature if you have an Adobe login and password. Acrobat.com uses Flash, a platform for animation and interactivity. It includes a self-contained cloud computing office suite with a word processor (Buzzword), presentation software (Presentation), and spreadsheet software (Project Mgmt). The other unique feature is that it includes webinar software. The free version allows up to three connections. The webinar includes all of the standard webinar features, such as ability to invite others, video conferencing, audio, screen sharing, remote control, and chat. The initial file size limitation was 100 MB.

Cloud Computing Office Suites

Web 2.0 cloud computing includes many tools that allow groups of users to work together virtually. Many of the tools are free and very easy to use. The only requirement is the use of a computer with an Internet connection. In addition to Acrobat. com, examples of online office suites that allow group collaboration are Google Docs™ and Zoho® Office. Google Docs™ (http://www.wikispaces.com/site/tour#introduction) includes word processing, spreadsheet, and presentation software. The documents are usually created offsite and then uploaded where they can be shared and edited by others. The documents can also be downloaded and saved. Zoho® (http://zoho.com) provides collaborative access to word processing, spreadsheets, presentation tools, and many other productivity tools. The website allows users to import files from other office applications. Joining either of these is free; all one has to do is create an account.

Sharing Media

The Sketchcast (http://sketchcast.com/) tool allows a registered user to draw and narrate an idea and then share it via a web page or blog. Slideshare (http://www.slideshare.net/) allows users to upload a slideshow presentation, embed it into a website or a blog, synch audio to slides, and join groups who share the same interests. Presentations can be downloaded to the user's computer or shared with others. The search terms "nursing" and "nursing research" at this site will find slideshows pertinent to the nursing profession. Slide (http://www.slide.com/) also allows you to create online slideshows including music videos as well as create a guest book for your site on which friends can share their pictures.

Evolving Collective Intelligence Applications

New collective intelligence applications are on the horizon. Freebase (http://www.freebase.com) is an open shared knowledge database. The website provides an introductory video designed to guide new users to efficiently search the database. To contribute, you must register and receive a login and password. The Google Image Labeler (http://images.google.com/imagelabeler/) uses a gaming strategy to improve the quality of Google images search term results. Users are randomly paired with an online partner. The players are shown a set of images over a 2-minute period and asked to describe the image with as many labels as possible. When the two players agree on a label, the players receive points.

Folksonomies and Tagging

Folksonomies taxonomies that "result from social tagging of diverse content such as documents, images, blog entries, links, and keywords" (Kaminski, 2009, p. 3). Folksonomies are another form of collective intelligence. The tags are word descriptors, often achieved by collaborative group consensus. The collection of **folksonomy** tags are known as "tag clouds." Their appearance varies on websites.

There are numerous tag cloud generators available for website authors. The generators provide options for either entering a universal resource locator (URL) of a website or entering specific tags and the associated links. Users may also have the option of choosing colors, fonts, and styles of the tag clouds and then copy the code to use on their websites so that the tag cloud is visible to others. The variety of visual representations of tag clouds is a feature of folksonomies.

Delicious (http://delicious.com/) and reddit (http://www.reddit.com/) are social bookmarking sites where people share and tag their favorite websites. At these sites, you can add your favorite websites to a tag and see those of others with the same tag. Digg (http://digg.com/) is a social news site that allows contributors to add links to articles. Other contributors can click a "thumbs up" icon if they like the link, make comments, share the link with others, or show their disapproval by clicking on "bury."

Folksonomies are present on healthcare websites. Online *Journal of Nursing Informatics* uses a cloud tag as a site map at http://ojni.org/ojni_sitemap_cloud.html. PatientsLikeMe® (http://www.patientslikeme.com/) is a free website devoted to individuals with a life-changing condition who want to share and learn from others. The site includes prevalent and rare disease categories, treatments, symptoms, and research. Participants share their experiences. Researchers who manage the site aggregate the rich data with statistical tools and output it with graphical representations.

Blogs

A blog is an online web log or discussion. Although blogs can be collaborative, more often, they are started by one person, known as a blogger, and although comments are usually allowed, they generally revolve around the blogger's posts. Blog has many definitions, but basically, it is a website on which the blogger, or bloggers, share ideas and thoughts, often about a given topic, with posts in reverse chronological order. It is, or should be, updated regularly. Their quality and content vary, from personal musings to those that are more serious and informative. Technorati (http://technorati.com/) is a search engine specifically for blogs. Users can search for information in blogs or posts. It is an interactive resource that allows users to make comments or blog preferences.

There are many different ways to use blogs in both education and healthcare. Because blogs are websites, nursing educators can easily incorporate their use into online course content. Family blogs that share experiences about care for a loved one with medical problems could be used as case studies for nursing students and provide insights into those affected by the illnesses. The teaching/learning effectiveness of patient-centered blogs is enhanced when readers are encouraged to participate in the conversation and to post personal reflections (Sandars, 2007).

Blogs can also be used to share information about a particular health topic. One example of this type of blog is the Scoliosis News (http://www.genengnews.com/blog/item.aspx?id=591), where news reports about scoliosis are posted. Health blogs have varying authors, including healthcare professionals, patients, and others who are interested in certain topics, read widely on the subjects, and want to share their knowledge. Nurses in both hospital and education settings use blogs to share learning. For example, the nurses at Saint Joseph Hospital (Orange, California) have created a nursing research blog (http://evidencebased-nursing.blogspot.com/search/label/ResearchatSt.JosephHospital0Orange) in which they communicate the research activities of their staff as well as the results of group discussions about research articles.

A blog is relatively easy to create by using free tools such as Google's Blogger (http://www.blogger.com/start), Live Journal (http://www.livejournal.com/), and Xanga (http://www.xanga.com/). Some of these tools also allow readers to post comments to the postings. Authoring a blog is not something to be taken on lightly; they can be time consuming and should be updated if others are to find them interesting. Like all web sources, information from a blog needs to be carefully evaluated.[2]

RSS Feeds

Because blogs are updated, but generally not on a fixed schedule, you can subscribe to an RSS feed, which will notify you when there is new information on a blog. RSS feed is an acronym for both **Real Simple Syndication and Rich Site Summary Feeds** (your choice). RSS feeds are not confined to blogs. You can have RSS feeds of new items from websites including electronic library searches, news, and blogs sent to your personalized web browser home web page, such as iGoogle or MyYahoo. The signal that a website is amenable to being subscribed to is the orange icon on the page itself or in the location bar (see **Figure 5-4**). The RSS icon became the industry standard denoting RSS feed availability in December 2005. By using the Help menu in your web browser or e-mail application, you can easily create an RSS feed for any site where you see the icon.

Mashups

A **mashup** is a web application that takes data from more than one source and combines it into a single, integrated tool (Skiba, 2007). There are several varieties of mashups. One type involves mapping, in which data are overlaid on a map. This type

---

2 Evaluating websites is discussed in Chapter 10.

Figure 5-4 The RSS icon.

of mashup was given a push with the advent of Google Maps (http://maps.google.com/), which, developers discovered, could be overlaid with current data from various sources. Google Maps allows users to add pictures and information about their business sites at no charge. Google Earth (http://earth.google.com/) is yet another example of a mashup that includes overlaid data. It involves associating videos or photos with the metadata about the picture such as who took the picture and the location where it was taken.

There are also search and shopping mashups, such as the comparative shopping tools that draw data from various sources. News mashups are another variety in which news from various sources is synthesized into personalized news. Personalized dashboard websites such as iGoogle (http://www.google.com/ig), MyYahoo!® (http://my.yahoo.com/), and Netvibes (http://www.netvibes.com/) are mashups.

Mashups are used in healthcare to place cases of infectious diseases on a geographical area. HealthMap (http://healthmap.org/en) allows users to create maps after selecting specific diseases and categories (international significance, new and ongoing outbreaks, and warnings). The map pins are color-coded according to disease incidence. Clicking on map pin leads the viewer to a news article or other types of reports.

Mashups could be patient centered and display information such as medical history, laboratory data as seen in the YouTube® video, "Creating a Healthcare Mashup with IBM Mashup," at http://www.youtube.com/watch?v=NX6Xr8gBLqo&feature=related. Hospital administration dashboards that display financial information, staffing, and patient outcomes (Frith, Anderson, & Sewell, 2010) are mashups.

Group Discussion Forums

There are many group discussion forums available on the web. Group discussion forums are similar to a wiki, but classified as a Usenet, a distributed discussion forum (Moraes, 2010). Google Groups™ (http://groups.google.com/) allows for sharing of documents as well as a group discussion. Google Groups users must register to create a login and password. Google Groups can be private or public or serve as an electronic bulletin board. Private Google Groups has a feature that alerts all the members when there is a change to the workspace. Google Groups are also used for collaborative work such as committee work, classrooms, and clubs. Yahoo!® Groups (http://groups.yahoo.com/) also provides the same service.

Grass Roots Media

The ability to share photographs and videos is a rapidly growing trend! The term **Grass Roots Media** refers to the widespread creation and posting to the web of media such as videos, slides, and blogs by nonprofessionals. There are multiple ways to create digital photos or videos that can be posted to the web. Most cell phones and digital cameras include both the ability to take photos and videos. Inexpensive but "good-enough" digital camcorders that record 60–120 minutes of video are also available. Video cameras complete with installation and video editing software and small enough to fit in a pocket are also available. Video files are transferred to the computer using a USB (universal serial bus) connection.

Online Photos

There are many photo-sharing websites. Photo-sharing sites allow photos to be shared privately and publicly. Websites such as Flickr™ (http://flickr.com/), Photobucket™ (http://photobucket.com/), Picasa™ (http://picasa.google.com/), Snapfish™ (http://www.snapfish.com/), and Shutterfly™ (http://www.shutterfly.com/) are designed for photo sharing. The sites all have a free service, but most charge based on the number of photos stored or folders that are maintained for file organization. Shared photos are an excellent way of sharing experiences from professional meetings and conferences.

Online Personal Videos

Video-on-demand websites, such as YouTube® (http://www.youtube.com/), allow users to upload, view, and broadcast videos to a worldwide audience at no charge. To find and view a video from YouTube®, enter a search term in the search box. Although free online videos vary in quality and length, users are guided to useful resources such as the ratings of other users.

To upload a video, register for an account, complete a short form where you indicate your account type, contact information, gender, and age, and agree to the website terms of use. Faculty and healthcare professionals are using the video-on-demand sites to deliver lecture material. When uploading video on healthcare topics, users must adhere to all privacy guidelines to protect patient confidentiality.

Podcasts and Vodcasts

Podcasts, or audio messages available online, and **vodcasts**, video and audio online, allow anyone with the appropriate hardware and software to create and publish audio and video contents on the web. Some developers publish these as a theme series on a specific subject that are available as an RSS feed. They can be identified by the orange icon with the word "POD." You can listen to a podcast by using a portable MP3/video player (including those built into mobile phones) or a computer with special software such as iTunes and Windows Media Player® (Little, 2007). Free podcatching software (the name given to software that allows users to play podcasts on their computer) is available from iTunes (http://www.apple.com/itunes/download/) and Juice (http://juicereceiver.sourceforge.net/). There are also many excellent resources for podcasts. To subscribe to a podcast, open the command to subscribe in podcatching software and then copy and paste the URL for the podcast.

Although podcasts and vodcasts are often referred to with only the term "podcast," they are in different file formats. Many MP3 players play both. Podcasts, like blogs, are available at just about every news website. Educators are taking advantage of podcasting by recording their lectures and then uploading them as a podcast to the iTunes store, iTunes University, or campus podcasting servers. Students are creating podcasts to display school learning projects. There are numerous online tutorials to assist learners to create their own podcasts and vodcasts.

Web 3.0

It's hard to believe, but the web is now thought of in context of generations. Web 1.0 provided information. Web 2.0, which was discussed in the last section, is characterized by websites that promote sharing and collaboration and is still a work in progress. How **Web 3.0**, the **semantic web**, will eventually look is not yet known, but the goal is to make it more of a guide and less of a catalog. To accomplish this, web scientists are trying to provide a level of web artificial intelligence that would understand relationships of information (Ohler, 2008).

In the semantic web, the data in documents will be processed, transformed, assembled, and even acted on, using tools that understand logic and structure to information (Ohler, 2008). Under this scheme, let's say that you have a patient who needs self-care information about a rare disease. It is one with which you are not familiar, so you search for this disease by using your favorite search engine. The results, however, are not satisfactory. You receive a list of 1,500 items, some of which are advertisements for questionable products, others are from non–English-speaking countries, and there are many long, involved, articles. After looking at a few, you realize that they are mostly concerned with the etiology and prevention and are not appropriate for self-care. The prospect of looking at each link to find what you need is daunting. In a semantic web-enabled environment, you would be able to search by using your specifications that this not be a commercial for a product and that the information be research based and about self-care for a person with this condition. Your results would be greatly reduced but would be more relevant to your needs.

E-mail

Sending and receiving e-mail on the computer is one of the primary uses of the Internet. E-mail offers many advantages to nurses and other healthcare professionals. Before 1995, only those who shared the same network connection could exchange e-mail. For instance, those using CompuServe as their **Internet service provider (ISP)** could e-mail only those who also used CompuServe. Today, with most computer networks being part of the Internet, the exchange of e-mail is possible with anyone in the world who has an Internet e-mail address. Being knowledgeable about how to use and manage e-mail makes you a more efficient professional communicator.

As seen in the introductory scenario, e-mail enhances communication with speed and convenience. Most messages arrive at their destination only a few moments after they have been sent, even if the destination is halfway around the globe. E-mail offers a way to avoid "telephone tag" and to create a written message that the receiver can read several times, convert into voice with special software, or save. To use e-mail, you need e-mail software (called an e-mail client) and an e-mail account.

E-mail Software

An e-mail client is software used to access e-mail from an e-mail server so it can be viewed and read. An e-mail server is simply a computer that uses server software to receive and make e-mail available for those who have an account on that server. Operating systems come with e-mail software such as Windows Mail® (formerly, Outlook Express®). Other free e-mail clients usable by both personal computers (PCs) and Macs can be found at Eudora (http://www.eudora.com/), or Mozilla's Thunderbird (http://www.mozilla.com/en-US/thunderbird/). There are similarities in the menus for all of the e-mail clients. **Figure 5-5** shows an example of the Microsoft Outlook 2007® window.

E-mail software can keep a copy of all messages that are sent and received; however, the default is to delete these messages when the e-mail software is closed. Many people like to be able to search and view these messages after more than one session. To accommodate this, the default is easily set to keep the messages. Because these folders can become huge, if the default is reset to keep the messages, one needs to open and delete the messages on a regular schedule, perhaps every month. E-mail software also provides a way to create folders so that incoming mail can be saved into a specific folder for future reference. E-mail is ideal for communicating across time zones, particularly those where night and day are opposite, not only because the sender and receiver can respond at times that are most convenient for them but also because it saves postage and telephone expenses.

E-mail Accounts

Access to the Internet is through an ISP, either a private one at home or through a college, work, or establishment that offers free Wi-Fi. There are many ways to create an e-mail account and get an e-mail address. ISPs provide e-mail accounts, usually two to five per account, for their customers. Colleges also provide e-mail accounts for their students, and many healthcare agencies create e-mail

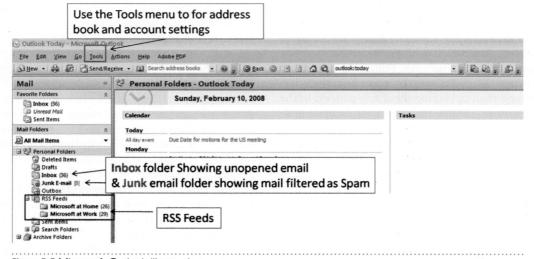

Figure 5-5 Microsoft Outlook illustration.

accounts for their employees. It is also possible to get a free e-mail account at Google, Microsoft, or Yahoo by visiting their home page and opening an account.

E-mail Addresses

Like postal mail, e-mail requires sender and receiver addresses. At first glance, an e-mail address may look forbidding, but a closer look at the address will reveal the formatting rules. An e-mail address has two parts separated by the @ sign. The first part, or the letters before the @ sign, is called the user name (sometimes called the **login name**) and identifies the sender. The part after the @ is the name of the e-mail server where the e-mail is received. The characters after the last dot in an e-mail address constitute the suffix that identifies the domain or main subdivision of the Internet to which the computer belongs (see **Figure 5-6**).

User Name

The computer name and domain suffix are dependent on which e-mail server you are using; these are assigned by the ISP that hosts the e-mail account. Most institutions assign a login name (**user ID**), which includes at least part of the user's name. If you create an account for yourself, remember that the user name reflects on you. E-mail messages can be forwarded anywhere, and the e-mail address of the person who created it, as well as anyone who receives it, is also forwarded. For this reason, healthcare providers should always select a user name that conveys their profession appropriately; cutesy names are never appropriate.

Configuring an E-mail Client

To configure an e-mail client that is on your PC to send and receive e-mail, you need just five pieces of information: the e-mail account type, the name of the incoming server, the name of the outgoing server, your login user name, and your password.

The account type and name of the incoming and outgoing server are assigned by the ISP where you have your account. The type of e-mail account is usually **POP3 (Post Office Protocol 3)**, but may also be **IMAP (Internet Mail Access Protocol)**. Outgoing servers use **SMTP (Simple Mail Transfer Protocol)**. In private accounts such as one from your own PC or one created with one of the free e-mail clients, you select your own login or user name and password when you open an account. The login user name and password allow you to retrieve your e-mail from your account. To simplify this process, Microsoft Outlook® 2007 and 2010 automatically configure the e-mail accounts by using the e-mail address and e-mail server password.

Planning E-mail Accounts

E-mail users should consider having several e-mail accounts, each with a different purpose. One e-mail account should be used for official communication with coworkers and colleagues. Students should use an account dedicated to official school communication with other students and faculty. A third e-mail account, using free online e-mail software or a home ISP, should be used for personal communication. In addition, a fourth e-mail account might be used for online shopping to trap potential resulting **spam**.

If you have more than one e-mail address, you may want to configure your e-mail client to download from more than one server. For example, if you create a free e-mail account at Google® or Yahoo®, you can set your e-mail client to download mail from there by using the account settings. Unless you are an expert, use only one outgoing server.

Creating and Sending E-mail

When you activate the Write feature of your e-mail client, your address will already be on the "From"

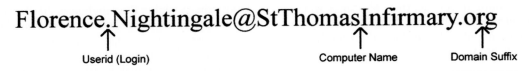

Figure 5-6 An e-mail address.

line. Your first step is to enter the address(es) of the receiver(s) on the "To" line. If you have put the recipient's name in your e-mail client's address book, when you start to enter the beginning of the name, the address book will automatically finish it for you. After entering the recipient's name, enter a brief word or phrase about the message on the subject line. E-mails with no subject line may be classified as junk mail by the user's e-mail server and not be received by the recipient. Finally, create your message and add a signature that clearly identifies you.

There may be times when you want to send the same message to more than one person. This is simple if the message is a reply to a message that was also addressed to others to whom you wish the reply to be sent; select "Reply All" to start your message instead of "Reply." If you routinely send e-mail to the same group of people, such as to members of a committee that you are on, you can use the address book to create a group. With a group, you then place the name of the group on the "To" line, instead of each name. Use Help to learn how to create a group of recipients. When sending a duplicate of a message to others, you have the option of using **"Cc"** or **"Bcc."** The acronym "Cc" is derived from earlier days of the typewriter carbon copy. The "Bcc" indicates a blind copy where the receiver is unaware that others have also received a copy of the message. Blind carbon copies should be used judiciously; the sender must consider the ethics of secrecy when using the function.

Sometimes you want to forward a message that you have received to someone else. Before forwarding a message, give thoughtful consideration to the sender and receiver. In consideration to the sender, send a copy of the e-mail to the original sender when forwarding the e-mail to others. When forwarding a message, edit the message to remove the e-mail addresses of prior recipients. Avoid passing on chain letters; most people do not want them, and many agencies will terminate your account if you do this. Messages warning about viruses or other dire things that will happen to your computer if you don't do something are generally hoaxes.[3]

---

3 See Chapter 3 for more information about viruses and hoaxes.

E-mail File Formatting

There are three main file formats for creating and sending messages: plain text (TXT), **rich text file (RTF)**, and **hypertext markup language (HTML)**. TXT files have no formatting, which makes them ideal for electronic mailing lists because any e-mail client can read them. RTF files allow for some formatting but not the robust features of a word processor. HTML files use HTML tags to display formatting of text. Not all e-mail software can read HTML messages, especially in less developed nations. For file formats that are either rtf or html, you can use the formatting functions, such as bold, italics, and bullets in your e-mail client.

The Do's and Dont's of E-mail Content

As convenient as e-mail is, it must be used appropriately. Care must be taken in deciding what is included in a message that is sent via e-mail; contents of e-mail must always adhere to common decency. E-mail should never be used to give bad news, such as a poor evaluation, work layoff, or pay decrease. A rule of thumb is to never include anything in an e-mail message that you wouldn't want to read on the front page of the newspaper. It is very easy for a recipient to accidentally or purposely forward your message to someone else. All messages carry headers that can be traced to the original sender. Even if the sender uses a remailer, a service that strips the identifying header so that e-mail can be sent anonymously, sender information can be traced by contacting the remailer service (Freeman, 2007).

E-mail Privacy Issues

There is no guarantee that e-mail that is sent using an educational facility or employer e-mail server or e-mail provider service will be private. A growing trend is for institutions to monitor e-mail to avoid potential litigation and investigations from government agencies (AMA/ePolicy Institute, 2008; Privacy Rights Clearinghouse, 2010). There is still no definitive case law on whether students or employees have the right to privacy in e-mail. This includes situations in which the institution has said that your e-mail is private because if the message can be construed as damaging to the institution, privacy promises may be legally invalidated. There are several court cases that have set precedence and ruled in favor of the employer ("Shoars v. Epson," 1994; Bourke v. Nissan," 1993; Smyth v. Pillsbury," 1996).

E-mail Etiquette

E-mail etiquette, like regular mail letter etiquette, is essential for professional communication. The rules for creating e-mail are important. First of all, always include a short pertinent subject line. When replying to e-mail, make sure to include appropriate information from the prior message in the reply. E-mail is a special form of communication, not as interactive as the telephone, but more interactive than written communication. Because it often seems very personal and quick, there is a tendency to regard it as a verbal conversation and forget that the recipient may have been involved in many complicated matters since he or she last sent you a message. For this reason, mailers provide an option to include the prior message with the original when you reply. To prevent messages that rapidly become too large and uncommunicative, edit the prior message so that only the parts pertinent to your reply are included. In general, e-mail should be short and to the point, but not too short. A message that is too short may be misinterpreted by the recipient, who may feel that the sender was being abrupt or curt.

There are some major differences between e-mail and letters sent by postal mail. Postal mail letters generally have the reader's full, undivided attention. In contrast, because of the sheer volume of e-mail, the reader may not read the message thoroughly, causing misunderstandings resulting in problems in relationships. If there is a chance for disagreement, or e-mail messages seem to be causing disagreements, use e-mail to set up a time for either a person-to-person meeting or a telephone conversation.

Use the appropriate font and case when writing e-mail. According to e-mail etiquette, use of all uppercase letters (all caps) indicates that the user is shouting, so all caps should never be used for sentence construction. Use of all lower case letters makes the writer appear as being lazy (Pagana, 2007). Use font colors thoughtfully. Depending on the message, a red-colored font may be interpreted as swearing (Cleary & Freeman, 2005). Finally, e-mail should always be signed. Professional e-mail should include a signature, title, and contact information, such as a mailing address of the agency, phone number, and home page URL (see **Box 5-1**).

E-mail Signature

E-mail written by professionals should always include a signature with the sender's name, title, company name, and geographical location. A signature is similar to the return address on a postal letter; however, personal information such as

---

BOX 5-1 Email Recommendations

Managing Accounts
- Be familiar with your employer's policy on the use of official e-mail.
- Use employer e-mail only for official business.
- Use several e-mail accounts – one for official e-mail, one for school e-mail, and the others for personal activities.

Sending E-mail
- Always check your e-mail for spelling, grammar, and punctuation before sending.
- Include a signature with contact information (title, organization, address).
- Be aware that all e-mails, even if deleted, are potentially discoverable.
- Be sure that your e-mail does not violate common decency laws.
- Never open attachments that you do not expect to receive.
- Never send confidential information in e-mail.
- Use e-mail appropriately – never use it to avoid face-to-face communication.

Managing E-mail
- Create e-mail filters to avoid spam and other unwanted e-mail.
- Never respond to spam.
- Organize your e-mail by using folders and alerts.
- Try to respond to e-mail within 24 hours.

street addresses and home phone numbers should be avoided. Most signatures are of one to five lines; a signature may be personalized by including a favorite quotation. Instructions for creating a signature for Windows Outlook®, Windows Mail®, Netscape®, or Mozilla Thunderbird® go to the web page for this chapter at http://dlthede. net/Informatics/Informatics.html. In Gmail, the signature can be created from the Settings window. In some e-mail packages, a user creates the signature as a "txt" file with a program like Notepad® and then, using account settings, tells the e-mail client where to find it.

Acronyms and Emoticons

E-mail is devoid of the nonverbal commands of face-to-face communication. Thus, expressions of subtle meaning and tone are easily lost. With the informality of much e-mail and the limited typing skills of many who send e-mail messages, it is only natural that common acronyms and icons have developed. They are only valuable when the recipients understand them. Acronyms use the first letter of words or word parts to communicate a common phrase (see **Table 5-2**). They are commonly used in informal e-mail and IM. Acronyms are not appropriate for professional communication.

To provide the appropriate body language tone, telecommunicators have devised icons called **emoticons** (emotional icons), sometimes called smileys, which can be created on the keyboard. For example, one that is frequently used is :-). When tilting your head to the left, which is the position for "reading" keyboard character emoticons, you can see a smiling face (see **Table 5-3**). Some e-mail clients include graphic emoticons. A classic graphic emoticon is a

Table 5-2 Common E-mail Acronyms

Acronym	Meaning
BTW	By the way
FAQ	Frequently asked questions
f2f	Face-to-face
FWIW	For what it is worth
<g>	Grin
IMO or IMHO	In my opinion or in my humble opinion
OTOH	On the other hand

Table 5-3 Common E-mail Emoticons

Emoticon	Meaning
☺ or :)	Smiley
☹ or :(	Frown
:O	Shock or disappointment
;)	Wink
> :(or > :O	Upset or angry

round, yellow button with two dots for eyes and half circle for a smile. Use emoticons sparingly, if at all, in professional business communication. See http:// netforbeginners.about.com/cs/netiquette101/a/ bl_emoticons101.htm for more information on emoticons (Gil, 2010).

Attachments

Many people use e-mail to send files created with other software, such as a word processor or spreadsheet. When including attachments in your e-mail, you should use the following guidelines. First, always alert the receivers before sending an attachment and verify that the receivers have the software that can view the attachment. For example, if a file is created and saved with Publisher® with the Publisher file extension ".pub," the recipients will not be able to view the file unless they have Publisher on their computer. Be sure that the recipients have the appropriate version of the software that you are using; many file formats from the same vendor's program are not **backwardly compatible**.

Attaching files to e-mail messages increases the size of the message, which in turn increases the time required to both send and receive it. If the attached file is large, consider "zipping" it to compress the file. An alternative for attaching a large file or **zipped file** is to use file transfer Internet websites. Examples include YouSendIt (http://www.yousendit. com/), SendThisFile (http://www.sendthisfile. com/), and LogMeIn (http://secure.logmein. com). The file transfer websites provide free as well as fee-based services; both require the user to register to receive a login and password. To send a file, go to the website, log in, enter the recipient's e-mail address and an e-mail subject, browse (find in your folders) to the file, select it, click open on that window, and click Send It. The recipient receives an e-mail with a web address (URL) to download the file. If you are in the habit of exchanging large files with someone whose e-mail account is limited in sending or receiving large files or if you are limited in this respect, one or both of you may want to get a free e-mail account where the size of attachments is not as limited.

Managing E-mail

Taking a few minutes to organize and manage e-mail can save you much time and energy later (see **Table 5-4**). Whether you use a stand-alone or web-based client, the e-mail management processes are similar. All e-mail clients have Help menus to guide you through the process of organizing e-mail. You can use e-mail alerts to assist in prioritizing e-mail. Alerts include flags, stars, and font colors. Use e-mail filters to automatically file incoming e-mail into designated folders and send you personal alerts for e-mail from certain senders. You can also use filters to filter unwanted mail such as spam (unsolicited commercial e-mail) to the deleted items folder.

Out-of-Office Replies

There are times when you will not be answering e-mail, such as when out of town. This, however, does not stop your e-mail. When you do not answer, your correspondents may become upset. To show consideration for them, it is smart to have an automatic response sent to them informing them that you are unable to read and respond to their message and letting them know when you will be able to do so. Most ISPs provide this service; to activate it, go to your account on their server and use Help to learn how to do this. If you are using Gmail, look for "Vacation Responder" in the Settings menu.

Filtering Spam

Spam (junk e-mail) is not only a nuisance, it is potentially harmful. As annoying as junk e-mail can be, it is important to recognize it to proactively limit or eliminate it. A first clue of junk is the sender's e-mail address. If you don't know the sender, the e-mail is probably junk. To proactively limit or eliminate junk mail, learn how to develop e-mail filters and rules. In Windows® Mail 2007 and 2010, using the junk e-mail options on the Tools menu can be used to filter spam to the junk folder to decide what to do with mail determined

Table 5-4 Managing E-mail: Tools May Vary According to the E-mail Agent

Tools	Function	How to Use
Folders and labels	Provide a way to categorize e-mail	Drag and drop e-mail into the folders or create a filter to automatically move the e-mail to the folder. Examples of categories are committees, school, and work.
		If using a filter to move e-mail into a folder, consider providing yourself an alert that the e-mail has arrived.
Flags or stars	Used to give a visual alert for importance and/or follow-up	After you have read the e-mail, you can click a flag or star to indicate importance and follow-up.
Colors	Provide a visual cue to help organize e-mail	Create rules to use color to categorize e-mail.
Sound	Provides an auditory alert for the arrival of e-mail	Use sound alerts to check e-mail as it arrives into the mailbox.
Filters	Provide rules to the software to perform actions on e-mail	Use filters to delete spam that escapes your Internet mail provider's spam filter. Filters can be used to apply rules to automatically perform an action on e-mail with identified senders, receivers, subject, and/or message words.

to be junk. In Gmail, the "Filters" window can be used to discard spam. Some online e-mail clients allow the user to report spam with the click of a button.

Spam is the electronic version of junk postal mail, except that it shifts the costs of advertising to the receiver; it exists because it is a cheap way to advertise. It also fills the Internet with unwanted messages. Usually, spam originates from a false address, so replying is a waste of time. If, however, you receive a spam message and you know from the e-mail address that the ISP exists, such as one of the online services, you can forward it to post-master@online.service (substitute the name of the service for online.service). Most services and ISPs take a very dim view of spamming and terminate the account of anyone who sends junk e-mail, or if someone's identity has been illegally assumed, the ISP will look for ways to prevent this from happening again.

All e-mail users must be knowledgeable about spamming practices and malware, such as **phishing** and **pharming**.[4] One of the best ways to avoid spam is to not give out an e-mail address to any website. An alternative is to acquire a free mailbox site and use that e-mail address when completing online forms, for example, when shopping online. Records of online shopping are then e-mailed to the free designated account along with any advertisements that they might send. When visiting the free e-mail account, legitimate e-mail can be forwarded to another address and spam can be deleted. Users should never open a known spam message! Finally, users should never purchase a product or service advertised from unsolicited e-mail (Pew Internet American Life Project, 2007).

Retrieving E-mail From a Remote E-mail Account

Perhaps you normally use a stand-alone e-mail client such as Outlook®, Windows Mail®, or Mozilla Thunderbird® to retrieve e-mail, but you want to check your e-mail when you are not at the computer that you usually use. Many ISPs will allow you to retrieve your mail directly from the server. Or, you can configure a web-based client such as Gmail, Hotmail, or Yahoo to retrieve the

e-mail from your server when asked. Web-based e-mail clients may also offer software designed for mobile devices. Mobile e-mail clients allow users to retrieve and download remote e-mail to hand-held devices such as personal digital assistants and smartphones.

E-mail Discussion Lists (Listservs)

An e-mail discussion list, sometimes referred to as a **listserv** (no "e" at the end) from the first software that was used to create one, is made up of a group of subscribers with a common interest. The software allows subscribers to receive discussion postings via e-mail. Subscribing, or joining, a list is generally free. Instructions for subscribing are specific to a list and are generally found on the website for the list or as a click at a place where you find information about the list. Once subscribed to a group, copies of any message posted to the group are sent to all members' mailboxes (see **Figure 5-7**). Members can reply to any of the messages or send an entirely new message to the group. The tasks of keeping track of subscribers and sending copies of messages are accomplished by a software program. Other kinds of e-mail list software include Majordomo®, Mailbase®, and Listproc®.

Once subscribed to a group, copies of any message posted to the group are sent to all members mailboxes. Members can reply to any of the messages or send an entirely new message to the group. Most lists are automated, that is, the software immediately sends out any messages posted to the group's posting address; some groups are moderated, that is, the message is first vetted by the list owner before posting.

Most mailing list software offer many options for subscribers beyond just sending messages. For this reason, there are two addresses for each group: one that manages the list, performing such tasks as subscribing a new member or evoking the available options such as temporarily suspending mail from the group; and another address that is used only when one posts a message to the group. This information is included in the information that is sent to all new subscribers. It is important to save this message because it not only provides you with the administrative

---

4 See Chapter 3 for a discussion on phishing and pharming.

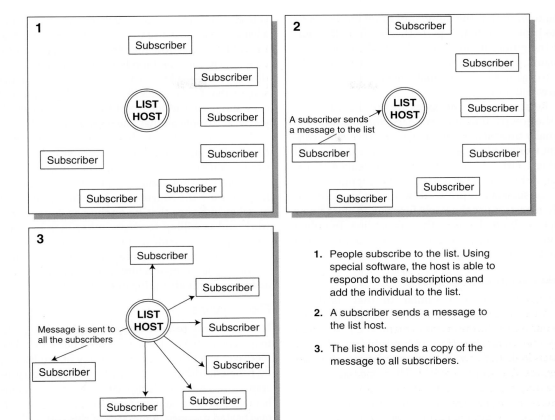

Figure 5-7 Listserv topography.

1. People subscribe to the list. Using special software, the host is able to respond to the subscriptions and add the individual to the list.

2. A subscriber sends a message to the list host.

3. The list host sends a copy of the message to all subscribers.

address but also tells you how to unsubscribe, find the names of other participants, digest your mail (so that you receive one message per day with all of that day's postings), and temporarily stop your mail from the list ("very" important if you are not able to check your mail for a while). The instructions for use of e-mail lists vary. When replying to a list message, pay particular attention to whether you need to use Reply or Reply All. With some lists, the Reply feature will permit you to reply to all list participants; with other lists, you need to use "Reply All" to send the reply to more than the person who wrote the last message. Make sure that you sign the e-mail posted to mailing lists with a standard "signature" that includes at least your name and e-mail address. Some lists "strip" the e-mail address of the participants in the header.

Finding a Nursing Discussion List

There are electronic mailing lists for just about every nursing and other healthcare specialty imaginable; finding the right one is not always easy. Although you can search the web by using the term "nursing discussion lists" or "nursing listserv," staying up-to-date on what mailing lists are active is almost impossible. Check the Book web page for current places where information about nursing mailing lists can be found. To find a nursing listserv, use a search engine and the term "nursing listserv."

Threaded Discussion List Messages

Threaded messages are organized by the topic of the message. The first message for a topic starts the thread followed by the other messages about the topic. Often the number of other messages on the topic is noted in parentheses after the topic of the group. If you receive list mail in the digest format, the messages are often threaded. You can also organize your personal e-mail by topic to have threaded messages.

Regular listserv messages are not threaded, but if the group has an archives page, the messages are usually threaded on that page. The threading concept works only when posters preserve the original subject, either by using the Reply or Reply All function or by copying and pasting the original subject on the subject line prefaced by "Re:." It breaks down when posters use the Reply function to start a new topic without changing the subject line. In online courses, messages are also threaded, so learning to use threaded messages is an important skill.[5]

Discussion List Etiquette

Listserv etiquette is similar to that used for standard e-mail. It is extremely important to be respectful of the other group members. Discussion list members represent an invisible number of individuals with a variety of experiences who may live anywhere in the world. Thus, messages need to be understandable to all. In messages, avoid acronyms, which are often not understood even by people in your own area. Keep messages on the topic of the list; information about the allowable topics is provided in the welcoming message.

Lists are maintained or "owned" by the person who is responsible for the list. It is a thankless task for which there is no payment. For this reason, as well as consideration of the other members, you should consider being a member of a list, a privilege that conveys responsibilities. Send nothing except messages to be posted to the group to the e-mail address that is used to send you group messages. For all other requests, like unsubscribing, use the administrative address or web page of the group; information about how to implement these features is in the welcoming message. If you are going to be away for a while, either unsubscribe from the list or set the mail to no mail (called noack in some list software). This is important to prevent a "full mailbox error," which is not happily received by the list owner who must then take the time to manually unsubscribe

you. If you want to receive only one message from a list a day, you can use the web page or administrative address to set the mail to digest. If you receive messages in the digest mode and use the reply function of your e-mail to reply to a message, delete the subject that is automatically on the subject line and copy and paste the subject of the message to which you wish to reply on that line prefaced by "Re:."

New list users may think that a list is a way to avoid doing a needed literature search. Don't expect other list members to do this for you. If you want information about a topic, when asking for help indicate the sources you have found. When a member indicates that he or she has done homework and is willing to share, other members are very happy to provide more help. Do remember to sign your e-mail and use a contact signature, which includes your e-mail address and the name and address of your affiliating organization.

Flame Wars

Messages sent to an electronic mailing list go to many people whom the sender does not know. The messages will be read under a variety of conditions, by people in different moods. Given these circumstances, it is not surprising that occasionally a member takes umbrage at what another says and posts an overheated message. A message of this sort, called a **flame**, can easily deteriorate into a **flame war** when others respond derogatorily with other positions on the disputed topic. In most groups, this ends on a conciliatory note when cooler heads prevail. Flame wars can happen in any group but tend to be more common in groups with controversial topics.

Summary

The WWW provides many opportunities for professional networking. As the web has matured, many new features have been added such as the interaction permitted by Web 2.0. Use of IM, Twitter, chat, Facebook, MySpace, LinkedIn, and Plaxo allow for communication with either a computer or a mobile device. Social networking sites provide a way for groups to interact with public and private notes, photos, and other media. From the sharing of documents to discussion groups, these features make possible a collective intelligence as many people from all geographical areas

---

5 Online education is discussed in Chapter 21.

and walks-of-life contribute their knowledge in such formats as wikis and blogs. Grass Roots Media has become a possibility with blogs and media-sharing facilities such as YouTube®, all of which can be useful in healthcare for providing both continuing education and patient education. E-mail has become a way of life, necessitating learning a new way of communicating that is between voice mail and letter writing. E-mail has also provided a method of networking through e-mail discussion groups often known as listservs. When healthcare professionals effectively use these new tools, they improve healthcare, both in the practice of the professional and for the patient.

APPLICATIONS AND COMPETENCIES

1. Examine the technology use policies and procedures for your educational or healthcare provider workplace facility for
   a. a procedure to set up an e-mail account,
   b. policies and procedures for use of the institution's e-mail server,
   c. a privacy policy for user e-mail,
   d. policies for use of social networking sites,
   e. policies and procedures for approved e-mail attachment file types, and
   f. policies and procedures for e-mail communication with patients and families (healthcare provider).

2. Discuss how the policies and procedures benefit e-mail users. Discuss any limitations that you noted. Compare your findings with those of your classmates.

3. Add three names and e-mail addresses to an e-mail address book and create a group for those three individuals.

4. Join a discussion list that relates to your nursing interest.
   a. Identify the address to be used to post a message to the group.
   b. Access the list's administrative website and experiment with the various options.
   c. Discuss advantages and limitations of the discussion list.

   d. Resign from the list by using the website when you no longer want to be a member or your e-mail address is going to be terminated such as when you leave a place of employment, graduate from school, or change ISPs.

5. Explore one or more of Web 2.0 social networking features that could be beneficial to you as a student/healthcare professional. Explain the benefits and compare your experiences with other students or nursing colleagues.

6. Open iTunes (or download the software at http://www.apple.com/itunes/) and then search for free nursing resources in the iTunes store. Discuss the pros and cons for two of the resources.

REFERENCES

AHC Media. (2009a). Facebook firings show privacy concerns with social networking sites: Remind staff about slippery slope with online postings. *Healthcare Risk Management*, *31*(5), 49–52.

AHC Media. (2009b). Search online for postings by employees, new hires. *Healthcare Risk Management*, *31*(5), 52.

Alana Shoars v. Epson American, Inc, No. B 073234 (Cal. Ct. App. Div. 1994). Retrieved April 2, 2010, from http://www.law.seattleu.edu/fachome/chonm/Cases/shoars.html

AMA/ePolicy Institute. (2008, February 28). *2007 Electronic monitoring & surveillance survey*. Retrieved March 28, 2008, from http://www.amanet.org/news/177.aspx

American Nurses Association now on Facebook, LinkedIn groups. (2009). *Colorado Nurse, 109*(3), 8.

Bonita P. Bourke et al. v. Nissan Motor Corporation in U.S.A, No. March 28, 2010 (Cal. Ct. App. 1993). Retrieved March 28, 2010, from http://www.loundy.com/CASES/Bourke_v_Nissan.html

Buckley, N. (2010). *The origins of Friendster*. Retrieved July 28, 2011, from http://social-networking.limewebs.com/friendster-history.htm

Cleary, M., & Freeman, A. (2005). Email etiquette: Guidelines for mental health nurses. *International Journal of Mental Health Nursing, 14*(1), 62–65.

Facebook. (2011). *Founder bios*. Retrieved July 28, 2011, from http://www.facebook.com/press/info.php?execbios

Freeman, E. H. (2007). Email Privacy and the Wiretap Act: U.S. v. Councilman. *Information Systems Security, 16*(3), 182–185.

Frith, K. H., Anderson, F., & Sewell, J. P. (2010). Assessing and selecting data for a nursing services dashboard. *Journal of Nursing Administration, 40*(1), 10–16.

Gil, P. (2010, January). *Emoticons and smileys 101*. Retrieved April 2, 2010, from http://netforbeginners.about.com/cs/netiquette101/a/bl_emoticons101.htm

Governors Highway Safety Association. (2010, March). *Cell phone and texting laws*. Retrieved March 29, 2010, from http://www.ghsa.org/html/stateinfo/laws/cellphone_laws.html

Harper, C., & Watson, K. (2008). Supporting knowledge creation: Using wikis for group collaboration. *Research Bulletin, 2008*(3), 1–13. Retrieved July 28, 2011, from http://net.educause.edu/ir/library/pdf/ERB0803.pdf

Johnson, L., Levine, A., Smith, R., & Stone, S. (2010). *The 2010 Horizon Report*. Austin, Texas: The New Media Consortium.

Kaminski, J. (2009). Folksonomies boost Web 2.0 functionality. *Online Journal of Nursing Informatics, 13*(2), 8. Retrieved from http://www.nursing-informatics.com/folksonomies.pdf

Little, J. K. (2007, July 4). Podcasting: A teaching with technology white paper. *Educause*. Retrieved March 28, 2010, from http://www.educause.edu/Resources/Browse/ELI%20Guide%20to%20Podcasting/33407

Michael A. Smyth v. The Pillsbury Company, C.A. NO. 95–5712 (Pa. District Court 1996). Retrieved from http://www.loundy.com/CASES/Smyth_v_Pillsbury.html

Moraes, M. (2010, February 14). *What is Usenet?* Retrieved April 1, 2010, from http://www.faqs.org/faqs/usenet/what-is/part1/

Neus, A. (2001). *Managing information quality in virtual communities of practice*. Paper presented at the Proceedings of the 6th International Conference on Information Quality at MIT. Retrieved July 28, 2011, from http://citeseerx.ist.psu.edu/viewdoc/download?doi=10.1.1.13.413&rep=rep1&type=pdf

O'Reilly, T. (2005). *What Is Web 2.0 - O'Reilly Media*. Retrieved July 28, 2011, from http://oreilly.com/web2/archive/what-is-web-20.html

Ohler, J. (2008). The semantic web in education. *EDUCAUSE Quarterly*, 31(4). Retrieved April 2, 2010, from http://www.educause.edu/EDUCAUSE+Quarterly/EDUCAUSEQuarterlyMagazineVolum/TheSemanticWebinEducation/163437

Pagana, K. D. (2007). E-mail etiquette. *American Nurse Today*, 2(7), 45–45. Retrieved from http://www.americannurseto-day.com/article.aspx?id=4584&fid=4538

Pew Internet American Life Project. (2007, May). *The volume of spam is growing in Americans' personal and workplace email accounts, but email users are less bothered by it*. Retrieved September 7, 2007, from http://www.pewinternet.org/Reports/2007/Spam-2007/Data-Memo/Findings.aspx?r=1

Privacy Rights Clearinghouse. (2010, March). *Fact sheet 7: Workplace privacy and employee monitoring*. Retrieved March 28, 2010, from http://www.privacyrights.org/fs/fs7-work.htm

Sandars, J. (2007). The potential of blogs and wikis in healthcare education. *Education for Primary Care, 18*(1), 16–21.

Skiba, D. J. (2007). Nursing education 2.0: Are mashups useful for nursing education? *Nursing Education Perspectives, 28*(5), 286–288.

Wikipedia Contributors. (2010a, February 12). *Wiki*. Retrieved February 25, 2010, from http://en.wikipedia.org/wiki/Wiki

Wikipedia Contributors. (2010b, March 29). *History of Wikipedia*. Retrieved March 30, 2010, from http://en.wikipedia.org/w/index.php?title=History_of_Wikipedia&action=history

CHAPTER 6
Mastering Word Processing

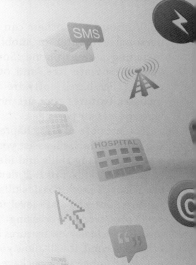

Objectives

After studying this chapter you will be able to:

- ▶ *Apply many common word processing features (headers, margins, hanging indents, changing fonts, using format painter, etc.).*

- ▶ *Compare free word processing features, with others requiring a fee.*

- ▶ *Compare cloud computing word processing features with desktop applications.*

- ▶ *List word processing features that are generic to word processing applications.*

- ▶ *Apply the use of new word processing skills.*

Key Terms

Attribute	Mail Merge
Endnote	Object
Font	Overtype
Footer	Page Break
Footnote	Page Orientation
Header	Typeover
Justification	Word Processor
Macro	

Software programs designed to help a user manipulate text, edit, rearrange, and retype documents on a computer are called **word processors**. The popularity of word processing attests to the fact that written communication, whether in the printed or electronic format, is still the primary means of spreading information and knowledge. Effective usage of a word processor is part of computer fluency and is necessary to advance in nursing. One of the benefits of mastering basic word processing skills is the transferability of these skills to other application programs that use the same basic editing features.

Word processing software packages vary in some of the features they offer, but all packages, even the text-editing software that comes with an operating system, offer the ability to insert, delete, cut, and paste text; search and replace words; and store and retrieve documents. With the exception of the Microsoft™ Windows Accessory program Notepad all others also offer word wrap (the automatic insertion of line breaks when text exceeds the width of the page). Even e-mail software offers many of these features. Word processors are available on the web as cloud computing applications, and others can be installed on the personal computer or mobile Internet device, including a smartphone. Some word processor applications are free, and others must be purchased. Fee-based software is very robust and includes features that are not available on free word processor packages.

The purpose of this chapter is threefold. First, the information will assist you to self-assess your word processing skills and identify opportunities to gain new skills. **Box 6-1** identifies three skill levels. Those of us with basic skills *use* word processing features. Intermediate-level users are competent *modifying* word processing features. Advanced level users *create* new features and are able to teach others. Second, it will allow you to compare different word processing packages. Microsoft Word® 2010 is featured with comparisons with Google Docs® and OpenOffice.org™. Google Docs® is an example of a cloud computing application. IBM Lotus Symphony, a free full-feature office suite product released in fall 2009, is an example of another free software download for the desktop computer. Finally, you will be introduced to free online learning resources that will allow you to learn new skills.

In order to demonstrate the use of competencies and applications at the three skill levels, the "APA 6th Template" created with Microsoft Word® is used. The template was designed to guide writers to easily format documents with *Publication Manual of the American Psychological Association* (APA), 6th edition citation style. Use of the template requires basic word processing skills. Modifications to the template require intermediate- or advanced-level skills. The template is available as a download from the textbook website. The template includes the four main sections of an APA paper: title page, abstract, main body, and references.

The Document

A word processing document is an electronic version of a blank piece of paper. The top of the screen has menus or tabs and icons that provide access to the features of the word processor. The bottom of the screen usually has what is called a status line, or a line that provides information about the document, for example, page number, zoom, and layout style (not available in Google Docs®). In the blank section of the screen, the user types a document, which often will be printed when finished.

Although typing skills are a great help in entering text, it is the only resemblance that a word processor has to a typewriter. In fact, thinking in terms of the printed page, as one does with a typewriter, interferes with maximizing word processing features. In word processing, a user should separate the tasks of writing from those of formatting the page. Concentrating first on writing and formatting later is a good rule for word processing.

The Word Processing Window

The word processing window uses windows, icons, menus, and a mouse. The menus for different software packages are very similar. **Figure 6-1** compares the menus of three popular word processing applications. Many of the features, such as file, preferences, insert, table, spell-check, and print options are similar, although you may need to use Help to discover their location in the menu. Microsoft Word® provides the capability to create a custom Quick Start menu. To customize the Quick Start menu, which by default includes the save and undo functions, click on the small black arrow just above the Home tab (see **Figure 6-1**) and then click on the items you want to have included, for example, spelling and grammar check.

The available layout views of a document that a user can access support the separation of formatting from writing. The draft view in Microsoft Word® shows just the text and is ideal for writing. In this view, when a new page becomes necessary, a solid or dotted single line appears to indicate a **page break**. The top and bottom page margins are not visible and do not interfere with one's thinking, nor is one tempted to paginate (create artificial page breaks) before editing is completed. In print view (page view in some word processors), one sees items that will appear on the printed page, such as **footnotes** or page numbers. The full-screen view shows two pages at a time for easy reading. Some word processors also have a web view, and most can be used to create web pages.

BOX 6-1 Word Processing Skills

Basic

Use word processors and word processing features
- Add basic text format – font size, color, style
- Alignment – center, left, right, justify
- Checking spelling and grammar
- Create a new document
- Create bookmarks
- Create headers and footers
- Customizing the quick access toolbar
- Demonstrate basic word processing skills with one application
- Format lines, words, and spaces – spacing: choosing and changing line spaces and bullets
- Identifying/correcting spelling and grammatical errors
- Insert clip art
- Insert hyperlinks (URL, e-mail addresses and other places in the document)
- Insert page numbers
- Make changes – undo/redo
- Move and copying text – cut/paste, copy/paste, drag/drop
- Name documents
- Obtain the word count information for a document
- Print documents – print preview, change printer settings
- Use "save as" to save a Microsoft Word® document to other file formats (.doc, .rtf, txt, PDF)
- Use Help
- Use search and replace
- Use tab key to indent
- Use the menu and quick access toolbar
- Use the ruler

Intermediate

Modify word processing features
- Create new documents from a template
- Design your own custom template
- Demonstrate word processing skills with two to four applications
- Modify text font style, color, size, and case
- Modify text using the format painter
- Modify text alignment
- Make changes – adding, deleting, moving text
- Create and format (styles, shadow effects, shape, and arrangement of) a textbook
- Format text with themes and styles
- Change paragraph setting – hanging indent
- Create a table with a table auto-header
- Change margins and bullets
- Use search and replace
- Use wizard – letter, envelopes, and labels
- Insert line breaks
- Modify the menus and toolbars
- Autocorrect and styles
- Add readability statistics to the menu

(continued)

BOX 6-1 Word Processing Skills *(continued)*

- Use readability statistics to modify a document
- Collaborate with others using the Review tool and Skydrive website
- Modify and position graphics in a document
- Create citations, insert citations into a paper, and to create an associated reference list with the citation and bibliographic manager
- Create a paper
- Use APA citation style, abstract, and a reference page
- Use mail merge

Advanced

Create new features and teach others how to use word processors and features
- Create forms
- Create lists of figures, captions, table of contents, index
- Create long documents – connecting several documents into one
- Create new functions with macros
- Create new style sets
- Create newspapers, brochures and other print media using desktop publishing tools
- Create templates
- Create word files with embedded multimedia, such as PowerPoint, video, and sound
- Demonstrate word processing skills with five or more applications

 Text Characteristics

The flexibility of entering and manipulating text in a word processor makes writing and editing very easy. Some basic word processing features that are common to many other programs such as using windows, word wrap, cutting, pasting, moving and erasing text, undo and redo, navigating a document, and default mode, discussed in Chapter 3, will not be discussed here.

Text-Entering Modes

Two modes are available for entering (inputting) text in a word processing program: insert and **typeover**. In many programs, users can toggle between these two modes by tapping the Insert key.[1] The Default mode is the insert setting. In this mode, when the user enters new characters, the original text automatically makes room for it. In typeover (may be called **overtype** or strikeover) mode, any new characters will replace those already in the document. Because the Insert key can be accidentally tapped, if you find that keys you type are overwriting text, tap the Insert key. There are times when one wishes to use overtype, such as when entering text into an electronic word processing form (not on the web). The insert text-entering mode is the default for the APA 6th Template. The template is found on the website for this textbook at http://dlthede.net/Informatics/Informatics.html

Changing the Appearance of the Text

The appearance of text can be changed in many ways. Changing the appearance of something is known as changing the **attribute**. An attribute is a characteristic that changes the appearance of an **object** (remember, an object is anything that can be manipulated). Attributes that can be applied to characters in most word processors include boldface, italics, color, and various types of underlines. Attributes can be turned on before or after characters are typed. To change an attribute before typing, choose the appropriate symbol from the toolbar, or click Format > Font (Home tab in Microsoft Word®). To make the change after typing, select the text and apply the attribute in the same manner.

---

1 In Microsoft Word® 2007, search help by using the word "overtype" to find out how to implement this feature.

Fonts (Typefaces) and Font Size (in Points)

A **font** is the name given to the typeface style that is used for the characters in the document. The font and its size can be changed for the entire document or for just a small section. Like other attributes, changes can be made before or after text is entered. A drop-down box for both fonts and size is generally found on the toolbox near the top of the screen, or they are available in the Font menu under Format on the menu line (Home menu in Microsoft Word®). Some programs use the term "point size" to refer to the size of the print. Font sizes, however, vary with the font and attributes (see **Table 6-1**).

The default font varies according to the software package. As seen in **Figure 6-1**, the default font in Microsoft Word® is Calibri (body) 11-point; in Google Docs®, it is Verdana 10-point; and in OpenOffice.org™, it is Times New Roman 12-point. The preference for APA typeface is Times New Roman, with 12-point font size. When designing the APA 6th Template with Microsoft Word®, the font was changed from Calibri 11-point to Times New Roman 12-point.

Styles and Headings

"Styles" are features that allow the user to create different fonts styles and sizes for use in documents. Styles include default fonts for body text and section headings. "Style Sets," unique to Microsoft® Word, are combinations of headings, font types and sizes, line spacing, and colors used in a document. Microsoft Word® allows the user to make customizations for different text "Styles" and then to save the combination of settings as a default "Style Set" for use in other documents.

A common mistake is overlooking the use of section headings. Section headings, an example of styles, provide a visual outline of the paper to readers, as can be seen in this textbook. The use of section headings is a common feature of most word processing packages. There are levels of headings, just as you might use to outline a paper. The abstract, title of the paper noted in the main body, and the references are examples of "heading 1." Sections and subsections in the main body of the paper would be heading 2, 3, 4, or 5. As in an outline, there should be at least two sections for a section subheading. Heading 1 is analogous to Roman numeral I, II, III, and so forth in an outline. Heading 2 is analogous to Roman number A, B, C, and so forth in an outline. Heading 3 is analogous to a, b, c, and so forth in an outline. The APA 6th Template, found on the textbook website, includes custom font styles for headings 1–3.

Headings provide more than a visual organization function in Microsoft Word®. Headings are used in the design of web pages. Headings also provide the basic structure for automatic generation of a table of contents. The "Table of Contents" feature is located on the References tab in Microsoft Word® (Insert menu in OpenOffice.org™ and Google Docs®). Microsoft Word® provides a gallery of choices for formatting the table of contents.

Format Painter

The format painter option is a commonly overlooked word processing feature that can be used to modify text styles. The option allows you to copy the text formatting from one place of the document to other places. In Microsoft Word®, the format painter is displayed as a paintbrush on the Home tab clipboard ribbon (default menu in OpenOffice.org™; not available in Google Docs®). To use the option, first, click anywhere on a text area with the desired formatting; second, click the

Table 6-1 Font and Point Size

Different Fonts and Sizes		
8 Point	12 Point	20 Point
Arial	Arial	Arial
Courier	Courier	Courier
Times New Roman	Times New Roman	Times New Roman

Microsoft Word 2010

OpenOffice.org Writer

Google Docs Document

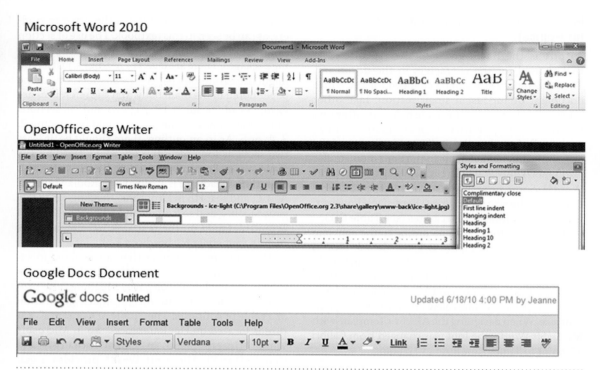

Figure 6-1 Word processing menus.

paintbrush, and then highlight the text you want to change. If you want to format text in more than one place in the document, double-click the format painter; when you are finished, tap the Esc key.

Paragraphs

Most word processors provide many options for formatting paragraphs. Line spacing, tab stops, line alignment, and margins were checked when designing the APA 6th Template. The icon to change line and paragraph spacing is located on the Home tab > Paragraph ribbon in Microsoft Word® (Format menu for OpenOffice.org™ and Google Docs®). APA citation style uses double line spacing. It does not require an extra line between paragraphs, although that is a Microsoft Word® option. Note that the Line and Paragraph Spacing menu also provides a way to modify the tab stops. Since the Microsoft Word® default tab stop is ½ inch, no changes were necessary when creating the APA 6th Template (found on the textbook website).

The APA template demonstrates the use of the hanging indent paragraph formatting for the reference list. The hanging indent feature is located in the paragraph dialog box in Microsoft Word® (manually created using the ruler in Google Docs and OpenOffice.org). To create a hanging indent use the Indents and Spacing window and select "hanging indent" from the dropdown menu next to Special in the Indentation section. An example of the hanging indent paragraph and indenting both paragraph margins is noted in **Box 6-2**.

All paragraphs, with the exception of the first paragraph of the abstract, should be indented to comply with APA style and line alignment should be left-justified. **Justification**, or text alignment, refers to how the left and right margins of the paragraph appear. Different justification can be applied to a paragraph, paragraphs, a page, or an entire document. Text can be justified in four ways (**Box 6-3**). Unless a very good printer and font are available, the easiest documents to read are those in which the text is aligned left, creating a straight left margin and even spacing between words.

BOX 6-2 Examples of Paragraph Formatting

Hanging Paragraph
Manually creating a hanging paragraph instead of using this feature not only wastes time but also creates problems when one needs to edit the text.

Indenting of Both Margins
Create page breaks only when it is imperative that the new text be on a fresh page and then use the forced page break (Ctrl + Enter). If it is necessary for all of a given set of text to always be on the same page, use the "Keep text together" feature found under Format (Paragraph in some word processors).

BOX 6-3 Justification (Alignment) Examples

Left justification (left margin straight)
Learning to use a word processor is not so much a factor of learning the commands, but of knowing what is possible. Once you know what is possible and can ask "How do you do x?" instead of being oblivious to the fact that it is possible to do x, you are 75% of the way to using a function effectively.

Right justification (right margin straight)
Few writers, even professionals, get it right the first time. Rewriting is as germane to writing as breathing is to staying alive. A word processor makes rewriting relatively painless, thus allowing a writer to appear at his/her best. Editing, however, leads to unintended results when one formats manually.

Center justification (text centered horizontally)
When an individual first moves from a typewriter to a word processor, and before one has learned to think "let the computer do it," some features in word processing can cause confusion, and yes, frustration! Much of the frustration new word processor users experience comes from ideas ingrained by the use of typewriters and a fixed page.

Full justification (both margins straight)
Those reared in the printed page world sometimes find it very anti-intuitive that they do not have to, indeed should not, use the Enter key to paginate. This results in unintended results when the document is edited. New pages created by using the Enter key are fluid and change their location as the text entered earlier is added or deleted. The result is that the text that was supposed to start in a "new page" is in the middle of a page with blank spaces above.

Page margins were also checked when creating the template. APA 6th edition specifies 1-inch margins on all four sides. In Microsoft Word®, you can change the margins from the Page Layout tab > Page Setup ribbon (Format menu in OpenOffice.org™ and Google Docs®). No changes were necessary since 1-inch margins are the default setting in Microsoft Word®.

Page Properties

The printed page is the ultimate focus of a word-processed document. A page has many properties that can be used to change its printed appearance. In Microsoft Word®, most properties are available from the Page Layout tab (Format menu in OpenOffice.org™ and Google Docs®). Like all programs that offer printing, including web browsers, pages can be printed in either portrait (default) or landscape view in word processors. The portrait view is the default in Microsoft Word®; therefore, no modifications were necessary when creating the APA 6th Template.

Centering a Page Vertically

Sometimes it is desirable to center the text on a page not only left to right but also vertically, or top to bottom. This can be useful in creating a title page. In many word processors, this feature is found on the File menu under the Layout tab in Page Setup. In Microsoft Word®, click the drop-down arrow on the Page Layout command box, then Layout, then change Vertical alignment to Center. This feature was not required when creating the APA 6th Template.

Page Breaks and Keeping Text Together

Page breaks work the same way as word wrap; the computer starts a new page when it finds that it is needed. When creating the APA 6th Template, page breaks were used to separate the title page, abstract, main body, and references. Like a line break caused by word wrap, this page break is fluid and will change as needed when the document is edited. If you want a hard page, that is one that will always start at a given location, tap the Ctrl + Enter keys at that location in the text.

Do not attempt to paginate, that is, determine where a new page will start as you write, unless you know that subsequent text must start on a new page, such as after a title page, an abstract, or when creating the first page in the reference section. Using a hard page break will ensure that no matter how much text is added or removed above it, the text on that page will always start on a fresh page. Under no circumstances use a soft page break or force a new page by using the Enter key. When a page break is forced by tapping the Enter key, editing by adding or removing text will cause it to move accordingly, because the computer regards tapping the Enter key as just creating a new line, not a new page.

Sometimes, although you may not necessarily need a new page, you want to be sure that a given block of text when printed will always be on the same page. This can be done by using the "keep lines together" feature. In Microsoft Word®, the feature is located in Home > Paragraph Dialog Box Launcher > Line and Page breaks tab.

Headers, Footers, and Page Numbers

A **header** is the text that is printed on the top of each page (see **Figure 6-2**), and a **footer** is text printed on the bottom of each page (**Figure 6-3**).

Some formal documents require headers on all pages. On others, the user may want to use a header as clarification for the reader. Headers were created for the APA 6th Template with a running head on the left and the page number right-justified. There are no APA specifications for footers.

Headers and footers should be inserted by using the word processor's Header/Footer function. Use the Insert tab in Microsoft Word® to access this function (Format menu in OpenOffice.org™ and Google Docs®). Right-click on a header or footer to make edits in Microsoft Word®. Headers and footers may have any attributes that can be applied to text and can be left, center, or right justified. A common error is to manually enter headers and footers on each page. This error results in their moving to a location other than the top of a page when there is any editing of the document that either adds or deletes a line.

A header or footer can include more than a title and page number. Many of those features are available from the Microsoft Word® gallery that displays selecting the header or footer on the menu. Check the application's Help option to learn the use of the functions, Header, Footer, or Page Numbers.

Saving and Retrieving Files

As with all computer applications, it is a good idea to save frequently when creating a document in a word processor. Files saved by a word processor are in a proprietary format, or one that is specific to the brand of the word processor that created it. Sometimes it is necessary to give a file to someone who uses a different type of word processor. To do this, you can save the file in a rich text file format that usually maintains all the font attributes when transferred from one application to another.

Running Head: "ABBREVIATED TITLE - LESS THAN 50 LETTERS - ALL CAPITALS"   1

Header -Section 1-

Figure 6-2 Example of a header in Microsoft Word®.

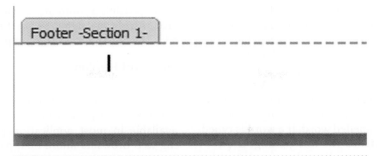

Figure 6-3 Example of a footer in Microsoft Word®.

Printing

In Windows-compliant programs, tapping Ctrl + P automatically starts the printing process. The File menu also contains a Print option. By using this option, a block of text, one page, a range of pages, or the entire document can be selected for printing. Although many features that improve the appearance of a printed page, such as a header or page numbering, can be applied anytime, others, such as entering page breaks to improve the cohesiveness of the pages, should not be introduced until all editing is finished and the document is ready to be printed.

Some Common Word Processor Features

Most people use only a very small portion of their word processor's capability, ignoring features that can save time, improve the quality of the document, and make a document more professional. Spelling and grammar check and page formatting options are examples of commonly overlooked features.

Spelling, Grammar Check, and Readability Statistics

A critical aspect for creating new documents is to use spell and grammar check. This feature is available on the Review tab > Proofing ribbon in Microsoft Word®, although it can be added to the Quick Access menu by using the drop-down menu (Tools menu in OpenOffice.org™ and spell-check only on main menu in Google Docs®). Many misconceptions exist about how spell-check works.

A computer does not think; it only makes comparisons (**Box 6-4**). When spell-check is used, the computer compares each set of characters between spaces with the words that are in its dictionary. If it finds a set of matching letters, it assumes that the word is spelled correctly.

Most word processors use a wavy red line at the point of entry to underline any words that are considered misspelled. When this line appears, to find out how the word processor thinks the word should be spelled, place the mouse pointer over the word and right-click. A list of suggestions will appear. If one of those words is the correct one, click it, and the spelling checker will replace the misspelled word. If No Suggestions appears, and the user knows the word is spelled correctly, the user can add that word to the dictionary. If one is engaged in writing for a specialty field for which many of the words are not part of the default dictionary, additional dictionaries, such as a medical dictionary, can be added.

> **BOX 6-4** Speller Peccadilloes
>
> I have a spelling checker
> I disk covered for my personal computer (PC).
> It plane lee marks for my revue
> Mistakes I cannot see.
>
> Eye ran this poem threw it.
> Your sure real glad to know.
> It very polished in its weigh,
> My checker told me sew.

One function related to the spelling checker is the ability of word processors to automatically change what is seen as a misspelled – or more usually mistyped – word to what it considers the correct format. This function is often referred to as AutoCorrect or Quick Correct. To provide for this function, the word processor stores a list of common misspellings together with the correctly spelled word. If a word is typed in a way that matches the misspelling, the correct word is automatically substituted for the misspelled one. New words can be added to this function, and those that may not be a misspelling in a certain context can be deleted, such as ADN, which the speller insists should be "AND." In Microsoft Word®, AutoCorrect features is found under File > Options > Proofing (Format menu in OpenOffice.org™; not available for Google Docs®). AutoCorrect options can be customized to best meet the writer's needs.

Grammar check errors are flagged with a wavy green line in Microsoft Word®. Once again, the writer must accept or reject the error flag. Microsoft Word® will flag many types of errors, including split infinitives, sentence fragments, subject–verb agreement errors, run-on sentence, and errors associated with the use of "that" and "which."

Readability statistics is a word processing feature that is commonly overlooked because the display is not a default setting in Microsoft Word® (not available for OpenOffice.org™ or Google Docs®). The feature is invaluable for nurses who create or review information for patients and family members. To turn on the feature in Microsoft Word® go to File > Options > Proofing and place a check mark by "Show readability statistics." Readability statistics will display after running spelling and grammar check.

Thesaurus

Although not as large, the Thesaurus is set up much like a printed one and is much quicker to use. Like spell-check, the Thesaurus is located on the Review tab > Proofing ribbon in Microsoft Word® (Tools menu in OpenOffice.org™ and Google Docs®). To use the Thesaurus, place the insertion point on the word for which a substitute is desired and click it. A window pops up that lists some possible synonyms. Some word processors also provide antonyms. Select the proper word and click the box that tells the computer to replace it.

Find and Replace

Find and Replace is another very useful tool. Find will locate every instance of a set of characters, which is usually a word or phrase. This feature is available in most application programs, including web browsers and e-mail packages. The Find and Replace feature can replace one set of characters with another. Suppose a user types the word "nurse" rather than "Registered Nurse." By accessing Find and Replace on the Home tab in Microsoft Word® (Edit menu in OpenOffice.org™ and Google Docs®), the word processor can be told to find every instance of "nurse" and replace it with "Registered Nurse." The replacement can be automatic or the user can decide which occurrences to replace.

Footnotes and Endnotes

Footnotes and **endnotes** are different features, but each is accessed and entered the same way. A footnote is a piece of text printed at the bottom of a page. It is usually additional information that may add to a reader's knowledge. An endnote is a piece of text that is printed at the end of a document, for instance, a list of references. Word processors automatically place these notes in the proper position and number them accordingly. The drop-down box to access this feature is found on the Insert menu.

Graphics

Graphical objects, any object other than a table or text, can be inserted in a document by using the Insert tab or by copy and paste. They can also be dragged from a web page opened with Microsoft Internet Explorer® into any program that accepts graphics. Once in a document, you can resize them just as you would any graphical object by dragging the edge.[2] Microsoft Word® includes a gallery of clip art, shapes, and SmartArt. Microsoft Word® 2010 also provides the ability to create and insert screenshots. This new feature is on the Insert > Illustrations menu (see **Figure 6-4**).

---

2 Chapter 7 discusses resizing a graphic in more detail.

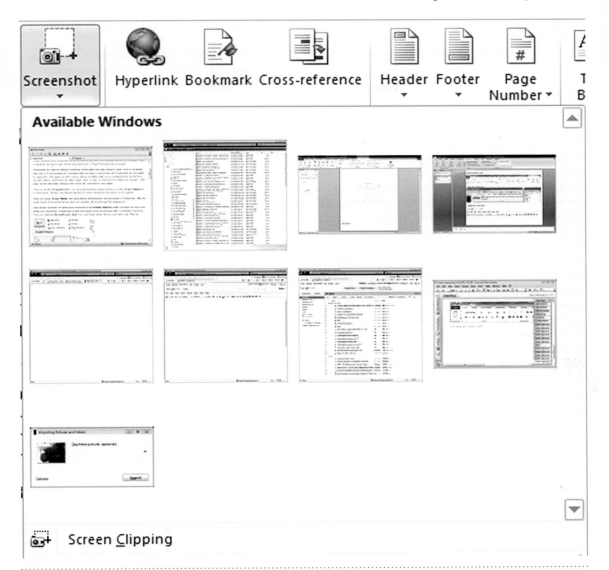

Figure 6-4 Screenshot menu in Microsoft Word®.

You may need to move the object in the word processor. In some word processors, you can easily accomplish this by dragging the graphic where you wish it placed or by selecting it and using the arrow keys to move it. In others, you will need to right-click the object, select Format Picture, then Layout from the next menu, and change to a square or tight format.

Columns

It is possible to split a document into two or more columns without using tables in Microsoft Word® (Use Table menu in OpenOffice.org™ and Google Docs®). Column creation is accessed from Page Layout tab > Page Setup ribbon in Microsoft Word®. Users are then asked to designate the number of columns and can either accept the default spacing between the columns or change it. Using a forced page break (Ctrl + Enter) in a column forces the text to the top of the next column.

Tables

Tables can be created by clicking the Insert tab > Tables ribbon (Tables menu in OpenOffice.org™ and Google Docs®) and dragging to create the desired number of rows and columns. Extra columns can be added or deleted at any time. If the default column size does not match a need, columns can be resized by placing the mouse pointer on the grid line between columns until it changes shape to an east–west arrow,[3] depressing the left mouse button and dragging the line. Microsoft Word® also provides the ability for users to draw a table. Microsoft Word® 2010 includes a gallery of "Quick Tables." To enter text into a table, simply type. The rectangle, or cell, will enlarge as needed. An often-overlooked feature in Microsoft Word® is "Repeat Header Row," which repeats the column headings for tables that are split between two or more pages. This feature is located in the Layout ribbon.

Many options for formatting a table are available. Although some word processors have more detailed features, all provide the following functions:

- Adding a row to the bottom of the table by placing the insertion point in the rightmost cell on the bottom row and tapping the Tab key.
- Navigating in the table by tapping the Tab key to go to the cell on the right, Shift + Tab to go the cell on the left, or using the arrow keys to move the insertion point up or down a row.
- Changing the appearance or style of a table. This includes removing all the borders, or changing their attributes. Several readymade formats are part of each word processor package. Table attributes can be accessed either by right clicking the table

or by clicking the Table icon on the menu line.
- Calculating by using elementary formulas.
- Changing cell sizes, either by a menu or dragging row or column borders.
- Joining and splitting cells either vertically or horizontally.

Selecting cells you wish to change and right-clicking will produce a menu of options.

Sorting

When typing a list of names, it is not always convenient to enter them in alphabetical order. The Sort function, however, can automatically alphabetize them based on the word (e.g., first, second) in the line that the user designates. Sort can be applied to a list, a table column, or paragraphs. The sorting function is useful in organizing references for a paper. Use the Help function to learn how to sort.

Mail Merge

Mail merge takes a set of data and places the different pieces into the desired place in a document (not just a letter). To use names and mail merge data in a form document, the user first creates a set of data that includes fields such as title, first name, middle name, last name, address, and so forth. The data for the document can be in a spreadsheet, a database, a table, or in some word processors created as a separate document. After the data are entered, a letter, or form, is then planned in which these items are placed appropriately (**Figure 6-5**). A mail merge wizard is available for Microsoft Word® on the Mailing ribbon (Tools menu in OpenOffice.org™; Google Docs® users can use Zoho [http://www.zoho.com] for mail merge).

Mail merge is not just for postal mail. It is an indispensable tool for personalized mass e-mail, for example, invitations to a conference or meeting. With Microsoft Word®, users can create a document on electronic stationery that includes the company name, logo, and address for e-mail. To use this feature, the data source must include e-mail addresses. After the e-mail is written and merged data is selected, "Send E-Mail Messages" is selected from "Finish & Merge." The e-mail will be sent from the default e-mail program.

---

3 An east–west arrow is a horizontal line with an arrow at each end. A north–south arrow is a vertical line with arrows at each end. A north–south–east–west arrow is horizontal and vertical lines crossed in the middle with arrows at all four ends.

```
(Title)Ms.
(First Name)Lucy
(Middle Name)X.
(Last Name)Caro
(Address)25 East Southwick Drive
(City)Anywhere
(State)Any State
(Zip)42424-1001
```

Sample of one record in a data set

```
(Title) (First Name) (Middle Name) (Last Name)
(Address)
(City), (State) (Zip)

Dear (Title) (Last Name):

        You have been selected from many people to
enjoy a special vacation at our new resort at the beautiful
seashore. (First Name), we know that you will not object
to paying a small fee of $2000 for this privilege. You need
to contact us by Friday at the latest to take part in this
great opportunity. Call us at 1-800-BELIEVE.

Sincerely,


Joe Barnum
A sucker is born every minute
```

Sample of a form letter

```
Ms. Lucy X. Caro
25 East Southwick Drive
Anywhere, Any State 42424-1001


Dear Ms. Caro:

        You have been selected from many people to enjoy a special vacation at our new
resort at the beautiful seashore. Lucy, we know that you will not object to paying a
small fee of $2000 for this privilege. You need to contact us by Friday at the latest to take part
in this great opportunity. Call us at 1-800-BELIEVE.

Sincerely,


Joe Barnum
A sucker is born every minute
```

Form letter after it has been merged

Figure 6-5 Dataset, form letter, and result of a merge.

Automatic Numbering and Bullets

If you need to outline something, or want a numbered or bulleted list, word processors will easily do this. Like most word processor features, you can select this one before you enter the text, or afterward. This feature is usually on the default toolbar that includes the ability to modify font style and size.

If you enter the number 1, a period, and a space and then enter text, some older word processors automatically assume that this should be a numbered list and will enter a number 2, a period, and space when you tap the Enter key. The maneuver to stop the numbering varies with the word processor, but tapping the Enter key twice will delete the unwanted number. The advantage to automatic numbering is that it saves the effort of entering the numbers when a list is wanted; but even more valuable is that if the items in the list are reordered, the numbers change automatically so they remain in sequence. That is, if item 4 is moved to the line after item 1, the number 4 automatically becomes number 2, and the former number 2 becomes number 3, and so on.

To create a hierarchal multilevel list, it is necessary to change the format of the numbering feature. Multilevel lists or outlines can be created either before one enters any numbers and text or afterward. The feature is on the Home ribbon in Microsoft Word® (Format menu in OpenOffice.org™, but not standard in Google Docs®). It is very useful for creating an outline for a paper or a multiple-choice test.

When the outline or bullet function is on, tap the Enter key to create the next numbered item. To move to the next lower level, tap the Tab key. To change to a level above, tap Shift + Tab keys. **Box 6-5** illustrates an outline format. The user can change the labels for each level (e.g., number 1, a). A regular outline format with Roman numerals as the top level and uppercase letters for the second level can be selected, or the user can select or create any desired style.

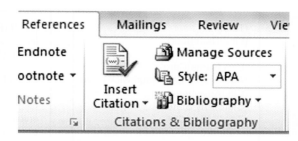

Figure 6-6 Personal reference manager in Microsoft Word®.

Personal Citation and Bibliography Manager

Microsoft Word® and OpenOffice.org™ documents include a personal reference manager (bibliography database). Both vendors allow users to type citation information into the database. OpenOffice.org™ does not currently have an easy way to use the bibliography database for citations and a reference list. Microsoft Word® does allow the user to select an output citation style, such as APA and to use the information to cite and create a reference list. The function is on the Reference > Citations & Bibliography ribbon (see **Figure 6-6**). Additional information on creating citations and reference lists is included in the APA 6th Template.

Cross-Referencing

With the popularity of the web, publishers of word processing software have added the ability to insert a web link into a document. Clicking the link, if the user is online, will retrieve the page in the link just as it does in a regular web page. Links within the document, known as cross-referencing, are also possible (e.g., "see page X–23"). The page number then is "generated" before printing to ensure its accuracy. It is also possible to use referencing or to mark items to be included in a table of contents.

Macro

A **macro** is a small program that automates a function. If the same functions are continually accessed, for example, a phrase or string of words, a macro can be created to perform this function automatically. Although complex macros are programmed, it is also possible to create a macro by

---

BOX 6-5 Example of an Outline

1. This is level one of an outline
   a. This is level two accessed by tapping the Tab key after the number 2 appeared.
   b. The "b." appeared automatically when the Enter key was tapped.
2. Shift + Tab moved back to the first level.
   a. Level two again
      i. Level three
         1. Level four
            a. Level five
3. After tapping Shift + Tab four times, back to level one again.

recording keystrokes as a function is performed. After creating a macro, it can be placed on the toolbar or assigned a key. To place a macro on the toolbar, place the mouse pointer on the toolbar and click the right mouse button, and then follow the directions. To record keystrokes to create a macro, click the View ribbon in Microsoft Word® (Tools menu in OpenOffice.org™; not a feature in Google Docs®), enter a name for the macro, implement the keystrokes, and stop the recording by clicking the square on the small window that is present when a macro is being created.

Forms

It is possible to create a form by using Microsoft Word®; although an Access database may be a better solution (OpenOffice.org™ requires the use of the database component of the office suite; Google Docs® uses the spreadsheet function for forms). A Microsoft Word® form is commonly used to provide uniform data input in a document that will be completed electronically, such as an application. The Developer ribbon in Microsoft Word® has the features such as check boxes and data entry boxes used on forms. To make the Developer tab visible on the ribbon, click File (Backstage in Microsoft Word® 2010) > Options > Customize Ribbon > Main tabs > and click the checkbox next to Developer. Click the Design Mode icon to switch to the design view. Controls commonly used on forms include Text Control Content (plain or rich), Drop-Down List Content Control, and the Checkbox Content Control. The next step is to create the form and insert the desired controls. Creating a form with tables is the optimal method for organizing and displaying the data. When the form is complete, simply click the Design Mode icon again to switch back to the normal view for data entry.

Desktop Publishing

Desktop publishing refers to creating newsletters, brochures, pamphlets, business cards, and similar other types of print media. Microsoft Word® provides access to a large assortment of templates that can be downloaded from the Microsoft website and modified for use. Customized templates can be saved as a template file type for reuse or saved in another file format, such as a Microsoft Word® file or an Adobe portable

document format (PDF) file. All you need is an idea and a little imagination to publish your own media.

Collaboration

The ability to collaborate with two or more authors on a document is a common word processing feature. One approach is to use the word processing review tool, and the other is to save the document to a shared work space. The traditional method is to use a review tool. The tool is on the Review ribbon in Microsoft Word® (Edit > Changes in OpenOffice.org™; not a feature in Google Docs®). This feature is used for formative writing assignments in the classroom, manuscript peer review process and in textbook editing. In Microsoft Word®, after the Track Changes icon is selected, changes are recorded. The Accept button allows the writer to accept or reject suggested document changes.

A Web 2.0 feature allows for online collaboration using a shared work. Users had the ability to share documents in Microsoft Word® after Microsoft™ introduced Windows Live®. Document sharing is included on the File menu (Backstage in Microsoft Office® 2010). Google Docs® also allows for online collaboration among multiple users. To initiate collaboration, the document is saved to the shared workspace (Skydrive in Microsoft Word®). Afterward, the owner of the document selects how the document is shared by choosing from categories, such as friends and coworkers, typing in an e-mail address, or selecting names from the contact list.

Learning New Word Processing Skills

Learning new word processing skills is a lifelong journey. The advent of new versions of software, the emergence of software from different vendors, and new delivery technologies as seen with cloud computing applications are challenging. If you are a novice, begin by gaining skills with a single software solution. This chapter has focused on comparing Microsoft Word® 2010, OpenOffice.org™ documents, and Google Docs®, the latter two of which are free. If you have intermediate or advanced skills, work on gaining expertise on multiple product platforms, mentor, and share what you know with others.

Using only a small fraction of the features that word processors offer limits output and results in time wasted. Manually entering things such as headers and page numbers renders it impossible to easily edit a document. The ability to edit is what makes a word processor superior to a typewriter. Few documents exist that cannot benefit from heavy editing. Learn to make your word processor work for you, not the other way around.

Online help gets better with every version of the office software suites and is a great source of assistance in increasing one's word processing skills. Face-to-face classes can help too, but they open a door only to the intricacies of the program; one must enter that door and try the features not only in class but in all settings. Microsoft Word® Help provides access to online tutorials with built-in quizzes, videos, and online courses. Becoming aware of what a word processor can do, then learning the features in a "just-in-time" manner, can keep the learning to a manageable level. Some examples of resources with free online courses on word processing are as follows:

- Microsoft Training (http://office.microsoft.com/en-us/training/FX100565001033.aspx)
- Goodwill Community Foundation International LearnFree.org (http://www.gcflearnfree.org/default3d.aspx)
- HP Learning Center (http://www.hp.com/go/learningcenter).

Language Translation

Given the global culture of today, there will be times when you want to translate something into another language. The web has programs that will do this to some extent, but they are far from perfect. Translating the occasional phrase is one thing, but translating an entire document is fraught with misunderstanding and misinterpretation. One example of a free translation program is AltaVista's BabelFish (http://babelfish.altavista.com/). Play with it, but go easy on using it except in very informal situations unless you have a native speaker of the foreign language who also understands your language and can rewrite the document for you (see **Box 6-6**).

BOX 6-6 Automatic Translations

English
The ocean shows signs of being windy, but we are sailing anyway.

Translated to Spanish
El océano demuestra muestras de ser ventoso, pero estamos navegando de todos modos.

Translated Back to English
The ocean demonstrates samples of being windy, but we are sailing anyway.

Microsoft Word® 2010 has a new language-translation function that allows you to translate a section or the entire document into another language by using machine translation. The function is located on the Review > Language ribbon. You must be connected to the Internet to use the feature. A simple wizard will walk you through the translation steps. Since the translation uses the computer to make the interpretation, it would be best if could speak and write the language fluently or, as noted above, have a native speaker of the language to assist you.

Word processors, however, do make it possible to write characters in another language, such as an "e" or an "a" with an accent (é or á, respectively) or adding an umlaut to a "u" (ü). If you need to constantly write in a language other than the default on your computer, use the Help feature to learn how.

Summary

Word processors have become very popular. You were introduced to the many of the basic word processing features with the APA 6th Template that could be downloaded from the textbook website. Features used in the template include page breaks, headers, fonts, font sizes, styles sets, form fields, and hanging indent line formatting.

The basic editing skills pioneered in word processors are used in most application programs, including e-mail programs. Once text is entered into a word processor, it can be altered in many ways. Attributes can be added; the font or font (point) size can be changed; and text can be deleted, copied, or moved. Learning to let the word processor perform such functions as line breaks and page breaks involves reconceptualizing the idea of a document from a fixed-page entity to a document that easily changes while it is being edited. Time spent learning to let the computer perform features such as centering a page vertically, formatting a paragraph, and entering headers and footers, and learning to cope with automatic numbering is returned many times over in creating future documents. Word processors have many other features that not only make tasks easier but also make them economically feasible, such as sorting, mail merge for personalizing notes, and cross-referencing to make it easier for a reader to locate information on another page of a document.

APPLICATIONS AND COMPETENCIES

1. Download the document "Multitasking.rtf" from Chapter 7 on the web page http://dlthede. net/Informatics/Informatics.html and open it in your word processor and do as follows:

   a. Select a paragraph and change the font and font (point) size. (If using Microsoft Word® 2007, before doing the next exercise, click the Microsoft Office® button, and on the drop-down menu in the lower right corner of the window, click Microsoft Word® Options and then Advanced. If the box before "Use the insert key to control the overtype mode" is blank, place a check in it and click OK. If you will never use overtype mode, you may want to go back and uncheck that after you do the following exercise.)

   b. Place the insertion point at the beginning of the first word in the second paragraph, tap the Insert key, and enter the letters "abc" and see what happens.

   c. Click the Undo icon (or tap Ctrl + Z) to undo this change.

   d. Tap the Insert key again to stop this mode of entering text.

   e. Boldface any one sentence.

   f. Create a hard page before the word References at the end of the document.

   g. Center the word "references."

   h. Make the reference a hanging paragraph (may be under Indent paragraphs in Help).

   i. Italicize the words and number "Nursing Assist 23."

2. Start a fresh page by making a hard page, and experiment with automatic numbering. If using Microsoft Word® 2007, before starting this exercise, on the Home ribbon, in the Paragraph commands, click the icon whose tip reads "numbering" when you rest the mouse pointer over it.

   a. Enter the number 1, a period, and tap the Tab key, and then enter the word "house."

   b. Tap the Enter key.

   c. What happened? (If you do not see the number 2, use the Insert or Format tab [word processor dependent] and select Outline/ Bullets and Numbering.)

   d. Enter the word "car" after the "2," and tap the Enter key.

   e. Type the word "boat," and tap the Enter key.

   f. Stop the automatic numbering.

3. Experiment with multilevel numbering.

   a. Find Bullets and Numbering on either the Insert or Format menu, and select outline numbered. (For Microsoft Word® 2007 select the Multilevel list icon from the Paragraph command on the Home ribbon.)

   b. Select any of the multilevel formats.

   c. After the "1" that appears on the screen,

      i. Enter the word "house," and tap Enter.
      ii. Tap the Tab key.
      iii. Enter the word "kitchen," and tap Enter.
      iv. Enter the words "family room," and tap Enter.
      v. Tap Shift + Tab.
      vi. Enter the word "car," and tap Enter.
      vii. Turn off the outline feature the same way the automatic numbering was turned off.

4. Copy the entire document to another document:

   a. Tap Ctrl + A to select the entire document.

There are three ways to place the selected text on the clipboard so that it can be copied. Select one and perform the activity.

   b. Tap Ctrl + C

or,

  c. On the toolbar, click the Copy icon (Home ribbon in Microsoft Word® 2007)

or,

  d. On the menu line, click Edit > Copy. (Home ribbon in Microsoft Word® 2007.)

5. Create a new document by tapping Ctrl + N, and paste the text into the new document by either of the following:

  a. Tap Shift + Insert

or,

  b. Tap Ctrl + V

or,

  c. Click the Paste icon on the toolbar in all word processors except Microsoft Word® 2007. (Home ribbon in Microsoft Word® 2007.)

  d. On the menu line, click Edit > Paste.

  e. Return to the original document by clicking its icon on the bottom of the screen. (If a line of icons is not seen there, place the mouse pointer there until one appears.)

  f. On the Page Setup screen (on the menu line click File > Page Setup or Page Layout ribbon):

    i. Change the **page orientation** to Landscape.

    ii. Change the margins to 0.75 inches (7 cm).

6. Insert a header that will automatically appear on each page that is right-justified and contains a left-justified running head, five spaces, and a page number. Use the Help feature to discover how to do this. You may have to experiment a little. (For Microsoft Word® 2007, see the instructions on Chapter 7 of the web page http://dlthede.net/Informatics/Informatics.html.)

7. Change the view of the document from the Print Layout to Normal (Draft) mode or the other way around if you are already looking at the document in the Normal (Draft) mode. (In the View menu in earlier Microsoft Word®; in the Document View command group on the View ribbon in Microsoft Word® 2007.) What happens to the header?

8. Create a table of three columns and two rows. Enter the following words:

  a. In the first cell in the first row, enter DATE.

  b. Tap the Tab key.

  c. Enter the word TIME, and tap Tab.

  d. Enter the word PROJECT, and tap Tab.

  e. In the DATE column, enter today's date, and tap Tab.

  f. Enter the present time, and tap Tab.

  g. Enter "Creating a table," and tap Tab. What happened?

  h. Create a header row in the table. First, select the top row in the table, leave your insertion point there, and ask help how to make this a header row. To search help, for some word processors, enter "header row" in the search bar; for others, enter "format table" and scroll down.

9. Identify one or two new word processing skills that you would like to learn. Practice the new skill(s) and then self-assess your experience. What problems did you experience? How might you use the new skill?

CHAPTER 7

Presentation Software: Looking Professional in the Spotlight

Objectives

After studying this chapter you will be able to:

▶ *Differentiate between information that can accurately be communicated with computer slides and information that needs a narrative.*

▶ *Compare the differences in design between a slide presentation that is used as an aid to a live presentation and one used as a stand-alone message.*

▶ *Apply principles of good slide design in creating a slide presentation.*

▶ *Employ appropriate principles in creating handouts.*

Key Terms

Attribute
Crop
Gradient Background
Lecture Replacement Model

Lecture Support Model
Progressive Disclosure
Storyboard

You skipped today's lecture because you could get the PowerPoint® slides from the course website. Now you are looking at these slides and wondering how the pieces of information fit together – should you memorize all these bullet points? However, how will you apply them? How can you make this information meaningful?

Many face this dilemma when reviewing class slides and handouts from online slideshow presentations, such as PowerPoint®. Most of us find ourselves frustrated in using information only from slides, or only from handouts of slides, even if we took notes along the sides of the slides. Slideshows may help us as presenters to outline our talk, but when they stand alone, do they help those on the receiving end understand the information that we are trying to communicate?

Nurses and students give many presentations, sometimes informally to one another, but often before a group. Feeling confident in this endeavor is something that comes with practice. Today the expectation of speakers is that they will use computerized slides. Not only knowing how to create these visuals, but also giving consideration to what the audience will take away from these slides is the key to developing useful visuals.

Visuals can be boring and distracting if not created and used appropriately. Most of us have been subjected to computer-projected visuals that either detracted from the speaker or upstaged him or her. The computer slideshow is your partner. It should not upstage you or detract from what you say or be expected to communicate a message alone.

This chapter first discusses the theoretical and pedagogical use of visuals in a presentation before discussing slideshow software. The terms presentation software and slideshow are used interchangeably. Understanding the educational purposes for visuals is essential to the design of an effective presentation. You will want to reflect on past presentations that you thought were excellent and compare those to ones that bored you. The information will assist you to self-assess your presentation skills. You should be able to identify opportunities to gain new skills. **Box 7-1** identifies a listing of skills for basic, intermediate, and advanced users. PowerPoint® slide examples that supplement the information in this chapter can be downloaded from the textbook website at http://dlthede.net/Informatics/Informatics.html.

Using Computer-Projected Visuals in Nursing

A question that has been asked about the February 1, 2003, explosion of the space shuttle Columbia was "Did PowerPoint® make the space shuttle crash?" Evidence proves that it was a contributing factor (Thompson, 2003, December 14). It seems that the National Aeronautics and Space Administration had become too reliant on using PowerPoint® to present complex information instead of narrative technical reports. The nesting and subnesting of complex points caused those who had to make decisions about the safety of Columbia to misunderstand the true picture. One then must ask, "Could depending on PowerPoint® slides to communicate information create a healthcare mistake?"

BOX 7-1 Presentation Skills

Basic Presentation Skills
- Design a simple presentation
- Apply a template
- Insert a new slide
- Apply the use of different slide layouts
- Use spell-check
- Save a presentation
- Add shapes to a slide
- View a slide show
- Print a presentation

Intermediate Presentation Skills
- Customize the presentation menu
- Create handouts
- Add clip art to slides
- Add SmartArt to slides
- Move and resize objects
- Incorporate multimedia (audio, graphics, animation, and video) into slide design
- Modify multimedia used for presentations, e.g.
  - Compress photos (right-click) to reduce file size
  - Edit photos/graphics for resolution, fit, and web use to use in a presentation
- Demonstrate competency using two presentation software applications
- Save a presentation in file formats for use with other software applications
- Share/collaborate with others on presentation design
- Apply pedagogical principles to presentation design (Purpose, visual clarity, consistency, readability)
- Print out a slide presentation handouts (more than 1 slide/page)

BOX 7-1 Presentation Skills *(continued)*

Advanced Presentation Skills
- Design on-screen navigation
- Customize presentation toolbars
- Embed/edit a spreadsheet
- Create a macro
- Add slide transitions
- Add slide sections
- Design slide animations
- Demonstrate advance text and graphic editing techniques
- Build custom slide masters
- Build custom handout masters
- Build custom notes masters
- Create a presentation template
- Publish and distribute presentations
- Demonstrate competency using more than two presentation software applications

Good slide design, as shown in **Table 7-1**, requires that one use only about 40 words per slide. The guidelines for graphics design apply to good slide design. Design principles such as balance, emphasis, movement, contrast, and repetition, as described by Carter (2003) for use in software development, should also be used in slideshow design. Visual literacy or the ability to interpret the meaning of visual images and to create messages with "culturally significant" images (Collins

Table 7-1 Basic Rules for Creating and Using Visuals

	Creating and Using Visuals
Text	• Limit to 6–7 words in a line and 6 lines on a slide
Fonts	• Choose a sans serif font for projected visuals. Limit the number of different fonts, to no more than three. Match font to reactions desired from the audience.
Font Size	• Transparencies ≥ 18 points
	• Slides ≥ 24 points
Colors	
Background	• Match to lighting of room where presentation will be given. Light for light rooms, dark for dark rooms.
Text and Background	• Contrasting – opposite sides of color wheel
For Emphasis	• Be consistent
Number Used	• Total of no more than 5–6.
Using Visuals	
Time on Screen	• At least 10 seconds and never more than 100; break up a slide if needed, use progressive disclosure, or blank out screen.
Coordinate	• Keep the talk focused on the slide in view.
Audience Reading	• If the audience need to read an entire slide, give them time!
Blank Screen	• To digress from the slides, tap the letter "w" to produce a white screen, or "b" for a black screen.
	• Hide mouse pointer: Tap the A key (toggle) to turn mouse on/off
	• Start Presentation: Tap the F5 key

Memorial Library, 2009; Felten, 2008) also applies to the design of slideshow presentations.

Oral presenters need to be aware that slides should only be used to help an audience keep track of ideas and occasionally illustrate a point, and not be used as the basis of understanding. Audiences also need to realize that slides alone are only an outline of a talk. Designers of self-running kiosks, tutorials, and video slideshows need to explain and elaborate on slide text and visuals. All presentations must have the purpose clearly stated, slides that provide additional details, and a summary.

Computer slides have two main uses: one as a guide for an oral presentation (lecture support) and another as a stand-alone information source (lecture replacement) such as for an online course. Common sense says that the design of each should be different (Springfield, 2007). The **lecture support model** can be effective to guide audiences to follow your presentation, while the **lecture replacement model** needs more than just bullet points.

Lecture Support Model

Lecture support slides should be used to communicate information that needs a visual backup such as body systems, or physiology (Springfield, 2007). During your lecture, use a question that is not easily answered with one or two words on a slide and get the audience involved in a discussion. If the question involves more than one point of view, help the audience to bring out all views. Questions with right answers can be explored with the audience in a way that gets them to think. Questions using polling software serve to both engage the audience participants and provide assessment feedback to the presenter. Examples of online polling software that can be integrated into slideshows are

- Micropoll **http://www.micropoll.com/**
- Poll Daddy **http://www.polldaddy.com/**
- Poll Everwhere **http://www.polleverywhere.com/**
- Toluna **http://www.toluna.com/**

Presenters do not have to tell the audience everything; letting the group figure out something on their own will result in greater retention and perhaps bring out points that you alone would never have considered.

Including too much information on your slides will lead the audience to read the slide and not hear what you are saying. Following the guidelines in **Table 7-1**, if you want to use a quote, place it on the slide and give the audience time to read it; do not hurry them. When images are included on a slide, make them convey information that would otherwise be difficult to communicate, not just fulfill an obligation to have X number of images or add interest that may upstage you.

Lecture Replacement Model

The first question to ask in this instance is, "Should I use slides, create a narrative with illustrations, or use the Notes section of the slideshow software to expand on the points on the slides?" Start by thinking about the nature of the information that needs to be communicated. Can it be made meaningful with just bullet points? Information that is 100% memorization can perhaps be communicated in this fashion, but it is doubtful if learning beyond Bloom's first level of learning (knowledge) can be accommodated with bullet points alone.

Creating a narrative with illustrations and interaction for learning at the level of analysis or evaluation is the best approach. When on the web, this information can be linked to other sources that are integrated into the narrative with discussion or questions. Alternatively, if the information to be communicated is at a low level, using the Notes section of slideshow software allows a designer to provide more information than just bullet points. Probably, the best method is to look at each objective and match the method to the objective. If the objective depends on learning from animation, the slideshow can be converted to a video format.

Slideshows can also be designed for self-learning as interactive tutorials. Because the tutorial replaces a lecture, the learning objectives should be explicit to the viewer. Citations and references to resources used to create the slideshow should be included. If the topic is broad and complex, such as congestive heart failure or chronic renal failure, chunk the learning into smaller components, each with a separate slide presentation that might be viewed in 5 or 10 minutes. To make the slideshow interactive, include multiple-choice questions that allow the user to select an answer and receive feedback on the answer using slide branching. Finally, make a decision about how the slideshow should be viewed. Will the user need to have the slideshow software? Do you want the slideshow to be self-running in a kiosk mode? Depending on how the particular slideshow application is viewed, the designer has several options.

Presentation Slides

A presentation slide is an electronic visual component of a slideshow. A slideshow, when effectively designed, conveys key points made by the speaker to the audience participants. Slideshow software shares many similarities to word processing software. The primary difference from word processing software is that the slides in a slideshow are designed to be projected one at a time onto a screen for viewing by an audience.

Slideshow software is commonly bundled with other office suite software. Like other components of office suite software discussed in this textbook, there are numerous types of slideshow software. Examples include Microsoft® PowerPoint, OpenOffice.org® Impress, IBM Lotus Symphony® Presentation, Apple iWord Keynote®, and Google® Docs Presentation. PowerPoint® is a full-featured slideshow included in the proprietary Microsoft® Office. OpenOffice.org® and IBM Lotus Symphony® are free full-featured office suites that can be downloaded to the desktop computer. Google® Docs Presentations are an example of a free cloud computing application. For the purpose of this chapter, PowerPoint® 2010 is discussed with comparisons to OpenOffice.org® Impress and Google® Docs Presentation software.

Commercial presentation software packages include features that may not be available with free versions. Examples include galleries of graphic samples, the ability to import and export presentations from other software programs, the ability to create custom handouts and interactive help files that include videos and tutorials. If you do not have PowerPoint® software on your computer, begin learning with a free version to visualize slideshow features and functions.

The Presentation Software Window

The presentation software or slideshow window is similar in all application programs using a graphical

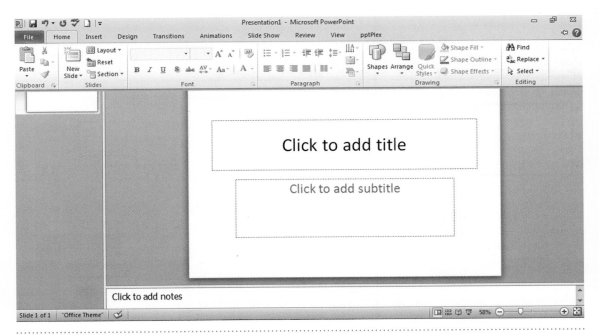

Figure 7-1 PowerPoint® 2010 menu.

user interface, which uses windows, icons, menus, and a mouse. The slideshow menu includes many of the same features of word processing menus, for example, font style and size options and ability to create tables and insert graphics and multimedia. Figures 7-1 through 7-3 compare the menus of three popular spreadsheet applications.

Basics of Slide Creation

With the understanding that slides, when properly designed and used, can be a useful aid in communications, we will look at some of the basics of slide creation. Each brand of presentation software, as well as specific versions within that brand, varies in how features are implemented, but all packages have more similarities than dissimilarities. They all have different views of the slides from the show view to handouts view. Additionally, they all operate with layers that are like pieces of transparent paper that are overlaid on each other, starting with the background layer, then the layout, and finally the content layer. In addition, they all treat images very similarly.

Views of the Slides

Slideshow creation programs allow users to look at their slides in many different ways. The view that audiences see is the Slideshow view. The default creation mode is called the Normal mode. In Normal view, the left-hand side of the screen has a column with thumbnail view of several slides. The right has a view of the slide under construction. PowerPoint® and Impress also provide an outline view. PowerPoint®, Impress, and Google® Docs Presentation have a Notes section that can be enlarged to enter notes and include a drawing menu with various drawing tools. The Normal, Outline, and Notes view allow the user to enter and edit information. The Slideshow view is used only for viewing, not editing.

The Slide Sorter view is useful for viewing many slides at once. The number of slides in the view can be changed using the Zoom feature. This view is especially useful for rearranging slides or for copying slides from one presentation to another. When slides are copied, the slides placed in the new environment will take on the style of the new

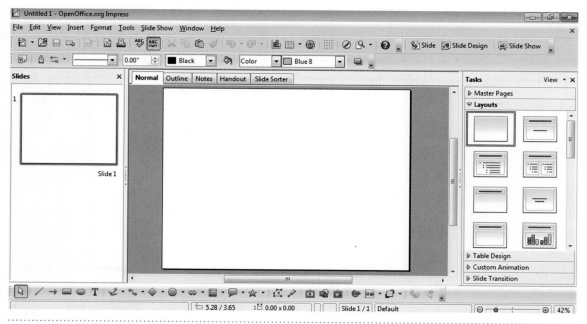

Figure 7-2 OpenOffice.org® Impress menu.

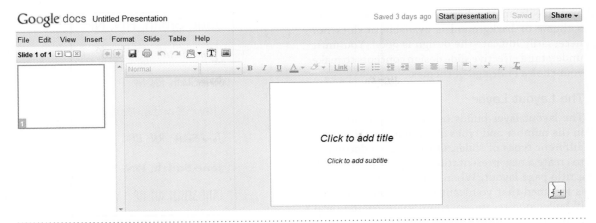

Figure 7-3 Google® Docs Presentation menu.

environment. Slides can be selected one by one by either clicking with the Ctrl key held down or as a contiguous group by selecting either the first or last slide or holding down the Shift key while left-clicking the slide at the other end. These principles of selecting objects either one by one or as a group is a Windows® principle that can be applied to objects on a graphical screen or while dragging files in Windows® Explorer.

The Background Layer

One of the first choices a user makes when creating a slide show is the background. This layer is often referred to as the master layer. Presentation programs all come with various background choices that the user can either accept or modify. More background designs are often available on the website of the vendor of the slide program, or you can create your own.

This layer is important because it keeps all the slides in the presentation consistent in looks. The background layer has place keepers for the title and subtitle for the title page, and for bullet points, graphics, and other items for subsequent pages. Because the place keepers are located in different places in different backgrounds, if you change the background layer after you have designed the slides, you need to check to be sure that all your slides are still intact.

When selecting a background, it is helpful to know the kind of lighting that will be used at the venue of the presentation. Borrowing from the days of 35-mm slides, when rooms were dark, many people still choose a dark background that is very appropriate with a dark room, but which allows content to get lost in a room that is lighted. Contrast is important, and having the background match the lighting in the room is a good principle to follow: light for light rooms and dark for dark rooms (Prost, n.d.).

To change the background for only one slide, right-click on a blank place in the slide and select Format Background from the menu. The Format Background menu provides the option of changing the background for all slides, too. Since consistency of colors and fonts is an essential component for good slide design, you should only change a slide background for an essential point of emphasis.

The Theme

A theme refers to a predesigned combination of background colors, font style, size, and color, and positions of the place keepers. Since consistency of colors is important in good slide design, slide-show software will change the theme for all slides by default. A gallery of themes is included with PowerPoint®. OpenOffice.org® Impress includes a gallery of themes called "Master Pages." Impress also includes backgrounds and components for users to design their own themes on the main menu. Google® Docs has a small gallery of themes available from the Format menu. Just because a theme or background is available, it does not necessarily indicate the design is good. You must understand effective slide design concepts to make your choice or design of themes.

The Layout Layer

The layout layer builds on the background layer in the number and types of placeholders it has for different types of slides. Opening up a document to create a new presentation will present you with a title page layout. When you add a new slide, it is assumed that you want to make bullet points. If bullet points are an appropriate communication method, use the Tab key to create a nested bullet point and the Shift+Tab to move back to a higher level just as in the outline feature of a word processor.

Explore some of the layouts beyond bullet points; they may very well be a better choice to communicate your information. For example, a layout has only a title on which you can place any objects you need to communicate your message; there are also blank pages and those that will allow placement of a graphic on one side and text on the other. Keep in mind that any graphics on your background layer will show through any of these layouts. To change the layout of a slide, click on Slide Layout in the Home menu or right-click on a blank spot on the slide (Tasks Layouts in Impress; can create new, not change in Google® Docs).

The Content Layer

Entering text or other objects is done on the top, or on the content layer. The layouts have boxes visible only in the Normal view that guide the user in placing text. All word processing principles apply to the content layer, including the use of the spell checker!

Text

A facet of presentation packages that can be both an advantage and a disadvantage is the number of fonts available, many of which are unsuitable for text in a projected visual. Even though one is always tempted to select a "jazzy" font in the hope that it will enliven a presentation, too often this choice creates readability problems. When selecting, remember that fonts can elicit an emotional response from the audience; thus, choose one that

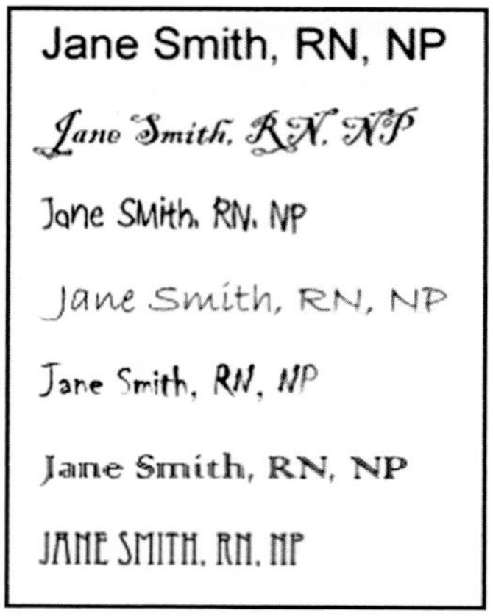

Jane Smith, RN, NP

Jane Smith, RN, NP

Jane SMith, RN, NP

Jane Smith, RN, NP

Jane Smith, RN, NP

Jane Smith, RN, NP

JANE SMITH, RN, NP

Which of the above fonts looks the most professional?

Figure 7-4 Different fonts elicit different emotional responses.

not only is visually appealing but also elicits the desired emotional response (see **Figure 7-4**).

The background templates for presentation programs have preselected fonts that are generally suitable for a presentation. These font styles can be changed either for an individual slide or for the entire presentation. However, changing a font after the completion of a presentation may disturb the layout on some slides because of the difference in size of the text in different fonts. For example, the font size in **Figure 7-4** is the same, yet you can see that the text is not all of the same size. The measurement unit for text size is points. Point size, as you can see, is not always an accurate guide. Some fonts at 12 points, despite being one sixth of an inch in height, are very difficult to read. This is because of what is called the x factor, or the height of lowercase letters. The smallest easily readable text size for computer slides is 24 points.

For projected visuals, use a sans-serif (i.e., without serifs) font such as Arial (**Figure 7-5**). This font follows the basic rule in choosing a display font – that the letters appear crisp and clean. Some fonts (e.g., Garamond and Times Roman) have projections from the type body called serifs that are fine strokes across the ends of the main strokes of a character. Serifs create softer edges to the characters, which add to readability on paper. When they are projected, however, they may have a tendency to look fuzzy.

Sans-serif font: Arial	Generally easier to read online
Serif font: Times New Roman	Easier to read in a print format

Figure 7-5 Comparison of sans-serif and serif fonts.

Identical to word processing, the appearance of text can be altered with **attributes** other than the type of font. Making a text boldface is one way to emphasize a point, as are underlining and italicizing. Italicizing, however, tends to make text more difficult to read; if it is used, give the audience more time to read the slide, a feature that can be used to advantage for a point that you wish the audience to read more slowly. If a point or points are emphasized with any of the above-mentioned attributes, be consistent throughout the presentation, that is, use the same attribute for the same type of information throughout.

When placing text on visuals, include only the essential elements of concepts. You should state ideas as though they were headlines. A visual is not meant to give the entire idea but rather to serve as a focus to assist the audience in following your presentation. Visuals can also be helpful to the presenter as a guide to the oral presentation.

Audiences should be able to get the point of the visual within the first 5 seconds after it appears. It is argued that a presenter should be quiet for those 5 seconds to allow the audience to grasp the point. To accomplish this, it is necessary to limit the text. One way to determine whether you have too much information on a visual image is to place the information on a 4 × 6 inches card and try to read it from a distance of about 5–6 feet. Never write the presentation on a series of slides that are intended to be read to the audience. Audience participants can read faster than a speaker can talk; therefore, they may become torn between reading ahead and listening. This practice leads the speaker to pay more attention to the slides than to the audience, and the audience to ignore the speaker.

Images

You should use pictures, graphs, or tables whenever it will illustrate better than words. Several sources of presentation quality images are available. One source of images in PowerPoint® is Clip art, or small drawings that have already been created; more clip art is available at Clip Art at Microsoft Office Online (OpenOffice. org® Impress and Google® Docs Presentation do not include sample images). Slideshow software packages provide a way to use an image file on your computer or to use a scanned image. Additionally, images that can be used for noncommercial presentations or in a class can be found on the web. Right-clicking on most images on the web will allow you to copy the image to the clipboard from where it can be placed in a presentation. You may even drag them into a Microsoft® program if using Internet Explorer® version 7+. If the presentation will be used commercially, check the copyright information[1] for any images, sound, or video. Many types of clip art and other web images have limitations on how they can be used. While buying a package of clip art, one should be sure to read the fine print before purchasing the software to be certain they are royalty free.

Images are placed on a slide the same way that they are inserted into a word processor; use the Insert tab and proceed from there. Dragging an image will easily move it to where you want it on the slide. To resize the image, you need to select the image, place the mouse pointer on either the square or the circle on its square border, and drag. Dragging when the mouse pointer is on a corner anchor will keep the proportions of the image; dragging while it is on a side will skew it.

Besides inserting images, slide creation packages provide drawing tools that allow one to create drawings, which can be used on slides or copied to another program. The drawing can also be saved, although in some presentation programs it will be saved as a slide. On a slide, images can be **cropped**; that is, the sides of the picture can be moved inwards to show only a smaller part of the image, a process that does not delete any of the images, but just makes the covered part invisible. If you want to use only a small portion of an image, use a screen clip tool.

---

1 Copyright and fair use are discussed in Chapter 25.

Occasionally, an image may not project well. To prevent this from marring a presentation, check the appearance of the slide in the Play or Show view before committing to using the visual in the presentation. Generally, if an image looks good in playback mode, it will project well, but if possible, check the image with the projection equipment and the version of the presentation software that will be used in the presentation.

Although using a scanned image, a clip art, or images from the Internet makes it possible to include very detailed pictures, these images can sometimes confuse the learner. For example, in presenting information about blood circulation through the heart, a detailed picture would probably not aid the understanding as much as a schematic drawing that only depicts the four chambers and the veins and arteries leading into and out of the heart.

When adding images, remember that the point of visuals is to communicate a message to the audience. Clip art can be appropriate if it emphasizes that message; when it is only used to enliven a slide, it seldom adds much to the presentation. A little variety, especially when it pertains to the message, can be helpful, but be careful not to distract the audience.

Charts and Tables

A table or chart is often clearer in communicating meaning than text. When using a table, one is limited in the size that can be created. Presentation software provides the ability to import a graph or data directly from a spreadsheet as well as the ability to copy and paste the graph. Be certain, when using either of these, that you use them to convey information accurately.[2] A detailed table or chart does not project well enough to be read by an audience. Instead, print the chart or table and use it as a handout.

Special Effects

Although one can add special effects independent of the visuals, those that are made possible by presentation software are often not available if the slides are put on the web, especially if they have been converted to a portable data file

---

2 The use of charts is discussed in Chapter 8.

(PDF) document. When doing a computer slideshow, especially when using special effects such as sound and video clips, the complete presentation should be tested on the equipment that will actually be used during the presentation itself. Moderation should be used with any special effects. Like images, special effects can be helpful to some messages, but they become distracting when used inappropriately. You want the audience paying attention to your message, not wondering what special effect they will be assaulted with next.

Color

Although color can be used to draw attention to a feature, it should never be used as the only distinguishing characteristic. As with fonts, it is important to be consistent in using color. When an audience grasps the implications of a given color, the visuals are more easily comprehended. Although the eye can perceive millions of colors, screen colors should be limited to about six, which is all that the eye can track in one glance (Faioloa & DeBloois, 1988).

Color, like text fonts, also has an emotional appeal (Paradi, 2009). Red can be seen as exciting or as the color of passion, excitement, or aggression, whereas green is usually interpreted as calming, health, or environment. The meaning of colors varies with cultures. Purple may indicate spirituality and physical and mental healing in some cultures; in others, it may symbolize mourning or wealth (Kyrnin, 2010).

Color combinations should be selected such that they are compatible but offer a contrast. When placed on top of one another, some colors, such as red on black, give a three-dimensional appearance that may make an object appear closer than the background. Additionally, objects sometimes appear larger in one color than in another. Reading accuracy is best when the colors used for background and text are on the opposite sides of the color wheel. Keep in mind that 9% of the population has some kind of color perception problem, usually a deficiency in discriminating red from green. When using a **gradient background** (Figure 7-6), it is imperative to use a very readable text and to test the slide for readability. Many of the backgrounds

Figure 7-6 A gradient background.

that are provided with presentation programs are gradient backgrounds.

Sound

Sound can be inserted into a slide with both PowerPoint® and Impress. Google® Docs Presentation allows only for sound associated with a YouTube video. PowerPoint® allows you to insert audio from a file, Clip Art sounds, or record narration (Insert > Audio). Narration can also be recorded from the Slide Show > Rehearse Timings menu. Of course, you will need a microphone that is built in or attached to the computer and a sound card to record narration. When recording narration, it is best to write out the information to be recorded first. You can use a separate word processing document or the Notes section.

There are pros and cons for using the narration-recording feature built into PowerPoint®. The pro is that recording is easily done using the narration menu. However, there are several cons. The narration menu does not allow for audio editing. If you want to make changes, you must rerecord the narration. The second con is that PowerPoint® may save records using an uncompressed file format. If you plan to save the file to a high-capacity flash drive or burn it to a CD, the file size may not be an issue. If you plan to use the file for podcasting and sharing with others on the Internet, the large file size would be a major issue and you should consider prerecording the narration and adding the audio to each slide.

There are a couple of software solutions that can be used to record narration with PowerPoint® and Impress. Both software applications allow

BOX 7-2 Sound File Formats

Sound File Formats Explanations
Uncompressed Formats
- WAV – used on Windows devices
- AIFF – used on Apple devices
- Au – designed by Sun Microsystems for use on LINUX systems

Compressed Formats
- MP3 – used on Apple devices
- WMA (Windows media audio) – a designed for Windows Media Player
- Ogg (Vorbis off) – open source sound format similar to MP3

Other
- MIDI (Musical instrument digital interface) for devices to play musical notes & rhythm

Source: Audio file formats explained in simple terms - http://www.makeuseof.com/tag/a-look-at-the-different-file-formats-available-part-1-audio/

you to import uncompressed and compressed file formats (see **Box 7-2**). On a Windows PC, you can use the Sound Recorder that is included in the Accessories folder. Narration recorded with Sound Recorder is saved as a WMA (Windows Media Audio) file, which is a compressed audio file. Sound Recorder saves to only the WMA file format and does not include a sound editor. A second solution is to use Audacity (http://audacity.sourceforge.net/), a free cross-platform sound recorder and editor. Audacity provides a means to export audio files in numerous formats. If you want to save the file in the MP3 format, be sure to download the LAME MP3 encoder. If the purpose of the slideshow is to allow users to view and listen to the slideshow on portable media player, record the narration saved in WMA or MP3 audio file formats. Since slideshows with graphics and compressed audio can still be quite large, creating several small 3- to 10-minute slideshows rather than one that runs 15–30 minutes.

Video

Video clips are equally easy to insert. PowerPoint® allows you to insert digital video from a file, from a website, or use Clip Art video. You can use digital video that was created using a camcorder, a webcam, or most digital cameras. PowerPoint® 2010 includes a video editor. Both PowerPoint® 2010 and Google® Docs Presentations allow you to insert video from YouTube; in fact, that is the only way you can add video with Google® Docs (Impress does not have a video insert feature). With PowerPoint®, you need to copy/paste the embed code from the YouTube website. With Google® Docs, you select the video from a YouTube search engine. Tutorials for inserting video from a website with PowerPoint® and Google® Docs can be downloaded from the textbook website.

If you are planning to add video for an oral presentation, limit its length to 45–60 seconds. Any length beyond that may distract the audience. As with sound, before using video in a presentation, check the equipment. Make a copy of the presentation without video available in case the video portion of the presentation equipment fails on the day of the presentation.

Transitions

A transition is the way a slide makes its entrance. Presentation programs have available many different types of transitions. Some cause a slide to fade in; some cause the slide to appear first at the center, and then expand the view; and yet others cause the slide to sweep across the screen. Transitions can be dramatic, enhance your message, or distract the audience. The best rule is to be consistent and use them sparingly. Avoid at all costs trying to dazzle the audience with multiple transitions.

Animation

The term animation, often referred to as Custom Animation, is used optimistically in the more well-known presentation software. Generally, animation takes the form of **progressive disclosure**, although some movement of objects is possible. Progressive disclosure is a technique in which one item at a time is revealed until all the items are displayed. When revealing bulleted points, those that have been discussed can be dimmed or converted to a different color while the current point takes center stage. The appearance of images can also be controlled with progressive disclosure. Additionally, using Custom Animation

you can make objects appear or disappear during a presentation.

Many options are available for how bulleted items will be progressively disclosed. Some of these options allow the item to slide in from any direction, bounce in, fade in, or even curve in. Like all options, this feature should be used judiciously. Animated gifs (a type of image files from the web that show movement) can be used with many presentation programs. If the animated gif will be on the screen for a long time, it is a good idea to cover it up after a given time period – something that can be set to happen automatically. Movement on a screen can become very distracting. If using animation, be sure to check the animation on the computer that will be used for the presentation before the actual presentation. Unless you are using your own computer, do not plan a presentation around the movement in the image.

A video simulation can be created with PowerPoint® using a combination of motion path animation and stop-motion, a technique where animation is simulated using a grouping of slides with progressive changes in the graphics (Stop Motion Works, 2008). Kuhlmann (2009) created a blog with the details about how to use this animation technique. The blog includes several narrated videos and graphics using the example, how to dissect a frog using a scalpel and scissors. This particular animation technique could be applied when creating nursing tutorials on topics like starting an IV (intravenous) infusion or inserting a nasogastric tube.

Speaker Notes

As mentioned earlier, speaker notes are entered as text in either the Normal or the Notes view. They can be very helpful to you as a speaker to remember what you had in mind when you created a given slide. Although the notes are not seen when the slide is presented, they are connected to the slide in a way that allows them to be printed for use. The notes can be used by participants during the presentation, for recording narration, or when rehearsing. If you use PowerPoint® and your computer is connected with two monitors, the Presenter's View can be used for a duplicate display, where the notes can be shown on the presenter's computer while the audience sees only the slides. To set up the Presenter's View, select Slide Show tab > Set Up Show.

Creating a Show that Allows for Nonlinear Presentations

When giving a presentation, you should be somewhat flexible. Some audiences may ask questions, others will not. A presenter can also misjudge the time needed for the presentation. By using the computer for the presentation, these eventualities can be handled easily. With PowerPoint® and Impress, the presenter can prepare a hidden slide to show if a specific question is asked or if time permits. PowerPoint® and Impress will allow you to advance (or retreat) to a specific slide when the number of the slide is typed followed by the Enter key. If using this feature, keep a list of slide numbers while presenting to allow you to show any slide in the presentation easily. Use the words "action settings" to search the Help contents to implement this feature.

Compatibility of Microsoft PowerPoint® Versions

Microsoft PowerPoint® 2010 is backward compatible with 2007. However, neither is compatible with earlier versions. Although you can open files created with earlier versions in the newer versions, you may lose some of the effects. If you create a slide show in Microsoft PowerPoint® 2010 or 2007, but need to show it in an earlier version, you will need to save it as an earlier version. Be certain, however, to look at it with the earlier version before show time. To avoid these problems, download one of the free viewers at http://www.microsoft.com/downloads/details.aspx?familyid=048dc840-14e1-467d-8dca-19d2a8fd7485&displaylang=en and place it along with the slides on the flash disk that you will use to transport the file.

The Presentation

Although creating good visuals is part of a good presentation, it does not alone ensure a good presentation. To achieve that, one needs to be sure that the visuals and the presentation reinforce

one another. To reach that goal, it is necessary to plan the visuals and the presentation together. A good presentation follows the rule of "tell 'em"; that is, give the audience an overview of what you will tell them, tell them or present the information, then tell them what you told them by presenting a summary of the important points. Keep in mind that people will remember no more than five points at the most (Feierman, 2010). One suggestion in preparation is to write out your conclusion slide first, emphasizing your most important points, and build the presentation around that.

Storyboarding

The concept of **storyboarding**[3] originated with film, but is valuable in any presentation that involves visuals. A storyboard is just a plan for the visuals. It forces you to organize your thoughts and allows you to assemble your ideas into a coherent presentation. As with all projects, planning saves time! With a presentation package, you can outline your thoughts using a title and text on a slide. After you complete the first draft, use the Slide Sorter view to look at the presentation as a whole. This will help you to see where a rearrangement of slides would be helpful and make it easy to rearrange the order by dragging the slides to a new position. When you think things are in the correct order, go back to each slide and develop it into a meaningful communication tool. Expect to switch between the Slide Sorter view and the Design view many times while working on the actual visuals!

Creating Handouts

As stated earlier, rarely is a printed copy of slides alone, even with space for the audience to take notes, a worthwhile reason to destroy trees. Preparing a word-processed document using your notes and inserting appropriate illustrations is a much better use of paper. Complex information cannot be reduced to bullet points! To keep the audience's attention focused on your message, rather than reading the handout, provide the handouts after the presentation.

---

3 Storyboarding has another meaning for standardized terminologies. In that context it means describing a case and pulling out the important points.

Transferring to the Web

Although it is actually possible to transfer a computer slideshow designed for an oral presentation to the web as an html or a PDF file, it may not be a good idea. Remember that every medium is different, and the difference between a live slide presentation and a stand-alone web presentation is huge. On the web, not only do the slides have to answer all questions, but they also need to be complete with all the information that readers need to have. Few slideshows meet this requirement. Bullet points do not! If the information needs to be posted to the web, think about how it will be best presented. You may need to add audio to the slides, or a narrative text with embedded illustration(s) for those who learn best by reading, or both. You may want to review educational principles in Chapter 22 when considering posting something to the web.

The Actual Presentation

The moment has arrived; you have rehearsed the presentation until you know it cold. Despite this, hundreds of butterflies are tap dancing in your stomach, and you are wondering, "Will I remember what to say?" The title slide opens; you give the audience 5 seconds to read it – an eternity when you are the speaker (count, e.g., from 1001 to 1005.). Then you read the title, and give the audience an icebreaker, maybe an anecdote about yourself or how you prepared for the talk, something light. Knowing that you want the audience to pay attention to the presentation, and not read ahead, you tell them that you will distribute handouts after the presentation. Your handouts are well thought out, are a narrative with occasional images, and will provide the reader with information months or years after your presentation is complete. With the introduction out of the way, you open the next slide and start to communicate your message.

By the third or fourth slide, the butterflies are ending their dance, and the points on the slide remind you of the information you need to communicate. You make eye contact with various people in the audience, and the presentation is going smoothly – you are beginning to enjoy it. A question is asked that requires you to diverge

from the planned presentation. If this is a point that you thought might come up, you switch to your nonlinear presentation. You can even take the time to jot down the present slide number to return to it before you do this – audiences do not mind. If the question is something not planned for, but to which you need to respond, tap the letter "w" to make the screen white, or "b" to make it black, answer the question, tap Enter to bring back the screen, and go on with the presentation. Then it is over! You made it – you are receiving thanks from the audience for sharing your knowledge.

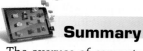 **Summary**

The overuse of computer slides has led some to believe that we are dummying down the message. Some believe that using bullet points forces presenters to "mutilate data beyond comprehension" (Thompson, 2003, December 14) and allows the speakers to not tie their information together. Nonetheless, they are a ubiquitous feature of most presentations. Avoiding these pitfalls means giving attention to the real message and using visuals to aid the message, not substitute for it. Even a small presentation given to a group of colleagues will be better received if well thought-out visuals are used. As a nurse progresses up the career ladder, knowing how to make presentations that convey a solid message is an aid to advancement.

Although there are several vendors of presentation packages, including OpenOffice.org® Impress and Google® Docs Presentations, they all have similarities. They facilitate the job of creating good visuals by providing a constant background for the visual and tailored layouts. Any of these things, however, can be modified at any time. Although there are many options available, such as adding images or special effects such as sound, video clips, animation, and progressive disclosure, they should only be used to enhance the message. In the same vein, select colors, fonts, backgrounds, and layouts to extend a message.

All presentations need planning and organizing. Handouts should reflect what the audience should take away from the presentation, not just the slides. Several issues are involved in creating a presentation: identifying key points, planning the visuals to be a partner, using good visual techniques, and preparing useful handout, and finally, rehearsing!

APPLICATIONS AND COMPETENCIES

1. Compare the slides of the Gettysburg Address with the actual address at http://www.norvig.com/Gettysburg/index.htm. Do the slides convey the actual message?

2. Watch a presentation using computer slides and analyze the slides for
   a. Whether the text is readable.
      i. Whether the background color shows text to best advantage.
      ii. Whether the font used is easily readable.
   b. Whether the content is enhanced or lost with the slides.
   c. Whether the presenter uses the visuals as a partner.
      i. Slides do not upstage the presenter.
      ii. Slides do not present a message different than what is being said.
      iii. Slides make the presentation easy or difficult to follow.
      iv. Images add to the message.
   d. Whether the slides could be used as handouts that would aid your understanding a month from today.

3. Open a presentation program, change the layout to blank, and insert one of the shapes or an illustration. Practice resizing it with the mouse. Try resizing it using a corner of the graphic, and then try resizing using one of the sides of the graphic. What happens to the image in each instance?

4. Experiment with different backgrounds and decide why or why not they would be effective in a specific type of presentation such as a research report, a class project, or a welcome speech. If they are not appropriate, how could they be modified to be more useful for your purpose?

5. How could you use a cartoon in a visual? What are some of the things that you would have to consider if you choose to do so?

6. You need to teach a class about a physiological process. On the web, find some illustrations that could be used in a noncommercial setting and insert it into a slide. (Search for "images of 'the process.")

7. Create a three- or four-slide presentation on a topic of your choice.
   a. Add a background and use more than the title and bullet layouts.
   b. Use progressive disclosure (Search for animation to learn how).
   c. Add an image.
   d. Add a video or sound.
   e. Use the principles of good design mentioned in Table 7-1.
   f. Create a handout that would be appropriate for an audience reference 6 months after the presentation.

8. Identify one or two new presentation skills that you would like to master. Create a 4- to 5-slide presentation employing the new skills. Self-assess yourself and summarize what lessons you learned.

REFERENCES

Carter, R. (2003). Teaching visual design principles for computer science students. *Computer Science Education, 13*(1), 67.

Collins Memorial Library. (2009, November 24). *Visual literacy*. Retrieved June 19, 2010, from http://alacarte.pugetsound.edu/subject-guide/30

Faioloa, T., & DeBloois, M. L. (1988). Designing a visual factors-based screen interface: The new role of the graphic technologist. *Educational Technology, 28*(8), 12–21.

Feierman, A. (2010). The art of communicating effectively: Tips from all aspects of pulling off the successful presentation! Retrieved April 9, 2010, from http://www.presentation-pointers.com/showarticle/articleid/64/

Felten, P. (2008, November/December). Visual literacy. *Change: The magazine of higher education, 40*, 60–64.

Kuhlmann, T. (2009, January 13). *Why dissecting an e-learning course will improve your skills*. Retrieved April 8, 2010, from http://www.articulate.com/rapid-elearning/why-dissecting-an-e-learning-course-will-improve-your-skills/

Kyrnin, J. (2010). *Visual color symbolism chart by culture*. Retrieved April 8, 2010, from http://webdesign.about.com/od/colorcharts/l/bl_colorculture.htm

Paradi, D. (2009). *Choosing colors for your presentation slides*. Retrieved April 8, 2010, from http://www.indezine.com/ideas/prescolors.html

Prost, J. (n.d.). *8 Mistakes made when presenting with PowerPoint® and how to correct them*. Retrieved April 8, 2010, from http://www.frippandassociates.com/artprost2_faa.html

Springfield, E. (2007). PowerPoint pedagogy: two usages, two pedagogical styles. *CIN: Computers, Informatics, Nursing, 25*(1), 15–20.

Stop Motion Works. (2008). *Frequently asked questions*. Retrieved June 19, 2010, from http://www.stopmotion-works.com/faq.htm

Thompson, C. (2003, December 14). Power Point makes you dumb. *The New York Times*. Retrieved July 30, 2011 from, http://www.nytimes.com/2003/12/14/magazine/14POWER.html

CHAPTER 8

Spreadsheets: Making Numbers Talk

Objectives

After studying this chapter, you will be able to:

▶ Identify differences between spreadsheet and word processing software.

▶ Use computer conventions to create mathematical formulas to analyze data.

▶ Develop basic competencies for use of spreadsheets to calculate numbers.

▶ Explore functions specific to spreadsheets.

▶ Design an appropriate chart to communicate a specific point.

Key Terms

Active Cell	External Reference
Area Chart	Freeze
Bar Chart	Line Chart
Cell	Pie Chart
Cell Address	Spreadsheet
Cell Range	Stacked Chart
Chart	Workbook
Column	Worksheet
Combo Box	

Numbers are often part of the information nurses need to manage. Computers, together with specialized software, provide freedom from the drudgery of manual calculations and make managing numerical information much easier. The first **spreadsheet** program, developed in 1979, greatly accelerated the acceptance of computers in the business world (Mattessich, n.d.). What is most remarkable about the first spreadsheet is that the design is so functional that few changes have been made to it over the years. Instead, many more features have been added, such as **charts** and components, which make it easier to enter formulas. The program design is intuitive and has remarkable similarities in spreadsheet vendor products.

Spreadsheets are not the only type of application program that simplifies managing numerical data. Other programs that assist in the management of numbers include financial management programs, tax preparation programs, and statistical software. Financial management software allows checkbooks to be balanced and the management of a personal budget, including providing help in categorizing items to facilitate tax preparation. Tax preparation software uses data from a financial manager or spreadsheet to create and print tax returns. Statistical software is designed with preset statistical functions to analyze data. While there are a variety of number-crunching software packages available, this chapter focuses specifically on spreadsheet competencies and applications.

Uses of Spreadsheets in Nursing

Spreadsheet skills are invaluable to all nurses. Because spreadsheet applications have many similarities with word processing and calculators, with a little practice, the use is almost intuitive. Spreadsheets can be used to capture postal and e-mail mailing addresses for use with the mail merge function in word processing. In clinical care, spreadsheets are used to monitor and analyze care processes and advents. Examples include adverse drug events (ADEs), sepsis, stroke, ventilator acquired pneumonia (VAP), and bloodstream infection (BSI). They are also used for administrative functions such as staff scheduling, time and attendance records, calculating nursing hours per patient day (NHPPD) for staffing decisions, budget analysis, and Failure Mode Event Analysis (FMEA). In the education setting, spreadsheets can be used for test item analysis, to calculate course grades, calculate grade point averages (GPAs), and prepare research data for statistical analysis.

Every student and practicing nurse should demonstrate basic spreadsheet competencies (see **Box 8-1**). Nursing educators, managers, and administrators should demonstrate intermediate or advanced spreadsheet competencies. Nursing informatics specialists should demonstrate advanced spreadsheet competencies because they are expected to develop new nursing applications and teach others.

As with any skill, learning the correct method is essential to maximize productivity and success. It is always easier to learn to do something correct than to unlearn and relearn. It is important to understand how to best display data for crunching, how to use the built-in powerful calculating functions, and how to display analyzed data with reports and charts. A self-assessment skills list

BOX 8-1 Essential Spreadsheet Competencies for Nurses

- Conditional formatting
- Copy data to other cells
- Create formulas using words
- Create charts (graphs) from data
- Create pivot tables
- Date/time
- Design a spreadsheet for efficient use
- Financial functions
- Format cell data using font styles, font sizes, and color
- Format cells using backgrounds and borders
- Insert graphics
- Manage text
- Merge cells
- Password protect
- Resize a cell
- Sort data
- Statistical functions
- Use templates
- Use wizards to guide you through complex calculation operations

and samples of spreadsheets with features used in this chapter can be downloaded from the textbook website at http://dlthede.net/Informatics/Informatics.html.

Nursing has lessons to learn from the business community. When searching the web on the topic of spreadsheets, results include articles that associate spreadsheets with "heaven" or "hell," which should alert us that while spreadsheets offer benefits, they might be associated with risks. The European Spreadsheet Risks Interest Group maintains a website with spreadsheet "horror stories" that include overpayment in thousands and millions of dollars to a miscalculated $5 million dollar deficit (European Spreadsheet Risks Interest Group, 2010). Panko (2008) reported that 20%–40% of all financial spreadsheets have errors. While it might be human to error, nursing needs to understand the nature of the errors and utilize solutions to mitigate them.

There are three types of quantitative errors in spreadsheets, which occur when data in a **cell** or formulas are incorrect: typing, logic, and omission errors (Panko, 2008). A typing error is a data entry error or a formula that addresses an incorrect cell. A logic error is a bug in the program, such as a cell formula, that causes it to work incorrectly. An omission error occurs when essential data are missing.

Tips for Better Spreadsheets

There is no doubt that spreadsheets have value in nursing practice, administration, and education settings. We need to leverage what we know from business and apply the knowledge in nursing by developing and using spreadsheets correctly. Follow the tips given in **Table 8-1**, take advantage of the built-in calculating capabilities of spreadsheet software, and avoid using a spreadsheet like a word processing document with tables.

As when working with other computer applications, it is important that the user be able to identify the problem to be solved first. Designing a spreadsheet that effectively communicates does not happen by adopting a casual approach. Spreadsheets should be carefully designed and organized to make them useful.

When beginning to use spreadsheet software, it's often most efficient to first draft out the design with a pencil and piece of paper. The paper and pencil design will assist the user to identify **columns** and field names and formulas. The computer should be used to calculate values from cell data. If the data need to be sorted for analysis, make sure that only one value is entered into the cell. For example, if you need to sort by last name, create separate headers for the first name and the last name. Increase the row height rather than leaving blank rows between data. This tip is particularly important when formulas are with a range of cells.

It is best to use a separate **worksheet** for each table in a **workbook**. If you design a worksheet to include more than one table, make sure that if you need to insert a new row or column, it does not change or corrupt other parts of the spreadsheet data. Name each spreadsheet to identify the purpose or topic.

While designing a complex spreadsheet or workbook, include a table of contents with

Table 8-1 Spreadsheet Skills

Basic Spreadsheet Skills

- Design a simple table
- Name a worksheet tab
- Apply a template
- Insert a new worksheet
- Create a simple formula (Add, subtract, multiply, divide)
- Use basic functions (SUM, AVG, MIN, MAX, COUNT)
- Resize columns and rows to display data
- Sort cell data
- Use search and replace
- Freeze rows and columns
- Use automatic data entry
- Use spell-check
- Use a chart
- Save a workbook
- Print a worksheet

Intermediate Spreadsheet Skills

- Customize the spreadsheet menu
- Design spreadsheets using data validation features
- Customize spreadsheets using conditional formatting features
- Use simple data analysis tools
- Create/modify a chart

- Import/export data in text format
- Link spreadsheet data from other sources
- Apply principles of effective spreadsheet design
- Create complex formulas
- Create/modify a pivot table
- Create a form
- Create a report
- Link and embed tables into word processing documents
- Use data protection
- Password protect a workbook
- Demonstrate competency using two spreadsheet applications
- Share/collaborate with others on a spreadsheet design

Advanced Spreadsheet Skills

- Create formulas that use logical and statistical operations
- Use advanced data analysis tools
- Create a dashboard
- Create a new template
- Create macros
- Create new functions using Visual Basic expressions
- Demonstrate competency using more than two spreadsheet applications

hyperlinks to the appropriate sections. Include explanations of any logic or assumptions on the first worksheet. Provide clear labels and instructions that all users will be able to understand. Other users rarely have the same viewpoint as the creator. When using a complex formula, especially one that references the results of other formulas, carefully test the formula with simple numbers. This is particularly important if the spreadsheet will be used with many different values (see **Table 8-2**).

Spreadsheets

A spreadsheet is an electronic version of a table consisting of a grid of rectangles (cells) arranged in columns and rows. Each cell can be uniquely formatted to display numbers, text data, and formulas. Spreadsheet software is similar to word processing tables, but spreadsheets are specifically designed to crunch numbers and analyze data. Competency in the effective use of spreadsheets is an invaluable skill for nurses and other healthcare providers. Anytime numbers need to be crunched and analyzed, the electronic spreadsheet is the software of choice.

Spreadsheet software, like word processing, is commonly bundled with other office software for purchase. Examples include Microsoft Excel, which is included with Microsoft Office, and Quattro Pro, which is included with Corel WordPerfect Office. Numerous free versions are also available such as OpenOffice.org Calc™ and Google Docs Spreadsheets™. What is the difference? Commercial software bundles are usually integrated, meaning that the various office products work together seamlessly. Vendor spreadsheet software includes features that may not be available in free versions. Examples include graphics samples, print formatting with custom headers and footers, formula wizards, dragging a cell data to copy data to other cells, and tools to expedite creating a series of numbers or words, such as the months of a year or a series of quarters of a year.

If you don't have spreadsheet software on your computer, begin learning with a free version to visualize the features and functions. **Figures 8-1** through **8-3** compare the menus of three popular spreadsheet

Table 8-2 Rules for Creating and Using Spreadsheets

1. Begin the spreadsheet development process with a clear purpose and carefully thought out design.
2. Use data validation tools with input and error messages for cells that might have repeating data.
3. Use conditional formatting tools to create assist users to interpret data.
4. Use charts to assist users to interpret aggregate data.
5. Treat the spreadsheet development as you would treat a major written paper, with footnotes and a bibliography (Ansari & Block, 2008)
6. Use formulas rather than entering precalculated numbers into cells to avoid data entry errors.
7. Check, recheck, and validate each formula and formula output.
8. If a formula needs to be reused, copy and paste the formula that has been validated and then recheck the results.
9. Write out and analyze complex formulas prior to entering them into cells.
10. Use cell protection to prevent users from inadvertently changing a formula or data.
11. If the spreadsheet is "mission critical," meaning it affects the financial or patient outcome bottom line, there should be explicit guidelines, rules, and testing policies for developers.
12. Be a smart consumer of spreadsheet information. Scrutinize the quality of the spreadsheet data; do not assume that it is correct.

applications. Microsoft Excel 2010 is discussed in this chapter with comparisons to free applications, OpenOffice.org Calc™ and Google Docs™.

The Spreadsheet Window

The spreadsheet window is similar in all application programs associated with a graphical user interface (GUI), which uses windows, icons, menus, and a mouse. At first glance, the main difference between a spreadsheet and a word processor seems to be that the document screen in a spreadsheet is only a table. Many of the features used in word processing are the same, such as file and edit. Some important differences, however, are,

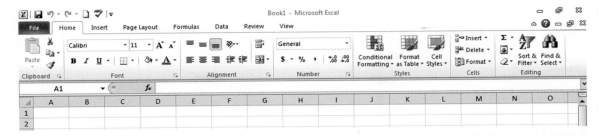

Figure 8-1 Excel 2010 ribbon menu (Microsoft product screen shot reprinted with permission from Microsoft Corporation).

for instance, formula and chart functions built into the menu options. By default, each spreadsheet file is actually a workbook containing one or more spreadsheets. The tabs at the bottom of each spreadsheet allow the user to provide meaningful names and differentiate between multiple spreadsheets in a workbook.

Spreadsheet Basics

The vocabulary of spreadsheets is simple. A cell refers to the rectangles in the table. A row is a horizontal group of cells, and a column is a vertical group of cells. **Cell address** is the name given to a cell, and it is derived from the letter of the column and the row where it is located (similar to a street map). The **active cell** is analogous to the insertion point in other programs. It is the location where any information entered will be placed. Besides being visible in the table by bold lines, the contents of the active cell are mirrored in the formula bar. A **cell range** is a group of contiguous cells, for example, B11:D13. The range of A2–B3 (**Figure 8-4**) would be expressed as A2:B3 or A2:B3; the formatting depends on the spreadsheet application publisher. Users can name ranges of cells and use this

name in commands instead of the cell location to create formulas.

Two terms that may, at first, seem confusing are worksheet and workbook. A worksheet refers to one spreadsheet, whereas a workbook consists of one or more worksheets. Workbooks allow the user to have many worksheets open at the same time. Worksheets are identified by editing the tab name at the bottom of the sheet. The user can change the order of the sheets, add, or delete sheets from a workbook. The number of columns and rows allowed in a worksheet varies according to the spreadsheet software publisher and version. For example, the size of a Microsoft 2010 Excel worksheet can be 16,384 columns by 1,048,576 rows for a 32-bit computer; the file size for a 64-bit computer is much larger (Decision Models, n.d.). In contrast, OpenOffice.org 3x Calc™ will allow for 1,024 columns by 65,536 rows with a maximum of 67,108,864 cells per sheet (OpenOffice.org Wiki Contributors, 2008). Google Docs Spreadsheets™ will allow for 256 columns or 200,000 cells or up to 100 sheets, with no limit on rows (Google, 2010). The size of a spreadsheet should be designed for optimum use.

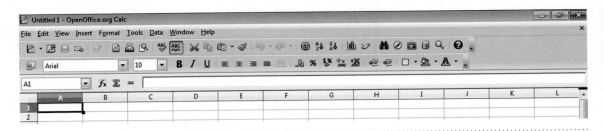

Figure 8-2 Open office.org Calc menu.

Google docs Unsaved spreadsheet   Save now   Share ▾

File   Edit   View   Insert   Format   Form   Tools   Help

🖶 ⟲ ⟳ 🖌▾ $ % 123▾   10pt▾   **B** Aʙᴄ **A**▾ ▦▾ ⊞▾   ☰▾ ▦ ⇥   Σ ▾

Formula: [   ] ⊠

	A	B	C	D	E	F	G
1							
2							

Figure 8-3 Google Docs Spreadsheet menu.

When working on a project, keep the spreadsheet size as small as possible. A worksheet with data in 256 columns may be more manageable if it is broken down into several worksheets. The content of a spreadsheet is not confined to a table. Microsoft Excel™, OpenOffice.org Calc™, and Google Docs Spreadsheets™ provide ways to include pictures (graphics). They provide a means to create charts (graphs) from data for analysis purposes. You have heard that a "picture is worth a thousand words"; charts can paint an impressive picture to assist in the analysis of complex data.

Excel and Calc spreadsheets designed for reuse can be saved as a template files (not available in Google Docs). A template provides a pattern of content for software applications. Excel is packaged with predesigned templates. Both Excel and Calc provide a means to download template files from their websites. For more information on the use of spreadsheet templates, check the software Help menu.

Spreadsheet Power

The real power of a spreadsheet is derived not only from the ability to organize and edit data but also from its ability to recalculate when a number in a referenced cell is changed. A referenced cell is the cell that is referred to in a formula. For example, in **Figure 8-5**, the cell F15 contains a formula. It references the cells C15, D15, and E15. Any changes made to the contents of either of these cells will cause the number in cell F15 to change. Notice that the formula is visible in the formula bar.

Formulas

A spreadsheet formula is a mathematical equation that provides instructions to the computer for processing the data. Formulas can be either relative

Spreadsheet Basics

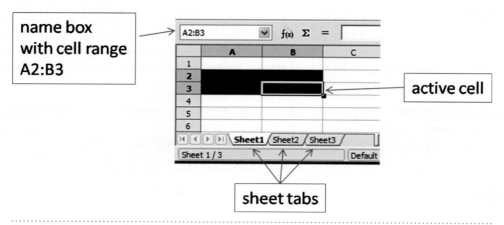

name box with cell range A2:B3

active cell

sheet tabs

Figure 8-4 Spreadsheet basics.

	A	B	C	D	E
1	Employee #	Hourly Salary	% Raise	Salary Increase	New Salary
2	4567	20	0.03	=B2*C2	=D2+B2
3	7865	22.3	0.03	=B3*C3	=D3+B3
4	9876	21.5	0.03	=B4*C4	=D4+B4

Figure 8-5 Relative formula.

or absolute. When a relative formula is copied to another cell or range of cells, it adjusts to the move by changing the referenced cells (see **Figure 8-5**). An absolute formula uses the dollar sign ($) to signify that it will retain the specific column and/or row cell when moved. For example, in **Figure 8-6** $F references column F; $2 references row 2; and F2 references the specific cell address F2.

The equals (V) sign is commonly used to indicate a formula in a cell. Errors can creep into a spreadsheet when entering formulas into cells. To prevent cell address entry errors, use the point and click method for entering cell addresses. After entering the symbol to indicate formula entry, put the mouse pointer on the first cell addressed by the formula and then click with the left mouse button.

The cell address will appear in the formula. Enter the necessary mathematical symbol, then point and click the next cell needed. When the formula is complete, tap the enter key. The formulas viewed in **Figures 8-5 and 8-6** demonstrate the symbols used to enter the formulas.

An expression refers to the algebraic formula that contains symbols and characters to complete the formula operation. Functions refer to common predesigned formulas used in spreadsheet applications. Both commercial and free spreadsheet softwares include functions to expedite the accuracy of the formula entry. Arguments are the specific values required by the formula. In computer terms, argument means the data that the user furnishes to calculate the formula value. To

Absolute Formulas

Values View

	A	B	C	D	E	F
1	Employee	Hourly Sal	Salary Inc	New Salary		% Raise
2	4567	20.00	0.60	20.60		3%
3	7865	22.30	0.67	22.97		
4	9876	21.50	0.65	22.15		

Formulas View

Press CTRL + ` (grave accent)

	A	B	C	D	E	F
1	Employee #	Hourly Salary	Salary Increase	New Salary		% Raise
2	4567	20	=B2*F2	=C2+B2		0.03
3	7865	22.3	=B3*F2	=C3+B3		
4	9876	21.5	=B4*F2	=C4+B4		

In this example, the % salary increase is 3% and noted in cell F2. The formula in C2 was copied to C3 and C4. The formulas in Column C reference the value in F2 using the $ sign (F2).

C2 is an example of an absolute formula. When the position of the cell that contains the formula changed, the absolute reference to cell F2 remained the same.

Figure 8-6 Absolute formula.

view or hide the formula view in the spreadsheet, tap the tilde key (~).

Creating Formulas

The principles and symbols of formula calculation are identical in all computer programs. The characters used to communicate that the computer should perform a specific calculation, such as multiplying or dividing, are not necessarily the same as used on paper. An asterisk (*) is used to denote multiplication; if the familiar x is used, the computer would be unable to distinguish the character "x" from a multiplication symbol. A computer formula for the multiplication of 5 times 50 is 5*50.

The forward slash (/) located under the question mark key is used to denote division. To use the computer to divide 10 by 5, the formula is 10/5. The results of division are not always a whole number (integer). Microsoft formats numbers as "general" in decimal format by default. To format a number as an integer (whole number), format the number with 0 decimal places. The integer is a rounded number, whereas a decimal provides accuracy to the specified decimal point.

The caret (∧) symbol located over the number 6 on the keyboard is used to represent an exponent (raises a number to another power). Calculation of body mass index (BMI) is an example for use of exponents in nursing. The formula for BMI when using pounds and inches is to divide the weight in pounds by height in inches squared and multiplied by a conversion factor of 703 (Centers for Disease Control and Prevention, 2009). For instance, if a person weighed 150 pounds and was 65 inches tall, the formula = ((150/65∧2)*703) would result in a BMI of 24.96. As seen in the formula for calculating a BMI, parentheses are used to identify and nest calculations. As in all mathematical formulas, the number of leading parentheses must balance the number of trailing ones.

Order of Mathematical Operations

In performing arithmetical computations, computers follow the order of operations for mathematics. Three factors determine the order in which mathematical procedures will be performed:

- The kind of computation required.
- Nesting or the placement of an expression within parentheses.
- Left-to-right placement of the expressions in the command.

The computer arbitrarily performs operations in the following order:

- Anything in parentheses is performed first.
- Exponentiation is done next.
- Multiplication and division follow in left-to-right manner.
- Addition and subtraction are performed last.

These rules, which follow algebraic protocols, are used in all application packages that allow calculations, including spreadsheets, statistical packages, and databases. When using the acronym (or mnemonic) given in **Table 8-3**, remember that when two mathematical operations are equal, such as multiplication and division, the calculations are completed from left to right. There are a number of excellent review sites about the order of mathematical operations. An example is the About.com: Mathematics website at http://math.about.com/library/weekly/aa040502a.htm (Russell, 2010).

Other Spreadsheet Features

Besides the normal functions that can be applied across the board in most application programs, such as changing the font style and size or changing the color of the background or text, spreadsheets possess some unique characteristics that require specialized functions.

Table 8-3 Acronym to Remember the Order in Which Computers Performs Calculations

Please	Excuse	My	Dear	Aunt	Sally
		Equal (Left to Right)		Equal (Left to Right)	
Parentheses	Exponentiation	Multiplication	Division	Addition	Subtraction

Formatting Cells

Spreadsheet software provides a number of ways to format cells. Contents in a spreadsheet cell are of two different types: numbers and text. Numbers, depending on what they reference, can be formatted in different ways and cell in a spreadsheet can be uniquely formatted. The default in all programs is no specific formatting; however, the cell will default to the type of data that is entered.

Format the font or content alignment of a particular cell using Excel or Calc by right clicking on any cell to view the options (use Format menu in Google Docs). To format a group of cells, row, or column, highlight the section using the mouse and right-click to use the format menu. The same technique can be used to merge two or more cells and to change the color or the border of a cell or range of cells.

Excel, Calc, and Google Docs Spreadsheets™ allow for the following formatting: rounded or decimal, financial, scientific (exponents), currency, percent, date, and time. To format a cell data type, right-click on the cell in Excel and Calc or click on the cell and then the 123 menu in Google Docs. Excel includes custom formatting for zip codes, telephone numbers, and social security numbers.

A rule of thumb is that a "number" is anything that could be used in a calculation, for example, added, subtracted, multiplied, or divided. Therefore, numbers used for medical record numbers (MRNs), admission numbers, zip codes, social security numbers, and telephones numbers can be formatted as text, since they are not used for calculations.

Spreadsheet software considers date and time as numbers, since they can be used in calculation. In fact, if you enter a date such as "4/3" (with no parentheses) into a cell, the spreadsheet will automatically display the data as a date defaulting to the current year. To enter a time, enter it using a colon, for example, 4:00 a.m. or 14:00. If you want to change the way that the date or time is displayed, right-click on the cell(s) and use the format menu (123 menu in Google Docs).

Spreadsheet software will also allow you to enter a date and time into a single cell. This data and time feature is very useful in nursing, when calculating a time difference for an event that begins one day and ends the next. For example, the visit time of a patient admitted to the emergency department (ED) on 1/2/2012 at 10:00 p.m. and discharged at 1:25 a.m. the next day. When you enter a formula calculating the difference into a cell, the calculation will appear as a number. In the example of ED's length of stay (LOS), the calculation is 0.14236111111. To get the decimal number to display as a time difference, format the cell as short time, meaning only hours and minutes. The reformatted cell will display 3:25.

Conditional formatting is a powerful spreadsheet feature that is often overlooked. Conditional formatting allows for a simple, quick analysis of data. For example, if you had a spreadsheet to monitor grades in a program of study, you could use a conditional format to highlight the font or background of a cell for a grade of "D" or "C" in a course. The conditional formatting feature is not case sensitive, meaning that the software will recognize both a "d" and "D" when entered. Conditional formatting can be used for numbers and text. An example of the conditional formatting display is shown in **Figure 8-7**.

Text to Columns

Consider this scenario. You created a spreadsheet with the names and addresses for all of the employees on your nursing unit before reading the section "Tips for Better Spreadsheets" in this chapter. The problem is that you included the first name and the last name in a single cell. You are unable to sort the names by last name because you entered the first name before the last name. Is there a solution? Yes, you can use the text to columns feature to separate the names. Simply insert a blank column next to the column that you want to change. If the name includes a middle name of initial, insert two blank columns. In the Excel and Calc menus, select Data > Text to Columns, and follow the wizard to make the changes (possible but not easily done in Google Docs). The text to columns feature is extremely useful for analyzing data that have been queried and extracted from a hospital information system. Data imported from other information systems may have complex data in column row cells, which need to be in separate row cells for analysis or an import into database software.

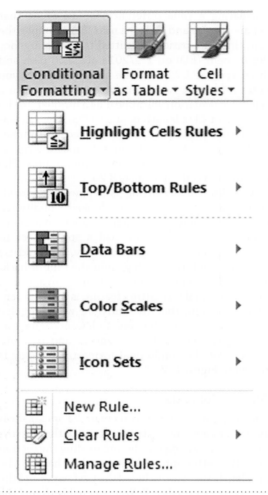

Figure 8-7 Conditional formatting.

Freezing Rows and Columns

When there are more rows or columns in a spreadsheet than can be viewed on a computer screen, it is difficult to know what information is represented. Spreadsheets provide a way to **freeze** either the rows or columns or both. The term "freeze" means that you can keep one part of the spreadsheet visible while scrolling to another area on the spreadsheet. Google Docs allows the user to freeze rows or columns, but not both at the same time, whereas Excel and Calc allow for both. This feature is important for accurate data entry when the data refer to a heading in a column or row. To learn how to accomplish this task, use the Help menu. The name of the feature varies slightly according to the publisher but usually refers to "freezing" rows, windows, or panes.

Using Automatic Data Entry

Sometimes spreadsheet design requires sequential data such as numbering 1–10, days of the week, months of the year, or quarters in the year. Excel includes a feature that allows the user to make a few entries and then have the computer complete the series (not available in Calc or Google Docs). This feature works with a series of skipped numbers such as 2, 4, and 6. The term for this feature varies according to the software publisher but usually refers to "fill."

Data Validation

Excel, Calc, and Google Docs Spreadsheets™ include features to assure that valid or correct data are entered into the cells. Data validation can be as simple as defining a rule for the spreadsheet software to verify that the text entered is the required number, text, or date. You can enter instructions and error messages to guide the user and ensure correct data entry.

Both Excel and Calc allow you to create a list to validate data that will appear from a drop-down menu (**combo box**). For example, you can limit data entry for a column heading of gender to two choices, male and female. To validate data with Excel, select Data Validation from the Data menu (Data > Validity in Calc, Tools > Data Validation in Google Docs). You can enter the values separated by a comma in Excel or point to the location of the unique values list.

As you learn new spreadsheet features, you may find that you have designed spreadsheets that include repeating data, such as unit names, or state abbreviations but with no data validation. You note typos, and so some data are omitted in error when you attempt to sort the data. You can use the Remove Duplicates feature in Excel (not an option with Calc or Google Docs) to create a unique list. Highlight the column with the repeating values and copy that data to another place on the spreadsheet or a new worksheet. With the data still highlighted, select Remove Duplicates from the Data menu. A listing of unique values will appear. Go back to the data validation menu and point to the location of the unique values to use for a validation list.

Forms

Excel and Google Docs softwares provide other spreadsheet features such as a Forms view of data (Not a menu option in Calc). Database features in spreadsheet software may not as robust as a true database, but they are functional for many simple operations. The forms view is not a default menu in Excel. To make it visible, click on the down arrow Quick Access menu > More Commands > Choose Commands from: Commands Not in the Ribbon > Forms. Excel will automatically attempt to determine the data used for the form.

The form feature in Google Docs is very different from Excel. The Google Docs form is not created from data in a spreadsheet; data entered in a Google Docs form create a spreadsheet. To create the form, click on Forms in the menu. A wizard guides you to create form questions and answers. Answers can be text, multiple choice, paragraph, list, check boxes, grid, or scale. The finalized form can be e-mailed or shared. The Google Docs Spreadsheet could be used for an online quiz or survey. Data that is entered into the form are aggregated on a spreadsheet.

Formatting a Spreadsheet for Use in a Database

A spreadsheet, or any range of cells, can be easily imported to most database software for more extensive data manipulation. Any data that are structured in a table listing format, whether a spreadsheet, a table in a word processor, a statistical package, or database, can be easily passed (imported/exported) from program to program. A listing format contains only column heading and the associated data.

Linking Cells and Worksheets From Other Sources

There are times when a user will want to reference (link) to a cell or a cell range in a spreadsheet located in another workbook. Use of an **external reference** to the workbook is less prone to error than trying to check the other sheet, copying the

value(s), and entering it into a formula. When cells are linked, if the value is changed in the linked cell, the change will be visible in the worksheet containing the referenced cell. Entire spreadsheet tables can often be linked in companion office software such as the word processor or database software. This feature is easy to use and is a very powerful tool to ensure data consistency. Use the spreadsheet Help menu for more information on this feature.

Data Protection and Security

In healthcare we often use spreadsheets to provide data protection and/or security. Data protection refers to locking cells to prevent the user from changing the cell value. This feature is very helpful to prevent accidental changes to cell text, numbers, or formulas. Security means that the user has to provide a password(s) to view and/or to edit the spreadsheet. Free online spreadsheets such as Google Docs Spreadsheets™ should not be used to store confidential data since the spreadsheets are stored online in a public domain. Use spreadsheets to enter confidential data only if there is a way to provide security. Only password-protected spreadsheets should be stored on public domains such as the shared healthcare agency or educational agency shared server. Check with your Health Insurance Portability and Accountability Act (HIPAA) security official if you have any questions about the security of your file(s).

Charts

A chart (graph), terminology used in spreadsheet software, is a graphical presentation of a set of numbers. They provide a means to interpret the relationships of quantitative and categorical data in a table (Few, 2004c). Charts are used to visually communicate meaning that can be difficult to understand from a raw set of numbers. That said, research has shown that the ability to interpret charts is strongly affected by the viewer's expertise and understanding of the purposes of the different chart formats (Ancker, Senathirajah, Kukafka, & Starren, 2006). Charts should be created, keeping in mind the user's ability to interpret the data. Distracting designs, fonts, and lines should be avoided.

Creating charts using a computer is relatively easy. A computer can create any type of chart, whether or not it communicates anything meaningful. Using charts appropriately involves knowing the message that needs to be communicated and selecting the type of chart that best accomplishes the goal accurately and efficiently (Few, 2004a). Although spreadsheets, word processors, databases, and presentation packages all facilitate the creation of charts, spreadsheets have the most powerful chart creation tools. Perhaps the biggest plus for creating charts in a spreadsheet is that if the numbers in the cells used to create the chart change, the chart automatically reflects the change.

Chart Basics

To construct a meaningful chart, it is necessary to understand the chart basics vocabulary. **Table 8-4** and **Figure 8-8** can assist with the task. It is important to use the types of charts appropriately. The chart should assist the viewer to understand data, but not ever distort the meaning of data.

Types of Charts

Spreadsheets take the drudgery out of creating charts. There are options for creating many different types of charts, including making them three dimensional, changing the orientation for the horizontal (x) axis to that of a vertical (y) axis position, and combinations of all these factors.

Each of these features can emphasize objects in the chart that may misconstrue the true meaning of the base numbers. Compare the two- and three-dimensional charts in **Figure 8-7**. In which does the figure for February stand out? Most of these variations can be used in all charts. When using these variations, be certain that they reflect the point that needs to be communicated. As a user of charts, be aware that these distortions exist. Although spreadsheet software provides many different chart types including pie, column, bar, line, stock, surface, doughnut, bubble, and radar; this section will focus on the four main types of charts: pie chart, column chart, bar chart, and **line chart**.

Pie Charts. **Pie charts**, classified as **area charts**, are used to communicate the proportion of various items in relation to the whole. They are "part-to-whole" charts designed to show percentages, not amounts. A pie chart may also be used to show a proportional relationship between a slice and a whole. To clearly communicate percentages, use six or less sectors. Color and shading of the pie sectors should emphasize the chart message (Duffy & Jacobsen, 2005). **Figure 8-9** illustrates different types of pie charts. All of the pie charts represent the same data, percentage of patient falls by shift. Notice how the exploded view chart looks

Table 8-4 Chart Basics	
Term	**Meaning**
x axis	The horizontal axis (line) of a bar, line, or scatter graph, generally represents time values, categories, or division.
y axis	The vertical axis (line) of a bar, line, or scatter graph, most often used to represent amounts.
Data	Numbers without meaning; those that are unprocessed.
Data series or set	A set of numbers that will be represented in the chart, usually on y axis, or a group of items that will be represented on x axis.
Axis title	The title for the information displayed on an axis.
Graph title	A description of the graph used to title the graph.
Legend	The visual representation of each item in the data series. Maybe a color, shape, or both.
Data point	The point where a number is plotted. It is the intersection of its value on the x and y axes.
Data labels	Labels that show the actual value of specific data, or the data points.
Two-dimensional chart	A chart that represents data on the x and y axes.
Three-dimensional chart	A chart that adds a third axis, referred to as the z axis. Can be very misleading, use only when there is need to communicate an added dimension.

2–Dimensional Chart

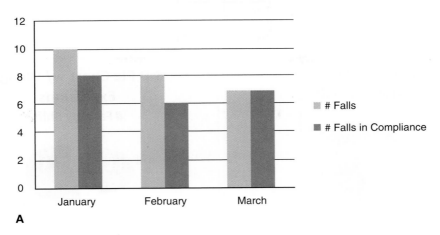

A

3–Dimensional Chart

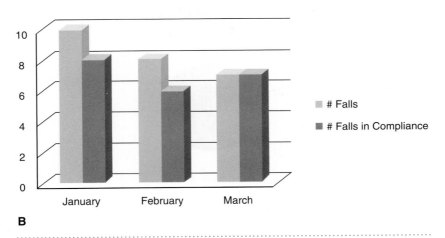

B

Figure 8-8 A,B: Two-and three-dimensional charts.

larger than the three-dimensional and simple pie views. The explosion view can distort the viewer's perception of the data. Without the percent values, it is difficult to determine which slice is largest in both the exploded wedge and the three-dimensional pie. Few (2004c), a well-known expert on information design, advises us to refrain from using pie charts, because our visual perception does not allow us to easily perceive the quantitative differences in the slices of the pie. If you believe that a pie chart does best depict your data, be sure to limit the number of slices and include percentages as labels.

Column and Bar Charts. Column charts are used to depict changes over time or to show comparisons. Placing amounts on the y axis meets the common expectation that an upward movement is associated with an increase in amount, whereas a downward movement indicates a decrease. When the horizontal x axis is used for the passage of time, the most effective form of communications is achieved when the earliest time is placed on the left and time elapses to the right. To prevent a distortion of value, it is best if the longitudinal y axis starts with a zero. If the y axis does not start with a zero, include an explanation in the chart.

Shift:	# Falls
Day	15
Eve	13
Night	25

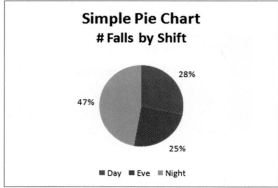

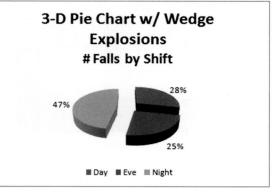

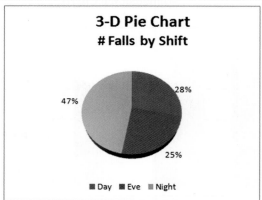

Figure 8-9 Pie charts.

If the **bar chart** is displayed in color, use bright and darker colors to emphasize key data. When possible, avoid the use of fill patterns, as they can distract from the data. If all of the bars are bright and/or dark, the message will be confusing (Few, 2004b)

Bar charts are generally associated with comparisons of amounts. They can be displayed either vertically or horizontally. A clustered bar chart provides a visual comparison of amounts for a given time period, such as a month or quarter. **Figure 8-10** depicts several types of bar charts that compare the percentage of all smokers, using 2-year intervals between 1997 and 2008. The simple bar chart compares smoking habit changes for all smokers. The clustered bar chart compares the percentage of smokers, aged 18 and older by income. It is clear that while the percentage of smokers decreased over the 12-year period, the percentages of persons in the poor and near poor income continue to be higher than nonpoor.

A stacked bar chart, like the pie chart, is classified as a part-to-whole chart. Percentage is usually the unit of measurement. In a **stacked chart**, each data set uses as its baseline the previous data set. For a 100% stacked chart, each data set is a percentage of the whole. Stacked bar charts can be used to compare differences in groups of clustered data, but they are not as easily understood as a simple bar chart or clustered bar chart.

	1997-1999	2000-2002	2003-2005	2006-2008
All	23.9%	22.7%	21.0%	20.3%
Poor	32.4%	30.7%	28.4%	28.8%
Near poor	29.7%	28.4%	26.0%	25.6%
Nonpoor	21.2%	20.2%	18.7%	17.7%

Source: http://205.207.175.93/HDI/TableViewer/tableView.aspx

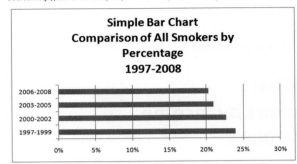

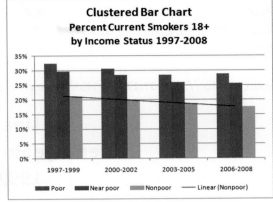

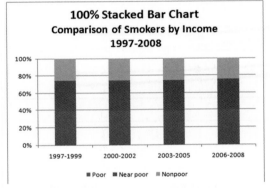

Figure 8-10 Bar charts.

Line Charts. There are two types of line charts, a line chart that communicates changes in data over an elapsed time period and one that shows trends in data. When communicating changes in data over time, lines are used to connect individual data points. **Figure 8-11** shows a line chart comparison of same smoking data used for the bar charts. When comparing more than one data set, consider using line colors or point markers to show differences in the data.

A chart with a trendline can be used for two-dimensional line or unstacked bar or column charts. A trendline can be straight, for example, showing a linear regression, or curved, such as a bell curve. The default trendline in Excel is linear regression. To learn more about trendlines in Excel, tap the F1 key for Help and type "trendline."

Sparklines. Sparklines are "simple, word-sized" graphics first described by Tufte (2004), a renowned American statistician and professor. Sparklines are a new chart feature introduced with Excel 2010. It is available as a free add-in for earlier versions of Excel from http://sparklines-excel.blogspot.com/. Sparklines show comparisons of data from individual data criteria in a single cell. **Figure 8-12** is an example of sparkline depicting glucose value variances for a hypothetical patient on an insulin drip. In other words, you could view data trends using a single spreadsheet cell. Sparklines could be used in the electronic medical record (EMR) to visually display variances in laboratory or vital signs. Like other standard chart features, you can add markers to depict specific periods.

	1997-1999	2000-2002	2003-2005	2006-2008
All	23.9	22.7	21	20.3
Poor	32.4	30.7	28.4	28.8
Near poor	29.7	28.4	26	25.6
Nonpoor	21.2	20.2	18.7	17.7

Source: http://205.207.175.93/HDI/TableViewer/tableView.aspx

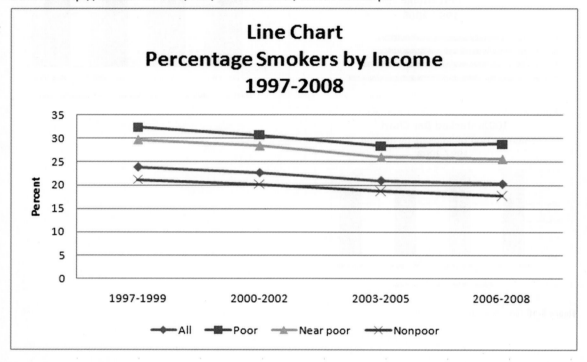

Figure 8-11 Line charts.

Creating the Chart

Computer applications programs allow the creation of many types of charts. The first task in creating any chart is to select the cells that represent the data to be charted. After the appropriate cells have been selected, click on the chart tool and select the types of chart that will best represent those data. Excel provides a preview of how the chart will look before the final selection is made. If you are using free software and do not like the chart, delete it and begin again. Both commercial and free spreadsheet softwares provide a way to create and edit the chart title and legends. Spreadsheet software includes the ability to modify fonts and colors used in the chart. Once you have clicked on the icon to indicate that you have finished, the chart appears on the spreadsheet. A completed chart can always be resized, moved, or edited (see **Figure 8-13**). To edit the chart, right-click the object that needs to be changed to obtain a drop-down menu of choices.

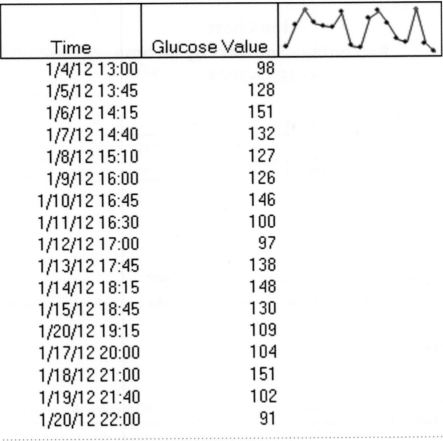

Time	Glucose Value	
1/4/12 13:00	98	
1/5/12 13:45	128	
1/6/12 14:15	151	
1/7/12 14:40	132	
1/8/12 15:10	127	
1/9/12 16:00	126	
1/10/12 16:45	146	
1/11/12 16:30	100	
1/12/12 17:00	97	
1/13/12 17:45	138	
1/14/12 18:15	148	
1/15/12 18:45	130	
1/20/12 19:15	109	
1/17/12 20:00	104	
1/18/12 21:00	151	
1/19/12 21:40	102	
1/20/12 22:00	91	

Figure 8-12 Sparkline example.

Dashboards

Dashboards provide a snapshot of trends from multiple data resources. Both Excel and Google Docs provide a way to display dashboards. A dashboard, similar to the control panel instruments used to drive a car, allows the user to visualize data from multiple sources to guide decision-making. Excel dashboards use charts and/or sparklines. Creating an executive looking dashboard may require advanced Excel skills. Camoes (2007) designed an easy-to-read tutorial on the topic at http://www.excelcharts.com/blog/how-to-create-an-excel-dashboard/.

A dashboard can be created in Google Docs Spreadsheets™ using charts and/or the gadget feature. Unlike Excel, Google Docs allows you to create a "gauge" using spreadsheet data. Select Insert > Gadget > Gauges from the menu, provide a name for the gauge, and data ranges for green, yellow, and red ranges, and then either select Apply and Close or Apply to view the gauges.

Pivot Tables and Pivot Charts

The term pivot tables is a good description of the function. A pivot table is used to pivot the data to view data in an aggregated format. It is an interactive view of aggregate data that allows the user to analyze the data in different views. It is especially useful to analyze very large data sets. For example,

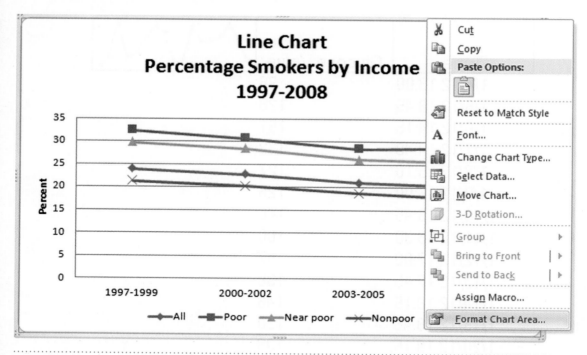

Figure 8-13 Editing a chart.

you could analyze numbers of infections by nursing unit, and then drill down to infection types. Data for pivot tables must be in the list formatting, which means that the data are organized using only column headings, which is not the standard way to display data in Excel. To create a Pivot Chart in Excel, choose Pivot Chart from the Insert menu (Data > DataPilot in Calc; not available in Google Docs). You may find the tutorial designed by French (2010) at http://spreadsheets.about.com/ helpful to learn this powerful data analysis tool.

Excel 2010 includes two new pivot table features, Slicer and PowerPivot. Slicer is an enhanced pivot table filter. PowerPivot is a free add-in that can be downloaded for use with Excel. It allows for integration of data from multiple sources and improved manipulation of very large data sets. To learn more about Excel features, including pivot tables and slicer, go to http://office.microsoft.com/en-us/excel/excel-skills-builderlearn-how-to-create-spreadsheets-and-workbooks-use-formulas-and-perform-data-analysis-FX102592909.aspx.

Pivot charts are charts that are generated from data sets. Pivot charts look identical to bar charts discussed earlier in this chapter. The difference is that pivot charts are interactive and allow you to filter the data and analyze differences. To develop skills with pivot tables and pivot charts, consider downloading one of the many data sets available from The Health Resources and Services Administration (HRSA) at http://datawarehouse.hrsa.gov/customizereports.aspx.

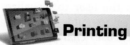 **Printing**

The printing function in Excel provides a number of alternatives. In Excel, if the printout is in multiple pages and there are columns and row headers, set up the pages to print both on every page using Page Layout > Print Titles (Format > Print Ranges in Calc). You can create page headers and footers from the Page Setup menu. Use print preview to set up and view the printout, especially if you are printing a large data set. Excel, Calc, and Google Docs allow you to print out a single spreadsheet or the entire workbook.

The Google Docs print function is slightly different. Google Docs Spreadsheets™ can be printed only to PDF or HTML file formats. To learn more about the print function in Google Docs, use the Help menu.

Summary

Spreadsheet programs have taken much of the drudgery out of calculations and deserve a place on every nurse's desktop. Nurses should all demonstrate essential spreadsheet competencies (see **Box 8-1**). Spreadsheets have much in common with other office application programs including word processing, presentation software, and database software. The basic structure in a spreadsheet is a table, with a column of numbers on the left side and a row of letters at the top. The letters and numbers provide a way for each cell to have a corresponding name. The principles and symbols for formula calculation are the same as all other computer programs.

Although spreadsheet software can make managing numbers easier, if spreadsheets are not carefully designed and used, they can create a great amount of misinformation. Users should use spreadsheets to perform calculations from data. Formulas should be scrutinized for accuracy to avoid misinterpretation of data. As with all computer use, nurses should use common sense when interpreting computer numerical and chart outputs; this includes understanding the assumptions that various models use. Given thoughtful use, spreadsheet software that calculates numbers can assist all healthcare professionals in managing information. Data protection and security features are especially important in healthcare. Users should be knowledgeable about how to protect cell data and formulas from inadvertent changes. Users should also know how to password protect confidential spreadsheet information. Spreadsheet competencies and skills are valuable assets for all nurses.

APPLICATIONS AND COMPETENCIES

1. Identify at least three differences between a word processor and a spreadsheet.

2. Use spreadsheet software to calculate a baby's gestational age at the time of the mother's prenatal visit. Copy the column headers and dates below. Type the formula in C2 and then copy the formula to cells C3:C5.

	A	B	C
1	Prenatal Checkup Date	Baby's Due Date	Baby's Gestational Age (Weeks)
2	1/1/2009	9/1/2009	=((B2–A2)/7)
3	9/2/2009	2/20/2010	
4	4/1/2010	9/1/2010	
5	1/20/2011	2/20/2011	

3. Calculate the BMI using the data in the table below. Copy the column headers and data below. Type the formula in C2 and then copy the formula to cells C3:C4. Format the BMI to one decimal point.

	A	B	C
1	Weight (pounds)	Height (inches)	BMI
2	67	110	=(B2/(A2)^2)*703
3	70	150	
4	75	200	

4. In a spreadsheet, create a formula to calculate the number of intravenous (IV) drops per minute when the IV tubing is calibrated to 20 drops per minute, the time for the infusion is 8 hours, and the total volume to be infused in 1,000 mL.

5. Calculate the ages of patients on admission to your nursing unit. Copy the data from the table below onto a spreadsheet. Format the cells C2:C4 as YY. Type the formula in C2 and then copy the formula to cells C3:C4. Type the formula noted in cell C5 to determine the average age of the patients.

	A	**B**	**C**
1	Admission Date	Birth Date	Age
2	9/16/2010	11/10/1985	=B2−C2
3	4/5/2011	11/17/1971	
4	4/27/2011	4/27/1950	
5			= AVERAGE(D2:D4)

6. You recently implemented a new intervention to prevent patient falls. Copy the data noted below on a spreadsheet. Use the Fill feature to create columns with the months of the year. Design a chart to show the changes in the number of falls. Use the Help feature when necessary.

	Jan	**Feb**	**Mar**	**Apr**	**May**	**Jun**
Number of Falls	25	31	35	10	12	30

7. You want to show the percentage of all visits to your emergency department during each shift. For the month of May, you had 600 visits on the day shift, 1,000 visits on the evening shift, and 400 visits on the night shift. Design a chart depicting the data.

8. You want to show the changes in the number of pounds gained each month of pregnancy from month 3 to month 5. You have the average number of pounds gained in each month (2 pounds in month 3, 5 pounds in month 5) for 300 pregnant women. Design a chart to show the changes over time.

9. Identify two new spreadsheet skills that you want to learn. Practice the skills and then self-assess what you learned. How easy or difficult was the experience?

REFERENCES

Ancker, J. S., Senathirajah, Y., Kukafka, R., & Starren, J. B. (2006). Design features of graphs in health risk communication: A systematic review. *Journal of the American Medical Informatics Association*, 13(6), 608–618.

Ansari, S., & Block, R. (2008, May 14). *Spreadsheet "worst practices."* Retrieved July 30, 2011, from http://cfo.com/article.cfm/11288290/1/c_2984312?f=search

Camoes, J. (2007). *How to create a dashboard in Excel.* Retrieved April 16, 2010, from http://www.excelcharts.com/blog/how-to-create-an-excel-dashboard/

Centers for Disease Control and Prevention. (2009, July 26). *About BMI for adults.* Retrieved April 9, 2010, from http://www.cdc.gov/nccdphp/dnpa/bmi/adult_BMI/about_adult_BMI.htm

Decision Models. (n.d.). *Excel memory limits.* Retrieved April 12, 2010, from http://www.decisionmodels.com/memlimitsc.htm

Duffy, M. E., & Jacobsen, B. S. (2005). *Organizing and displaying data. Statistical methods for health care research* (5th ed., pp. 16–27). Philadelphia: Lippincott Williams & Wilkins.

European Spreadsheet Risks Interest Group. (2010). *EuSpRIG original horror stories.* Retrieved April 12, 2010, from http://www.eusprig.org/stories.htm

Few, S. (2004a). Common mistakes in data presentation. *Perceptual Edge.* Retrieved July 30, 2011, from http://www.perceptualedge.com/articles/ie/data_presentation.pdf

Few, S. (2004b). Elegance through simplicity. *Intelligent Enterprise*, 7(15), 35.

Few, S. (2004c). *Show me the numbers: Designing tables and graphs to enlighten* (1st ed.). Oakland, CA: Analytics Press.

French, T. (2010, April 9). *Excel 2007 pivot table tutorial.* Retrieved April 16, 2010, from http://spreadsheets.about.com/

Google. (2010). *Size limits: Getting to know Google Docs – Google Docs help.* Retrieved April 9, 2010, from http://docs.google.com/support/bin/answer.py?hl=en&answer=37603

Mattessich, R. (n.d.). *Spreadsheet: Its first computerization (1961–1964).* Retrieved July 30, 2011, from http://www.j-walk.com/ss/history/spreadsh.htm

OpenOffice.org Wiki Contributors. (2008, November 26). *What's the maximum number of rows and cells for a spreadsheet file.* Retrieved April 9, 2010, from http://wiki.services.openoffice.org/wiki/Documentation/FAQ/Calc/Miscellaneous/What%27s_the_maximum_number_of_rows_and_cells_for_a_spreadsheet_file%3F

Panko, R. (2008, May). *What we know about spreadsheet errors.* Retrieved April 12, 2010, from http://panko.shidler.hawaii.edu/SSR/Mypapers/whatknow.htm

Russell, D. (2010). *Order of operations.* Retrieved April 9, 2010, from http://math.about.com/library/weekly/aa040502a.htm

Tufte, E. (2004, May 27). *Sparklines: Theory and practice.* Retrieved April 22, 2010, from http://www.edwardtufte.com/bboard/q-and-a-fetch-msg?msg_id=0001OR&topic_id=1

CHAPTER 9

Databases: Creating Information From Data

Objectives

After studying this chapter, you will be able to:

- ▶ *Describe a database.*
- ▶ *Use Boolean tools in searching a database.*
- ▶ *Explain the role of databases in improving patient care.*
- ▶ *Describe methods of discovering knowledge in both relational and large databases.*
- ▶ *Differentiate methods of viewing data in a database.*
- ▶ *List some steps in creating a database.*

Key Terms

Aggregated Data
Atomic Level
Attribute
Boolean Logic
Child Table
Data
Database
Database Management System (DBMS)
Database Model
Data Mining
Data Warehouse
Entity
Field
Flat Database
Form

Hierarchical Database
Knowledge Discovery in Databases (KDD)
Lookup table
Network Model
Query
Record
Relational Database
Report
Scope Creep
Secondary Data Use
Sort
Structured Query Language (SQL)
Table
Virtual

Does hospitalization of patients whose diabetes is newly diagnosed prevent future hospitalizations for diabetic complications? Do certain approaches to pain management shorten hospital stays? Is the incidence of preventable illnesses lower in children whose mothers received postpartum visits from a nurse? The literature can provide some answers to these questions, but true evidence-based practice requires clinical **data**. The clinical data that could be used in conjunction with the literature to answer these questions are recorded, but are very infrequently used to answer these questions.

This chapter provides an overview of **database** concepts as well as software that is available for the personal computer. The first part of the chapter discusses how you can use Microsoft® Access to find meaning in clinical data. The second part of the chapter discusses concepts common to all databases including web-based databases and the electronic medical **record**.

Uses of Databases in Nursing

As nurses, we are concerned with improving patient care. In the past, we have looked to experience and experts to help us in this area. The electronic patient record, however, allows us to add patient documentation data to this equation. Although a paper medical record provides a wonderful individualized record for one patient, because most of the data lack structure, retrieving the data is difficult, which makes comparisons with similar patients exceedingly difficult. As a result, we are not aware of the richness that lies embedded in patient care data.

When we think about documentation and patient care, we think of one patient. We carefully record patient care information in the proper place in the patient's record and use it to care for this patient at this time. Any thought of using data aggregated[1] from many medical records to answer clinical questions and gain a broader understanding of a condition is generally discarded because the location of most of the data in paper records makes this type of data retrieval difficult.

The electronic patient record, however, changes this equation. With electronic records, we can retrieve data that will provide answers to the questions at the beginning of this chapter and many others. Given the long history of the use of paper records, it is not surprising that even when data are in an electronic format and could be used to answer clinical questions, we are unaware of the possibilities for using these data. This picture will change only when we gain an understanding of how a database works and how one can manipulate data to provide information. This chapter will provide a beginning view of the principles behind storing, retrieving, and manipulating data that could be used to create knowledge from data in an electronic record. Experimenting with, and expanding on, these ideas in a real database will further your ability to employ evidence-based care.

---

1 Aggregated data are discussed in detail in Chapter 1.

Learning about databases will also guide you to see a use for databases in the many **reports** that modern healthcare demands. To illustrate some of the potential, we will present an example of a current use for a database in nursing. As you know, as of October 1, 2008, the Center for Medicare & Medicaid Services (CMS) no longer paid for care for patients with nosocomial urinary tract infections (UTIs). To be a successful hospital, it will be necessary to develop and implement protocols to keep these infections to a bare minimum. To do this requires data. UTIs are sometimes caused by indwelling catheters and may or may not be associated with the agency that treats them.

For our example, let's pretend that your agency is a tertiary care hospital and admits patients from other hospitals, long-term care facilities, and directly from home. Your nurse manager wants to find out how many patients arrive with UTIs and how many develop them after they arrive. She assigns you to do a monthly report with these data.

To do this, you will need to track the data. You could do this with a word processing **table**, a spreadsheet, or a **relational database**. The tool that you use to create this database, however, determines the answers that you can get from the data. A word processing table will allow you to count instances as will a spreadsheet. A spreadsheet will also permit some searching and reordering of the records. Both of these, because there may be the same data entered in more than one place, may lead to errors. A well-designed relational database, however, not only prevents data duplication but also provides maximum searching with multiple variables. It allows processed, selected data to be exported into a spreadsheet, a statistical package, or word processing software and to be presented in many different ways – all without reentering a piece of data more than once. Experience has also shown you that once the data are collected and reported, the nurse manager will want more answers. Therefore, you decide that the best choice is a relational database.

Tips for Database Design

You should have mastered basic spreadsheet skills prior to embarking on database design. Many of the spreadsheet functions, such as formula construction, sorting, and data formatting, can be applied to database design. In fact, a spreadsheet is an example of a "**flat database**." Database software provides a way to link two or more related tables.

Although a database table looks like a spreadsheet formatted as a list with only column headings, there are distinct differences. A spreadsheet is good for crunching numbers, while a database is best for analyzing data that may include numbers (Microsoft, 2010b). Data in a spreadsheet are displayed in different cells, whereas data in a database are connected with records (rows) and **fields** (columns). Spreadsheet workbooks can contain a variety of unrelated worksheets, but the objects in a database are related.

There are three important steps in the database design process. The first is to identify the purpose. Consider what data will be included as well as data that will be excluded. The next is to identify the questions or queries that **aggregated data** can answer. Third is to make a listing of data requirements. It is often helpful to write out the purpose, questions, and data requirements before constructing the database. A common error that novices make when designing a clinical database is to replicate the patient record. The database should contain only the data that will be aggregated for analysis.

A database is a collection of related objects: tables, **forms**, queries, and reports. Tables contain all of the data. Forms are used to add, edit, and view data from a table or **query**. A query is used to ask questions of one or more related tables or other queries. The output of a query looks identical to a table. A report is used to display data from a data or query.

Another common mistake is to design forms before the table design is complete. Since a form is based upon a table or query, the tables must be designed first and include at least some sample data. Designing a database without data is a plan for disaster. It is impossible to see that the components are working correctly.

The relationship of tables in a database is important. You will see the terms, "one-to-many" and "parent/child" used. For example, one patient can have many hospital admissions and one hospital admission can include bed locations on many nursing units. Each record (row) of data table has a unique key to identify the location. Each table is identified with a primary key. The primary key is represented in the related table as a foreign key to link related tables.

Use of consistent terminology (naming conventions) is required for efficient database design. This applies to column headings and names of tables, forms, queries, and reports. Consistent terminology also applies primary and foreign keys. For example, the medical record number (MRN) is the primary key of a patient table and represented as the foreign key in the admission table. If the term MRN is used for the patient table's primary key, MRN, not MR#, should be used for the foreign key in the admission table.

Databases use normalization rules to organize, aggregate, and display data (Microsoft, 2010a). Each table represents a category of data, and each field should be unique to the database. For example, the patient's name is located in the patient table, but no other table. The keys allow the name to be associated with the data in related tables.

Learning the correct database design method is essential to maximize productivity and success. It is important to understand how to best design the database for efficient analysis, how to use the built-in powerful query functions, and how to display analyzed data with reports and charts. Samples of databases with features used in this chapter can be downloaded from the textbook website at http://dlthede.net/Informatics/Informatics.html.

 Databases

A database is a collection of data that are organized or structured in such a way that data from it are retrievable, singly or as a group. Paper databases are organized, or indexed, by only one bit of data (e.g., a name in the phone book). With indexing only on the last name field, finding a name connected with a number is not an easy process. When a phone book is in an electronic format, one can easily either re-sort the records by number or request that the database produce the record that contains the desired number. Electronic databases, however, have many more capabilities than reordering records or finding an isolated piece of information.

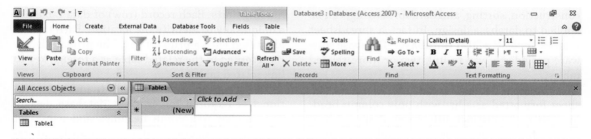

Figure 9-1 Microsoft Access menu.

With the pervasiveness of technology in our lives, we used electronic databases daily, often without awareness. E-mail software, mobile phone applications, digital libraries, and Internet search engines are all electronic databases. Many of the principles discussed in this chapter apply to all types of databases.

There are two main categories of database software, enterprise and desktop. Enterprise database software is used to deploy databases across an organization. Examples of enterprise software include Oracle® and Microsoft® SQL Server®. Examples of desktop database software include Microsoft® Access and OpenOffice.org Base. Google Docs does not include a database, although another cloud computing application, Zoho Creator (http://www.zoho.com) does. Since the design principles for enterprise and desktop database software are similar, this chapter will focus on use of Microsoft Access. Since cloud computer databases are not appropriate for a use with patient information, they are not discussed in this chapter.

If you don't have database software on your computer, begin learning with a free version, such as OpenOffice.org Base, to visualize the features and functions. Base can be used to open Access database files. **Figures 9-1 and 9-2** compare the menus of two popular database applications.

The Database Window

When you start Microsoft Access, you have a choice of creating a blank database or using a template. When you select a blank database, you are prompted to give it a name and choose where it will be filed. The default is to open Table1 in a datasheet view, which looks identical to a spreadsheet grid, but without the row numbers or column letters. As noted earlier, each row is called a record. All data entered into a row should relate to that specific record. It is best to switch from the datasheet view to design view when creating a new table. Use the Access menu and click View icon to toggle between design view and datasheet view. The design view allows you the ability to provide explanations for the field names and to customize the way data should be entered.

Creating a Database

Databases are a tool that can assist nurses and other healthcare personnel in uncovering knowledge in data from an information system or in managing information such as tracking UTIs. A relational database is one in which data from more than one table can be integrated as if it were in one table. For the purpose of this example, we

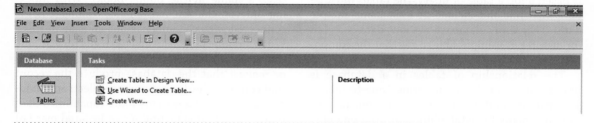

Figure 9-2 OpenOffice.org Base menu.

will work together to create and use a database to accomplish these aims.

The very first step in creating a database, identifying the question that the data needs to answer, has been done for us. The nurse manager wants to know each month how many patients arrive with a UTI and how many develop one after they arrive. Once the question or questions have been decided, you can identify the data needed to answer them. After conferring with the nurse manager, we developed a purpose for the database and identified what data we would want to provide the needed information. The result of our efforts can be seen in **Box 9-1**.

Our job now is to identify the pieces of data that will answer these questions. Using the written purpose we realize that we need to collect data about where the location from which the patient was admitted, if they had an indwelling catheter on admission, whether they had a UTI on admission, if they were on antibiotics when admitted, and how long they were in our facility.

Our first plan envisions creating two tables. One table for the patient data and the second table for the admission with UTI data. The patient table (tblPatient) will have the following fields: MRN, LastName, FirstName, StreetAddress, City, State, ZipCode, HomePhoneNumber, Birthdate, Gender, and Race. The UTI (tblUTI) table will have CaseID, MRN, AdmittedFrom, AntibioticsOnAdm, CatheterOnAdmission, UTIOnAdm, AdmDt, and DischDt. Use of the field names are brief text words with no spaces is an example of a naming convention. You certainly want your database to be people friendly, so use Field Properties > General tab > Caption to write out the meaning for each field name. The caption will be displayed in the datasheet view and for all forms and reports. Also write a short description for each field.

Because a database can do "date arithmetic," we decide to have a field for the date admitted and the date discharged and let the computer calculate the length of stay (LOS). Then we create a table, the design view of which is seen in **Figure 9-3**A. Notice that in this view, we have named each field, designated its type, and provided a description of the data that this field will contain. The data entry view is seen in **Figure 9-3**B. Note that each table name is preceded by the suffix "tbl." It is good

BOX 9-1 Purpose of our Database

The purpose of this database is to provide the data for a monthly report of patients that arrive on our unit with UTIs, and how many develop one after they are admitted.

To answer this question, we need data for those patients with UTIs about:

• Where the patient was admitted from;
• Whether the patient had a UTI on admission

After conferring with the nurse manager we found that we needed the answer to some other questions:

• Did the patient have an indwelling catheter when admitted?
• Was the patient with a UTI on admission already on antibiotics?
• What was the LOS in our agency?

practice in a database to precede each object with a prefix designating its type.

After completing the design of the table, to test our theories of the data that we will need, we enter some data into the table itself. As we do this, we realize that for the patients who are on antibiotics, we would like to know what the antibiotics are and the dosage. We also realize that a patient may be on more than one antibiotic. In the original table, we have a field that just answers the question of whether the patient is on antibiotics.

How should we structure the data to accommodate this? There are several possibilities, but only one is desirable. What most beginners will do in these cases is say, "Let's just add a few extra fields to accommodate this data." How many extra fields? This is unknown. In addition, putting the same data in more than one field reduces searching and sorting capabilities. Others will say, "Let's just create an extra record for those patients who are on more than one antibiotic." This, however, requires duplicate information in the new record, an approach that is prone to error. The best solution is to create another table to be used if the patient is on antibiotics when admitted, which will be "related" to the master table, but will have data only when it is necessary. This will accommodate

tblUTI

Field Name	Data Type	Description
⚷ CaseID	AutoNumber	Primary key used for relating tables
MRN	Number	Foreign key which is the same of the tblPatient Primary Key
AdmittedFrom	Text	Where the patient was admitted from
AntibioticsOnAdm	Yes/No	Was the patient on antibiotics when admitted?
CatheterOnAdm	Yes/No	Did the patient have a foley catheter on admission?

Field Properties

General	Lookup		
Field Size	50		
Format			▼
Input Mask			
Caption	Admitted from where?		

A

tblUTI

CaseID ▾	MRN ▾	Admitted from ▾	Antibiotics c ▾	Catheter on ▾	UTI on admi: ▾	Admission d ▾	Discharge da ▾
⊞ 1	1111	Another acute ca	☑	☐	☐	2/7/2013	2/10/2013
⊞ 2	2222	Emergency depar	☐	☐	☐	2/8/2013	2/18/2013
⊞ 3	3333	Home	☐	☑	☐	2/8/2013	2/11/2013
⊞ 4	2222	Emergency depar	☐	☐	☑	2/12/2013	2/15/2013
⊞ 5	4444	Long-term care fa	☑	☑	☐	2/18/2013	2/22/2013
✱ (New)			☐	☐	☐		

B

Figure 9-3 Master UTI table in (**A**) datasheet view and (**B**) design view.

the patient who is taking more than one antibiotic and will preserve space when a patient is not taking any antibiotics. We then design the antibiotics table (tblAntibiotics) for which you see the design view in **Figure 9-4**.

In the design view of the tables, there is a column labeled "Data Type." Notice that the information in this column is not the same for all fields. The data type tells the database how to process or

handle the data in that field and limits the type of data that the field will accept. The first data type in both tables is AutoNumber. For this type of field, the computer generates a number for each new record that is automatically entered into the table each time a new record is created. This field has been made a primary key field; a unique field for which there will never be an identical entry in that field (column) in that table. Using the

tblAntibiotics

Field Name	Data Type	Description
⚷▸ AntibioticID	AutoNumber	Primary key for antibiotic table
CaseID	Number	Foreign key from tblMasterUTI used to connect to this information
Antibiotic	Text	Name of antibiotic
Dose	Text	Prescribed dose amount and frequency
DateStart	Date/Time	Date that the patient started taking the antibiotic

Field Properties

General	Lookup	
Field Size	Long Integer	
New Values	Increment	▼

Figure 9-4 Design view of antibiotics table.

AutoNumber type of field ensures this. Letting the computer number the records saves the data enterer from the trouble of entering the data for a key field as well as preventing any duplication of key field data. Notice that in the antibiotics table there is a field for the data, which is in the key field of the UTI table with the description, "foreign key." When these data are identical in both the tables, the information from the records in them is tied together, or related.

Notice that the field type in the foreign field that matches the AutoNumber field is numeric. Fields that are related must be of the same type, and a numeric field that contains only long integers matches the AutoNumber type of field. Numeric fields serve other purposes too. Among many things, they can be used in calculations the same as in a spreadsheet and added for totals for a report page or the entire report. A text field can contain any type of data, but is limited to 255 characters, including spaces. If a field will contain more than 255 characters, use a Memo field. Date/Time fields allow "date calculations." In this database, the date fields will allow us to calculate the LOS when the time and the date are entered in this field. The "Yes/No" field type is a logical field, that is, only yes or no can be entered.

By looking at the table in **Figure 9-3**B again, we realize that the data that we want in the field "Where the patient is admitted from" are limited to four possibilities: long-term care facility, emergency department, home, or another acute care facility. To make data entry easier we create a lookup list (Data Type > Lookup Wizard > I will type in the value that I want) that has these entries and relate this table to that field in the design view. When this is done, a data enterer selects from a list instead of typing in an entry. Whenever possible, the designer should create a list of possible data entries to be used as a **lookup table**. This makes it easier for the data enterer and ensures that correct, identical, data will be entered in the field. An alternative to creating a lookup list is to create a lookup table. You would still create the relationship using the Data Type Lookup Wizard.

Full table relationships, as opposed to lookup table relationships, are created in the relationship window by dragging the key field in the Master Infections table to the matching field in the Antibiotics table, which is the table that may or may not contain a record that matches a record in the Master Infections table. This type of relationship that you see pictured in **Figure 9-5** is a one-to-many relationship. That is, a record in

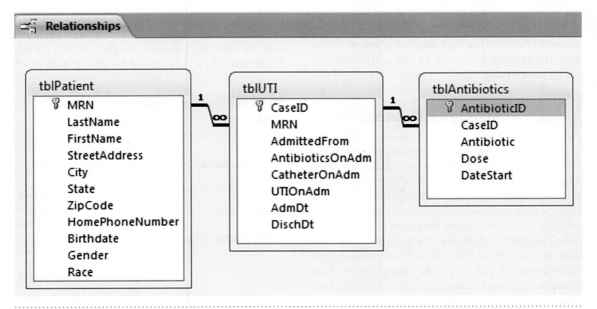

Figure 9-5 Relationship between tables.

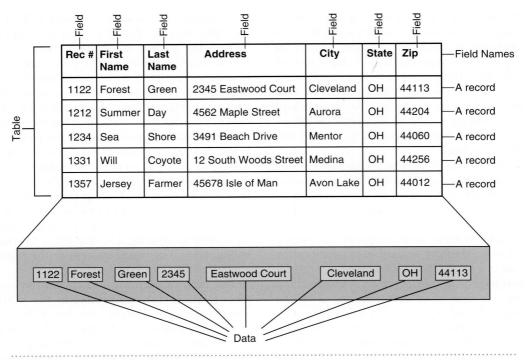

Figure 9-6 Anatomy of a database.

the main, or Master Infections table, may have none, or an infinite number of matching records in the antibiotics table. This type of relationship is symbolized in the relationship window by the infinity symbol (∞) next to the antibiotics, or subordinate table.

 Anatomy of Databases

Let's digress for a minute and use a different example to reiterate some important points and look at the overall anatomy of a database table. **Figure 9-6** shows the names of the objects in a database table and **Table 9-1** provides the terminology that database professionals use for these objects. Data are always stored in a table; other views as well as data manipulations are **virtual** and use data from the tables. This makes it possible to use a piece of data many times, even though it has only been entered once. This concept also underlies healthcare information systems, although data storage is more complex.

Forms

Although stored in a table, data entry is not confined to the table view. Data entry can be made easy by creating a form view that shows all the fields related to that record for which data must

Table 9-1 Database Phenomena

Database Term	Definition
Data	Facts without meaning, e.g., the number 37.
Field (**attribute**)	Smallest structure in a database.
Field name	The label applied to a field.
Record (tuple)	All the information about a single "member" of a table
Table (**entity** or file)	A collection of related information. A table consists of records, and each record is made up of a number of fields.

Words in parentheses are the names that database professionals use for these items.

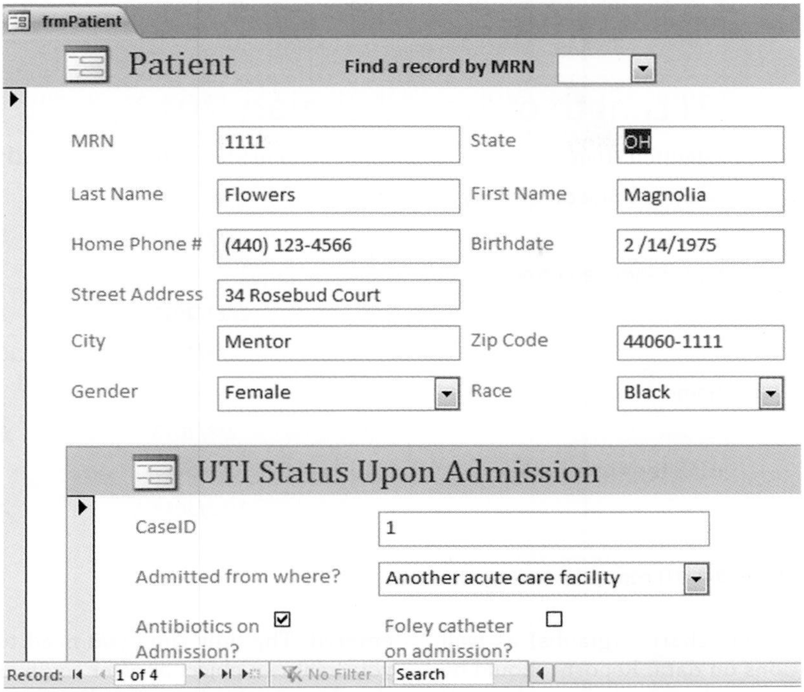

Figure 9-7 Data entry form.

be entered, regardless of the base table in which this data will be stored. To ease data entry in our UTI Infections database, we create the data entry form seen in **Figure 9-7**. Notice the "drop-down" list for the field "Admitted from where?" When the data enterer clicked the black triangle at the end of the blank field, this list, which is from a lookup table, appeared. Now all the data enterer does is to point and click the correct choice. Notice that the logical fields all have checkboxes for data entry, again forcing answers to conform to given choices and making data entry easier. Because we knew that different people would be entering data, we included instructions on the form for the data enterer. Forms are not only useful for data entry, but can be used to view or print data for one record.

In the upper left corner of the entry form is a box that allows a data enterer to search for a case by number. It is strongly suggested that the person in charge of this database have some way of finding the data that belongs to a specific case.

This could be a separate table with the name of the patient, or the MRN, or this information could be included in the master table. This information, of course, needs to be kept locked up to comply with Health Insurance Portability and Accountability Act (HIPAA) regulations. Tables can be locked so that a password is required to open them.

Reports

Reports are another view of data and, like forms, can present information from more than one table as well as from queries. **Figure 9-8** shows one report that is possible from the data that were gathered in the UTI database. By using "date arithmetic," the computer calculated the LOS for patients. We also organized the report by reporting the data for the type of facility from which they were admitted. Once this report is constructed and saved, when run, it reports the data that are currently in the table, not the data that were there when it was created. Thus, time spent creating a well-designed report is paid back many times.

Length of Stay Report

UTI Length of Stay - February 2013

Admitted From	Admission Date	LOS
Another acute care facility		
	2/7/2013	3
Emergency department		
	2/12/2013	3
	2/8/2013	10
Home		
	2/8/2013	3
Long-term care facility		
	2/18/2013	4

Figure 9-8 UTI report by facility admitted.

Reports may include charts[2] (graphs) as well as permit calculations on data. Reports should be designed in such a way that the information will be easy for the person who needs the report to understand. If a person is used to a given format for paper reports, the data from a database can be presented in a report styled to match that format even when the data input screens do not match the old paper input.

Saving Data in a Database

Unlike other office application programs, Access saves a data entry as soon as the insertion point is moved from the record in which the data was entered. This has several implications. Once you make a change to a record and leave it, consider the change permanent. It is possible to undo one change, but only the last change made. Deleting a record, however, is permanent; there is no undo. When using a database, the only things that you need to save are objects such as a table, query, or form after you create them. Entering data into a table or form does not change the basic design; hence, they do not need to be saved after data are

entered. The only time you need to save is after you create an object or after you make a change to the object in the design mode. When you close this object, you will be prompted to save. Some databases, such as Access®, save all the objects such as tables, forms, and reports as one file. If you want to send a piece of a database that you have created, such as just a table, to someone, you will need to send the entire file, or copy the piece to another database and send that.

Queries

We've looked at all the basic objects in a database except a query. Queries are one of the characteristics that give databases their power. The ability to create information from the data in a database is limited only by the ingenuity of the query creator. Because querying is such a powerful and important tool in all electronic databases, not just relational ones, we will leave our example and look at searching, which is a type of querying.

With the progression from paper to electronic library catalogs as well as Web search tools, most of us have had experience with some type of database searching. You have probably searched the Web for something or needed references on a specific

---

2 See Chapter 8 for information about graphs. Graphs can be used in spreadsheets and databases as well as pasted or linked into a word processing document.

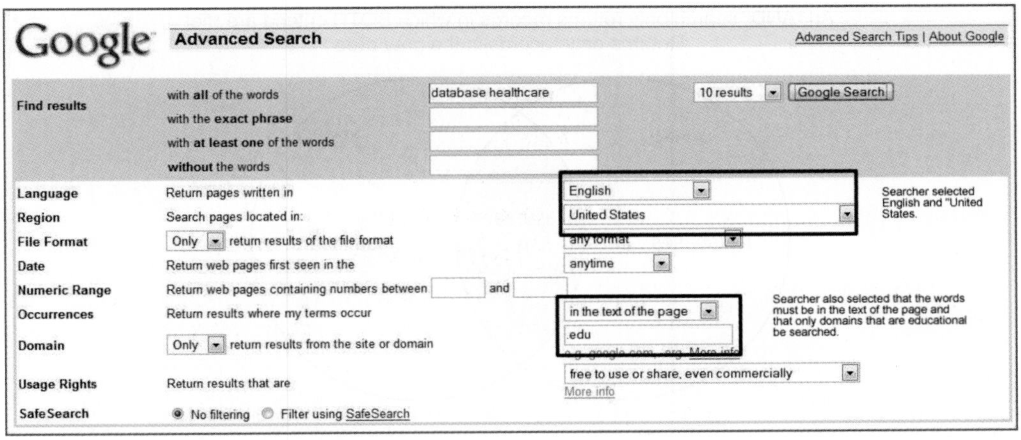

Figure 9-9 Google Advanced Search.

subject and used an electronic bibliographic catalog to find them.[3] In asking for this information, you created a query, or a set of conditions that the located records should meet. When you clicked the Search button, the search tool looked for references that met the criteria you stated in the query.

Boolean Logic Querying

Sometimes simple queries produce too many results. To refine a search further, it is necessary to use the advanced features of a search tool. For example, one searcher was told that there was a Web page[4] from an educational institution that described the use of databases in healthcare. Because using just those two words retrieved too many links, she narrowed her search using the Google™ Advanced Search tool. In the illustration in **Figure 9-9**, you can see that she set criteria to return pages with the words "database" AND "healthcare." When two words are entered in the Search box, Google, and many other catalog search tools including many bibliographical ones, assume that the searcher means to find sources that have both words, even if separated. (This does not apply to searching in a relational database.) To

locate links in which these two words appeared as a phrase, the user would have put quotation marks around them.

Searching in any database uses what is called **Boolean logic**, which is named after the 19th century mathematician George Boole. It is a form of algebra in which matches are either true or false. That is, the data in the field either match or not. There are three concepts that make up Boolean logic: "AND," "OR," and "NOT." "And" searches require that all specified terms be returned. By specifying that both database AND healthcare needed to be present, our searcher was using the Boolean "And" to narrow the search. If the user had selected the choice "At least one of the words," this would have been an "OR" search and would have returned not only records with both terms but also those in which only one term appeared. What criteria would you use and where would you enter it in **Figure 9-9** if you wanted to see Web pages for healthcare, but NOT databases?[5] Searching a database created with Microsoft Access or any other database from an office suite has the same feature of stating the criteria for the records you wish see; however, they add many other query abilities (**Figure 9-10**).

---

3 An in-depth look at searching bibliographical databases is seen in Chapter 11.

4 A Web page is not peer reviewed. Information there should be carefully evaluated using the information in Chapter 10.

5 You would enter "database" in the field "without the words" on the upper-left side of **Figure 9-7** and delete it from the "with all the words" field.

An "AND" search only returns records in which BOTH criteria are met
Returns only records in the gray area

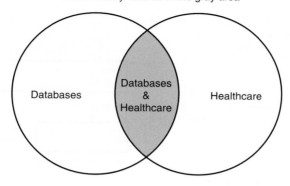

An "OR" search returns any record with either criteria
Returns all records in the gray area

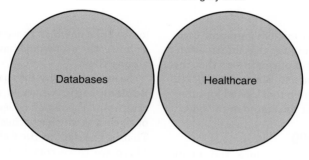

A "NOT" criteria returns records that do NOT have the designated criteria
Finds records with the term Database that do NOT contain Healthcare
Returns only records in the gray area

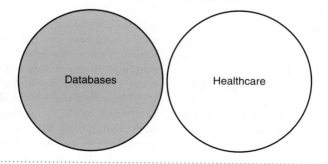

Figure 9-10 Boolean Logic.

Record Requirements

If data are to be searchable, there are several requirements that it must meet. The data must be structured, there must be a category for the data that is to be searched, and the terms used for a given meaning must be standardized.

Structured Format

To allow specialized searching, data must be organized in a way that allows criteria to be matched to the data in a given field such as title. If a bibliographical database were just full text with no organization, you would not be able to state that you wanted to search only in the author or title areas. When data are organized by categories, it is said to be structured data. In a structured format, labels such as the field names that we used in our UTI database identify the categories into which data are placed. Additionally, there must be agreement about exactly what data match the label. In bibliographical databases, or the phone book, these decisions are easy because there are universal definitions for each category and it is not difficult to determine what data they should contain. This is not always the case, which is why in the design view of the tables we created in the UTI database, we wrote a description of the data that belongs in each field.[6]

In the example of Google™ Advanced Search tool given earlier, the searcher entered criteria limiting the search to sites in which database and healthcare were in the text field. When searching, the search engine ignored the other fields and searched only the data in the text field, ignoring the title and links fields. The more structure to a database, the easier it is to set search criteria. For example, if a demographic database contains only one field for name and it holds all the parts of a name, for example, first name, middle name (or initial), and last name, it is more difficult to specify search conditions that will bring up just the correct record. Well-designed databases would include at least two fields for name, first and last names and often one for the middle name and another for the salutation. If you have ever filled out a form on the Web that asks for demographic information, you will have noticed that you are asked to enter the different parts in different boxes. Each piece of data that you enter is then stored in the field with that label. For example, first name is stored in the first name field.

Contains a Field for the Data. You can search for data only in the fields that the database contains. For example, an electronic record for an obstetric labor and delivery unit would probably contain a field for data about the type of birth, such as vaginal, cesarean, and forceps. It would also contain fields, or probably fields in related tables, to record any complications such as postpartum hemorrhage as well as date and time fields. From this database, you could learn how many Cesarean births occurred in the month of October 2008. You could not, however, answer the question, "Do women with red hair have more postpartum hemorrhages than brunettes or blondes?" because there is no field to record the color of a patient's hair. In the UTI database, you could not find out which units the patients were on because these data are not in the current form of the database. (In real life, it certainly would be, but we wanted to keep this simple to make understanding easier.)

Terminology Used to Enter Data Is Standardized. You may have experienced frustration in searching an electronic database or for help in a software program using a term that has meaning to you, but that returns no results. Computers, as you remember, are black-and-white instruments. When your term is not one used by the database that you are searching, it cannot find it. For this reason, in electronic databases it is necessary to use terminology that has been agreed on by all to have the same meaning. For example, if the agreed upon term for aspirin is acetylsalicylic acid, if you enter the term "aspirin" or ASA, all synonyms for acetylsalicylic acid, as a search word, you will not be able to find any references.

To meet these criteria, when entering data, the terms used must be standardized. To provide this standardization, many electronic databases limit the terms that can be used to enter data just as we did in the UTI database. In the example of aspirin given above, if you try to enter aspirin when the agreed upon term is acetylsalicylic acid, the computer may tell you that this term is not acceptable and ask you to enter another term.[7] In the UTI database we decided that there would only be four

---

6 In some databases, when in the data entry mode and the insertion point is in a field, the information in the description column for that field can be seen in the lower-left corner of the screen.

7 Standardized terminology is discussed in Chapters 15 (national and international) and 16 (nursing).

entries allowed in the "admitted from where" field and limited those by using a lookup table. We also decided to limit entries in the "date admitted" and "date discharged" fields to dates so we could do date arithmetic. The database program accomplished this limitation when we made the field type a Date/Time field.

Today, many regulatory agencies from The Joint Commission to the government require that hospitals submit electronic data about their patients. These data, which must be standardized, are used for many things, including identifying healthcare needs. When an electronic patient record does not contain fields for the independent actions of nursing, nursing care cannot be analyzed, and there is no indication that nursing care is part of hospital care. Reaching conclusions on incomplete data often results in poor decisions.

Manipulating Data

We have discussed different ways of viewing data in a table and some requirements for searching a database including Boolean Logic searching. Relational databases also provide the ability to reorder records, a process known as sorting as well as additional ways of searching, or querying.

Sorting

When data are entered in a database, a record is created. The records are often not entered in the order in which they need to be viewed. This can be overcome by sorting the records on a given field, either alphabetically or numerically. Sorting is just rearranging the records in a table based on the data in a field or fields in a table. The simplest **sort** is a primary sort; that is, the records are resorted based on one field. An example would be reordering records in a database based on last name to produce a table similar to the records shown in **Figure 9-11**.

Databases, however, are not limited to sorting on just one field. One can have primary, secondary, tertiary, and even further levels of sorts, each built on the groupings provided by the sort one level above it. In a tertiary sort, the records will first be sorted in a primary sort so that those that have similarities in the sort field are listed together. Then another sorting is done on another field on records in each group created from the primary sort (the secondary sort); finally, a tertiary sort on another field of each group from the secondary sort. For example, a primary sort is performed on all patients in a hospital by the type of surgery; then, the records are reordered within each type of

PtID	Last Name	First Name	Unit	Surgery Type	Site	LOS	Cl
1	Bright	Star	2 West	ORIF	Rt Hip	6	
2	Coyote	Will	2 East	Arthroscopy	Lt Hip	7	
3	Day	Summer	2 West	Arthroscopy	Rt Hip	4	
4	Farmer	Jersey	2 East	ORIF	Rt Hip	3	
5	Flower	Spring	2 West	ORIF	Lt Hip	3	
6	Green	Forest	2 East	ORIF	Rt Hip	4	
7	Light	Tiffany	2 West	Arthroscopy	Lt Hip	3	
8	Mountain	Misty	2 West	Arthroscopy	Rt Hip	6	
9	Night	Tuesday	2 West	ORIF	Lt Hip	4	
10	Shore	Sea	2 West	Arthroscopy	Lt Hip	3	
11	Springs	Glen	2 East	Arthroscopy	Lt Hip	3	
12	Time	Mark	2 East	Arthroscopy	Lt Hip	4	
13	Wave	Storm	2 West	Arthroscopy	Rt Hip	4	
14	White	Caspar	2 East	Arthroscopy	Rt Hip	3	
15	White	Pearl	2 West	Arthroscopy	Rt Hip	4	

Surgery Patients

Figure 9-11 Patients, surgery, and LOS sorted on last name.

Unit	Surgery Typ	LOS	PtID	Last Name	First Name	Site
2 East	Arthroscopy	3	14	White	Caspar	Rt Hip
2 East	Arthroscopy	3	11	Springs	Glen	Lt Hip
2 East	Arthroscopy	4	12	Time	Mark	Lt Hip
2 East	Arthroscopy	7	2	Coyote	Will	Lt Hip
2 East	ORIF	3	4	Farmer	Jersey	Rt Hip
2 East	ORIF	4	6	Green	Forest	Rt Hip
2 West	Arthroscopy	3	10	Shore	Sea	Lt Hip
2 West	Arthroscopy	3	7	Light	Tiffany	Lt Hip
2 West	Arthroscopy	4	15	White	Pearl	Rt Hip
2 West	Arthroscopy	4	13	Wave	Storm	Rt Hip
2 West	Arthroscopy	4	3	Day	Summer	Rt Hip
2 West	Arthroscopy	6	8	Mountain	Misty	Rt Hip
2 West	ORIF	3	5	Flower	Spring	Lt Hip
2 West	ORIF	4	9	Night	Tuesday	Lt Hip
2 West	ORIF	6	1	Bright	Star	Rt Hip

Figure 9-12 Primary, secondary, and tertiary sort.

surgery in a secondary sort so that those from the same unit within each type of surgery are together. The records, for a tertiary sort, are further reordered so that the records on a given unit for each type of surgery are reordered by the primary surgeon. In the example shown in **Figure 9-12**, the primary sort is the patient unit, the secondary sort is the type of surgery, and the tertiary sort is the LOS. This type of grouping is most useful in producing reports that need to look at a given characteristic within various groups. The report shown in **Figure 9-8** was produced by a primary sort of the records into the type of facility from which the patient was admitted.

Using Math in Queries

A query is the most powerful tool in a database. You have seen the results of a Boolean query in databases. There are many other ways that queries can be used to manipulate data. Queries can produce a subset of records based on fields that meet given criteria, or they can report on the entire database. Additionally, queries can be performed on the results of another query. The only limiting

factors are the data available, the user's imagination, and the ability to use the criteria selectors of Boolean algebra and the symbols referred to as mathematical operators. (This is not as complicated as it sounds, keep reading! ☺.

The mathematical operators in **Table 9-2** may be used in combination with each other or with Boolean Logic. The patient table that is part of **Figures 9-9 and 9-10** has another related table that contains the nursing diagnoses for each patient. This allowed the nurses on that unit to see how many times each nursing diagnosis occurred in this given set of patients. To accomplish this, they used the "count" function and created the table shown in **Figure 9-13**. They also wanted to see the average LOS and standard deviation for each of these patients. Using those functions on the LOS field, they created the table in shown **Figure 9-14**. On finding the average LOS to be a little over four days they became curious about what the nursing diagnoses were for those patients whose LOS was greater than four days. Using the greater than operator, with the number 4 (>4), they created a query that produced the table you

Table 9-2 Mathematical Operators for Querying

Operator	Query Criteria in Age Field	Returns from a Table with Data in the Age Field
> (greater than)	>50	Records in which the entry in the age field is greater than 50.
< (less than)	<50	Records in which the entry in the age field is less than 50.
<> (not equal to)	<>50	Records in which the entry in the age field is any number but 50.
≥ (greater than or equal to)	≥50	Records in which the entry in the age field is greater than or equal to 50.
≤ (less than or equal to)	≤50	Records in which the entry in the age field is less than or equal to 50.
Between	Between 30 and 40	Records in which the entry in the age field is between 30 and 40 (inclusive).
Null, or blank (field is empty)	Null (or blank)	Records in which the entry in the age field is empty.
Count, sum, average, standard deviation, minimum, maximum, and others	Make a selection from a drop-down list.	Does a calculation based on the term selected. For text fields, only the count function, which counts the number of times a given term appears, is available. Numeric fields are open to all types of calculations.

see in **Figure 9-15**. They used this information to study their care plans and see if they could improve care for these nursing diagnoses.

It is possible to have data downloaded from a large information system in a way that it can be manipulated to answer questions such as those above. Although some of the examples used in this chapter included identifying information about fictitious patients to help clarify the examples, data downloaded from a healthcare agency database should not contain any data that would allow individual patients to be identified.

Effective querying involves not necessarily the technical skill to construct a query, but instead the cognitive component that allows us to see the possibilities. When we can communicate exactly what information we want from data, a technical person can construct the query. One way to get this cognitive component is to create and use small databases. Using data that you have entered, or a database that you have designed, creates a situation in which you can see more of the possibilities for getting answers.

One caveat, when you design a query, always test it with a subset of data for which you know the answers to test if it actually works as desired. Include in this subset, outliers that might or might not conform to your query. The best way to learn

how to query is to play with the data by querying. You may have to try several different times to get the desired answer. This is not unusual; this author has seen database professionals work hard to enter just the right criteria to produce the answers they needed. Because ultimately the database designer is responsible for answers that are produced, testing a query with a small subset of data holds true especially when someone else, unfamiliar with the data, constructs the query.

Database Models

In our UTI example, we used a relational **database model**. The term "database model" refers to the way in which the data/tables in a database are organized. Several models exist: hierarchical, network, flat, relational, and object oriented. Each has advantages and disadvantages. The choice of which model to use is based on the tasks that the database must perform. Today, many operational databases, instead of belonging to one class, have characteristics from more than one model.

Flat Database

A flat database is a database in which the data are all in one table. As noted earlier, it is exemplified

Nursing Diagnosis	CountOfNur
Altered role performance - work	1
Altered tissue perfusion	1
Colonic constipation	4
Fear	1
Impaired home maintenance management	3
Impaired physical mobility - Level 1	4
Impaired physical mobility - Level 3	9
Impaired physical mobility - Level 4	2
Ineffective breathing pattern	5
Ineffective management of theraupeutic regin	1
Pain	4
Potential for impaired tissue integrity	1
Potential impaired tissue integrity	2
Powerlessness - Low	2
Risk for altered parenting	1

Figure 9-13 Number of patients with each nursing diagnosis.

by a spreadsheet worksheet and is the simplest database model. The address book in a word processor is another example of a flat database. Flat databases are very simple to construct and use, but they have limitations when it comes to tracking items that belong in a record when there are more than one of the same item. For example, if one wanted to track the infections that occurred in a unit using a flat database, one would need to enter two records for each patient that had more than one pathogen causing the infection. This duplicates data and wastes memory, but more importantly, creates errors in data manipulation when the person doing data input does not enter identical information for the same field in the new record.

Unit	AvgOfLOS	StDevOfLOS
2 East	4.00	1.55
2 West	4.11	1.17

Figure 9-14 Average and standard deviation.

Hierarchical Database

The **hierarchical database** was an early database model. This type of database (see **Figure 9-16**) is a database with tables that are organized in the shape of an inverted tree like taxonomy or the file structure of a disk as described in Chapter 4. In this organizational plan, often called a tree structure, records are linked to a base, or root, but through successive layers. In **Figure 9-16**, the Record Number table would be the root table. The Demographics table would be a child of the root, as would the LOS table. Nursing Diagnosis and Surgery would be the children of the parent LOS table and the grandchild of the Record Number. Each child in a hierarchical database can have only one parent, whereas a parent may have none, one, or many children. The difficulty with the hierarchical structure is that it is hard to link data from one branch of the tree with another (e.g., Nursing Diagnoses with Demographics). Because of its structure, this model results in redundant data and cannot support complex relationships (Hernandez, 2003).

LOS ▼	Nursing Diagnosis ▼
7	Colonic constipation
7	Impaired physical mobility - Level 4
7	Pain
6	Impaired home maintenance management
6	Impaired physical mobility - Level 1
6	Pain
6	Risk for altered parenting
6	Impaired physical mobility - Level 3
6	Pain

Figure 9-15 Nursing diagnosis patients LOS greater than four.

Network Model

The **network model** of database organization was developed in part to address some problems with the hierarchical model (Hernandez, 2003). The basic structure is similar to that of the hierarchical model, but the trees can share branches. If **Figure 9-14** were a network database, you would see a line indicating a relationship between demographics and all the tables at lower levels. Additionally, the Demographics table would be able to connect with both the Nursing Diagnosis and Surgery table.

Relational Database Model

To review, in a relational database model there can be two or more tables that are connected by identical information in fields in each table that

are called key fields. This allows the data in a record from one table to be matched to any piece or pieces of data in records in another table. How the tables are related can be clearly seen in **Figure 9-15**. The number 1 in the key field of "ID#" from the master, or Demographics, table is matched to the number 1 in the records in the drug reactions table; likewise the number 2. Thus, data from the record with 1 in the key field in the demographics table are connected with the data having the number 1 in the ID# field of the reactions table.

In **Figure 9-17**, the key field for the reactions table is not shown because it is automatically populated when a new record is entered. Fields that populate themselves do not need to be visible in a form view of a record. However, including one in the table design for **child tables** is an excellent

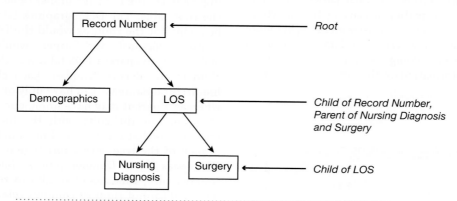

Figure 9-16 Hierarchical database model.

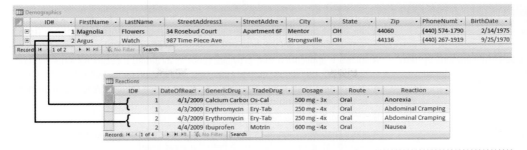

Figure 9-17 Relational database model.

idea because it preserves the ability to develop the database. Databases have a habit of "**scope creep.**" That is, when those who want information see what they can learn from the data, they ask for more information. A good database designer will anticipate this reaction and provide for expansion in the original design (see **Table 9-3**).

The table shown in **Figure 9-18** is an example of a query that matched the UTI infections table and the antibiotics table from the UTI database using the key fields. Notice that there are two entries for case number 6. This is because, although there is only one entry in the master infections table for this case, there are two entries in the antibiotic table. This query created a flat table from the two tables to provide an answer of what antibiotics the patients were taking.

In the relational model, queries can be used as a basis for a report. Queries, like reports, always produce their information based on the current data in the tables, not the data that was there when they were created. It is often desired to routinely, such as monthly, have a query answer a question using specific criteria in a given field; for example, what were the medical diagnoses for a specified nursing diagnosis in January 2011. To meet this need, a query can be designed so that when run, it asks the user to specify criteria for a field, such as the month and year for the date field. These are called parameter queries. To print out monthly reports in our UTI database, we will create a parameter query that when run, asks us for the dates for which we wish information. Then we will design a report to be based on the results from only the query data – a report that will ask for desired parameters when run. In this way, the same report can be used every month, but instead of

showing all the data in the table, it will only show the information in which the date match the information entered when the report is run.

When designing a database, it is imperative that each field contains **atomic level** data. Atomic level data are data that cannot be reduced any more. First name is at the atomic level, as is the systolic blood pressure. When the systolic and diastolic are in one field, the data are not at the atomic level, nor is a combination of the first and last name in one field. This is one aspect of a guide to database design that is called normalization. The complete process involves what are termed "five forms," each one building on the one below it. At the level of our UTI database, we need to be concerned only with the following:

1. Each value in a table is to be represented once and only once. With the exception of the key fields, a piece of data should never be repeated in another table.
2. All data should be at the atomic level.
3. Each row in a table having a field should have unique data in the form of a key field, that is, it is not repeated in that table in that field.

Remember how we created another table for the antibiotics? Anytime it is possible for data that belongs in a field to have more than one entry for a field, another table should be created. Given the fact that many people have more than one phone number, cell, home, and business, designers of databases that contain demographic data need to create a special table for phone numbers with fields designating the type of phone and the number. Anticipating when this is possible is often

Table 9-3 Relational Database Terms

View	A look at the data; these vary according to the requirements of the user. Tables, forms, queries, and reports are all different views of data.
Database Management System (DBMS)	A software application that provides tools for creating a database, entering data, retrieving, manipulating, and reporting information contained within the data.
Form	A view of data that often shows only fields from one record. Very useful for data entry. Can be printed.
Query	Search function for a relational database.
Parameter query	A query that when run asks the user to specify data for a given field so that only records that match that "parameter" are returned.
Report	Often used for printing information from data in a table(s) or query, it provides data organized to fulfill user need.
Primary key	The key field in the master (parent) table.
Foreign key	A field that contains data identical to that in the master table, but is in the detail (child) table.
Validation table (lookup table)	A table that provides a list of allowable entries for a field that is linked to that field. The data in the drop-down boxes in the Google™ Advanced Search are an example.

a difficult task and requires people to have input who actually enter, use, or ideally, both enter and use, the data.

To summarize, the relational database model consists of two or more tables that are related through a key field. When the datum in a key field of a record in one table matches the datum in a key field in another table; the data in the records are related, that is, able to be looked at as if they were one record. It is this principle that makes possible using one piece of data in many different ways. A rule of database design is that users are never required to enter the same piece of data more than once. One entry of the data, many uses!

Object/Relational Model

The object/relational database model is essentially a refinement of the relational model. In simplest terms, this model allows various objects in the database, such as the query that produced the table shown in **Figure 9-18**, to be treated as one object. Objects contain data as well as any actions that might be taken on this data. An object includes all its characteristics and behaviors. Doing this allows the execution of complex processes to be simplified by applying them only once.

Object-Oriented Model

The true object-oriented model combines database functions with object programming languages making a more powerful tool (Barry, 2010). It provides better management of complex data relationships, hence is more suited to applications such as hospital patient record systems, which have complex relationships between data. To create such a database requires knowledge of programming languages and is not suited to the application software in an office suite. Data from this type of

qryAntibiotics

Case ID	Admitted from where	Antibiotic
1	Another Acute Care Facility	Trimpex
6	Long-Term Care Facility	Bactrim DS
6	Long-Term Care Facility	Amoxicillin

Figure 9-18 Query from two tables.

database, however, can be exported and used in a relational database from the professional version of office suites to analyze data.

Database Management System

A **database management system (DBMS)** is an application program that provides the tools for creating a database, entering data, retrieving, manipulating, and reporting information contained within the data. The tools available within a DBMS vary. A simple address book requires very few tools, whereas a clinical information system requires a DBMS with many tools. Examples of middle of the road DBMSs are Corel's Paradox® and Microsoft® Access. These tools are quite powerful and can be used by noninformatics and informatics healthcare professionals.

Secondary Data Use

In this chapter, we have looked at the use of health information for purposes beyond direct patient care, a process known as **secondary data use** (Safran et al., 2007). This usage permits the analysis of all aspects of care for which data are available. Secondary use of healthcare data can greatly improve healthcare by increasing our knowledge of diseases and treatments. It can improve nursing care by enabling us to have empirical evidence to support our practice. The use of secondary health data, however, has ethical implications.[8] It is imperative that before this is done, safeguards are in place to be sure that the data is fully de-identified (Safran et al., 2007). That is, all identifiers such as the name of the patient, record number, or social security number are removed.

Ideally, a statistician will determine that there is only a very small chance that secondary data can be combined with public sources of information to identify an individual. If clinicians are to be able to learn answers to clinical care questions, it is necessary that agencies create policies that safeguard patients' rights while also providing for the secondary use of data within their walls. Before this happens, clinicians will need to be able to communicate the importance that secondary

data can have in improving patient care. A first step toward this goal is to become knowledgeable about the questions that can be answered using secondary data.

Discovering Knowledge in Large Databases

The methods described in this chapter are very useful for gaining answers from a relational database. Relational databases, however, are limited to a relatively, that is compared with a hospital information system, small set of data. In the relational database example, we had limited fields (could be thought of as variables), and we knew what type of questions that we wanted answered. To answer these we can engage in ad hoc querying, or querying in a situation in which we know enough about the data to know what questions to ask. Electronic healthcare records contain huge number of records and variables. Although we can ask for a subset of this data to analyze with a relational database, to find more information requires more powerful tools such as **data mining**.

Data Mining

Large clinical databases possess an inordinate amount of information that is not amenable to this type of relatively simple querying. To uncover this knowledge requires what is called "**knowledge discovery in databases**" **(KDD)**. Using a process known as data mining, it is possible to extract from data potentially useful information that was previously unknown. Like ad hoc querying, data mining can only find relationships between the data to which it has access (Vararuk, Petrounias, & Kodogiannis, 2008). Data mining can be used to predict diseases, understand the relationships of symptoms, and identify where to target treatment.

For example, Massachusetts Institute of Technology (MIT) has a research partnership with a hospital to predict patients who are likely to crash in order to allow early intervention and thwart the bad outcome (Healthcare Data Management, 2010). Data analysis is done with data from the critical care monitoring system and the electronic

---

8 The ethics of secondary data use is explored more fully in Chapter 25.

medical record. This is a strong incentive for nurses to use standardized terminology to ensure that not only medical information but also independent nursing actions and outcomes are included in data that will be analyzed.

Data mining requires the use of specialized software. Two data mining software packages that you may be familiar with are SAS® Business Analytics and IBM® SPSS. Both are statistical software packages commonly used in statistics and nursing research courses.

Originally developed to process corporate sales and production data, data mining is very relevant to healthcare. It has been successfully used to uncover fraud in many areas including healthcare and is useful in uncovering hidden relationships in patient care. There are three types of data mining applications: classification, regression, and clustering (StatSoft Inc., 2010a). Data mining is a form of research, but research in a retrospective manner using existing data to see what, if any, relationships are present. It uses complex statistical techniques to uncover hidden relationships that are predictive of some outcome.

Although it is possible to do data mining against a regular large electronic database, it is more effective when done on a "**data warehouse**." A data warehouse is a comprehensive collection of clinical and demographic data on large populations (Harrison, 2008; Lyman, Scully, & Harrison, 2008). Developing a data warehouse involves processes that extract the data, then clean and date it. It is not a process that is done in a vacuum. It is imperative that this be done with someone who is familiar with the data. Barriers that impede the large-scale use of data mining in healthcare are the lack of integrated medical data repositories, such as those that can be made possible by regional health information organizations (RHIO),[9] guidelines for the secondary use of medical data (Harrison, 2008), and differing work processes among healthcare facilities that make it difficult to maintain clean and useful data.

Online Analytical Processing

Online Analytical Processing (OLAP), or Fast Analysis of Shared Multidimensional Information (FASM), performs real-time analysis of data stored in databases. Despite the name, one does not have to be online to use it. Not nearly as powerful as data mining, it is a faster way of analyzing information. OLAP provides a multidimensional analysis of various types of data as well as the ability to do comparative or descriptive summaries of data (StatSoft Inc., 2010b). For example, OLAP can be used with patient records to discover degree of disease within sets of patient groups (Ordonez & Chen, 2009). OLAP when combined with geographical information system (GIS) can analyze climate changes and the effects on the associated population health (Bernier, Gosselin, Badard, & Bedard, 2009). The final result can be as simple as frequency tables, cross tabulations, or descriptive statistics, or more complex such as the removal of outliers, or other forms of data cleansing (StatSoft Inc., 2010a).

Structured Query Language

Structured Query Language (SQL) is the name of the coding that is used for querying in many databases. It is an ANSI (American National Standards Institute) standard computer language for retrieving and updating data in a database. It is used by Microsoft® Access as well as with the more powerful Oracle™ relational DBMS. Many different versions of SQL are available, but to comply with the ANSI standard they must support such major query keywords as Select, Update, Delete, Insert, Where, and others (w3schools. com, 2010).[10]

 Summary

Databases are the underpinning of all healthcare information systems. Data at the atomic level are the basis for the tables that are the structure on which a database is built. There are several different database models: hierarchical, network, object oriented, flat, and relational. The databases that come in the professional version of Office software suites are a hybrid combination of the object-oriented and relational

---

9 RHIOs are discussed in Chapter 14.

10 In Microsoft® Access if you click View when Queries are the active object, one of your choices is SQL View. Clicking that will show you the code that is executed when you run that query.

models, but they primarily use the relational model. In a relational database, the records in tables are related by a key field that is present in both tables. Getting data into a database, including a healthcare information system, is one of the most difficult tasks involved with databases. This is why a database designer should try to make it as simple as possible with forms and entry selections.

Information is produced from a database by querying. Boolean and mathematical operators can be used with criteria either singly or in combination. Before trusting query outcomes, results should always be tested with a subset of data for which the answers can be visually determined. When conclusions are drawn from data, it is advisable to consider whether all the data needed for that conclusion are present in the database.

Effective databases are planned on paper before being created on the computer. The first step is to identify what outcomes the database should provide. By using that information, the data necessary to meet these needs are determined, along with the methods for manipulating and reporting those data. These steps are iterative; it is often necessary to make corrections or additions to a prior step as planning progresses.

A well-designed database, whether a small one such as the UTI example or a large electronic patient record system, can perform many tasks. When electronic patient records become more prevalent, we will move beyond just using patient care data in a primary way, that is, only for the care of one patient, and use it in a secondary way, or for purposes other than the primary one for which it was collected. To use this data we will need the skills for effective querying.

One difficulty with today's electronic patient records is the lack of identifiable, retrievable in an aggregated form, nursing data in which we can link problems, interventions, and outcomes. This puts nursing at a disadvantage in improving our practice as well as preventing nursing data from being considered in planning healthcare. As was pointed out in this chapter, if data are not in the database, the database cannot be used to answer questions. Missing data lead to erroneous conclusions.

APPLICATIONS AND COMPETENCIES

1. Analyze the table shown below in the design view. Keeping data types in mind what is wrong with this design? What problems do you think this might create?
2. Search Google using the Advanced Search tool and specify
   a. files only in English,
      i. files from the country where you live,
      ii. where the terms are in the text of the page that the pages returned only be from websites in the ".edu" domain.
3. You are searching a Web database with Boolean Logic searching. The returns are very few and you wish to expand the search. Which Boolean term will you use? Why?
4. With what database functions will terms with the same meaning, but that are synonyms instead of identical, interfere?
5. List some clinical conditions that it would be possible to investigate by importing data from a healthcare information system. What data would you need?
6. In the database below, identify a field, field name, and record.

Patient	Unit	Pathogen
Sylvia Forest	2A	*Streptococcus*

7. What is a function of a key field?
8. What fields would be needed in a database that has data at the atomic level to record the five (include pain) vital signs?
9. You have a table with the fields in the table below. Reduce the fields in this table to atomic level and create a new design that would accommodate BPs taken at hours other than those in the present design.

Name	Date	8a BP	12p BP	4p BP	8p BP

10. What questions could you ask of a database with the following data? Which of the Boolean or mathematical operators would you use for the query?

First Name	Last Name	Primary Diagnosis	Medical Diagnosis	Nursing Diagnosis

11. Plan a database to provide information for a topic of your choosing. Keep it simple!

12. Discuss the limitations of a database.

13. Evaluate the data that are collected by an information system for identifiable nursing-sensitive data.

REFERENCES

Barry, D. (2010). *Object-oriented database mangement system (OODBMS)*. Retrieved August 10, 2011, from http://www.service-architecture.com/object-oriented-databases/articles/object-oriented_database_oodbms_definition.html

Bernier, E., Gosselin, P., Badard, T., & Bedard, Y. (2009). Easier surveillance of climate-related health vulnerabilities through a Web-based spatial OLAP application. *International Journal of Health Geographics, 8*, 18.

Harrison, J. H., Jr. (2008). Introduction to the mining of clinical data. *Clinics in Laboratory Medicine, 28*(1), 1–7, v.

Healthcare Data Management. (2010, May 1). *Mining ICU data for early-warning signs*. Retrieved April 27, 2010, from http://www.healthdatamanagement.com/issues/18_5/mining-icu-data-for-early-warning-signs-40168-1.html

Hernandez, M. J. (2003). *Database design for mere mortals: A hands-on guide to relational database design* (2nd ed.). Boston: Addison-Wesley.

Lyman, J. A., Scully, K., & Harrison, J. H., Jr. (2008). The development of health care data warehouses to support data mining. *Clinics in Laboratory Medicine, 28*(1), 55–71, vi.

Microsoft. (2010a). *Description of normalization*. Retrieved April 26, 2010, from http://support.microsoft.com/kb/100139/en-us

Microsoft. (2010b). *Using Access or Excel to manage your data*. Retrieved April 28, 2010, from http://office.microsoft.com/en-us/help/HA010429181033.aspx

Ordonez, C., & Chen, Z. (2009). Evaluating statistical tests on OLAP cubes to compare degree of disease. *IEEE Transactions on Information Technology in Biomedicine, 13*(5), 756–765.

Safran, C., Bloomrosen, M., Hammond, W. E., Labkoff, S., Markel-Fox, S., Tang, P. C., et al. (2007). Toward a national framework for the secondary use of health data: An American Medical Informatics Association White Paper. *Journal of the American Medical Association, 14*(1), 1–9.

StatSoft Inc. (2010a). *Data mining techniques – OLAP. Electronic Statistics Textbook*. Tulsa, OK. Retrieved April 27, 2010, from http://www.statsoft.com/textbook/data-mining-techniques/#olap

StatSoft Inc. (2010b). *Statistics glossary: On-Line Analytic Processing (OLAP) (or Fast Analysis of Shared Multidimensional Information – FASMI)*. Retrieved April 27, 2010, from http://www.statsoft.com/textbook/statistics-glossary/o/button/o/

Vararuk, A., Petrounias, I., & Kodogiannis, V. (2008). Data mining techniques for HIV/AIDS data management in Thailand. *Journal of Enterprise Information Management, 21*(1), 52.

w3schools.com. (2010). *Introduction to SQL*. Retrieved April 27, 2010, from http://www.w3schools.com/SQL/sql_intro.asp

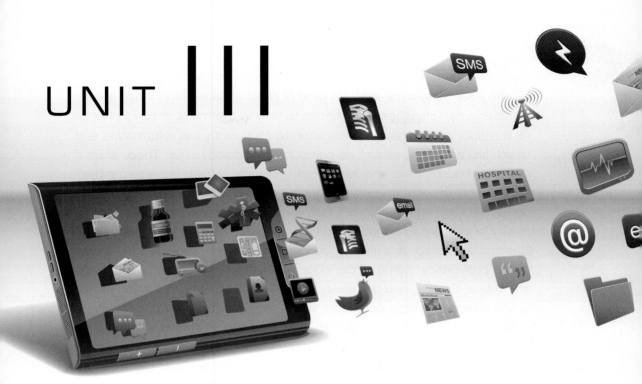

UNIT III

Information Competency

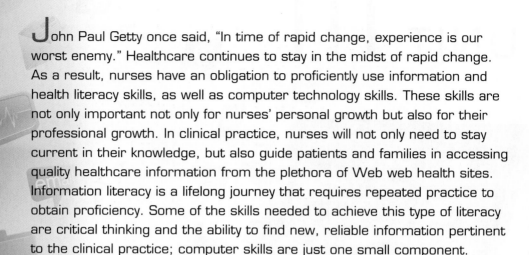

John Paul Getty once said, "In time of rapid change, experience is our worst enemy." Healthcare continues to stay in the midst of rapid change. As a result, nurses have an obligation to proficiently use information and health literacy skills, as well as computer technology skills. These skills are not only important not only for nurses' personal growth but also for their professional growth. In clinical practice, nurses will not only need to stay current in their knowledge, but also guide patients and families in accessing quality healthcare information from the plethora of Web web health sites. Information literacy is a lifelong journey that requires repeated practice to obtain proficiency. Some of the skills needed to achieve this type of literacy are critical thinking and the ability to find new, reliable information pertinent to the clinical practice; computer skills are just one small component.

Chapter 10 opens this unit with an exploration of evidence-based practice (EBP) using the untold millions of resources found on the Internet while focusing on the essential skills for discovering valid and reliable health information in the literature and on the Internet. Chapter 11 guides the user to develop the essential information search competencies necessary to discover knowledge embedded in online library resources and digital databases. Chapter 12 focuses on the use of handheld mobile devices, such as PDAs and smart phones in educational and healthcare settings.

CHAPTER 10

The Internet: A Road to Evidence-Based Practice Information

Objectives

After studying this chapter, you will be able to:

▶ *Interpret the relationships between information literacy, health literacy, and information technology skills.*

▶ *Discuss the impact of health-care consumer information literacy on patient care and education.*

▶ *Identify the essential elements for validating nursing knowledge on the Internet.*

▶ *Differentiate a scholarly nursing article, from an article in a magazine, newspaper, newsletter, or website.*

▶ *Compare and contrast the quality and quantity of evidence-based nursing resources found on the Internet with those in library databases.*

▶ *Discuss how to identify evidence-based practice nursing resources on the Internet.*

▶ *Identify three stumbling blocks that interfere with the adoption of evidence-based resources in nursing practice.*

Key Terms

Evidence-Based Nursing
Evidence-Based Practice (EBP)
Ezine
Flesch–Kincaid Grade Level
Flesch Reading Ease
Health Literacy
Information Literacy
Information Technology Skills
Nursing Knowledge
Peer-Reviewed Article
Readability
Scholarly Nursing Journal

There was a time when scholarly health information was found only in printed journals, textbooks, and brick and mortar libraries. The nonprofessional healthcare consumers were dependent on healthcare providers for all their information needs. The advent of the Internet in the 1990s leveled the playing field so that the consumer had access to much of the same information as the healthcare professional. The caveat is that the Internet has empowered consumers to take ownership of their health but without the benefit of advanced education and training to interpret the meaning of most of the information. The brick and mortar libraries continue to be essential resources for healthcare knowledge and **evidence-based practice (EBP)**, but now include access to the Internet as well as digital library catalogs. This chapter will focus on the essential skills for discovering valid and reliable health information on the Internet for nursing and other healthcare professionals.

According to reports from the Pew Foundation, 75%–80% of Internet users and 62%–68% of people with chronic illnesses have searched for health information (Fox, 2008; Fox & Purcell, 2010). Of the 85 million Americans who searched for health information, only 15% stated that they always check for the source and date of the information (Fox, 2007). In essence, the public is turning to the Internet for health information but most need assistance to evaluate and effectively use the information. If the public is learning to be information literate, it behooves those of us in the healthcare profession to stay one step ahead. We must be able to guide the healthcare consumers to make decisions about the care that they receive. Healthcare providers must develop **information literacy**, **health literacy**, and **information technology skills** to identify valid and reliable health information on the Internet and interpret the findings to improve patient care outcomes.

Information and Health Literacy

Information literacy refers to the awareness that there is "a need to know" information, the ability to find it, analyze it for validity and relevance, and interpret it for use. Health literacy is a subset of information literacy. Health literacy is "the degree to which individuals have the capacity to obtain, process, and understand basic health information and services needed to make appropriate health decisions" (Nielsen-Bohlman & Institute of Medicine [U.S.], Committee on Health Literacy, 2004). Both information and health literacy are learned competencies that require repeated practice over time to develop expertise. According to the American Library information, literate individuals should be able to demonstrate the six competencies listed in **Box 10-1** (Association of Colleges and Research Libraries, 2000).

Healthcare Professional Information and Health Literacy

Because of the rapid changes in healthcare developments and information technology, information and health literacy skills are necessary for nurses and other healthcare professionals to continue lifelong learning. The American Association of Colleges of Nursing (AACN) recommends that nursing curricula include information seeking, sorting, and selecting; critical

---

BOX 10-1 Information Literate Competencies

The information literate individual is able to:
- Determine the extent of information needed
- Access the needed information effectively and efficiently
- Evaluate information and its sources critically
- Incorporate selected information into one's knowledge base
- Use information effectively to accomplish a specific purpose
- Understand the economic, legal, and social issues surrounding the use of information, and access and use information ethically and legally.

Source: Reproduced with permission from American Library Association (2008).

---

thinking; and information and healthcare technologies (American Association of Colleges of Nursing, 2005). The National League for Nurses has issued a position paper supporting the use of information and healthcare technologies (National League for Nursing, 2008). The Joint Commission standards emphasize the importance of every patient receiving information in a way that they can understand it as a fundamental right (Joint Commission, 2007). Information literacy skills are addressed in the Technology Informatics Guiding Education Reform (TIGER) report (Technology Guiding Education Reform, 2007) as well as the Quality and Safety Education for Nurses (QSEN) (Quality and Safety Education for Nurses, 2010). Because of these recommendations, nursing programs are beginning to focus on teaching these essential skills.

Faculty members have chosen to teach literacy skills using specific learning modules in various ways. Courey, Benson-Soros, Deemer, and Zeller (2006) reported findings of research done with 57 first-semester associate-degree nursing students. They reported a comparison of evaluation of students' skills at the beginning of a semester, before a 1-day interactive collaborative module, and at the end of the semester. At the end of the semester, the associate-degree students expressed increased knowledge about the access of professional nursing literature; however, they also expressed a less positive attitude toward the need to stay current.

Ku, Sheu, and Kuo (2007) reported a similar study conducted with 77 RN–BSN students studying women's health in Taiwan. The program was conducted over a 4-month period and integrated into the course content. Their study focused on changes in the following skills: searching and screening, integrating, analyzing, applying, and presenting. With the exception of presenting skills, the researchers found a significant difference between the group that had information literacy education and the one that did not.

Grant and Brettle (2006) reported a study conducted with 13 masters and PhD students studying nursing, occupational therapy, and physiotherapy in England. They used interactive web-based tutorial delivered over a 12-week period to teach information skills as part of an EBP module. Although the study was very small, there was a significant difference between pretraining and posttraining scores.

Perhaps, the associate-degree first-semester students did not have enough domain knowledge about nursing to appreciate the need to stay current with nursing literature. The RN–BSN and graduate students would have had both domain knowledge and nursing experience to appreciate the importance of nursing information literature. Moreover, the learning content for the RN–BSN and graduate students was delivered over time, providing opportunities for skill building, feedback, and practice. The results of the studies indicate that information and health literacy skills cannot be learned by reading a book or listening to a lecture. Nursing and other healthcare professionals must have domain knowledge, clinical experience, functional understanding of search skills, and be able to analyze, integrate, and apply knowledge to practice. The skills are best learned with repeated practice using a variety of search settings over time.

Pluses for Healthcare Professional Information and Health Literacy

Synthesizing the results of a literature search is an important tool for improving the quality of patient care as well as the first step in any research study. Research has shown that the information provided by literature searches changes clinical decisions. Literature findings provide information to justify, question, and improve patient care. Synthesis of literature leads to new knowledge, design of solutions, implementation, and evaluation methods. Knowledge from literature findings allows the nurses to empower the healthcare consumers so that they can be partners in their own care. The positive patient care outcomes from nursing and medical research support the Joint Commission requirements for access to knowledge-based information resources. Information literacy is essential for **evidence-based nursing** practice.

Critical Thinking

Critical thinking supports information literacy. It is a difficult concept to define. It is a little like good nursing care, we know it when we see it, but defining it in objective terms is complex. Consequently, it has been defined from several different perspectives. Some say it is thinking about thinking. Others believe critical thinking is purposeful, goal directed, and that it requires the use of cognitive strategies to increase the probability of a desired outcome. Breivik (1991, p. 226) related information literacy as an initial component to the continuum of critical-thinking skills stating, "In this information age, it does not matter how well people can analyze or synthesize; if they do not start with an adequate, accurate, and up-to-date body of information, they will not come up with a good answer." Critical thinking is a tool that does not exist until it is used. It has two components: skill sets to process and generate information and the intellectual commitment to use those skills to guide behavior. Critical thinkers approach a problem from multiple angles and in a logical manner. A vital part of critical thinking includes asking questions, knowing when one needs more information, developing and applying a plan for acquiring this information, and using the plan to generate knowledge. This plan can encompass searching for information in established databases, creating a database for information and knowledge, or both. Either way, the result is directed toward improved outcomes based on information and knowledge.

Knowledge Generation

Integrating evidence-based literature with clinical information results in new knowledge. Knowledge generation has two parts. In terms of clinical informatics, it refers to the knowledge that is developed from converting nursing data into information and reinterpreting it. Some clinical information systems are designed with decision support systems that automate knowledge generation from clinical data. From the research perspective, knowledge generation starts with the application of the steps of information literacy – identifying, retrieving, appraising, and synthesizing nursing literature to solve nursing problems in new and better ways. Recognition of the nurse's role as a knowledge worker evolves from understanding both parts and their relationships to nursing practice. Information literacy and informatics are keys to knowledge work and generation.

Knowledge Dissemination Activities

When nurses change data from information into knowledge, it maintains value only if it is also shared among the others in the profession so that it makes an impact across practice settings. Knowledge sharing allows nurses to influence not only nursing but also drive health policy and influence interdisciplinary health practices. The computer is a tool that facilitates knowledge dissemination in multiple ways. In a broad sense, raw data can be transferred between settings to facilitate use in different ways by different nurse groups.

Once data are changed into information and interpreted, the findings can be published for dissemination across the profession. This can be accomplished by desktop software:

- Word processing to create a manuscript
- Presentation and graphics programs to develop drawings or create a presentation or poster presentation
- Spreadsheets to aggregate data and create graphs

- Databases to query, aggregate data, and create reports
- Web development software to create web documents
- Statistical software to analyze quantitative data
- E-mail to collaborate and share **nursing knowledge**
- Wikis and blogs to interact using web-based professional collaboration on nursing knowledge.

The maturation of professional nursing practice is dependent on the development and dissemination of nursing knowledge. Whether information is shared between two nurses or more widely shared across the members of the profession, information technology can speed the dissemination process.

Healthcare Consumer Information and Health Literacy

The information literacy level of the healthcare consumer is a significant factor for the nurse providing patient education and discharge planning for acute and chronically ill patients. Noncompliance with treatment and care regimes is often a sign of literacy problems. Noncompliance is associated with higher costs of healthcare that is particularly associated with treatment and medication errors (National Network of Libraries of Medicine, 2010). Patients with literacy problems are often embarrassed and hide their problems. In addition to gaining personal information and health literacy, the nurse must be able to assess those same skills with the patient to plan and implement effective care and teaching.

In a 2003 study of health literacy of 19,000 adults, the U.S. Department of Education found that 36% of the adults had only basic or below basic literacy skills. Adults who were 65 or older had lower average literacy skills than any of the other age groups; 29% had below basic skills and 30% had basic skills (Kutner, Greenberg, Jin, & Paulsen, 2006). To address the literacy issue and improve patient outcomes patient education materials be written at no higher than a fifth-grade reading level ("Communicating with patients who have limited literacy skills. Report of the National Work Group on Literacy and Health," 1998; Wilson, 2009). In addition, healthcare providers should incorporate nonwritten materials into patient education.

Initial patient assessments often include questions about learning styles and educational levels. One research study found that a straightforward approach for clinicians to identify those with limited or marginal health literacy skills was to ask how confident the patients were completing medical forms on their own (Wallace, Rogers, Roskos, Holiday, & Weiss, 2006). Limited skills were defined as reading at sixth grade or lower and marginal skills were defined as reading at the seventh- to eighth-grade levels.

The Pfizer Clear Health Communication Initiative (Pfizer, 2008) provides a website at http://www.pfizerhealthliteracy.com/ with comprehensive information about the health literacy problem. The website includes a white paper "Eradicating Low Health Literacy: The First Public Health Movement of the 21st Century," references, a health literacy quiz, and a checklist for providers. Although Pfizer is a commercial pharmaceutical company, the website was developed with the purpose of improving patient outcomes. The site references the National Assessment of Adult Literacy Study, published by the National Center for Education Statistics, and the National Patient Safety Foundation, a nonprofit organization.

Readability

The ability to read and understand is an important component of the health literacy problem. Nurses and other healthcare professionals may attempt patient care teaching using printed educational literature or websites that the patients and families cannot understand. Fortunately, there are a number of methods to test written information for **readability**. For example, Microsoft Word can calculate readability statistics with the **Flesch Reading Ease** and the **Flesch–Kincaid Grade Level** tests. The Flesch Reading Ease calculates a value from a formula using the average sentence length and the average number of syllables per word. The recommended score is between 60 and 70; higher scores correlate with easier readability. The Flesch–Kincaid Grade Level test also uses the average sentence length and average number of syllables to calculate a U.S. school grade level. An online solution to test readability is the Online Utility tool available at http://www.online-utility.org/english/readability_test_and_improve.jsp. The user can copy and paste text into a window and then click a button to process the text to obtain readability statistics. The website How to write

easy-to-read health materials (http://www.nlm.nih.gov/medlineplus/etr.html), published by Medline Plus, outlines a four-step process for writing health materials and includes links to additional readability resources.

To visualize how readability statistics work, consider the problem of asthma. Asthma is a common health problem affecting millions of people in the world. Nurses frequently need to teach patients and their families about the condition starting with a definition of asthma. The definition of asthma from Medline Plus website at http://vsearch.nlm.nih.gov/vivisimo/cgi-bin/query-meta?v%3Aproject=medlineplus&query=asthma was copied and pasted into a Microsoft Word document and readability statistics were calculated. The same definition was copied and pasted into the Online Readability Test and Improve website to process the text (see **Box 10-2**).

A comparison of the results from the two tools shows similarities and differences. Although both tools provided identical information for the word and sentence counts and the average characters per word, the Reading Ease and Flesch–Kincaid Grade Level differed slightly. According to Word, the Flesch Reading Ease was 72.6 and the Flesch–Kincaid Grade Level was 6.8. According to the Online Readability Test and Improve site, the Flesch Reading Ease was 63.28 and the Flesch–Kincaid Grade Level was 7.94. The Online Utility tool provided recommendations for rewriting two sentences. It is important to understand that the results of the two tools were generated by a computer and must be further analyzed by the nurse. Most professionals would agree that the Medline Plus definition of asthma could be used in a teaching plan. The result of the readability statistics serves to alert the nurse that further explanation of the definition may be necessary.

Information Technology Skills

Information technology skills are necessary to support the application of information literacy. Information literacy is concerned with information seeking, access, content, communication, analysis, and evaluation, while information technology is concerned with an understanding of the technology and skills necessary for using it productively. Information technology skills require three kinds of knowledge: current skills, foundational

BOX 10-2 Tests Document Readability and Improve It

This free online software tool calculates various readability measurements such as Coleman Liau index, Flesch–Kincaid Grade Level, ARI (Automated Readability Index), SMOG. Document readability is the indication of number of years of education that a person needs, to be able to understand the text easily on the first reading. Comprehensions test and skills training.

This tool is made primarily for English texts but might work also for some other languages.

It displays also complicated sentences (with many words and syllables) as suggestion what you might do to improve its readability.

Number of characters
(without spaces):   589.00
Number of words: 127.00
Number of sentences: 9.00
Average number of characters per word: 4.64
Average number of words per sentence: 14.11

Indication of the number of years of formal education that a person requires to easily understand the text on the first reading.
Gunning Fox Index: 7.53

Approximate representation of the U.S. grade level needed to comprehend the text:
Coleman Liau index: 9.39
Flesch–Kincaid Grade level: 7.94
ARI: 7.47
SMOG: 7.47

Flesch Reading Ease: 63.28

List of sentences that we suggest you should consider to rewrite to improve readability of the text:
- That makes them very sensitive, and they may react strongly to things that you are allergic to or find irritating.
- In a severe asthma attack, the airways can close so much that your vital organs do not get enough oxygen.

concepts, and intellectual abilities (Association of Colleges and Research Libraries, 2000).

Current skills imply the ability to use up-to-date computer applications such as desktop applications and searching tools. Foundational skills refer to understanding the underlying principles of computers, networks, and information. Current and foundational skills provide insight into the abilities as well as limitations of this technology in information management. The skills also provide the raw material for adapting to new information technology. The ability to apply information technology for problem solving requires intellectual capabilities that encompass abstract thinking about information and how it can be manipulated to produce new understandings. Information technology skills combined with information literacy enable individuals to cope with unintended and unexpected problems when they occur.

Discovering and Evaluating Health Information on the Internet

Health information on the Internet is growing in abundance. Unfortunately, many of the websites have misleading and incorrect information. All Internet users must approach searching for health information through a systematic analytical review process. The evaluation process for a health information website should use the same basic principles for evaluating general websites, but since health information can involve life and death issues, health information websites must be held to a higher standard of review. **Table 10-1** shows essential information that must be validated when using a website for health information. Health information on the Internet should

Table 10-1 Health Information Website Check List

• Source	Who is the website sponsor? Who is the website owner?
• Funding	Who is the author? Are the author's credentials noted? Is the author an expert in the subject area? Is the author qualified to write the information?
	What is the author's affiliation?
	Is there a link that will allow the user to contact the author?
	Is the site a not-for-profit site?
	Is there any commercial funding?
	Are there any potential conflicts of interest?
	Are there any advertisements on the site, if so, are they clearly labeled?
• Validity and quality	Is the date that the site was last updated clearly specified?
	Is the purpose of the website clearly stated?
	Is the information accurate and referenced to current scholarly nursing and medical resources?
	Is the information up-to-date?
	Is the information peer reviewed or verified by a qualified editor?
	Is the site free from content and typing errors?
	Is the information free from bias and opinion?
	Are all the links to quality reputable resources?
	Are all the links functioning?
• Privacy	Does the site include a privacy statement that is easily understood?
	Does the site meet a recognized privacy standard such as "Health on the Net" (http://www.hon.ch/)?

always be approached with a certain amount of skepticism. If the information sounds too good to be true, it is probably not true. The National Library of Medicine has a variety of resources including links to tutorials and journal articles to assist the consumer in navigating health information websites. These resources can be found at http://www.nlm.nih.gov/medlineplus/evaluatinghealthinformation.html.

Nursing Knowledge on the Internet

Nursing knowledge on the Internet is a subset of health information. Nursing knowledge addresses resources that enhance professional nursing expertise. Examples of nursing knowledge include websites that involve laws, rules, and regulations related to nursing practice, nursing care, healthcare agencies, and nursing education programs; government sponsored and not-for-profit health and disease specialty organizations; nursing professional organizations and continuing education resources; and evidence-based nursing resources. This list is not meant to be all-inclusive, but serves to provide the wide scope of resources designed to enhance nursing practice.

Laws, Rules, and Regulations

Several sites relate to laws, rules, and regulations. The National Council of State Boards of Nursing (NCSBN) (https://www.ncsbn.org/index.htm) includes links to all U.S. state boards of nursing and includes information about the National Council Licensure Examination (NCLEX). Each state board of nursing site includes clearly stated laws, policies, and rules and regulations. The state boards of nursing websites also provide services for license verification and license renewal online. Other regulatory websites include the Joint Commission (http://www.jointcommission.org/), the Centers for Medicare & Medicaid (CMS) (http://www.cms.hhs.gov/), and individual state departments of health and human services.

Government and Not-for-Profit Health and Disease Specialty Organizations

Government sponsored and not-for-profit health and disease specialty organizations include quality information that enhances nursing knowledge. The National Institutes of Health (NIH) (http://www.nih.gov/) has links to the associated 27 specialty institutes and centers providing information to the latest research, clinical trials, and grants to promote health. The Centers for Disease Control and Prevention (CDC) (http://www.cdc.gov/) provides statistical data, information about diseases and disease control, and online disease control and prevention journals. CDC Wonder (http://wonder.cdc.gov/) provides searchable online databases with public health data, morbidity tables, and Healthy People 2010. The Agency for Healthcare Research and Quality (http://www.ahrq.gov/) provides information on EBP, grants, research, and quality and patient safety issues.

Scholarly Journals and Journal Articles

Although libraries provide the most comprehensive nursing and medical knowledge, some nursing and medical journals and full-text scholarly journal articles are also available on the Internet. True online journals publish all of their articles online with no print version. They feature **peer-reviewed articles** and maintain an archive of the articles. Some online journals are indexed in nursing bibliographic databases such as Cumulative Index to Nursing and Allied Health Literature (CINAHL) and Medline. Most feature articles in HTML format, but some use portable document format (PDF), which requires Adobe Acrobat Reader to use.

Online Journals

There are a small but growing number of free online nursing journals. The *Online Journal for Issues in Nursing* (OJIN) at http://nursingworld. org/OJIN/, first published in June 1996 by Kent State University College of Nursing Faculty in conjunction with the American Nurses Association (ANA), is now sponsored by the ANA. The focus of OJIN is to provide different views on current topics relating to nursing practice, research, and education. OJIN is peer reviewed and indexed in both CINAHL and Medline. The *Online Journal of Nursing Informatics* (OJNI) at http://www.ojni.org/current. html focuses on topics relating to nursing informatics. OJNI is peer reviewed and indexed in CINAHL. BMC Nursing, at http://www.biomedcentral.com/bmcnurs/ is a peer-reviewed open-access journal that publishes research on topics relating to nursing research, training, practice, and education.

Open access journals have limited copyright/licensing restrictions and allow anyone with an Internet connection to download, copy, and distribute the articles. Access to full-text articles from other medical journals is available from Free Medical Journals at http://freemedicaljournals.com/ and BioMed Central at http://www.biomedcentral.com/browse/journals/. The MERLOT Journal of Online Learning and Teaching (JOLT) at http://jolt.merlot.org/ is a peerreviewed journal, with articles about the scholarly use of multimedia resources in education. All BioMed Central journals and JOLT are classified as open access.

Factors Affecting Online Journals

Several factors are associated with online journals. One difficulty with online journals is the perception that the quality of their content is lower than that of print journals. Some bibliographic indexes still categorically refuse to index such journals. Part of this perception may result from the great variability in online journals; part is a belief among some academics that only print journals have peer-reviewed articles. This perception is changing as the realization that online journals can be and are peer-reviewed permeates faculty.

Writing for publication in an online journal can present a dilemma, given that most writers are members of academic faculties who need publication in recognized journals to gain promotion and tenure. Promotions are made on both the number of articles published and the reputation of the publishing journal. This makes publishing in an online journal risky for faculty who are seeking tenure. These perceptions can affect the quality of writers and therefore the quality of the articles these writers produce.

Another difficulty with online journals is nurses' lack of awareness that the journals exist. Although nurses in all specialties need to be information literate, many are not. A person who has not learned how to use the web is limited to print journals. In addition, search engine results do not necessarily make a distinction between a scholarly print journal with a web presence, a true online journal, **ezine**, or newspaper. Ezine is a term for an electronic magazine; however, ezines may also be newsletters. The user might simply conclude that no online journals exist because the results of an Internet search are overwhelming and lead to many false links.

Unlike print journals, which are the product of a publishing company, most online journals have been started with little financial or organizational support. This has resulted in many being started, but not nearly as many being able to display staying power. It is not unusual to find that an online journal has not had a new article for several years or that it has completely disappeared. Although it may look easy to run an online journal, a large amount of work is involved in producing one of high quality. The journal staff must find writers, reviewers, and persons to coordinate the progress of articles; someone to convert the articles to a web format; and staff to market the journal. The journal overhead includes staff salaries and office expenses. All these tasks take time and money. Without a strong financial backing, sustaining publication of the journal can become insurmountable.

Web Presence for a Print Journal

Full-text digital versions of print journal articles are often available online as a personal subscription benefit of the printed journal or a small fee for nonsubscribers. For more information on how to download full-text articles, go to the print journal website. Users with a personal subscription will be instructed on how to activate their online subscription accounts to receive a login and create a password. Nonsubscribers will be prompted to set up an account where they can purchase and download journal articles.

Articles from Internet Search Engine Results

Internet search engines such as Google™ Search or Google Scholar™ scholarly text search may reveal free full-text journal articles from websites such as Medscape (http://www.medscape.com/) and FindArticles (http://findarticles.com/). Medscape®, sponsored by WebMD®, is free but requires a login and password. The FindArticles website includes a few nursing journal articles and some from ezines. Most ezines are delivered without charge and supported by advertising. Generally, they address current topics such as career information, jobs, and news items of interest to their audience. Few ezines maintain archives; thus, information on these sites has a very short life. Users must be extremely cautious when using a search engine because many of the results link to ezines and websites that are not scholarly resources.

Scholarly Article Versus Ezine, Newspaper, or Website

It is critically important for nurses to be able to differentiate a scholarly nursing article from an article in an ezine, a newspaper, or a website. A scholarly article is written by a qualified nurse with expertise in the subject area and published in a **scholarly nursing journal**, and it is subjected to a complex peer-review process before publication. Once received by the editorial office, the article is screened by the journal's editor. If the editor considers the subject matter appropriate for the journal readers, a copy with the author(s) name(s) removed (sometimes called a blind review) is sent to two or more nurse experts for review to assure the validity, quality, and reliability of information. If the article is approved for publication, the author(s) is/are allowed to make final editing changes based on the reviewers' and editors' comments.

In contrast to the peer-review process, reporters write ezine and newspaper articles. They are not required to be nurses or to have any expertise in nursing practice. Content is reviewed and approved by editors prior to publication. Magazines and other news media do not cite specific references. Examples of ezines include ADVANCE for Nurses (http://nursing.advanceweb.com/), ADVANCE for Nurse Practitioners (http://nurse-practitioners-and-physician-assistants.advanceweb.com/) and ALLnurses (http://allnurses.com).

Many websites, at first glance, appear to be a scholarly article or ezine. Websites, such as ezines, need not be authored by a qualified nurse. Unlike journals, magazines, or newspapers, websites are not necessarily updated on a regular basis. Generally, information on websites is not archived. The information on websites varies in quality, which is why nurses should carefully scrutinize websites using a checklist such as the Health Information Checklist (see **Table 10-1**).

Professional Nursing Organizations

Each professional nursing organization has a website with general information for the public and password-protected information for its members. For example, the ANA website, http://nursingworld.org/, includes membership information and links to purchase the nursing code of ethics and the scope and standards of practice for nursing specialties. The ANA also includes links to information on continuing education modules, individual and Magnet certification; ANA-sponsored nursing journals and books; healthcare policy and much more. Sigma Theta Tau International (STTI) honor society for nursing (http://www.nursingsociety.org/) has membership information, links to STTI-sponsored journals and books, and continuing education modules. One distinctive factor for the STTI website is the link to the Virginia Henderson International Nursing Library. The library includes an online list of comprehensive nursing resources including grants, research, journals, and evidence-based nursing.

Clinical Practice and Informatics

Information literacy, knowledge generation, and knowledge dissemination activities are an integral part of all nursing roles. Few nurses will become informatics nursing specialists, but all nurses need an awareness and general understanding of the potential of the various applications. The nurse as a knowledge worker should embrace role-appropriate activities and processes.

Evidence-Based Nursing

STTI defines evidence-based nursing as "an integration of the best evidence available, nursing expertise, and the values and preferences of the individuals, families, and communities who are served" (Sigma Theta Tau International, 2005).

The Institute of Medicine identifies use of EBP as a core competency for healthcare professionals (Greiner & Knebel, 2003). The Internet includes many resources that explain evidence-based nursing as well as evidence-based care guidelines. The Internet, however, must never be used as a primary source for evidence-based nursing research. Although there are several excellent evidence-based nursing websites, STTI is striving to become a global leading source of information on evidence-based nursing. The "Find Resources" section of the STTI website http://www.nursinglibrary.org/portal/main.aspx?PageID=4013 is an excellent place to begin searching the Internet for evidence-based guidelines and other evidence-based nursing resources.

Nursing Evidence-Based Practice and the Star Model of Knowledge Transformation©

The Star Model of Knowledge Transformation© seen in **Figure 10-1** (Stevens, 2005) depicts EBP as a cyclical process of moving knowledge from original research into patient care. In the first step of this process, original research studies are synthesized

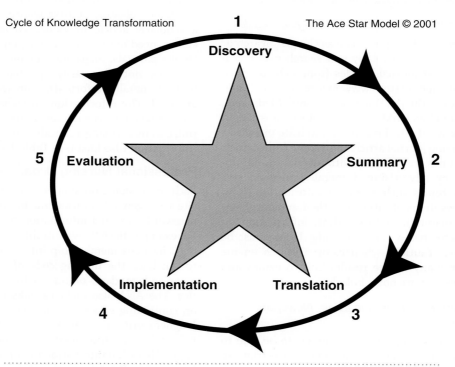

Cycle of Knowledge Transformation   **1**   The Ace Star Model © 2001

1 Discovery
2 Summary
3 Translation
4 Implementation
5 Evaluation

Figure 10-1 Star model of evidence-based practice.

to produce an evidence summary. The goal of an evidence summary is to provide the best evidence of effectiveness by summarizing an entire body of studies. The process involves identifying pertinent research evidence through a critical appraisal of original studies using defined questions. The evidence is then translated into practice guidelines for use in the clinical setting and is often combined with clinical expertise to produce a set of recommendations of best practice. These best practices are then implemented into practice and evaluated in terms of patient outcomes, health status, efficiency,

satisfaction, and economic factors. Conclusions from the evaluation stage may lead to more research.

Online Evidence-Based Resources

The Internet has an abundance of information about evidence-based care resources. As with other healthcare information found on the Internet, the variation in quality is tremendous. The first step toward approaching a search for evidence-based care is to determine what you want to learn. Some of the most comprehensive websites are found in libraries and educational EBP centers. Clinical practice guidelines

Table 10-2 Evidence-Based Practice Information on the Internet

Evidence-Based Practice Topic	Websites and URLs
Evidence-Based Practice • Definition • History • Recommendations • Terminology	*Crossing the quality chasm: A new health system for the 21st century* http://www.nap.edu/openbook.php?isbn=0309072808 *Health professions education: A bridge to quality* http://www.nap.edu/catalog.php?record_id=10681 EBP (Interactive Tutorial) http://www.biomed.lib.umn.edu/learn/ebp/ Center for Evidence-Based Medicine http://www.cebm.utoronto.ca/ NOAH http://www.noah-health.org/en/ebm/
Evidence-Based Nursing • Definition • Challenges • Other Resources	Sigma Theta Tau International http://www.nursingsociety.org/default.aspx Academic Center for Evidence-Based Nursing http://www.acestar.uthscsa.edu/ Evidence-Based Nursing http://www.hsl.unc.edu/services/tutorials/ebn/splash.htm Joanna Briggs Institute: Evidence-based nursing http://www.joannabriggs.edu.au/
Evidence-Based Care Competencies	*Health professions education: A bridge to quality* http://www.nap.edu/catalog.php?record_id=10681

Clinical Practice Guidelines	AHRQ Clinical Practice Guidelines Online http://www.ahrq.gov/clinic/cpgsix.htm
	CDC: The Community Guide http://www.thecommunityguide.org/
	Nursing Best Practice Guidelines (Registered Nurses of Ontario)
	   http://www.rnao.org/Page.asp?PageID=861&SiteNodeID=133
	Canadian Medical Association: INFOBASE http://mdm.ca/cpgsnew/cpgs/index.asp
	Joanna Briggs Institute: Best Practice Information Sheets
	   http://www.joannabriggs.edu.au/Access%20Evidence/Best%20Practice%20Information%
	20Sheets

Research
Types of research
• How to read
 	
• How to evaluate
• How to use
	Evidence-based nursing http://www.hsl.unc.edu/services/tutorials/ebn/splash.htm
	
	What is critical appraisal?
	   http://www.medicine.ox.ac.uk/bandolier/painres/download/whatis/What_is_critical_appraisal.pdf
	Nursing research: Show me the evidence (blog)
	   http://evidencebasednursing.blogspot.com/

Online Databases	The Cochrane Collaboration (abstracts) http://www.cochrane.org/index.htm
Handheld Computer	National Institute of Nursing Research: Video/Audio/Podcasts http://www.ninr.nih.gov/NewsAndInformation/PodCastMultimedia/
Evidence-Based Care Resources	Center for Evidence-Based Medicine http://www.cebm.utoronto.ca/

are available from government and educational websites in the United States, Canada, England, and Australia. **Table 10-2** was designed to provide a starting point for nurses and healthcare professionals beginning to learn about EBP.

Summary

Nurses and healthcare providers have an obligation to become proficient in the use of information and health literacy skills as well as information technology skills for several reasons. Nurses should be able to guide the patients and their families to obtain health information using the Internet. Health information on the Internet should be held to a much higher standard than any other information because inaccuracies have the potential to impact patient injury, illness, and death. Nurses must be able to assess patient and family information literacy skills, including their ability to read and understand information. To match written health teaching learning materials with the patient's health literacy skills, nurses need to be able to test written resources using readability statistics.

Information literacy is a skill that must be introduced in the undergraduate nursing program. As with all skills, it must be practiced in a variety of settings over time. Expertise in health literacy depends on the development of nursing domain knowledge, experience, information technology skills, critical thinking, and knowledge dissemination skills. Information literacy is an integral component of evidence-based nursing practice.

EBP is recommended by the Institute of Medicine and by professional nursing organizations to improve patient care outcomes. In theory, EBP is widely accepted, but practice of EBP is not universal in all education and clinical practice settings. Knowledge deficits about how to access, search, and synthesize literature findings has slowed implementation. Moreover, nurses in some clinical settings prefer to consult colleagues seen as having clinical expertise rather than analyze clinical and literature findings.

The good news is that abundant health information and EBP resources are available on the Internet. The Internet opens endless learning opportunities to nursing and healthcare providers who use analytical skills to scrutinize online resources for value.

APPLICATIONS AND COMPETENCIES

1. Discuss the differences between the relationships between information literacy, health literacy, and information technology skills. Give examples of each and describe the significance to nursing.

2. Identify the impact of healthcare consumer information literacy on patient care and education in one of your local healthcare agencies.

3. Analyze a patient education brochure using readability statistics. After completing the analysis, would you recommend continued use of the brochure for patients? Why or why not?

4. Identify a website with nursing knowledge and identify the essential elements for validating the knowledge.

5. Find healthcare examples for each of the following and discuss the differences:
   a. online scholarly nursing article
   b. article in a nursing magazine
   c. newspaper
   d. newsletter
   e. Website

6. Identify one EBP nursing resource you found by searching the Internet. Explain how you were able to determine the quality of the website.

7. Identify any obstacles that interfere with the adoption of evidence-based resources in nursing practice in your clinical or healthcare agency work setting. Discuss how those obstacles could be successfully addressed.

REFERENCES

American Association of Colleges of Nursing. (2005). *Position paper: Nursing education's agenda for the 21st century*. Retrieved May 17, 2010, from http://www.aacn.nche.edu/Publications/positions/nrsgedag.htm

Association of Colleges and Research Libraries. (2000). *Information literacy competency standards for higher education*. Retrieved May 18, 2010, from http://www.ala.org/ala/mgrps/divs/acrl/standards/standards.pdf

Breivik, P. S. (1991). Information literacy. *Bulletin of the Medical Library Association, 79*(2), 226–229. Retrieved from http://www.pubmedcentral.nih.gov/picrender.fcgi?artid=225527&blobtype=pdf

Communicating with patients who have limited literacy skills. Report of the National Work Group on Literacy and Health. (1998). *Journal of Family Practice, 46*(2), 168–176.

Courey, T., Benson-Soros, J., Deemer, K., & Zeller, R. A. (2006). The missing link: Information literacy and evidence-based practice as a new challenge for nurse educators. *Nursing Education Perspectives, 27*(6), 320–323.

Fox, S. (2007, October 8). *E-patients with a disability or chronic disease.* Retrieved July 30, 2011 from, http://www.pewinternet.org/Reports/2007/Epatients-With-a-Disability-or-Chronic-Disease.aspx

Fox, S. (2008). *The engaged e-patient population.* Retrieved July 30, 2011, from, http://www.pewinternet.org/Reports/2008/The-Engaged-Epatient-Population.aspx

Fox, S., & Purcell, K. (2010). *Chronic disease and the Internet.* Retrieved May 17, 2010, from http://www.pewinternet.org/Reports/2010/Chronic-Disease.aspx

Grant, M. J., & Brettle, A. J. (2006). Developing and evaluating an interactive information skills tutorial. *Health Information and Libraries Journal, 23*(2), 79–86.

Greiner, A. C., & Knebel, E. (Eds.). (2003). *Health professions education: A bridge to quality.* Washington, DC: National Academy Press.

Joint Commission. (2007). *"What did the doctor say?:" Improving health literacy to protect patient safety.* Retrieved July 30, 2011, from http://www.jointcommission.org/What_Did_the_Doctor_Say/

Ku, Y., Sheu, S., & Kuo, S. (2007). Efficacy of integrating information literacy education into a women's health course on information literacy for RN-BSN students. *Journal of Nursing Research, 15*(1), 67–77.

Kutner, M., Greenberg, E., Jin, Y., & Paulsen, C. (2006, September). *The health literacy of America's adults: Results from the 2003 National Assessment of Adult Literacy.* Retrieved May 18, 2010, from http://nces.ed.gov/pubs2006/2006483.pdf

National League for Nursing. (2008). *Position statement: Preparing the next generation of nurses to practice in a technology-rich environment: An informatics agenda.* Retrieved May 18, 2010, from http://www.nln.org/aboutnln/PositionStatements/informatics_052808.pdf

National Network of Libraries of Medicine. (2010). *Health literacy.* Retrieved May 17, 2010, from http://nnlm.gov/outreach/consumer/hlthlit.html

Nielsen-Bohlman, L., & Institute of Medicine (U.S.), Committee on Health Literacy. (2004). *Health literacy: A prescription to end confusion* (pp. xix, 345 p.). Retrieved from http://www.nap.edu/openbook.php?record_id=10883&page=1

Pfizer. (2008). *What is clear health communication?* Retrieved May 18, 2010, from http://www.pfizerhealthliteracy.org/

Quality and Safety Education for Nurses. (2010). *Project Overview | QSEN – Quality & Safety Education for Nurses.* Retrieved May 17, 2010, from http://www.qsen.org/overview.php

Sigma Theta Tau International. (2005, July 7). *Evidence-based nursing position statement.* Retrieved May 18, 2010, from http://www.nursingsociety.org/aboutus/PositionPapers/Pages/EBN_positionpaper.aspx

Stevens, K. R. (2005, June 23). *ACE: Learn about EBP: ACE star model.* Retrieved July 30, 2011, from, http://www.acestar.uthscsa.edu/acestar-model.asp

Technology Guiding Education Reform. (2007). *The TIGER initiative: Evidence and informatics transforming nursing: 3-year action steps toward a 10-year vision.* Retrieved May 17, 2010, from http://www.aacn.nche.edu/Education/pdf/TIGER.pdf

Wallace, L. S., Rogers, E. S., Roskos, S. E., Holiday, D. B., & Weiss, B. D. (2006). Brief report: Screening items to identify patients with limited health literacy skills. *Journal of General Internal Medicine, 21*(8), 874–877.

Wilson, M. (2009). Readability and patient education materials used for low-income populations. *Clinical Nurse Specialist CNS, 23*(1), 33–40; quiz 41–32. doi: 10.1097/01.NUR.0000343079.50214.31

CHAPTER 11

Finding Knowledge in the Digital Library Haystack

Objectives

After studying this chapter, you will be able to:

- ▶ *Compare nursing knowledge found in online library databases with that found using the Internet.*

- ▶ *Discuss library bibliographic databases useful to nurses.*

- ▶ *Demonstrate effective literature search strategies to support evidence-based practice.*

- ▶ *Describe the use of personal reference management software.*

Key Terms

Advanced Search	Meta-Analysis
Evidence-Based Care	Personal Reference
Factual Database	Manager
Federated Search	Randomized Controlled Trials
Index	Research Practice Gap
Keywords	Seminal Work
Knowledge-Based Database	Subject Heading
Medical Subject Headings	Systematic Review
(MeSH)	

Given the vast amount of published information, it is impossible to know everything applicable to nursing practice. According to Barnard, Nash, and O'Brien (2005, p. 505), "the amount and complexity of information nurses are expected to manage continues to increase exponentially." Library online resources provide a pivotal gateway to knowledge discovery. All nurses and healthcare providers must proactively develop and practice information search competencies to improve patient care and promote the scholarship of nursing. Without effective information search competencies, knowledge remains embedded in the digital haystack.

To assist with information searches, librarians created digital **index guides** to the literature. The index guides are produced as bibliographic databases, which can be searched electronically. Bibliographic databases have replaced print card catalogs and annual print indexes of the periodical literature. Electronic databases, not limited by paper, are generally more flexible and provide more information than print indexes. A user can retrieve information from electronic databases in the form of citations, abstracts, and in some cases, even full-text journal articles or full-text books. Many types of information and media resources are indexed in online databases.

Digital Library Basics

There are two types of digital databases: knowledge based and factual. **Knowledge-based databases** index published literature. **Factual databases** replace reference books with searchable and updatable online information, for example, drug and laboratory manuals. Knowledge-based databases focus on areas such as health sciences, business, history, government, law, and ethics. Furthermore, each database is specialized by the number and type of resources (e.g., journal or book names) indexed, the span of years indexed, and the words that the database uses to describe the resources for searching purposes.

Libraries purchase electronic databases from library vendors. Library vendors market and package their databases into bundles containing two or more separate databases. Libraries, therefore, may offer different electronic resources depending on the vendor and the database bundle that the library purchased. Each bundle of databases comes with a search interface window that identifies the vendor name. A few examples of library venders that package health science databases are EBSCO, Ovid, and ProQuest. Access to databases is essential for clinical nurses, nursing students, and faculty to stay current in the profession and to provide **evidence-based care**. Nurses should discuss their needs with their librarian to ensure access to the specific health science databases that allow them to improve clinical practice.

Searching online bibliographic databases is a skill demanded of all healthcare professionals. An index system used to file or catalog references provides the mechanism for library searches. Electronic databases are indexed, or searchable, by many different attributes such as title, author name, and year. Given that, unlike print catalogs, only one entry for a source is needed; there are many other ways to search an online bibliographic database. **Keywords** are used, and searchers may designate if this word or words should be searched for in a title, abstract, often even the text, or all of these. Searchers can also limit searches to finding

sources by language, by age of subjects of a research article, by type of article, and by years of publication, and in some databases to finding only those sources that provide full text. There may be times when it is helpful to search more than one database at a time; this is called a **federated search**.

Most library vendor search windows allow users to select a citation format and to save the search results. If there is an option for saving with a specific citation format, there will be a drop-down menu with the common formats such as the American Psychological Association (APA), the Modern Languages Association, and the American Medical Association. Search findings can be printed, e-mailed, exported to a **personal reference manager**, and/or saved as a file onto the personal computer (PC).

Personal Reference Managers

Library database search findings can often be exported into a personal reference manager. A personal reference manager refers to database software that allows the user to create a personal collection of citations. Most library database interfaces include an export feature that allows the user to download citation information into a personal reference manager. There are a number of commercial products available, for example, EndNote®, ProCite®, Reference Manager®, and RefWorks. The citation information saved in commercial software can include hyperlinks to the associated resources on the PC, such as digital versions of articles, websites, or graphics.

Personal reference managers that include the import/export feature provide an efficient means of managing citation information. However, reference managers integrated into word processing software may not be capable of importing citations from a digital library database. For example, Microsoft® Word 2010 and OpenOffice.org Writer 3.2X both include personal reference manager features; however, each citation must be keyed in separately.

Personal reference managers are also available free online. Zotero (http://www.zotero.org/) is a very powerful open-source personal reference manager. Once downloaded it is an extension in the Firefox 3.6 web browser (Zotero, 2010). Zotero allows the user to save citation information from most library bibliographic databases and certain websites, such as Amazon.com and the New York Times. Other features include note-taking, the ability to hyperlink to files and images, and automatically capture screenshots of web pages. Zotero personal libraries can be imported into EndNote and RefWorks. Zotero works with Microsoft Word as a plug-in so that users can cite while writing and create reference lists in a Word document. Once the plug-in is installed, Zotero will be visible from the Add-In tab in the Word Ribbon menu. Zotero is also compatible with OpenOffice.org after downloading and installing the OpenOffice. org extensions. Zotero also works with Google docs. **Figure 11-1** shows a screen shot of Zotero.

Zotero can be used online or offline. Besides the benefit of importing citations from the web and digital libraries, using Zotero online provides cloud computing file synchronization. The service is free and simply requires the user to register and create a login and password. The online service provides a social networking feature that allows users to collaborate. Although Zotero is embedded in the Firefox web browser, users can edit citation information when offline because Firefox can be used offline.

CiteULike at http://www.CiteULike.org/ is a free online personal reference manager service that allows users to store, organize, and share citation information (CiteUlike, 2010). Users must register for an account with a login and password. Building an online library of personal citations is easy using Bookmarklets. Bookmarklets allow you to import book and journal article citation metadata into your personal CiteULike library. For additional information on Bookmarklets, go to http://www. citeulike.org/bookmarklets.adp. Once you have navigated to a website or a digital library article, click on the *Post to CiteULike* on your web browser bookmarks or links toolbar to add the metadata. You can also import and export references from CiteULike to other personal reference manager software. Like Zotero, CiteULike includes a social networking feature.

Library Guides and Tutorials

Even the most experienced library patrons can benefit from library guides and tutorials because the technology development for library resources continues to change rapidly. Lifelong learning for professional nursing must begin with demonstrated competencies in the use of digital library searches to discover new nursing knowledge. Nursing knowledge, including evidence-based practice (EBP) findings, should be quickly integrated into clinical practice to improve patient outcomes. Fortunately, there are numerous library guides and tutorials available on the Internet. The most efficient way to develop/improve library competencies is with the assistance of a librarian. Qualified librarians have a master's or doctoral degree with a specialization in an area of library science. The focus of their expertise and continuing education is to assist users in accessing and utilizing library resources.

Just-in-time learning using online library guides and tutorials is also an efficient way to develop/improve library information competencies. The

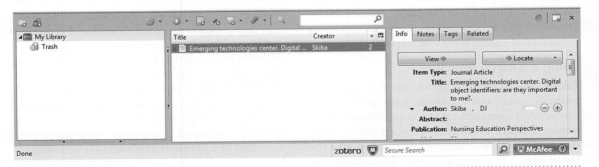

Figure 11-1 Zotero citation detail.

guides and tutorials address how to use the specific library facility, how to search using **medical subject headings (MeSH)**, how to use a vendor search interface, and how to use a specific database. To learn how to use a library facility, use the Internet to find the library's homepage. Information on a library web page generally includes the hours of operation, links to services and departments, information on how to find books and journals, and links to help resources such as guides and tutorials.

Subject Headings

Subject headings refer to standardized terms used to index or catalog reference materials. Each library chooses a standard subject authority or thesaurus for all of its cataloging. Libraries using the National Library of Medicine (NLM) classification use the "medical subject headings" or MeSH (http://www.nlm.nih.gov/mesh/).

Searching Using Mesh Terms

Each library database also uses a "controlled vocabulary" of terms (subject headings) to index the materials so that the database can be searched. MeSH refers to the controlled vocabulary of terms used to index materials in PubMed and MEDLINE databases. Cumulative Index to Nursing and Allied Health Literature (CINAHL) subject headings follow the MeSH structure (CINAHL, 2010). Since CINAHL and MEDLINE are two primary databases with nursing literature, it is important to understand the search term structure. MeSH differs from many other subject-heading lists because it is based on a hierarchal structure, as shown in **Box 11-1**. Because of this structure, searches on a broad subject can be constructed to include the narrower subjects in the MeSH tree structure. This is known as "exploding" the broader term to include all of the terms in the hierarchy.

Using a Search Interface

Taking time to review a search interface guide and tutorials before embarking on a literature search may prevent hours of frustration and disappointing results. Guides and tutorials for how to use a vendor search interface are commonly embedded into the Help menu. It is very important to understand that the search features for each library vendor differ.

BOX 11-1 The Mesh Tree Structure

....

Neoplasms
Neoplasms by Site [C04.588]
   Abdominal Neoplasms [C04.588.033] +
   Anal Gland Neoplasms [C04.588.083]
   Bone Neoplasms [C04.588.149] +
   Breast Neoplasms [C04.588.180]
     Breast Neoplasms, Male
     [C04.588.180.260]
      Carcinoma, Ductal, Breast
      [C04.588.180.390]

From http://www.nlm.nih.gov/mesh/mbinfo.html

The EBSCOhost includes a link to Help in the main menu at the top of the search window. The Help website has a very comprehensive listing of Help files that range from general information on database searching to online Flash videos and PowerPoint tutorials. The Ovid search window help provides training specifically for Ovid users, using interactive one-hour web-based workshops on numerous topics. Ovid also provides an online self-paced tutorial. **Table 11-1** provides the web pages for the tutorials for some of these bibliographic search tools.

When searching for nursing knowledge, be familiar with the way the vendor search engine handles Boolean terminology (AND, OR, and NOT).[1] Truncation and wildcards with the asterisk (*) and question mark (?) can be used with some search engines. Truncation is used for searching spelling variations. For example, a search for nur* would result in citations with the words nurse and nursing. The question mark with a wildcard is used to replace a single unknown character or letter anywhere in the word. For example, a search for hea? would result in citations with the words heat and head. Users should be aware of stop words ignored by the search engine (see **Box 11-2** for examples). Search engines generally do not search for stop words such as articles and prepositions unless they are a part of a phrase that is enclosed with quotes.

---

1 See Chapter 9 for more information on Boolean searching.

Table 11-1 Online Search Help Resources

Interface Help	URL
EBSCOhost	EBSCOhost research databases – http://support.ebsco.com/help/
	Tutorials – http://support.epnet.com/training/tutorials.php
Ovid	Training and documentation – http://www.ovid.com/site/help/ovid-tutorial.jsp
	Self-paced tutorial – http://www.ovid.com/site/help/ovid-tutorial/index.html
ProQuest	Advanced search – http://proquest.umi.com/i-std/en/hsp/advanced/adv.htm
	Top questions regarding advanced search – http://proquest.umi.com/i-std/en/hsp/advanced/adv_faq.htm
	Search tips – http://proquest.umi.com/i-std/en/hsp/searchtips/searchtips.htm

Some vendor search engines, such as EBSCOhost, Ovid, or ProQuest, allow the user to restrict online searches to peer-reviewed articles in scholarly journals, articles with references, articles with abstracts, research articles, or full-text articles. Peer-reviewed articles are excellent resources to support nursing knowledge. A journal is a scholarly publication that provides peer-reviewed articles.[2] In contrast, articles in magazines, newsletters, and newspapers should serve as points of information and entertainment, but should never be used to support nursing knowledge.

Bibliographic Databases Pertinent to Nursing

There are numerous databases with information pertinent to nursing. Essential ones with a focus on nursing and health-related topics are CINAHL, MEDLINE/PubMed, Cochrane Library, and PsycINFO. Although there may be some overlap in the journals and resources these databases index, there are important differences that may affect the search outcome. Furthermore, there are variations for each of the

databases for each library system: Some include only citations and abstracts and others contain varying numbers of full-text documents. Unless you are an experienced researcher, consult with a reference librarian to assist with refining your search question and selecting the best databases to search. See **Table 11-2** for a list of databases according to nursing topic. The databases discussed in this table are commonly available through most medical and academic libraries.

Using a Specific Library Database

Most vendor search interfaces and online libraries provide links to guides and tutorials for specific databases within the collection. Unfortunately, currently there is no universal standard for indexing health science search terms; each library database is unique. Unless you have expertise in using a particular library database, it is critical that you review a guide and tutorials first. The nuances in the search terminology and methods can be very tricky, especially for novice student nurses who are in the process of learning terminology. **Table 11-3** provides the location of the tutorials for many of the bibliographic indexes that nurses need.

CINAHL

When researching a nursing topic, the CINAHL database is an excellent place to start. This database includes citations and abstracts for more than 500 nursing journals and 400 allied health journals dating back to 1982 (CINAHL, 2010). CINAHL Plus with Full-Text database includes full-text articles in addition to citations and abstracts. The subject headings use the NLM MeSH structure. To identify search terms, click CINAHL Headings in the Menu bar and enter the word or phrase you are

BOX 11-2 Examples of Stop Words

After	Be	Like	Said	Through
Also	Do	Make	Should	To
An	Each	Many	So	Use
And	For	More	Some	Was

2 See Chapter 10 for more information on the peer-reviewed process.

Table 11-2 Discovering Nursing Knowledge in Library Databases

Topic of Search Question	Examples of Databases to Search	Topic of Search Question	Examples of Databases to Search
Nursing	CINAHL	Patient teaching	MedlinePlus
	Cochrane Library		HealthSource: Consumer Edition
	ProQuest Nursing and Allied Health Source		Consumer Health Complete
	PubMed/MEDLINE		Micromedex CareNotes™
Biomedical research	PubMed/MEDLINE		CINAHL
	EMBASE	Psychosocial	PsycINFO
	CINAHL		PsycARTICLES
Education	ERIC		Sociological Abstracts
	CINAHL		Sociological Collection
Legal/ethical	LexisNexis Academic		Cambridge Scientific Abstracts
	CINAHL		
	PubMed/MEDLINE		CINAHL
Management	ABI/INFORM®		
	CINAHL		
Oncology	PubMed/MEDLINE		
	National Cancer Institute & Physician Data Query (PDQ®)		
	CINAHL		

searching to get a list of the associated subject headings. CINAHL may also include selected full-text documents such as nursing journal articles, evidence-based care sheets, book chapters, newsletters, standards of practice, and nurse practice acts.

MEDLINE

When researching a biomedical research topic that crosses healthcare disciplines, use MEDLINE in addition to CINAHL. MEDLINE, a service made available through the NLM, is unique from proprietary library databases because it is also a free service that is accessible on the Internet through PubMed. The NLM is the largest medical library in the world. MEDLINE provides access to over 5,400 journals worldwide and includes a comprehensive collection of citations from biomedical articles dating back to 1947 (National Library of Medicine, 2010). You can access MEDLINE through PubMed on the Internet at http://www.ncbi.nlm.nih.gov/PubMed/. PubMed includes citations to literature not yet included in MEDLINE in addition to other services. PubMed Central allows access to free full-text articles (PubMed Central, 2010).

PubMed provides a variety of free services. NLM Mobile at http://www.nlm.nih.gov/mobile/ provides software applications for Palm™ and Pocket PC handheld computers. PubMed on Tap is an application for the iPhone.[3] PubMed for Handhelds at http://pubmedhh.nlm.nih.gov/nlm/ is a website designed specifically for use with handheld computers. My National Center for Biotechnology Information at http://www.ncbi.nlm.nih.gov/entrez/cubby.fcgi? provides the ability to save user information and preferences and store searches, and automatically e-mails the search information (National Center for Biotechnology Information, 2010) on designated topics to users after they register and receive a login and password.

Cochrane Library

In 2001, the Institute of Medicine (Institute of Medicine & National Academy of Sciences, 2001) challenged healthcare providers to implement "systematic approaches to analyzing and synthesizing

---

3 See Chapter 12 for more information on handheld computers.

Table 11-3 Online Help for Specific Library Databases

Online Help for Specific Library Databases	URL
CINAHL	http://support.ebsco.com/training/tutorials.php
Cochrane Library	http://www.thecochranelibrary.com/view/0/index.html
PsycInfo	http://scientific.thomson.com/tutorials/psycinfo2/
PubMed/MEDLINE	http://www.nlm.nih.gov/bsd/disted/pubmedtutorial/
	http://www.nlm.nih.gov/bsd/viewlet/search/subject/subject.html
	(MeSH) http://www.ncbi.nlm.nih.gov/sites/entrez?db=mesh

medical evidence for both clinicians and patients." The Cochrane Collaboration, founded in 1993 by Dr. Archie Cochrane, was recognized by the IOM as a model for synthesizing evidence to inform healthcare decision-making. The Cochrane Library, available through Wiley InterScience, is considered a gold standard for **meta-analysis** of medical research (Sackett, Rosenberg, Gray, Haynes, & Richardson, 1996). Access to the library may be through the library digital database listing or by using a login and password provided by your local library. The Cochrane Library is online at http://www.thecochranelibrary.com/view/0/index.html. The Cochrane library is available free in certain locations (The Cochrane Library, 2010). For example, it is available free for residents of the state of Wyoming in the United States and all low-income countries.

Cochrane reports are useful to nursing students, practicing nurses, and nurse researchers. Nursing students and practicing nurses may not have the confidence and experience to analyze research without assistance of faculty or nurse researchers. The Cochrane Library provides access to **systematic reviews** of the best research evidence. A systematic review is designed to reduce three types of bias inherent in individual research studies: selection, indexing, and publication (South African Medical Research Council, 2008). Selection bias is based on a person's point of view. Indexing bias is caused by limited searches to limited databases or search

terms. Publishing bias results when searches are limited to certain publications or languages. The process of systematic reviews is known as meta-analysis, which means that the results of multiple, similar research studies are carefully reviewed and analyzed.

PsycINFO

Because nursing is a holistic profession, some questions are best answered with information from searches of psychosocial databases, such as PsycINFO and PsycArticles. PsycINFO, a service of the APA, provides citations and abstracts for psychology and psychosocial aspects of other disciplines dating back to the 1600s and 1700s for psychology and psychosocial aspects of other disciplines (American Psychological Association, 2010). PsycArticles provides access to full-text articles.

Embarking on the Quest for Knowledge

The quest for knowledge is a five-step process (**Figure 11-2**). The process is cyclical and iterative rather than linear. In other words, the researcher may go back and forth through the steps. The process never stops because new knowledge is continually being generated.

Step 1: Questioning Practice: Recognize an Information Need

The first step in the quest for knowledge is recognizing an information need. Questioning practice may be difficult, but a new means of providing cost-effective care must be found. A case in point is Medicare nonpayment for higher costs of care resulting from preventable hospital-acquired injuries such as patient falls and infections from medical errors (Centers for Medicare & Medicaid Services, 2010). Healthcare practices must change to make patients safe, and nurses must be involved in searches for solutions to improve care practices.

As an example of a quest for knowledge, consider conducting a literature search for information on prevention of patient falls. The search question is "How can patient falls be prevented in nursing?" Notice that the broad topic, patient falls,

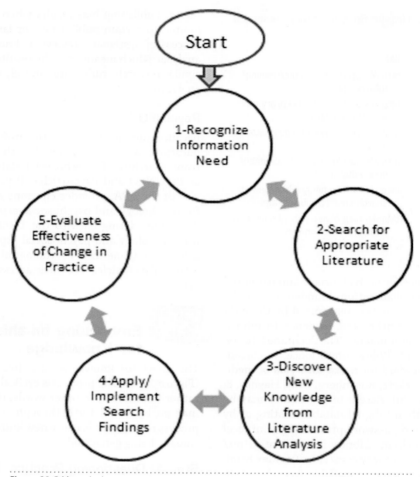

Figure 11-2 Knowledge quest.

is narrowed using the terms prevention and nursing. A common search mistake is that the search topic is too broad. Take a few moments to write out the search question to focus on the topic. Although it is best to carefully define the information need before beginning the search, it is possible to allow the search engine to assist by allowing you to choose terms from a list of search terms.

Step 2: Searching for Appropriate Evidence

The literature search process is an essential skill that nursing professionals must learn and practice. It is a vital step in discovering nursing knowledge and developing EBP. The quest for new nursing knowledge involves discovering, understanding, analyzing, and applying findings from literature. The process for conducting a literature search must be systematic and comprehensive. Subject headings are used to develop search strategies that will lead you to the most useful information on your search question. Although ideas for changes in clinical practice may come from regular reading of the literature, it is still necessary to search for more information to determine whether the information in the original article is supported by other articles and warrants a change in clinical practices (Price, 2009).

New Search | Publications | CINAHL Headings | Evidence-Based Care Sheets | More ▾

Searching: **CINAHL Plus with Full Text** | Choose Databases »

"patient falls" in Select a Field (optional) ▾ | Search | Clear | ?

AND ▾ prevention in Select a Field (optional) ▾

AND ▾ nursing in Select a Field (optional) ▾ Add Row

Basic Search | Advanced Search | Visual Search | ▶ Search History/Alerts | Preferences »

Figure 11-3 Advanced search – selecting search terms.

While searching, first determine the library databases that are most appropriate for the evidence for which you are searching and then identify the search terms that match that database. Selecting the most appropriate database(s) is just as important as the search strategy. If you are looking for peer-reviewed scholarly literature, use the online databases for libraries serving populations engaged in healthcare and education, and search databases and indexes such as CINAHL, MEDLINE, Cochrane Library, and Education Resources Information Center (ERIC). If you are looking for patient teaching resources, use the online library databases and the Internet, especially MedlinePlus (http://www.nlm.nih.gov/medlineplus/), an NLM resource, which is designed for consumers. It is important to remember that a comprehensive search must never be limited to the Internet or online library full-text resources. Although a wide range of information resources may be found online, libraries, librarians, and bookstores are vital to help borrow or purchase the knowledge-based resources needed for nursing education and practice. If a search finds resources that your library does not have, it is often possible to obtain these from interlibrary loan.

For the patient fall example, we used the CINAHL Plus with Full-Text database and EBSCO search interface window. After opening the database, the **Advanced Search** tab was selected (see **Figure 11-3**).[4] The phrase advanced search is misleading because the search tools allow users to define the search clearly. The Subject Terms checkbox (if it is available) or CINAHL Headings can be used for assistance with search terms. In this example, patient falls was entered with double quotes to find only "patient falls" as a phrase. A goal for an effective search is a return of about 50 results.

The search was run in 2010. There were 76 results; the most recent article was published in 2010. Using the option of further narrowing the search by clicking Risk Assessment in the "Narrow Results by Subject" (see **Figure 11-4**) window produced 11 citations. The first four citations were published between 2003 and 2007. A rule of thumb is to use the most current citations for sources published within the past three to five years. A search

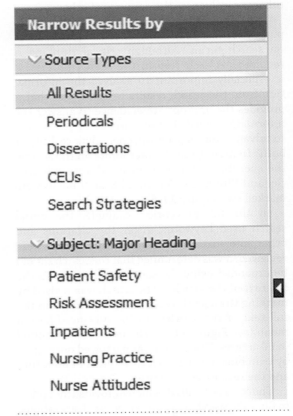

Narrow Results by

⌄ Source Types

All Results

Periodicals

Dissertations

CEUs

Search Strategies

⌄ Subject: Major Heading

Patient Safety

Risk Assessment

Inpatients

Nursing Practice

Nurse Attitudes

Figure 11-4 Narrowing the search.

4 See your librarian if you need help gaining access to the database.

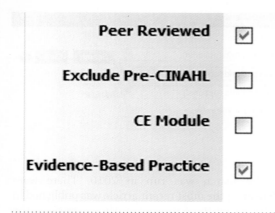

Figure 11-5 Advanced search checkboxes.

for a classic journal article, for example, one that documents **seminal work** on a particular topic, may require searching into much older resources. Seminal work refers to work frequently cited by others or influences the opinions of others.

It is important to remember that a computer determined the results of the search based on search terms. Although critical thinking is required for each step in the search process, it is especially important to analyze the information from the search results to make sure that it provides the appropriate evidence to answer the information need. Is the purpose of the search to advance nursing knowledge, advance EBP, or both? In order to set further limits on the search, the checkboxes for peer-reviewed, research article, and EBP in the Advanced Search menu were marked (see **Figure 11-5**).

In the fall prevention example, the initial search used keywords. After the citations and other information from the initial search were reviewed, it was determined that the search should be expanded using the same search terms in the full text of the articles. The search was revised by marking the checkbox for "Also search within the full text of the articles" in the Advanced Search menu (see **Figure 11-6**). The new search resulted in 60 articles. The search was narrowed once again by searching only the past three years of literature and the result was 23 articles.

The *Narrow Results By* window provided the option to filter the search to view periodicals, dissertations,

or articles offering Continuing Education Units (CEUs) (see **Figure 11-3**). Filtering does not affect the search results. It provides a quick method to assist with analysis of the findings.

In the final step of the search process, the citation information is saved or downloaded for use in the analysis and summary of the literature search. The EBSCO search window allows the user to save results of searches to a search folder. Once the search is completed, the search folder should be clicked for options (see **Figure 11-7**). When the search folder is opened, the user can print, e-mail, save, and/or export the selected citations from the results of the search (see **Figure 11-8**).

Personal Reference Manager Software

The Export Manager in EBSCO can be used to format the search findings for export into a commercial product personal reference manager (e.g., EndNote, ProCite, or Reference Manager) by clicking the Save tab.[5] For the patient fall example discussed in the preceding text, clicking the Save tab prompted the file format export option. Use the default setting, "Direct Export to EndNote, ProCite, CITAVI, or Reference Manager" to export to Endnote or Zotero or choose another more appropriate file format (see **Figure 11-9**). Click the Save button to automatically export the citation metadata.

Step 3: Critical Analysis of the Literature Findings

Critical analysis of the literature findings is the point in the process where new knowledge is discovered. The first step is to select citations for articles that are possibly relevant to the information need and then obtain a full-text version of the articles. Review of the article abstract, reference list, and journal name are helpful to determine which articles to read. Consult a librarian if you need assistance in finding full-text printable versions of the articles.

The next step is to read each article to analyze the findings critically. Highlight key points pertinent to the search question. Identify any gaps in knowledge. For example, what age groups of

---

5 If using the Zotero extension in the FireFox Web browser, clicking the folder icon to the right of the URL will prompt the user to select citations for download in the Zotero personal reference manager.

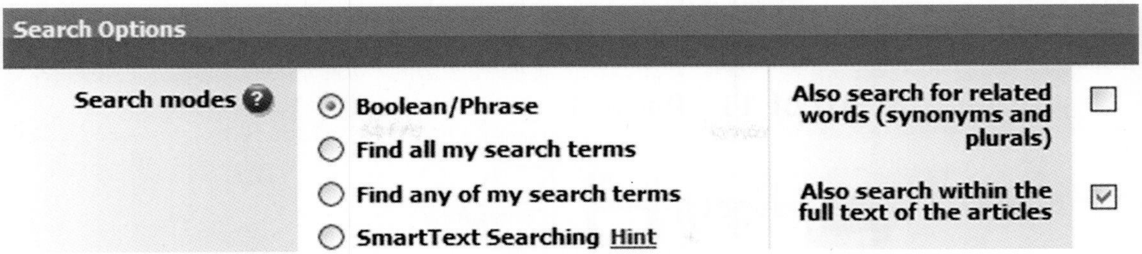

Figure 11-6 Further modifying the search.

patients were not addressed? What practice settings were omitted? Look for agreements and differences in research findings using the literature review, discussion, and conclusion sections of the research articles. Assess whether or not the literature findings are current and relevant to answer your search topic question.

Finally, assess the quality of the evidence. Analyze the literature using the seven-level rating system for hierarchy of research evidence (Melnyk & Fineout-Overholt, 2011) (see **Box 11-3**). The highest priority or evidence should be derived from meta-analysis of **randomized controlled trials** (RCTs) and evidence-based clinical guidelines based on systematic reviews of RCTs. When searching and reviewing the literature, look for the search terms systematic review and meta-analysis.[6] Be aware that the lowest forms of evidence are from the opinion of authorities and/or reports from expert committees.

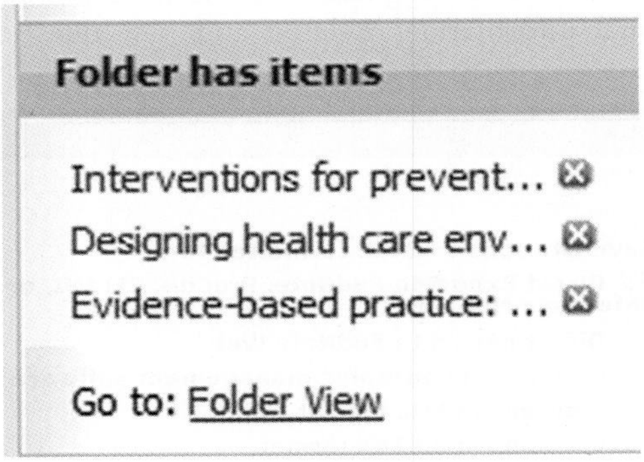

Figure 11-7 Saving the search.

Step 4: Apply/Implement the Search Findings

EBP is about using rather than doing research. It is an outcome-focused tool for clinical decision to improve healthcare delivery. Its purpose is to bridge the gap between research and clinical practice. In EBP, clinical observations are systematically recorded without bias and synthesized with original research that has been subject to a systematic review. The healthcare team with a patient-centered focus should practice EBP collaboratively.

BOX 11-3 Rating System for the Hierarchy of Evidence

Level I: Evidence from a systematic review or meta-analysis of all relevant randomized controlled trials (RCTs) or evidence-based clinical practice guideline based on systematic review of RCTs.

Level II: Evidence obtained from at least one well-designed RCT.

Level III: Evidence obtained from well-designed controlled trials without randomization.

Level IV: Evidence from well-designed case–control and cohort studies.

Level V: Evidence from systematic reviews of descriptive and qualitative studies.

Level VI: Evidence from single descriptive or qualitative study.

Level VII: Evidence from the opinion of authorities and/or reports of expert committees.

---

6 See Chapter 24 for more detailed information on research.

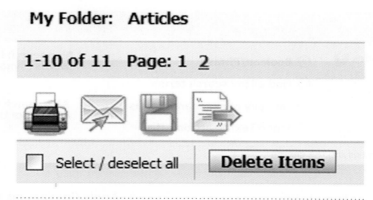

Figure 11-8 Saving options.

The IOM recommends that EBP be applied to healthcare delivery to reduce the time between the scientific discovery of effective forms of treatment and their implementation (Institute of Medicine & National Academy of Sciences, 2001). Sackett (1996, p. 71), credited for one of the earliest definitions of EBP, said, "Evidence-based medicine is the conscientious, explicit, and judicious use of current best evidence in making decisions about the care of individual patients." Current definitions of EBP recognize the importance of clinical expertise to assess, diagnose, and plan care. They also emphasize the importance of patient-centered care that encompasses the patient's values, beliefs, concerns, and expectations.

The emphasis on outcomes and efficiency in the healthcare changes the focus from data gathering to the use of data (evidence) from both the literature and the clinical documentation.

According to Valente (2003), the "discrepancy between research on effective clinical practice and the direct care provided to patients is called the research practice gap." Nurses must expedite closing the **research practice gap** in order to make dramatic, needed improvements to our healthcare delivery system.

Step 5: Evaluate the Result and Effectiveness of Practice Changes

Although expedient implementation of quality search findings is vital, it is not the final step in the quest for improved care based on knowledge and research evidence. The result and effectiveness of practice changes must be evaluated. The process of evidence-based care is cyclical and iterative (Dobbins, 2007). Once changes are implemented, nurses must be cognizant of the need for additional information. Related and new questions

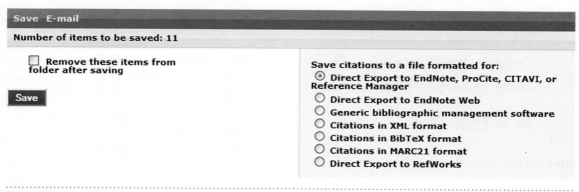

Figure 11-9 Using the export manager.

will emerge from the practice change. The new questions must be explored.

Challenges to the Adoption of Evidence-Based Nursing

Although EBP is widely accepted today, originally the concept was criticized. Those critical believed that it was impractical to implement and served to only reduce costs and limit clinical freedom (Sackett, Rosenberg, Gray, Haynes, & Richardson, 1996). Critics believed that EBP was a cookbook approach to medicine that eliminated their clinical decision-making skills. Findings from nursing research suggest that challenges to wide adoption of EBP in nursing persist. The problem is complex, ranging from access to knowledge resources, attitudes toward research, and information literacy knowledge and skills (Pravikoff, Tanner, & Pierce, 2005). Other barriers to evidence-based nursing include lack of time, lack of sufficient staff, and difficulties in interpreting statistics and research writings (Hannes et al., 2007; Thompson, McCaughan, Cullum, Sheldon, & Raynor, 2005).

Access to resources is a challenge. Joint Commission requires facilities to have knowledge resources available in the healthcare facility; however, access to digital libraries resources is not universally available 24 hours a day, 7 days a week. Recommendations from the IOM and professional nursing organizations are unified in the definition of EBP as being the best evidence currently available, yet there is no universal recommendation about what constitutes resources (e.g., library databases) of best practice. As a result, the available library resources for nursing programs and healthcare providers vary. Access to information and knowledge resources is improving, but is not yet universal for all nursing programs and clinical settings (Penz & Bassendowski, 2006). The Cochrane Library is recognized as the gold standard for systematic reviews and meta-analysis research findings, but Wyoming is the only state in the United States that has free access.

The culture of clinical practice settings may not support or value information-seeking practices and current research (Mohide & King, 2003). Culture of clinical practice refers to situations in which management, physicians, and other nurses do not value or support information seeking and research. Another challenge to the adoption of EBP is that nurses prefer to obtain their information from another colleague, especially if they see that person as a nursing expert (Penz & Bassendowski, 2006). Often in the fast pace of providing healthcare, nurses prefer to ask another nurse whose opinion they value rather than search for answers themselves.

Nursing research on the challenges for adoption of evidence-based care reveals the complexity of the problem. A Sigma Theta Tau International (STTI) 2006 quantitative survey of 568 nurses (Sigma Theta Tau International, 2006) revealed unsettling results. Twenty-four percent of the nurses reported a low familiarity with EBP. The majority (66%) stated that the primary challenge for finding and using EBP is time to search and analyze findings. Almost half (45%) of the nurses indicated that finding and using EBP was difficult because they have difficulty interpreting and analyzing the findings because of the way they are written.

A study by Pravikoff et al. (2005) revealed 10 personal barriers to the adoption of EBP; the most significant was the lack of value in clinical settings for research. The other nine barriers related to access of research resources, lack of research skills, lack of information literacy skills, and lack of information technology competencies. The study revealed six different institutional barriers; the primary one was the presence of goals with a higher priority. Other organizational barriers related to staffing issues, budget, organizational perceptions about nurses preparation for EBP, and organizational perceptions about the unrealistic use of research.

A qualitative research study done in Belgium indicates that the barriers to evidence-based nursing may be universal (Hannes et al., 2007). The study revealed characteristics related to five themes: doctors, patients, families, management, and supervisors. There were two subthemes for nurses' discomfort: (1) Nurses did not feel comfortable questioning doctor's opinions and (2) they were uncomfortable making suggestions that conflicted with the wishes and preferences of patients and families. Nurses who were concerned with quality of care found themselves at odds with management/supervisors that were perceived to be more concerned with reducing costs. The Belgium study finding, lack of knowledge and skills, was very similar to the research reported by STTI and Pravikoff.

Summary

The two types of library databases – knowledge based and factual – provide an essential gateway to knowledge discovery. Information search competencies and the use of a personal bibliographic reference manager are essential skills for all nurses who use online library databases to extract nursing knowledge. Effective use of online library databases provides unlimited opportunities to discover knowledge that will improve patient care.

The CINAHL, PubMed/MEDLINE, Cochrane Library, and PsycINFO databases are just a few knowledge-based databases vital to nursing knowledge discovery. The process of searching for knowledge is a skill that is learned only with repeated practice. The process is cyclical and iterative but not linear. There are five steps in this process: (1) defining a search topic based on an information need, (2) searching for evidence embedded in the literature, (3) critically analyzing and summarizing the literature, (4) implementing the findings into practice, and (5) evaluating the results of implementation by asking additional questions or discovering new questions.

Improving patient care and reducing healthcare errors require that nursing and hospital administrators, clinicians, educators, and nursing students adopt a culture of care that uses evidence-informed nursing practice. To this end, nurses must be proactive in breaking down the challenges and barriers to adopting EBP. It also requires that nurses self-assess their knowledge needs in locating and evaluating research and identify strategies for gaining the skills needed for competency in this area. Additionally, administrators must see that clinicians have the necessary time, training, support, and access to knowledge resources needed for EBP.

APPLICATIONS AND COMPETENCIES

1. Indexing an article:
   a. Find a peer-reviewed nursing journal article, either online or in your library or personal collection.
   b. Create an electronic document using word processing software or spreadsheet software. (Use a piece of paper if a computer is not available.) At the top of the document note the author's name, date, article title, journal title, and source. Create a four-column table using the following column headings: My Subject Terms, CINAHL Subject Terms, MEDLINE Subject Terms, and Cochrane Library Subject Terms.
   c. Read the article and write the subject terms you think it includes in the first column.
   d. Do an author/title search in each of the three databases and note the subject terms in the corresponding columns.
   e. Discuss your analysis of similarities and differences of subject terms for the three databases.

2. Finding databases:
   a. Look for five databases that are pertinent to nursing knowledge in your library and health system websites.
   b. Create an electronic document using either word processing or spreadsheet software.
   c. Develop a five-column table using the following column headings: Library Databases, Bibliographic Database, Bibliographic With Full-Text Database, Factual Database, and How Information Can Support EBP.
   d. Complete the matrix noting the database name, type(s), and EBP implications.
   e. Discuss your findings.

3. Searching a database:
   a. Choose a search topic related to a current patient care question.
   b. Plan a search strategy for CINAHL, MEDLINE, and one of the other databases described in this chapter. Note the subject headings on a worksheet similar to the one used in the first exercise.
   c. Execute the search in each of these databases.
   d. Compare and contrast your results.

4. Searching for EBP:

   a. Identify a nursing outcome that needs improvement in your health system.

   b. Plan search strategies to identify relevant translation literature, evidence summaries, and original research.

   c. Execute these searches and evaluate results.

   d. Discuss how the cited publications might help you prepare a clinical guideline to facilitate needed changes in practice.

5. Searching for personal reference (or personal bibliographic) management software:

   a. Conduct an online search for personal reference management software.

   b. Read recent articles and reviews discussing personal reference management software, both online and in journal articles that you retrieve through searching.

   c. Investigate the availability of online tutorials and support for specific products.

   d. Based on your research, designate a personal reference management software package that best meets your needs and discuss the rationale for the choice.

REFERENCES

American Psychological Association. (2010). *PsycINFO*. Retrieved June 4, 2010, from http://www.apa.org/pubs/databases/psycinfo/index.aspx

Barnard, A., Nash, R., & O'Brien, M. (2005). Information literacy: Developing lifelong skills through nursing education. *Journal of Nursing Education, 44*(11), 505–510.

Centers for Medicare & Medicaid Services. (2010, January 11). *Hospital-acquired conditions*. Retrieved June 4, 2010, from http://www.cms.gov/HospitalAcqCond/06_Hospital-Acquired_Conditions.asp

CINAHL. (2010, January 19). CINAHL databases. Retrieved June 4, 2010, from http://www.ebscohost.com/cinahl/

CiteUlike. (2010, March 4). *CiteULike Help and FAQs*. Retrieved June 4, 2010, from http://wiki.citeulike.org/index.php/Main_Page

Dobbins, M. (2007). Journey to evidence-informed nursing practice: Understanding the process as an iterative loop. *Reflections on Nursing Leadership, 33*(2). Retrieved from http://www2.nursingsociety.org/RNL/2Q_2007/columns/dobbins.html

Hannes, K., Vandersmissen, J., De Blaeser, L., Peeters, G., Goedhuys, J., & Aertgeerts, B. (2007). Barriers to evidence-based nursing: A focus group study. *Journal of Advanced Nursing, 60*(2), 162–171.

Institute of Medicine & National Academy of Sciences. (2001). *Crossing the quality chasm: A new health system for the 21st century*. Washington, DC: National Academies Press.

Melnyk, B. M., & Fineout-Overholt, E. (2011). *Evidence-based practice in nursing & healthcare: A guide to best practice* (2nd ed.). Philadelphia: Wolters Kluwer Health//Lippincott Williams & Wilkins.

Mohide, E. A., & King, B. (2003). Building a foundation for evidence-based practice: Experiences in a tertiary hospital. *Evidence-Based Nursing, 6*(4), 100–103.

National Center for Biotechnology Information. (2010). *Welcome to NCBI*. Retrieved June 4, 2010, from http:/ www.ncbi.nlm.nih.gov/

National Library of Medicine. (2010, June 2). *MEDLINE fact sheet*. Retrieved June 4, 2010, from http://www.nlm.nih.gov/pubs/factsheets/medline.html

Penz, K. L., & Bassendowski, S. L. (2006). Evidence-based nursing in clinical practice: Implications for nurse educators. *Journal of Continuing Education in Nursing, 37*(6), 251–254; quiz 255–256, 269.

Pravikoff, D. S., Tanner, A. B., & Pierce, S. T. (2005). Readiness of U.S. nurses for evidence-based practice. *American Journal of Nursing, 105*(9), 40–51; quiz 52.

Price, B. (2009). Guidance on conducting a literature search and reviewing mixed literature. *Nursing Standard, 23*(24), 43–50.

PubMed Central. (2010, June 3). *Pubmed Central homepage*. Retrieved June 4, 2010, from http://www.ncbi.nlm.nih.gov/pmc/

Sackett, D. L., Rosenberg, W. M. C., Gray, J. A. M., Haynes, R. B., & Richardson, W. S. (1996). Evidence based medicine: What it is and what it isn't. *British Medical Journal, 312*(7023), 71–72. Retrieved July 30, 2011, from http://www.bmj.com/content/312/7023/71.long

Sigma Theta Tau International. (2006). *2006 EBP study: Summary of findings*. Retrieved January 3, 2008, from http://www.nursingknowledge.org/Portal/CMSLite/GetFile.aspx?ContentID=78260

South African Medical Research Council. (2008, June 24). *What is a systematic review?* Retrieved June 4, 2010, from http://www.mrc.ac.za/cochrane/systematic.htm

The Cochrane Library. (2010). *Free online access through funded provisions*. Retrieved June 4, 2010, from http://www.thecochranelibrary.com/view/0/FreeAccess.html

Thompson, C., McCaughan, D., Cullum, N., Sheldon, T., & Raynor, P. (2005). Barriers to evidence-based practice in primary care nursing – Viewing decision-making as context is helpful. *Journal of Advanced Nursing, 52*(4), 432–444.

Valente, S. M. (2003). Research dissemination and utilization improving care at the bedside. *Journal of Nursing Care Quality, 18*(2), 114–121.

Zotero. (2010, May 31). *Quick start guide [Zotero Documentation]*. Retrieved June 4, 2010, from http://www.zotero.org/documentation/quick_start_guide

CHAPTER 12

Mobile Computing: Finding Knowledge in the Palm of Your Hand

Objectives

After studying this chapter, you will be able to:

▶ *Discuss the uses of mobile computers in healthcare.*

▶ *Describe the strengths and weaknesses of personal digital assistants and smartphones.*

▶ *Discuss data security issues associated with the use of mobile computers.*

▶ *Identify mobile software appropriate for nurses to use in the clinical setting.*

▶ *Identify mobile software appropriate for students to use in the learning setting.*

Key Terms

Beaming
Bluetooth
Cell Phone
e-Book
Flash Memory
Handheld Computer
Hotspot
Personal digital assistant (PDA)

Personal information management
Piconet
QWERTY Keyboard
Random-access memory (RAM)
Read-only memory (ROM)
Smartphone
Synchronization
WiFi

The development of wireless technology has radically changed the way we do business worldwide. Communication devices are no longer tethered to a cord in the wall. Batteries supplement electricity requirements. As a result, nurses and other healthcare providers can use mobile Internet devices (MIDs) such as the **smartphone**, personal digital assistant (**PDA**), and tablet computers at the point of need.

Most MIDs come with an assortment of personal information management software, such as contact information, a calendar, and a clock. The large storage capacities of mobile devices allow for storage of electronic books (**e-books**) reference material, graphics, videos, and other data files. Connectivity using **synchronization** software, **beaming**, **Bluetooth**, **WiFi** (wireless fidelity), and cellular phone lines allows for transfer of information from mobile devices to personal computers (PCs) or health information clinical systems.

The possibilities for effective use of handheld mobile computing in education and healthcare are endless.

Mobile Computing Basics

Mobile computers, such as smartphones, PDAs, netbooks, and tablets are all small computers. All mobile devices use an operating system (OS), and most allow the use of third-party software applications. The **cell phone** is a shortwave wireless communication device that has a connection to a transmitter. The word "cell" refers to the area of transmission. Cell phones, like landline phones, require a paid subscription to the transmission service provider. Smartphones are a combination of a PDA and a cell phone. This chapter focuses on mobile devices. The common term "**handheld computer**" is used in this chapter to refer to all handheld mobile devices. The information includes differences in features for each device, as well as examples of the use of these devices in educational and healthcare settings.

History of PDAs and Smartphones

The PDA concept was developed in the early 1980s with the Psion (Medindia, 2010). The first PDAs were designed primarily as personal information managers (PIMs) that included electronic telephone books and appointment calendars. The Newton MessagePad, developed by Apple in 1983, was the first popular PDA that featured a touch screen and handwriting capabilities. However, the Palm Pilot, introduced by U.S. Robotics in 1996, was light, fit in the palm of the user's hand, and featured Graffiti handwriting recognition software. It also had much better handwriting recognition than the Newton. As a result, it quickly dominated the market by 1999. Apple discontinued production of the Newton in 1998. The Pocket PC, introduced by Microsoft in 2000 (Tilley, 2009), offered a compact version of the Windows OS. It gave users the privilege of having more than one application open at the same time. They could also view or edit Microsoft Office documents. The Pocket PC grew in popularity with users, capturing the market with 54.2% of the OS shipments

in the second quarter of 2006 (Cellular News, 2006). PDAs began to lose popularity beginning in 2007 with the introduction of the Apple iPhone and later, the Google Android smartphone.

The first smartphone, known as "Simon," was introduced by IBM in 1993. The smartphone combined features of the cellular telephone and personal information management software. In 1999 (3Com Public Relations, 1999), Palm released the QUALCOMM pdQ, which featured a cell phone and the Palm organizer. The smartphone of today is a miniature computer that includes multiple software programs, documents, music, video, Internet access capability, and a telephone. The smartphones of today provide Internet access using cellular phone connections, or WiFi, or both. All smartphones require a subscription to a cellular phone provider. They are popular with users who do not want to carry a PDA and phone as separate devices. They are growing in popularity because cellular providers offer them at substantially discounted rates over stand-alone PDAs with the same features. A variety of PDAs and smartphones are available through manufacturers including Palm®, Hewlett-Packard Company, Research in Motion Limited, and Apple®. Smartphone features are very similar. Some smartphones, such as the iPhone, allow for scrolling using a finger and on on-screen keyboard (see **Figure 12-1**). Others include a keyboard either below the viewing screen or as a slideout. In 2010, Blackberry and iPhones had the majority of the smartphone market share (see **Figure 12-2**).

The iPod®, a PDA introduced by Apple in 2001, dominated the music player market with more than 100 million devices sold in less than six years (Apple, 2007). The iPod® uses Apple iTunes software to transfer music, video, or other applications quickly to the device. In a short time since the iPod's® inception, a number of generations have been released. The iPod® Touch and the iPhone™ were both released in 2007. The iPod® Touch provides a screen size close to the width and length of the device including touch screen icons and WiFi access to the Internet. The iPhone™ looks almost identical to the iPod® Touch, but it is smartphone. The size of the storage drives and the simplicity for transferring audio, video, and data have made the iPod®

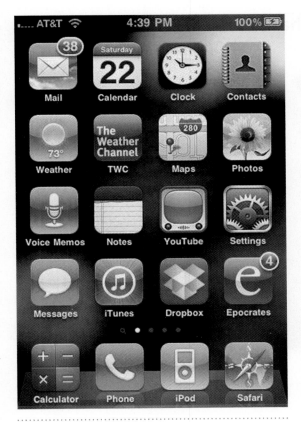

Figure 12-1 iPhone.

and iPhone favorite media devices for users of all ages. The iPad (**Figure 12-3**) was released in 2010. The iPad looks like a large (7.8 inch × 5.8 inch) iPod Touch. The first device released in 2010 did not include a camera or phone capabilities. The iPad sold two million units less than 60 days after it was first released (Apple, 2010b).

 ## Understanding Mobile Computer Concepts

There are similarities and differences between PCs and mobile computers. Mobile computers do not necessarily have the same OS as the PC. Even if the OSs differ, mobile computing software is designed for interoperability (the devices work together). There are hardware differences between mobile computers and PCs, and it is important to understand these differences. Hardware variations

include display, battery, memory, synchronization and connectivity, and data entry devices. Synchronization and connectivity using beaming, Bluetooth, WiFi, and cellular phone line connections are data transfer functions common to mobile computers.

Mobile Computer Operating Systems

The smartphones and other mobile devices OSs determine the functions and software capabilities. The OSs include Blackberry Research in Motion (RIM), Apple iPod® and iPhone™, Palm webOS™, Windows Mobile Compact Edition (CE), Google Android, Symbian, and Linux.

The Palm OS has been popular in the healthcare arena because it is simple to use. Many electronic nursing and medical reference resources and free and shareware (available for a small fee) medical software applications have been developed for the Palm. Windows CE has been popular among healthcare providers because it resembles the Windows desktop OS. Numerous nursing and medical reference software applications are available for Windows CE, though less freeware and shareware. A growing number of medical software applications are available for the RIM Blackberry OS, although commercial, free, and shareware applications trail behind the Palm and Windows CE OSs.

There is nursing and medical software for the newest OSs, the iPhone OS, and Google Android. The iPod (integrated with the iPhone), originally designed to allow sharing of music, provides access to numerous free audio and video podcasts through the iTunes store or any iPod® server for the iPod®. The Google Android OS, released in 2008, is a modified version of Linux kernel – an open software platform designed to rival the Apple iPhone™. Numerous mobile device manufacturers use Android OS. Unlike the Apple OS, the Android OS supports the use of Adobe Flash for streaming audio and video.

Display

Mobile computers have a liquid crystal display like laptop PCs. Many mobile computers also provide a touch screen for data input. The screen display size and resolution differ from PCs. The diagonal screen display size on mobile computers ranges from 3.5 to

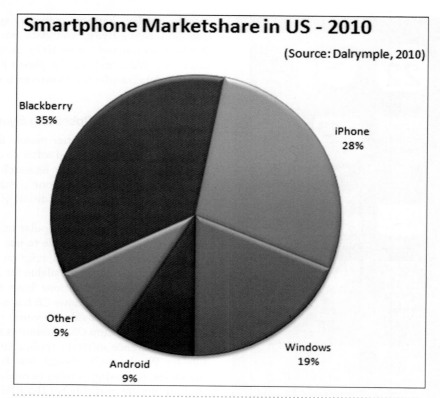

Figure 12-2 Smartphone market share.

9.7 inches (see **Table 12-1**). Resolution is an important consideration – the higher the numbers, the sharper is the image. A sharp screen image is a factor to consider if the user needs to view video, for example, of physical assessment or nursing procedures.

Table 12-1 Examples of Screen Resolution and Display Size Differences for Mobile Devices

Operating System	Mobile Device	Screen Resolution	Display Size (Inches)
iOS4	iPhone	960 × 640	3.5
Android	Motorola Droid	480 × 854	3.7
Palm WebOS	Palm Pre	480 × 320	3.2
Research in Motion	Blackberry Storm 2	480 × 360	3.25
Windows Mobile	Samsung Omnia II	480 × 800	3.7
Linux	Kindle DX	600 × 800	6
Android	Nook	600 × 800	6
Modified iOS	iPad	1024 × 768	9.7

Battery

All mobile computers operate using battery power.[1] Earlier Palm devices used replaceable alkaline (AAA) batteries that lasted several weeks. Most mobile devices now use rechargeable (nickel–metal hydride, nickel–cadmium, lithium ion) batteries. Factors that shorten battery life are multitasking features (Pocket PC), increased memory, a color display, audio, backlight display, and Bluetooth/WiFi connections (Cornelius & Gordon, 2007). If the battery is removable, a second one should be charged and made available as a replacement.

Memory

Mobile devices use three types of built-in memory – read-only memory (**ROM**), random-access memory (**RAM**), and built-in **flash memory**. Flash memory is also available as expansion cards, as shown in **Figure 12-4**. The ROM stores the

---

1 See Appendix A for more information about batteries.

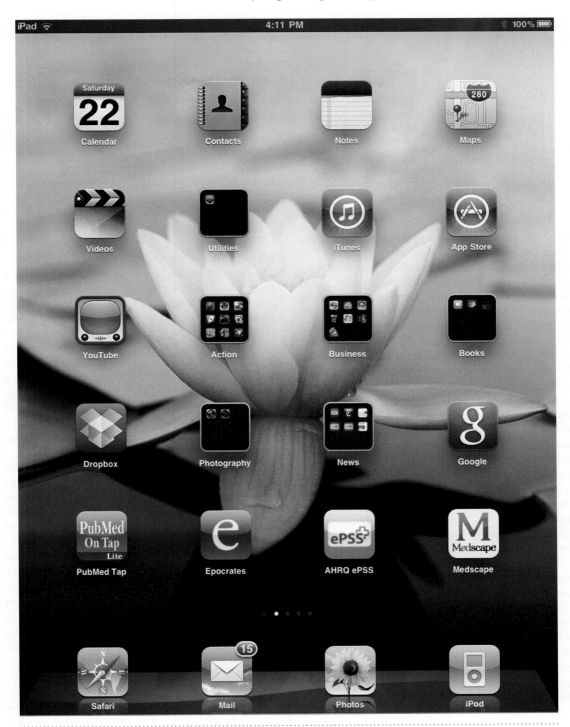

Figure 12-3 iPad.

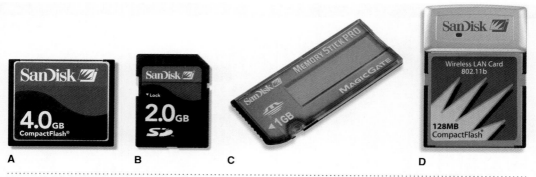

Figure 12-4 A–D: Flash memory cards.

OSs and standard applications such as contacts, calendar, and notes. The RAM stores all of the add-on applications and data files and requires a small amount of continuous battery power. RAM memory is volatile; hence, if the battery power is depleted, all of the data stored in RAM are lost. Some devices use flash memory instead of RAM because flash memory is nonvolatile, meaning that the applications and data will not disappear if the battery power is depleted.[2]

Unlike the PC, most PDAs and smartphones do not have a hard drive. Many mobile digital devices have expansion slots for removable flash memory cards for software and data storage. Removable memory, commonly used by mobile devices, includes Secure Digital (SD) cards, Compact Flash cards, and Memory Sticks. A few PDAs also accept a universal serial bus flash drive. Flash memory cards are useful for storing e-books, photographs, video, and music. The price of flash memory has plummeted. Today a 4-gigabyte (GB) SD card can be purchased for less than $10.

In contrast to Palm and Windows Mobile devices, the Apple iPod® Classic comes equipped with a very large hard drive. In fact, the iPod® Classic is available with a 160 GB hard drive. The Apple devices were designed primarily to deliver music and video; so it makes sense that they are designed with large storage capacities. The iPod® Nano, iPod® Touch, iPhone™, Kindle, and Nook use flash memory instead of a hard drive (Apple, 2010a; Carnoyon, 2009a, 2009b).

Data Entry

Many devices, such as iPod® Touch, iPad, iPhone™, and Nook, allow for data entry using the touch of a finger on a screen. Some devices allow the use of a stylus. **QWERTY keyboard** data entry is available in all smartphones and many PDAs (see **Figure 12-5**). QWERTY refers to a keyboard layout common to the PC and typewriter and comprises the first six letters on the top row of letters. Depending on the mobile device, data entry is enhanced using a navigation button and thumbwheel for scrolling. Mobile devices may also include a microphone and an audio recorder. Smartphones usually include a camera with a zoom lens that can be used to capture pictures and video clips.

Unless there is a separate keyboard especially designed for the mobile device, it is easier to enter large amounts of data using a PC, rather than the mobile device, and then synchronize the file with the mobile device. It is simple, however, to enter data such as a new appointment or contact on a mobile device. Office software such as Documents to Go (http://www.dataviz.com/) or Windows Office Mobile (bundled with some versions of Windows Mobile 6) allows users to create or edit Microsoft Word or Excel files on the mobile device. Google Docs allows for word processing and spreadsheet solutions (http://docs.google.com/m) on mobile devices.

Synchronization

Mobile devices are designed to synchronize with the PC using proprietary software so that all of the files on the two computers coincide. The Palm devices use

---

2 See Appendix A for more information about Flash memory.

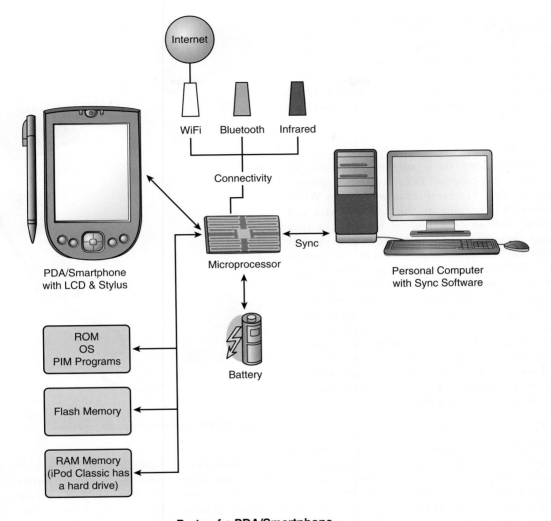

Parts of a PDA/Smartphone

Figure 12-5 Parts of a personal digital assistant/smartphone.

HotSync and Windows Mobile devices use Windows Mobile for data transfer between the mobile device and the PC. The Apple devices use iTunes, a free download, to transfer data. PIM contact information (names, phone numbers, and addresses) is transferred to mobile devices using software such as Microsoft Outlook or Palm Desktop.

Connectivity

Depending on the mobile device, these devices can connect in several ways with other devices or the Internet. Connectivity features include beaming, Bluetooth, WiFi, and cellular phone line. Bluetooth and WiFi expansion cards are available for those devices that have an expansion card slot but do not have this built-in feature of connectivity.

Beaming

Beaming allows for wireless, very short-ranged (3 feet), infrared (IR) transmission of information to other beam-enabled devices with the same OS. The beaming feature is used to share files, such as contact information and calendar, or documents such as Word or Excel, with another mobile device. To use beaming, both mobile devices must have an IR port and the beaming feature enabled.[3] You select the file that you want to share and then select beam from the menu (see **Figure 12-6**). Check your user's manual for the exact procedure to use with your device.

Bluetooth

Bluetooth allows for a wireless, short-ranged (32 feet), low-powered radio frequency connection to other Bluetooth-enabled devices. When Bluetooth is enabled on the mobile device and paired with another Bluetooth device, a personal area connection or a **piconet** is created (Franklin & Layton, 2007). There are several uses of Bluetooth. Bluetooth can be used to synchronize a mobile device with a PC or print to a Bluetooth-enabled printer. Bluetooth headphones allow the user to listen to music, podcasts, and other audio media. Bluetooth headsets provide hands-free use of smartphones for phone calls. Security is always a potential issue for wireless use, and so it is a good idea to have the feature turned off when it isn't necessary to have the mobile device discoverable.

WiFi

WiFi networking is another means of mobile device connectivity. WiFi is an acronym for wireless fidelity, and it is an industry standard (Brain & Wilson, 2007; Mitchell, 2010). It uses a router that supports WiFi standard 802.11 a, b, g, or n to form a local area network. The 802.11 b g standard is very common and inexpensive. The newer 802.11 n is the most recent standard that improves the range and speed of the wireless connection (Brain & Wilson, 2007). WiFi networking is popular with family homes because it allows multiple users to access wireless printers and the Internet. WiFi networks are simple to set up using a software wizard that comes with the purchase of a wireless router.

"**Hotspot**" is a term used to identify a WiFi-enabled area so that you can use your WiFi-enabled mobile device to connect to the Internet. You can

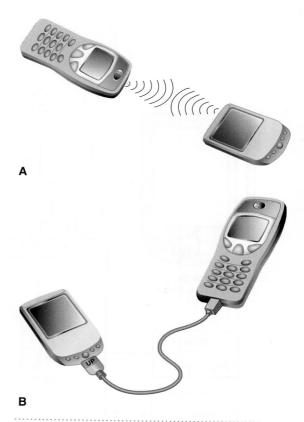

A

B

Figure 12-6 A,B: Beaming data using infrared.

find Hotspots at public libraries, most colleges and universities, coffee shops, airport terminals, and hotels. Not all Hotspots are public; many are encrypted for security reasons and require the user to enter an access code or pay a fee for access. WiFi security, like Bluetooth, is an important issue. For example, hospitals that use WiFi have very secure encrypted systems. Setup information for routers used in home wireless networks includes methods to address security issues.

Smartphones can connect to the Internet using regular cell phone networks. Smartphone users who use this connection should be aware of their "connection package" agreement to avoid paying high fees for large data downloads. Users who need to access the Internet using the cellular phone network, as opposed to WiFi, should have unlimited minutes as part of their cellular service agreement.

---

3 See Appendix A for more information about IR ports.

Uses of PDA in Nursing

There are benefits and shortcomings for the use of handheld computers in nursing, although many argue that the benefits far outweigh the short-falls. Time saving and time management are often mentioned in the literature as positive outcomes after infusing PDAs in nursing education and clinical settings. Instead of looking up information in several printed textbooks, the nursing students can query the handheld mobile device, which can hold numerous textbooks. Patient safety and error reduction are also benefits. The ease of looking up reference information (see **Table 12-3**) improves confidence and prevents errors in the clinical setting. Unlike the printed counterpart, reference e-books can be updated and subscriptions renewed. Finally, the PDAs are easy for nursing students and other healthcare professionals to use when answering patient questions at the point of care (Farrell & Rose, 2008).

Concerns about patients having a negative perception of nurses' use of PDAs have not been validated by research. A qualitative study of patients in Taiwan indicated that patients perceived that nurses' use of PDAs could improve work efficiency and facilitate accuracy of data recording (Lee, 2007). Patients did suggest that nurses be willing to explain the use of the digital tool and provide computer access to patients and families. The most important finding of this research is that patients value the quality of care more than any tool, such as a PDA, that a nurse uses to provide the care. As patients become more aware about the benefits of accessing online and e-book resources with handheld devices, they may have an expectation that we use mobile devices at the point of care.

The benefits of handheld computer use are tempered by a few shortcomings. The rapid change in technology is a concern. There is no guarantee that the manufacturer of a given handheld computer will continue to manufacture and support a specific device. The expense of the PDA is a common concern. Some nursing programs require the students to purchase the device, while others use grant money or incorporate the cost as a laboratory fee. The time involved with the selection and preparation of the devices for use is another concern. Finally, there are occasional issues with faulty devices and short battery life. Despite the shortcomings, advances in technology are easing the adoption of mobile devices for students in nursing education, and for students, registered nurses (RNs), and advanced practice RNs in clinical practice settings.

Use of Handheld Computers in Nursing Education

Imagine the scenario in which the nursing student, with his instructor, is preparing to administer a combination of regular and NPH insulin. The student removes the small mobile device from his uniform pocket and taps the screen several times to pull up insulin on the drug e-book. He verifies the procedure for mixing the two types of insulin before proceeding to prepare the injection. This type of use of mobile devices in education is a growing trend. Some of the issues that have prevented widespread adoption of mobile devices include faculty and nursing students' attitude toward technology, costs, and rapid change of technology. Despite the issues, nursing, medical, and dentistry programs are using mobile devices in the classroom and clinical settings.

Nursing students' attitudes about the use of technology have a direct effect on their "willingness to learn computer systems and ultimately the use of technology to improve patient safety" (Maag, 2006). Although use of technology has not been widely adopted as a tool in nursing curricula, nursing students are expected to have proficient technology skills in the delivery of patient care. For example, nursing students learn how to set up intravenous administration pumps, administer medications using barcode patient identification, and record patient care using the electronic health record. Nursing students are also expected to have proficient technology skills for use of computers to write care plans using a word processor, draw concept maps with concept map software, use online learning management systems to submit assignments, take quizzes, and participate in online discussion forums.

Drexel University nursing students were early innovators in the use of PDAs for classroom and clinical settings (Donnelly & Rockstraw, 2003; Skyscape, n.d.). The purpose of introducing PDAs was to incorporate the use of technology to improve patient outcomes. Drexel piloted the use of PDAs in 2001 and now requires their use for all undergraduate and graduate nursing students. Students are introduced to the PDA in an informatics course in which they learn how to download and use nursing reference programs. Initially, the students could choose their own PDA; the program has now standardized the PDA configuration. Undergraduate students are provided an iPod Touch and an e-book bundle with point-of-need resources to use in class and clinical settings (F. Cornelius, personal communication, June 8, 2010). Graduate students are required to have a PDA but may use their own device since they often already use a PDA or a smartphone.

Both Duke and Auburn Universities adopted the use of PDAs for their accelerated degree nursing programs. Auburn University initiated the project based on alumni feedback that expressed concern about limited exposure to the use of technology in nursing practice (Smith & Pattillo, 2006). Duke University adopted the use of PDAs to support the leadership and technology thread in the curriculum. To address concerns about confidentiality and security of patient data, Duke nursing students are taught how to de-identify patient data and use a password to access the device. Faculty at Duke identified several benefits of PDAs, including mobility of the PDA data and improved time management (White et al., 2005).

Ball State University piloted the use of PDAs for baccalaureate nursing students in 2005 in an effort to assist students to develop the essential technology skills necessary for the workplace environment (Hodson Carlton, Dillard, Campbell, & Baker, 2007). The project implementation team included the nursing program associate director, Curriculum Committee faculty representatives, Learning Resource Center faculty and staff, and the University Computing Services (UCS) staff. The team made the decision to standardize the PDA with the Hewlett-Packard iPAQ hx2790 using a Windows Mobile 5.0 OS. The team also identified standard software requirements for the PDA. Prior to training, the UCS staff prepared a series of video tutorials (http://cms.bsu.edu/About/AdministrativeOffices/HelpDesk/

TechClips). The tutorials covered information on how to get started, access e-mail, use web browsers, and download software.

The use of PDAs at Ball State University was implemented in 2006 with sophomore students enrolled in physical assessment and nursing foundations courses. Students were required to purchase the PDA and nursing reference software. Technology specialists provided classroom orientation for use of the PDAs. To assist students in the use of the PDA, nursing faculty prepared various instructional resources and classroom assignments that required the use of PDA software. Examples of assignments included use of case videos and PDA software to find answers to questions about medical terminology, nursing diagnoses, disease processes, and medications. After using PDAs in the first semester, nursing students reported that the greatest benefits were portability of information and efficient use of time.

Use of Handheld Computers for Library Searches

Your smartphone rings; when you glance at the screen you note that you have received a text message – from the virtual librarian answering your question about when the library closes. Yes, libraries have changed from bricks and mortar to include websites, digital catalogs of books and journal citations, e-books, e-mail notification, blogs, really simple syndication (RSS) feeds, chat, and text messaging. Libraries are lending more than books; they are also lending music CDs, movies on DVDs, and computer equipment, such as laptops and iPods®. Many college and health science libraries have extensive handheld mobile resources designed to assist healthcare students and professionals.

Handheld computers can be used to assist in finding and storing literature citations used for library searches. For example, users can download their reference library to a Palm device using Endnote™ bibliographic software. The portability of the references could save time when visiting the library to search for journal articles and books, or storing the call numbers for the book locations in the library.

Most libraries have websites on the Internet, but only a few of those websites are PDA and smartphone friendly (see **Table 12-2**). Mobile-computing

Table 12-2 Library Websites Designed for Handheld Computers

Library Sites Designed for Mobile Computers	Website Address
American University Library	http://www.library.american.edu/mobile/
Ball State University Libraries	http://www.bsu.edu/libraries/mobile/
New York Public Library	http://m.nypl.org/
Boston University Medical Center Mobile Library	http://medlib.bu.edu/mobile/
Harvard College Library	http://hcl.harvard.edu/mobile/
National Library of Medicine	http://pubmedhh.nlm.nih.gov/nlm/
University of Richmond Library	http://library.richmond.edu/m/
Fondren Library, Rice University	http://m.library.rice.edu/

websites need to be specifically designed for handheld computers (Cuddy, 2006; W3C, 2008) by designing the content so that it fits the screen size and does not require horizontal scrolling. Additionally, the URL should be as short as possible to facilitate input, and the content should address what the mobile user needs.

The number of resources for mobile devices is growing exponentially every day. To discover new resources, search the Internet using the terms "mobile learning resources." The value of mobile learning is now recognized by many universities. For example, the Tennessee Board of Regents, a system responsible for forty-five institutions, hosts an innovative website designed to assist users with mobile devices at http://www.tbrelearning.org/.

Use of Handheld Computers in Clinical Practice

General Nursing Clinical Practice

When nurses discover better ways to deliver patient care, they quickly adopt the new ways. The nursing literature has an abundance of information on how to purchase and use handheld computers. Nurses find handheld computers affordable and indispensable in various nursing practice clinical settings including the medical-surgical nursing unit, the operating room, and the emergency department. A growing number of clinical information systems incorporate the use of handheld computers for point-of-need documentation. Wireless synchronization allows for real-time documentation in the electronic medical record.

Personal Handheld Computers for Clinical Use

Many nurses in clinical practice purchase their own handheld computers to use electronic references to provide point-of-need information for decision-making in practice (**Box 12-1**). References commonly used by a clinical nurse include a nursing drug book, a medical dictionary, a nursing procedures manual, a handbook of diagnostics tests, and a health assessment handbook (see **Table 12-3**). The cost of the electronic references is comparable to the print version. The advantage of the electronic format is that when updates are available, they can be downloaded and saved to the mobile device so that the information is available at the point of care.

The American Association of Critical Care Nurses (AACN) offers a variety of critical care software, including the AACN Medicopeia and Critical Care Nurse Edition for the PDA. Nurses can choose to purchase a PDA with software already installed or to purchase and download software packages to install separately (American Association of Critical Care Nurses, 2008).

BOX 12-1 PDAs and Nursing: Words From a User

"When you use a PDA while providing clinical care, you have a remarkable resource in your hand." Edward Stern, RN. [From Hodson Carlton, K., Dillard, N., Campbell, B. R., & Baker, N. (2007). Personal digital assistants in the classroom and clinical areas. *CIN: Computers, Informatics, Nursing, 25(5),* 253–258.]

Table 12-3 Examples of Mobile Computer Reference Resources

Examples of Handheld Reference Resources	Website Address
Skyscape Drug books, medical dictionaries, laboratory and diagnostic test books, NCLEX (National Council Licensure Examination for Registered Nurses) review manuals, and nursing procedure manuals	http://www.skyscape.com
Handango Many healthcare and office applications	http://www.handango.com/
Centers for Disease Control and Prevention Podcasts and sexually transmitted disease (STD) treatment guidelines	http://www2a.cdc.gov/podcasts/ http://www.cdcnpin.org/scripts/std/pda.asp
Epocrates Rx Drug database (free)	http://www.epocrates.com/
Pepid Reference resources for clinical nursing, oncology, and critical care	http://www.pepid.com/
Critical care American Association of Critical Care Nurses' Personal Digital Assistant Center	http://aacn.pdaorder.com/welcome.xml
The Group on Immunizations of the Society of Teachers of Family Medicine Shots (free)	http://www.immunizationed.org/
Statcoder Coding and billing tools (free)	http://www.statcoder.com
iPad apps iPhone apps	http://www.apple.com/ipad/apps-for-ipad/ http://www.apple.com/iphone/apps-for-iphone/

The AACN PDA website empowers new PDA users with multimedia tutorials on PDA basics, clinical software, Adobe Acrobat, and PowerPoint. After completing the tutorials tests, AACN members can obtain free continuing education credit.

Handheld Computers for Clinical Information Systems

The use of PDAs for bar code administration of medications is becoming more prevalent. Visualize a scenario. The nurses arrive for report from the 7 a.m. to 7 p.m. shift on the cardiac nursing unit. After the walking rounds report, each nurse picks up a wireless PDA, logs into the device, and uses a stylus to select assigned patients from the list of patients on the nursing unit. While planning medication administration for the shift, the nurse uses the real-time electronic medication administration record (MAR) to review the scheduled medications for each patient in preparation for organizing care. When administering the medication, the nurses follow the six rights of medication administration (right drug, right patient, right dose, right time, right route, and

right documentation) using bar coding technology by first scanning the bar code on the drug. In addition to asking the patients their names, the nurse also scans the identification band to verify that the correct patient is administered the medication. Afterward, the nurse charts the drug administration by clicking a checkbox on the PDA MAR.

PDAs with a secure wireless connection to the clinical information system are used in many healthcare facilities for medication administration. Because the PDA is wireless, the patient data are always up-to-date. As soon as a patient is admitted to a room, the patient's name shows up on the list of patients for that unit. When a medication is ordered and verified by the pharmacy, it shows up on the list of scheduled medications for administration. The medication name and information disappear when discontinued. The PDA eliminates the need to push heavy drug carts with attached computers or other computers on wheels. If the physician or advanced practice nurse checks the electronic chart on a remote computer, they can view the medication charted seconds ago.

Advanced Practiced – Nurse Practitioner's Use of PDAs

Nurse practitioners have quickly adopted the use of handheld computers into their practices. In addition to references used by the clinical nurse, nurse practitioners can monitor and evaluate patient progress. Patient Keeper (http://patientkeeper.com) and Patient Tracker (http://www.patienttracker.com/) are two programs used by physicians and nurse practitioners for patient care management. HanDBase software (http://www.ddhsoftware.com/medical.html) has numerous software handheld mobile computing solutions for the practitioner.

The practice setting for nurse practitioners can be extremely busy. Prescription writing and coding for reimbursement of care can be automated with handheld software. Prescription writing software such as Allscripts ePrescribe (http://www.allscripts.com/eprescribe) is available for handheld computers in addition to patient care management software. There are also numerous software packages to identify ICD-9 (International Classification of Diseases, Version 9) and CPT codes for billing of care. Examples of coding software are noted on MeisterMed (http://www.meistermed.com/) and StatCoder (http://www.statcoder.com) websites.

Data Security Issues

Data security is a minimal issue if the mobile device is used only for reference resources. However, data security is always an issue with small wireless devices, and it can and must be addressed by the user. Because handheld computers are small, it is inevitable that they fall out of pockets, be misplaced, or stolen. All handheld computers with any type of clinical data must be secure or encrypted using a password or biometrics, such as fingerprint recognition. If passwords are used, they must be one that cannot be easily hacked (Microsoft, 2010). Other password considerations are as follows:

- Prefer longer passwords (7–10 characters).
- Use words or characters easily remembered, but that are not personally identifiable.
- The misspelled name of a fruit or flower, rather than the name of a family member or pet.

- The first letter of each word in a phrase.
- Replace letters of the word with number or other keyboard characters. For example, the letter A might be replaced with the @ sign and the letter O with the number 0. Also include other keyboard symbols.
- Be familiar with password strategies to avoid at http://www.microsoft.com/protect/fraud/passwords/create.aspx.
- Check the strength of the password using an online tool such as https://www.microsoft.com/protect/fraud/passwords/checker.aspx?WT.mc_id=Site_Link.

Most important of all, if there is a need to store patient data, users must follow the policies and procedures outlined by their healthcare agency. Check with the agency's Health Insurance Portability and Accountability Act (HIPAA) officer for questions.

Use of Handheld Computers in Nursing Research

Handheld computers are useful for the research process. Users can take web-based research surveys with a handheld computer. The data from the surveys are stored on the researcher's web server for aggregation and analysis. Researchers can use the audio recorder on the handheld computer to record focus group interviews and then later download the recordings for data analysis. The camera on the handheld computer could be used to take pictures to document changes that occurred as a result of a research treatment.

The mobility of a handheld computer makes it an excellent tool for accessing and collecting research data. Many online evidence-based resources are designed specifically for handheld computers.[4] The Agency for Healthcare Research and Quality includes the National Guideline Clearinghouse (http://www.guideline.gov/resources/pda.aspx), which has links to evidence-based clinical practice guidelines specifically designed for Palm-based devices. The website also has a comprehensive listing of links to pocket guidelines from multiple medical societies, such as the American

---

4 See Chapters 10 and 24 for more information.

College of Cardiology, the National Institutes of Health, and the Centers for Disease Control and Prevention (CDC).

Future Trends

We need to have a crystal ball to predict the future of handheld mobile devices in education and clinical settings; however, history has already set trends that we can expect to continue. We can expect mobile devices to be easier to use. The software will be more intuitive. Voice commands currently available to operate handheld computers can be expected to improve and become a primary method of data input. Mobile broadband, for high-speed transfer of data, will be an accessible and affordable feature for smartphones. We can expect smartphones to become the norm. There will be a much smaller market for the stand-alone PDA. The PDA will continue to be appropriate for use in education and the classroom. As the popularity of mobile devices increases, the pricing will continue to drop. Flash memory or a nonvolatile equivalent will be a standard feature for mobile devices.

As the future unfolds, healthcare will harness the use of technology to improve patient care and save lives. All healthcare agencies will ask the providers to log in to their human resources information systems to input a cell phone contact number. In the event of a disaster, team notification will be done primarily using text messaging to smartphones. Clinical information systems will "push" text messaging alerts to healthcare providers, advising them to log in to the system to retrieve reports of critical values.

Summary

Once technically savvy students and nurses learn how to use a handheld computer, the small mobile device becomes an essential clinical tool just as valuable as their stethoscope and patient care devices. Handheld computers allow nurses to discover essential knowledge in the palms of their hands. Synchronization software makes it very easy to update the handheld computer from the PC with calendar appointments, contact name, e-mail, phone numbers, and addresses. Users can store digital e-book nursing references to use in the classroom and clinical practice. Handheld computers with access to the Internet provide real-time access to e-mail, news, and other essential information resources.

Handheld computers provide added value to nurses in all settings. Nursing students should be expected to use handheld computers in the classroom and the clinical setting. Development of proficient technical skills improves time management and work efficiency. Knowledge gained from up-to-date information improves decision making and patient care outcomes and prevents unnecessary errors. The handheld computer, designed to integrate with clinical information systems, has the potential to improve accuracy of documentation and shorten the time between the delivery of care and documentation in the electronic medical record. Future uses of handheld computers in the nursing are limited only by our imaginations.

APPLICATIONS AND COMPETENCIES

1. Use a search engine, such as Google, to search for health science library PDA websites.

2. Check with your local library to see if they lend out mobile computing devices such as PDAs, iPads, and/or iPods®.

3. If you have access to a PDA or a smartphone, discuss the connection resources. Does the device have Bluetooth, beaming, or Internet capabilities? Explain the advantages and disadvantages of each type of connection.

4. Enter your name and contact information on a handheld mobile device and then beam the data to the device of a classmate.

5. Download a trial version of nursing reference software from the Internet. Use a search engine, such as Google, and enter the search terms: "nursing mobile software trial downloads."

6. Use the Internet to preview software that you might use on a mobile device. Discuss the similarities and differences between the printed book view and the electronic view.

REFERENCES

3Com Public Relations. (1999). *Press release: 3Com Corporation acquires Smartcode Technologie*. Retrieved June 5, 2010, from http://investor.palm.com/releasedetail.cfm?releaseid=338041

American Association of Critical Care Nurses. (2008, August 24). *Welcome to AACN's PDA and Mobile Resources Center*. Retrieved June 5, 2010, from http://aacn.pdaorder.com/welcome.xml

Apple. (2007, April 9). *100 million sold*. Retrieved June 5, 2010, from http://www.apple.com/pr/library/2007/04/09ipod.html

Apple. (2010a). *Apple*. Retrieved June 5, 2010, from http://www.apple.com/

Apple. (2010b, May 31). *Apple sells two million iPads in less than 60 days*. Retrieved June 5, 2010, from http://www.apple.com/pr/library/2010/05/31ipad.html

Brain, M., & Wilson, T. V. (2007). *How WiFi works*. Retrieved June 5, 2010, from http://computer.howstuffworks.com/wireless-network1.htm

Carnoyon, D. (2009a, February 24). Amazon Kindle wireless reading device (U.S. wireless). *CNET Reviews*. Retrieved June 6, 2010, from http://reviews.cnet.com/e-book-readers/amazon-kindle-wireless-reading/4505-3508_7-33517190.html?autoplay=true&tag=rtcol;relnews

Carnoyon, D. (2009b, December 6). Barnes & Noble Nook. *CNET Reviews*. Retrieved June 6, 2010, from http://reviews.cnet.com/e-book-readers/barnes-noble-nook/4505-3508_7-33786175.html?tag=rnav

Cellular News. (2006, August 9). *PDA shipments reached record high in second quarter of 2006*. Retrieved June 5, 2010, from http://www.cellular-news.com/story/18733.php

Cornelius, F., & Gordon, M. G. (Eds.). (2007). *PDA Connections: Mobile Technology for Health Care Professionals*. Lippincott Williams & Wilkins.

Cuddy, C. (2006). How to serve content to PDA users on-the-go. *Computers in Libraries, 26*(4), 10.

Donnelly, G. F., & Rockstraw, L. (2003). *The personal digital assistant (PDA) – A tool for minimizing risk and error in nursing care*. Retrieved November 5, 2007, from http://www.nso.com/newsletters/advisor/2003_11/pda.php

Farrell, M. J., & Rose, L. (2008). Use of mobile handheld computers in clinical nursing education. *Journal of Nursing Education, 47*(1), 13–19.

Franklin, C., & Layton, J. (2007). *How Bluetooth works*. Retrieved June 5, 2010, from http://electronics.howstuffworks.com/bluetooth1.htm

Hodson Carlton, K., Dillard, N., Campbell, B. R., & Baker, N. (2007). *Personal digital assistants in the classroom and clinical areas*. CIN: Computers, Informatics, Nursing, 25(5), 253–258.

Lee, T. T. (2007). Patients' perceptions of nurses' bedside use of PDAs. *CIN: Computers, Informatics, Nursing, 25*(2), 106–111.

Maag, M. M. (2006). Nursing students' attitudes toward technology: a national study. *Nurse Educator, 31*(3), 112–118.

Medindia. (2010). *History of PDA*. Retrieved June 5, 2010, from http://www.medindia.net/pda/pda_history.htm

Microsoft. (2010). *Create strong passwords*. Retrieved June 5, 2010, from http://www.microsoft.com/protect/fraud/passwords/create.aspx

Mitchell, B. (2010). *Wi-Fi – wireless fidelity*. Retrieved June 5, 2010, from http://compnetworking.about.com/cs/wireless80211/g/bldef_wifi.htm

Skyscape. (n.d.). *Skyscape references in pockets of Drexel nursing students*. Retrieved June 5, 2010, from http://www.skyscape.com/group/Drexel_testimonial.pdf

Smith, C. M., & Pattillo, R. E. (2006). *Technology. PDAs in the nursing curriculum: Providing data for internal funding. Nurse Educator, 31*(3), 101–102.

Tilley, C. (2009, October 11). *The history of Microsoft Windows CE – Index & humble beginnings. HPC Factor*. Retrieved June 5, 2010, from http://www.hpcfactor.com/support/windowsce/

W3C. (2008, July 29). *Mobile web best practices 1.0*. Retrieved June 5, 2010, from http://www.w3.org/TR/mobile-bp/

White, A., Allen, P., Goodwin, L., Breckinridge, D., Dowell, J., & Garvy, R. (2005). Infusing PDA technology into nursing education. *Nurse Educator, 30*(4), 150–154.

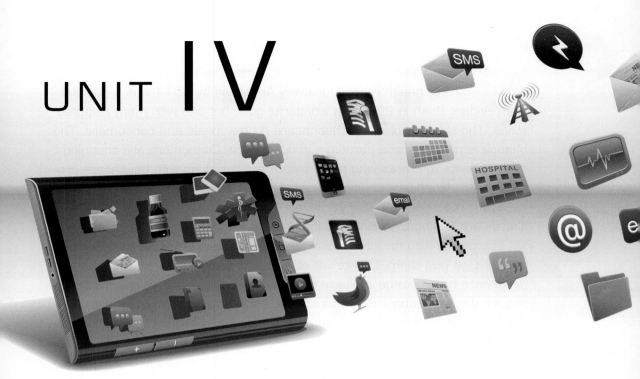

UNIT IV

The New Healthcare Paradigm

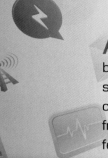

AN electronic health record for every American by 2014 was a goal set by President Bush in 2004 – a wonderful goal, but one with many required steps. The steps involve both healthcare professionals and consumers. The change is part of a new paradigm in healthcare. Consumers are changing from patients to clients who make treatment decisions with healthcare professionals. Healthcare consumers are challenged to take an active responsibility for their care. As this paradigm makes its perspective felt, professionals are finding that clients want reasons for treatments and that they will search the web for information to either support or refute the information that we give them. Clients will also expect designated parts of their healthcare history to be available to all their healthcare providers. This will require decisions about who should have access to what information, what terms to use for this information, and the protocols needed to electronically exchange it.

This unit begins with Chapter 13 in which consumer usage of electronic health records in the form of personal health records is explored. Benefits, current availability, and barriers to personal health records are examined along with the use of e-mail in patient communication. Chapter 14 looks at all aspects of the empowered patient, the good, the not so good, and the healthcare professional's part in implementing this role. Interoperability, an elusive characteristic, is explored in Chapter 15 as it applies at both the international and national levels. The last chapter in this unit, Chapter 16, looks at nursing's efforts to make nursing information interoperable through standardizing our data.

CHAPTER 13

The Consumer and the Electronic Health Record

Objectives

After studying this chapter you will be able to:

► *Differentiate between an electronic patient record, an electronic health record, and a personal health record.*

► *Describe the various forms of a personal health record.*

► *Discuss barriers to the establishment of personal health records.*

► *Describe healthcare smart cards.*

► *Construct a plan for electronic communication with patients.*

Key Terms

Confidentiality
Consumer Informatics
De-identified Data
E-Encounter
Electronic Health Record
Electronic Medical Record
Encryption
Flash Drive
Health Insurance Portability and Accountability Act (HIPAA)

Interoperable
National Health Information Network (NHIN)
PIN
Privacy
Protocol
Readability
Smart Card
Unique Patient Identifier
USB Port

As you help the paramedics wheel the unconscious patient into the emergency room, you notice something around his neck. Upon closer inspection, you see that it is an identification device with a USB connection. Quickly you remove the device and plug it into the **USB port** of a nearby computer. Immediately information appears on the screen that tells you his name and other identifying information including that he is on Coumadin® and that he has congestive heart failure. You print this information and communicate it to the rest of the team. Sounds far-fetched? It is not. Such a device, a **flash drive**, exists today and it can be seen in

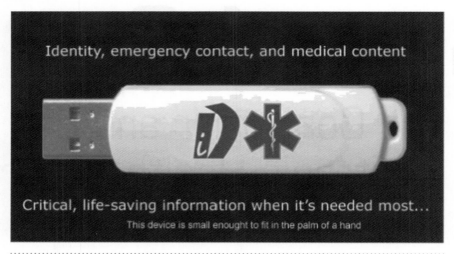

Identity, emergency contact, and medical content

Critical, life-saving information when it's needed most...

This device is small enought to fit in the palm of a hand

Figure 13-1 Identification device. (Printed with permission of Identification Devices, LLC, Sandy, UT 84093; http://www.identificationdevices.net/)

Figure 13-1. Information technology is changing the face of healthcare. Between a public demanding more participation in their healthcare, providers looking for ways to improve the quality of healthcare, and communication technology that can access and transmit health information, we are seeing a transformation of healthcare. The **Internet** is at the heart of this revolution. In less than a decade, the percentage of the U.S. population who are online has increased to almost 80% (see **Figure 13-2**). Worldwide usage has also increased, with 21.5% of Asians and 54.4% of Europeans now online (Miniwatts Marketing Group, 2010). With this trend, the pressure on healthcare providers to use the Internet for healthcare communication has increased. Additionally, consumers are starting to take more responsibility for their healthcare as the patient in the above scenario did when he purchased, entered data into, and wore the identification device. Further, as more and more "patients" use the Internet to learn about their conditions, you will see the relationship between patient and healthcare providers change and healthcare providers become more of an advisor while patients become clients or consumers.

Implementing the Promise of the Internet in Healthcare

Before the full promise of the Internet in healthcare becomes a reality, all healthcare records must be integrated. Many other countries are ahead of the United States in this endeavor, particularly those with a nationalized health service; however, none has yet reached the full potential. Many of the reasons, such as **privacy** issues and the development of a national network of healthcare records, are shared by all countries, although some, such as the Netherlands and the United Kingdom, are ahead of others.

In the United States, the **National Health Information Network (NHIN)**[1] serves as a foundation for secure information exchange over the Internet (Department of Health and Human Services, 2010). The effectiveness of the secure information exchange is dependent on each healthcare provider using electronic patient care records, these records being accessible by those designated by the patient anywhere in the United States, and patients having access to their healthcare records. The components for the information exchange are built gradually, with full interconnectedness being

---

1 The NHIN are addressed in Chapter 14.

Growth of U.S. Population Online 2001-2009

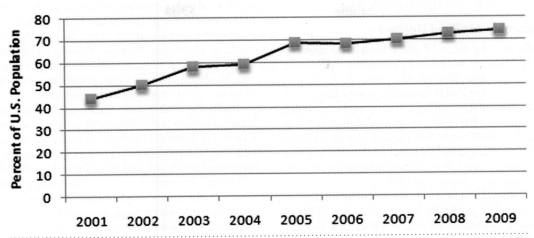

Figure 13-2 Growth of U.S. population online. Data from Internet Usage and Population Growth. (2010). Retrieved November 27, 2010, from http://www.internetworldstats.com/am/us.htm

the last step. Agreement for terms used to identify the three parts of the patient's record was reached in 2008 and continues to be used by the Office of the National Coordinator for Health Information Technology (ONC) (National Alliance for Health Information Technology, 2008; Office of the National Coordinator for Health Information Technology, 2009). The terms are used in this book. A diagram depicting the health information record integration is shown in **Figure 13-3**.

- An **electronic medical record** (EMR) is a healthcare record created by healthcare providers or agencies, such as a hospital. EMRs that meet national standards for interoperability will be able to share health information with the electronic health record (EHR).
- An **electronic health record** (EHR) is an **interoperable** healthcare record that can contain data from multiple EMRs and the personal health record (PHR). The EHR provides real-time information and includes evidence-based decision support tools (Office of the National Coordinator for Health InformationTechnology, 2009).

- A **personal health record** (PHR) is cre- ated when users can communicate with authorized providers and maintain/manage their own health information. If the PHR conforms to interoperability standards, it can contain data from the EHR, but still controlled by the individual. PHRs

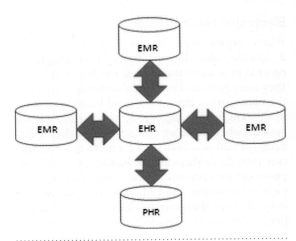

Figure 13-3 Integration of health information with the EMR, EHR, and PHR.

that communicate with EHRs are private, secure, confidential, and protected by the **Health Insurance Portability and Accountability Act (HIPAA)**. Stand-alone PHRs are not HIPAA protected.

Electronic Medical Record

EMRs are the focus of most healthcare agencies today. They are owned and managed by the institution or provider that creates them. As healthcare agencies merge and form large corporations, these EMRs are often combined so that information from all member agencies and providers is accessible by those with the required authorization. Many agencies refer to their EMR as EHR, but an electronic record that cannot interface with outside agencies is not a true EHR.[2]

Consumers' access to their own health information is being gradually introduced into EMRs. A person's healthcare record, whether in a hospital or clinic, used to be regarded as the property of the agency providing the care. Patients were not allowed to see their records; in fact, in the past even providing patients with knowledge of their own temperature was regarded as improper. HIPAA, passed in 1996, changed this by mandating that patients be allowed to see their own healthcare records (U.S. Department of Health and Human Services, 2010a, 2010b). Difficulties arise however because in most cases, pieces of a patient's medical history are scattered in many different locales.

Electronic Health Record

When babies born in the United States are 2 months old, they probably have healthcare records in at least two places: the hospital where they were born and in the pediatrician's office. As the babies grow, the number and location of their healthcare records also grow. The current record system, whether paper or electronic, makes it difficult for individuals to have access to their healthcare records. Additionally, it handicaps healthcare providers by preventing them from having complete information about a person. Individuals who have not kept their own health records find it difficult to remember details. Try to remember what

your last immunization was, where it was given, or if you have ever been immunized against a disease such as yellow fever. Even trying to remember all one's surgeries becomes difficult as one grows older, let alone being able to remember one's medical history. These problems can be life threatening in an emergency situation, as was seen in the aftermath of Hurricane Katrina. Paper records were either destroyed or inaccessible, making it impossible to obtain any past medical information or list of medications of people in need of care.

Under the EHR model, one's health information is available from any location where there is Internet access. The accessibility makes it easier for patients who visit multiple providers to supply each one with an up-to-date record, and the information available will usually be more than what a referring provider sends. It also provides safer care in the advent of an emergency when regular records may not be available. With a record of all the prescriptions that a consumer has, adverse drug effects can be minimized. Additionally, those who use different sources to gain drugs will be identified and can be helped. Having healthcare data in an electronic format also means that **de-identified data** can be used in an aggregated form to assess patterns of disease, quickly identify potentially dangerous side effects of medications, and detect disease outbreaks.

Although change is evolving, the results of a 2010 Harris Interactive poll revealed that less than 10% of Americans use electronic health information or e-mail communication with their providers (Harris Interactive, 2010). Many Americans still do not understand the rationale for use of electronic health information. Only 78% thought their physicians should have access to the electronic information. Twenty-eight percent thought that their physicians used an electronic record (see **Figure 13-4**).

Personal Health Record

A PHR provides clients access to their healthcare information and may allow clients to enter data into their records. If it communicates with the EHR, it can provide information from healthcare encounters along with information about the medications the client is taking, the results of various tests, and healthcare information designed for the consumer. The term PHR may refer to a health record kept only by the consumer, although the

---

2 EMRs are discussed in Chapter 17.

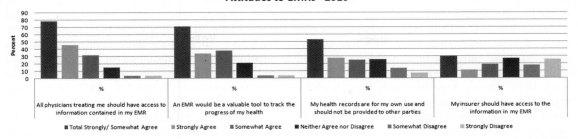

Figure 13-4 Percent of Americans attitudes to EMRs – 2010.

full benefit cannot be realized until it communicates with the EHR.

Initially, computerized PHRs were in a state of evolution, with no one agreeing on exactly what they were (Halamka, Mandl, & Tang, 2008). PHRs that are certified and meet the national interoperability standards can share data with the EHR. A study conducted by the Consumer Education and Engagement Collaborative (Daniel, Posnack, & Consumer Education and Engagement Collaborative, 2009) identified three main formats for the PHR:

1. Software applications for the computer or portable drive, such as a flash drive.
2. Web-based services that store the information on another computer remotely.
3. Hybrid PHRs that allow for remote storage of the health information as well as the ability to store the information on a personal computer or portable drive.

The researchers identified five classifications for the company affiliation associated with the PHR:

a. Humanitarian, in which the developer is a person who identified the need, based on personal experience. The humanitarian PHR may be supported through a foundation. Examples include Full Circle Registry and the ER-ID(SM) Card.
b. Government, in which the federal or state government identified the need to share information. The U.S. Department of Veterans Affairs is an example.
c. Healthcare organizations, such as health systems, provider offices, health plans or insurers create websites or portals for information access. Kaiser Permanente® is an example.
d. Core business, in which a company recognizes the need for the population it serves. The core business could be for profit or not for profit. An example is Microsoft HealthVault.
e. Business expansion, where a company develops a PHR to compete in the marketplace. Cerner Health and Dossia are examples.

A 2008 Markle Foundation poll (Markle Foundation & Westin, 2008) reported 42.7% of 1,580 Americans surveyed keep some type of PHR; however, less than 3% keep them electronically. About 80% recognized the benefit of an online record. A little over half (57%) expressed concerns about privacy and security of the PHR. Other concerns reported in the Markle poll were in regard to the record not meeting their healthcare needs, discomfort with computers, and the amount of time necessary to transfer data from paper to the computer.

Benefits of PHRs

PHRs will further collaborative care, that is, care in which there is a partnership between the patient and their healthcare providers. When an individual's PHR is viewed together by both a healthcare provider and a consumer, instead of the healthcare provider giving orders, which the patient may or may not understand or accept, the healthcare provider can help the patient to understand his or her condition and work together with this individual to achieve an agreed-upon goal. Consumers can also collaborate in the creation and maintenance of the healthcare record.

Another benefit of PHRs is the ability to manage one's disease treatment more effectively. For example, those suffering from a chronic disease, such as diabetes or hypertension, can be able to track their disease together with their healthcare provider, which can lower the communication barrier between consumer and provider and empower the consumer (Curtin et al., 2008; Kaissi & Parchman, 2009). A PHR also permits the provider to link individualized information to the client, thus providing more personalized as well as higher-quality care. The improved communication that results will lead consumers to a better understanding of their healthcare responsibilities and disease management. A study done by the Dartmouth Cooperative Practice-Based Research Network (Wasson, Johnson, Benjamin, Phillips, & MacKenzie, 2006) studied the effects of various levels of collaborative care on chronic diseases. To judge the level of this care, they asked participants to evaluate the information given to them by their doctor, the explanation of the problem, along with the patient's confidence in their self-care ability. They found that when the provider and patient had a high exchange of information instead of a one-way flow, the patient's confidence in their self-care ability increased and outcomes improved.

Barriers to Implementation of PHRs

As can be imagined, there are several barriers that must be overcome before the full PHR becomes a reality. The technology to create a full PHR is here, but the agreements, **protocols**, and procedures are still evolving.

Provider Reluctance and Responsibility. A PHR and an EHR can threaten the autonomy of some healthcare providers who still want to practice in the traditional model (Tang, Ash, Bates, Overhage, & Sands, 2006). That said, the reluctance should dissipate with the rollout of reimbursement incentives (and eventually penalties) associated with the 2009 Health Information Technology for Economic and Clinical Health (HITECH) Act "meaningful use" plan. Despite the fact that patients can now

get copies of their healthcare records, traditional agencies and healthcare providers may still see themselves as owners of this information, instead of guardians. Historically, healthcare practitioners have had concerns about providing client access to information not designed for lay interpretation or that may contain information inappropriate to divulge to patients (Ross & Lin, 2003), such as psychiatric problems or diseases. Providers are also concerned about the effects on the patient, on the provider–client relationship, and on healthcare itself. There have been questions about a client's interest in reading and contributing to a healthcare record. Other concerns are that the patient for litigious reasons may use access to healthcare records. In addition, there are concerns about problems with client understanding of information in the records.

Some of the decisions that providers must make when implementing electronic client access to healthcare records include

- deciding which problems should be shared;
- whether or not to share the entire medication and allergy list;
- which laboratory and diagnostic tests should be shared;
- whether or not to share clinical notes, how to authenticate patient access; and
- whether minors should be allowed to access their records (Halamka et al., 2008).

Some of the challenges that may become apparent as the building of the full EHR and PHR occurs are

- whether to provide a single PHR that works with all agencies;
- if data input from other agencies should be permitted to other agencies' record;
- how to integrate web-based information with a PHR, allowing patients with specific diseases to connect with others with similar diseases; and
- how to permit clients to participate in clinical trials, pharmaceutical evaluation, and public health surveillance via their PHR.

Unique Patient Identifier. Besides an EMR, in theory, a full PHR requires that each citizen have a **unique patient identifier** (UPI) for his or her healthcare information regardless of where it is stored. Today, individual providers have their own method of identifying EMRs. This despite the fact that the 1996 HIPAA required the UPI. The Rand Corporation, a nonprofit research group, published a report noting that use of the UPI would improve efficient use of the electronic record and reduce errors (Hillestad et al., 2009). The RAND report also indicated that the cost for a UPI would be as much as 11 billion dollars. Privacy groups immediately rejected the report (Lauer, 2008). Privacy groups have lobbied against the use of the UPI vociferously since HIPAA was passed, citing privacy and security concerns. The National Alliance for Health Information Technology (NAHIT) was another very strong proponent of the UPI. However, once NAHIT disbanded in September 2009 (Monegain, 2009) with the nation experiencing a deep recession, there has been little further discussion.

Data Security. For consumers to feel comfortable with exchanges of their healthcare information, there must be assurances that their data will be protected from those without permission to access it. This will require not only that individual healthcare providers and agencies have the state-of-the-art security but also that there are protocols that govern access to data.

Data Standards. Another barrier has been the lack of data standardization.[3] It is necessary for all agencies involved in healthcare, including pharmacies, to agree to record a defined set of data in a defined manner. That is, there must be decisions made about what information will be recorded and the protocols used to record and transmit it. Identification of this core set of data elements requires participation by representatives of all healthcare record users including consumers. This barrier is currently being resolved by using the ONC certification process.

Data Presentation. It is one thing to provide consumers with access to their healthcare data and it is another to present this in a useful, understandable manner. How will information be grouped? What should one screen present? This area is one of the primary focuses in the new field of **consumer informatics**. This area is also of concern for healthcare providers and often falls into the category of usability.

Consumers. There are also consumer changes that need to be considered. Patients need to start thinking of themselves as healthcare consumers with a responsibility to actively in their healthcare actively (Tang et al., 2006). We are still in the beginning stages of this transition. As nurses participate in these changes, they will find a need for reeducation with some clients. Many were raised in an era in which one is a passive patient and therefore have developed security in placing responsibility for health with others. Consumers may need assistance to understand new roles and responsibilities. One suggestion for helping the population make the transition is to start education about the responsibilities and use of PHRs in grade school (Tang et al., 2006).

Costs. Financing of EHRs and PHRs is another barrier. Although the U.S. government is offering financial incentives to adopt electronic records for healthcare providers, like so many informatics advances, the expectation is often that healthcare agencies and healthcare providers will pay for them. Yet, the majority of advantages accrue to payers and patients. It is easy to say that electronic records will save money; these savings, however, generally come from the pocket of the healthcare agencies and healthcare providers who will lose business as patients do not require as many office visits, laboratory tests, or hospitalizations. Thus, a method of financing healthcare that does not reward hospitalizations and procedures is required. Managed care, theoretically, can offer this, but in many cases there have been implementation and patient acceptance difficulties. Incentives such as pay for performance, in which access to aggregated data is imperative for improving care, are an approach to motivating healthcare providers to find a business case for EMRs, EHRs, and PHRs.

Current PHRs in Use

Given the many barriers to creating EHRs, let alone a full PHR, along with the demand by

---

3 Data standardization are explored in Chapter 15.

consumers for a PHR, it is not surprising that consumers and providers have started on the road to a PHR. There are also some healthcare providers that permit client access to at least parts of their healthcare record.

Self-Created. One approach used by consumers is to keep their own healthcare record. It may be on paper or on their computer with or without special-purpose software. With this approach, the consumer needs to carry an updated printout with them at all times if it is to be useful in an emergency. There are many free and fee-based web services available that allow consumers to create their own Internet-based PHR. However, there are many variations in these services, especially in the data that the consumer records. Some of these services permit healthcare providers, with permission of the record owner, to use a personal identification number (**PIN**) created by the consumer to interact with the records by phone, fax, or online. Less useful but helpful is the provision of a printed format that allows the consumer to take a hard copy to his or her physician. Those that only provide consumers with a view of their data have a limited value. Search the web by using the term "personal health record" to find PHR resources.

Potential users should always investigate the fine print in the privacy policy of the organization sponsoring a consumer-created and consumer-maintained PHR. A review requested by the ONC about the privacy and security of online PHRs found that of the 30 privacy policies reviewed, none included more than 18 of the 31 criteria used in their review (Lecker et al., 2007). These criteria included such items as **readability** (of the privacy policy), details of how the information is shared, and definition of critical terms. It would also be wise to check the organization with the Better Business Bureau.

One of the difficulties with this model is the time-consuming task of entering data and deciding what data to enter. Medical personnel can access a web-based record if the patient is conscious and able to provide the website address, login, and a password. Currently, an online PHR record that delivers on its promises is still in its infancy, but evolving. There are many PHR websites available on the Internet. A few examples include AHIMA (American Health Information Management Association) MyPHR, and Microsoft HealthVault. When choosing a PHR platform, consumers should look for statements regarding information privacy and security. Often the websites will include accreditation seals and logos, such as the HONcode, URAC Accreditation, and/or EU Trust seal. Consumers should consider choosing PHRs that have EHR connectivity, whether or not they choose to use the EHR because it indicates that the PHR platform has addressed interoperability standards.

Some PHRs can be saved to a flash drive that plugs into USB ports on a computer, such as the one that the patient in the introductory scenario had. Flash drives are affordable and small enough to carry on a key chain. Consumers plug them into their computer, fill in the labeled fields, and save the information. Some flash drives are preconfigured with PHR software. The flash drive PHR information is then available to any emergency medical service (see **Figure 13-1**).

Smart Cards. **Smart cards** are devices that are created by providers for use by their patients. A smart card looks like a plastic credit card and, like a credit card, is embedded with information that can be read by a reader. In a smart card, however, the embedded data are on a computer chip that cannot only be read but can also be written to with the appropriate computer system and access code. Functioning similarly to the central processing unit of a computer, smart cards contain RAM, ROM, and an operating system (see **Box 13-1**). They were first introduced in France to combat fraud in telecommunications and banking (Cagliostro 2005; Smart Card Alliance, 2009) and since then have found use in many industries including healthcare.

BOX 13-1 Contents of a Smart Card

A CPU for managing data
ROM to store the operating system
RAM for temporary storage

A smart healthcare card is defined by the International Standards Organization as a card containing computer-readable data that is issued to a person or healthcare provider to facilitate providing healthcare (Smart Card Alliance, 2009). They are used as identification by patients when making contact with the healthcare system to transmit information that will assist healthcare providers in their treatment. A healthcare smart card has four subsets of data: data necessary to operate the card including privacy protection, data unique to the consumer, administrative data such as insurance carrier, and clinical data. Access, however, is not automatic; users must provide a password, a PIN number, or both. These cards can also be designed to allow access by a biometric feature such as a thumbprint.

Smart cards are now in use in several places across the United States. Mount Sinai Hospital joined with nine other healthcare institutions in the greater New York city area to form a regional smart card network (Smart Card Alliance, 2009). All members of the network accept a common healthcare smart card. The University of Pittsburgh Medical Center with over 19 hospitals and 400 doctors' offices, following a 2-year pilot project, has also implemented smart cards (Smart Card Alliance, 2006). Another example is Inland Northwest Health Services, serving 38 in Washington and Idaho, which uses healthcare smart cards for healthcare consumers (Smart Card Alliance, 2009).

The biggest concern with health smart cards is security. However, using intelligence embedded in the card, as well as its processing capability and standards-based cryptography, it can be designed to ensure adherence to the privacy requirements of HIPAA (Smart Card Alliance, 2009). Additionally, the card has built-in tamper resistance and the ability to store large amounts of data. Health smart cards also aid in the portability provision of HIPAA. This provision is concerned with the ability of healthcare data to be portable, that is, to be able to be electronically sent and received in an understandable format while the **confidentiality** of the data is protected. The objective is to simplify the administration of healthcare data.

There are many advantages to health smart cards such as providing information management that ensures that security practices are followed, simplifying hospital admissions, and providing emergency healthcare data (Smart Card Alliance, 2009) (see **Box 13-2**). Having patient information such as allergies, prescribed medications, and medical conditions such as diabetes or congestive heart failure readily available in emergency rooms and ambulances can greatly facilitate care. Additionally, smart cards can provide patients with the knowledge in situations where their healthcare data are not readily available.

Practitioner Instituted. Practitioners have instituted client access to their healthcare records as will be seen in the discussion about **e-encounters**. Electronic access falls into four different categories (Halamka et al., 2008):

1. Vendor created and clinic hosted, such as MyChart and eClinicalWorks.
2. Self-built and provider hosted, such as MyActiveHealth and HealthProfiler.
3. Self-built research system that is agency neutral such as the one developed at Boston

---

BOX 13-2 Advantages of Healthcare Smart Cards

Require user identification and authorization.
Require employee credentials for strong authentification for HIPAA compliance and network security.
Provide immediate access to lifesaving information.
Provide data portability.
Guard against healthcare fraud, abuse, and misuse.
Resolve language issues associated with health record information.
Reduce administrative costs.
Support the NHIN standards.

From Smart Card Alliance. (2009, February). *A healthcare CFO's guide to smart card technology and applications.* Retrieved November 26, 2010, from http://www.smart cardalliance.org/resources/lib/Healthcare_CFO_Guide_to_Smart_Cards_FINAL_012809.pdf

Children's Hospital with open source code using a subscription model that integrates data from different hospital EMRs and enables patients to maintain collated copies of their own records electronically wherever they choose.

4. A system that links an EMR with a PHR. In this model, information can also be imported from other sources such as pharmacies, healthcare providers, and even devices such as home blood pressure monitors.[4] The PHRs from Google Health and Microsoft Health Vault are of this type, but they vary in the services they offer.

E-Encounters

An e-encounter (or e-visit) is a two-way exchange of healthcare information between a healthcare provider and a client/patient, which may be initiated by either the provider or the client. Most of the focus to date has been on the use of e-mail, but with both healthcare providers and clients looking for more efficient and less costly methods of healthcare, other uses of e-encounters will be seen. Several vendors offer applications that support secure e-mail and other web messaging services with clients.

Electronic Encounters

A Mayo clinic study reported the results of providing online care to 4,282 patients over a 2-year period ending in 2009 (Adamson & Bachman, 2010). As a result of the electronic encounter, there was a reduction of 40% face-to-face office visits. Patients demonstrated the ability to upload digital images and the ability to refill prescriptions online. As a result of the study, the Mayo Clinic was able to bill for a large number of the e-visits. The study reported that Medicare and Medicaid visits were billed, but not reimbursed. The Clinic absorbed the expenses of the Medicaid visits, but billed the services for Medicare visits to the patient. The study demonstrated that e-visits are feasible alternatives for face-to-face visits. As seen

in the Mayo study, secure messaging is emerging as the method of choice for e-visits.

Tasks such as making an appointment, obtaining test results, or refilling a prescription lend themselves well to e-mail. E-mail communication can be used in multiple ways, both for tasks that are often done by telephone or regular mail and, in some cases as noted in the example above, to substitute for an office visit. Instituting electronic communication that is a substitute for telephone and regular mail tasks is by far the easiest to justify and to institute.

Benefits of E-Mail Communication with Providers

E-mail can be found useful to facilitate retention and clarification of information provided during visits. Patients who may be stressed during a visit often forget to ask important questions. Additionally, they often may not fully understand information provided about their self-care or the need for further healthcare. When a patient is referred to other facilities, addresses and telephone numbers can easily be included in e-mail, saving the patient from having to write them down or decipher someone else's handwriting.

E-mail communication with a healthcare provider avoids telephone tag. Waiting by the phone all day for a healthcare provider to return a call and having to use voice mail are frustrating for consumers. For providers, trying to return a phone call can be equally frustrating. E-mail can also be used for such things as sending patients' information or providing links to relevant information on the web. Patients can also use e-mail to ask for further clarification after an office visit. E-mails do not need to be transcribed; they can be printed and placed in a patient's record or, if the record is online, filed electronically. When properly implemented, e-mail communication can result in time and cost savings.

Barriers to E-Mail Communication with Providers

With more and more people using e-mail, it may seem surprising that electronic communication with healthcare providers has not become more prevalent. Reasons that healthcare providers give for not instituting e-mail are lack of time, lack of office staff, lack of interest in

---

4 See Chapter 21 for more information about home monitoring.

electronic communication, concerns about privacy and confidentiality (Gerstle, 2004), increased workloads (Baker, Rideout, Gertler, & Raube, 2005), reimbursement concerns, and potential malpractice liability (Roter, Larson, Sands, Ford, & Houston, 2008). One last barrier relates to computer literacy issues. For patients who are not technologically savvy, computer communication can be compounded by technology issues, such as forgotten login information and web browser configurations. These concerns are valid, but with some planning, they can be overcome.

Privacy of E-Mail. Perhaps the biggest concern is privacy. Healthcare providers have a responsibility, both under HIPAA and ethically, to maintain confidentiality about their patients. They must be certain that the person requesting information is entitled to receive it and that it is accurately transmitted and received. Additionally, in electronic communication, healthcare providers must be assured that the messages are not able to be intercepted by others. Most standard e-mails are not so protected. However, secure e-mail is encrypted so that if intercepted by a third party it cannot be easily read.[5] Nothing, of course, is foolproof, and this includes mail and telephone calls. When a patient's voice mail message does not identify the person, there is no way of knowing if a wrong number was reached.

In e-mail, to assure that the e-mail is going to the correct recipient, it is necessary to be certain that the correct e-mail address is being used. If e-mail is integrated with a person's EMR and messages sent from the record, the correct e-mail address could be assured. E-mail needs to be both encrypted and sent with careful checking of the e-mail address of the recipient. Without an EMR, protocols should be instituted to assure that the correct information is being sent to the correct patient. Just as paper information can be inadvertently slipped into the wrong envelope by harried office staff, so can information be e-mailed to the wrong patient. A suggested procedure is to use an address book with a previously tested address and carefully check the name in the address line.

Liability. Liability, although expressed as a concern, is not as big an issue as one might think. If one compares e-mail liability with that for telephone calls, one finds that e-mail is safer. E-mails can be printed and filed in the patient's record, providing a written record of what was asked, as well as the answer. Healthcare providers, so familiar with telephone calls, may not realize that these calls expose them to liability, especially because they are so seldom documented (Sands, 2004).

BOX 13-3 Nationally Recommended Policies for Healthcare Providers' Use of E-Mail

Print e-mail communication and place in patients' chart.
Inform patients about privacy issues with respect to e-mail.
When e-mail messages become too lengthy, notify patients to come in to discuss or call them.
Establish a turnaround time for messages.
Request patients to put their names or identification numbers in the body of the message.
Send a new message to inform patient of completion of request.
Establish types of transaction.
Explain to patients that their message should be concise.
Remind patients when they do not adhere to [e-mail] guidelines.
Develop archival and retrieval mechanisms.
Instruct patients to put the category of transaction in subject line of message (e.g., schedule an appointment, refill a prescription).
Configure an automatic reply to acknowledge receipt of patients' messages.
Request patients to use autoreply features to acknowledge a clinician's message.

From Brooks, R. G., & Menachemi, N. (2006). Physicians' use of email with patients: Factors influencing electronic communication and adherence to best practices. *Journal of Internet Medical Research, 8*(1), e2. Retrieved November 27, 2010, from http://www.ncbi.nlm.nih.gov/pmc/articles/PMC1550692/?tool=pmcentrez

---

5 **Encryption** is discussed in Chapter 3.

Policies that protect healthcare providers from liability with e-mail communication can be seen in **Box 13-3**.

Workload. Increased workloads, especially without additional reimbursement, are another concern. One method of alleviating time demands for both the client and the provider is to develop structured forms accessible on a website that limit patient requests as well as facilitate a quick reply. For example, there can be forms for renewing a prescription, requesting an appointment, referrals, or follow-up communication with one's healthcare provider. Interestingly, where e-mail communication has been instituted, an increased workload for healthcare providers has not materialized (McDonald & California Healthcare Foundation, 2003). For example, ConnectiCare found that online communication increased productivity by reducing administrative tasks. It has also been found that participating physicians were able to spend more time with patients because it is easier to integrate online communication than telephone calls into their daily work. Anecdotal reports during a study of patient–physician e-mails found that physicians believed that web messaging reduced their telephone calls and that they required less time than phone calls (Liederman, Lee, Baquero, & Seites, 2005). It was also reported that office visits triggered by e-mails are more efficient because the history is known.

Implementing E-Encounters

Clearly, the ability to perform many tasks electronically such as making an appointment will

Table 13-1 Tasks Patients Would Like to Do Online

Task	Percentage of Clients Who Want
Ask questions with no visit	77
Make appointments	71
Get new prescriptions	71
See results of medical tests	70

From Harris Interactive Inc. (2002, April 10). *Patient/physician online communication: Many patients want it, would pay for it, and it would influence their choice of doctors and health plans.* Retrieved November 27, 2010, from http://www.harrisinteractive.com/news/newsletters/healthnews/HI_HealthCare-News2002Vol2_Iss08.pdf

save patients and providers time (see **Table 13-1**). Implementation of responding to patient questions and reporting of tests online, however, requires thoughtful planning. The first hurdle may be winning over healthcare providers. Some may respond that "Patients can't handle this information" or fear that they will be deluged with "worried well" questions. E-mail can be used to create a therapeutic relationship or partnership between the provider and the patient. It can mimic the traditional face-to-face dialogue. The use of e-mail allows the provider to respond to the patient worries and concern questions in a patient-centric manner (Roter et al., 2008).

Substitution for an Office Visit

Using e-mail instead of an office visit is a complex subject. Dartmouth-Hitchcock Clinic has instituted what they call "e-visiting" between a client and a provider with whom the client has a relationship (Wasson et al., 2006). The client, who, using a secure website, can request the e-visit and provide an outline of the reason for the e-visit such as asking for advice, requesting a diagnosis, or therapy, tasks that previously required an office visit, sets up an e-visit. The request is reviewed by a clinical person who brings it to the attention of the provider who determines whether the reason meets the criteria for an e-visit. When the e-visit is complete, the provider enters information into the EHR and provides an ICD-9 code, which generates billing.

Triaging E-Mail Messages

Other planning that needs to occur is how to respond to and triage e-mail messages. If web form requests are used, they can be slotted to the correct box for attention. If e-mail is used without a web form, patients can be instructed to use given subject lines for various requests. It must be realized, however, that patients will not always adhere to this. In many ways, triaging e-mail can follow methods used for telephone calls. It is important that a method be devised that assures a reply within a given time period and that this period be communicated to the patient. If a patient sends an e-mail and does not receive a reply within this period, he or she will conclude that their provider is not serious about using e-mail. When properly instituted, e-mail communication with patients will save time now spent on the telephone by both the patient and the provider.

Who Pays?

Healthcare providers still need to be paid for the healthcare they deliver, whether through an office visit, through a telephone call, or electronically. Some considerations for payment are having either the payer or patient pay as for an office visit, or charge the patient an annual fee for these services. Given that patients have expressed a willingness to pay for e-mail messaging (Harris Interactive, 2002) any of these solutions may be feasible. E-mail messaging may be able to save money. One researcher has reported that supporting online patient–provider interaction could save up to $12 million in annual health costs (McDonald & California Healthcare Foundation, 2003). The question again becomes "Who should pay for a service that will benefit mostly patients and payers?"

Summary

As the Internet and web features are used increasingly in healthcare, there will be a change in the relationship of the provider and the client as client access to information previously held only by the practitioner increases. EMRs that provide healthcare records for only one provider will morph into EHRs that provide access to records from many different agencies from one access point. Subsequently, a PHR that permits and encourages client access to their healthcare information will emerge. Before this becomes a reality, many barriers must be overcome including gaining provider compliance, a UPI, and a change in consumer behavior.

E-encounters, the exchange of information between a healthcare provider and a client, will become an expected mode of communication, one that nurses, particularly those involved in telephone consultations of private practice, will be involved. This will not happen without overcoming provider reluctance and planning that includes decisions such as what information to provide to clients and when. The final step of having an e-encounter substitute for an office visit will be sometime in the future for most agencies. Nevertheless, e-encounters and PHRs will become a normal part of healthcare delivery.

APPLICATIONS AND COMPETENCIES

1. Differentiate between an EMR, an EHR, and a PHR, as described in this chapter.

2. List the benefits of a PHR.

3. Find an online PHR by searching the web and evaluate their privacy policy by using the criteria on page 5 of the government report at http://www.hhs.gov/healthit/ahic/materials/01_07/ce/PrivacyReview.pdf. Based on this evaluation, make a recommendation to a client about whether to use this service.

4. Would you use a healthcare smart card? Why or why not?

5. Write a proposal for instituting e-mail communication with clients in a specific practice such as primary care, obstetrics, or cardiology.

6. Examine the pros and cons of a unique patient identifier.

7. Appraise the various methods of electronic communication with patients.

REFERENCES

Adamson, S. C., & Bachman, J. W. (2010). Pilot study of providing online care in a primary care setting. *Mayo Clinic Proceedings, 85*(8), 704–710.

Baker, L., Rideout, J., Gertler, P., & Raube, K. (2005). Effect of an Internet-based system for doctor–patient communication on health care spending. *Journal of the American Medical Informatics Association, 12*(5), 530–536.

Cagliostro, C. (2005, February 26). *Smart cards primer.* Retrieved August 17, 2011, from http://www.kis-kiosk.com/casestudies/assets/smartcardhandbook.pdf

Curtin, R. B., Walters, B. A., Schatell, D., Pennell, P., Wise, M., & Klicko, K. (2008). Self-efficacy and self-management behaviors in patients with chronic kidney disease. *Advances in Chronic Kidney Disease, 15*(2), 191–205.

Daniel, J., Posnack, S., & Consumer Education and Engagement Collaborative (2009, March 31). *Personal health record (PHR) website inventory, analyses and findings.* Retrieved November 16, 2010, from http://

healthit.hhs.gov/portal/server.pt/document/872291/
cee_tool_special_phr_analysis_pdf

Department of Health and Human Services. (2010,
September 3). *Nationwide health information network.*
Retrieved November 11, 2010, from http://healthit.
hhs.gov/portal/server.pt?open=512&objID=1142&p
arentname=CommunityPage&parentid=25&mode=2
&in_hi_userid=11113&cached=true

Gerstle, R. S. (2004). E-mail communication between pediatricians and their patients. *Pediatrics, 114*(1), 317–321.

Halamka, J. D., Mandl, K. D., & Tang, P. C. (2008). Early
experiences with personal health records. *Journal of the
American Medical Informatics Assocation, 15*(1), 1–7.

Harris Interactive. (2002, April 10). Patient/physician online
communication: Many patients ant it, would pay for it,
and it would influence their choice of doctors and health
plans. *Healthcare News, 2*(8). Retrieved from http://
www.harrisinteractive.com/news/newsletters/health-
news/HI_HealthCareNews2002Vol2_Iss08.pdf

Harris Interactive. (2010, June 17). *Few Americans using 'e'
medical records.* Retrieved June 29, 2010, from http://
www.harrisinteractive.com/NewsRoom/HarrisPolls/
tabid/447/mid/1508/articleId/414/ctl/ReadCustom%20
Default/Default.aspx

Hillestad, R., Bigelow, J. H., Chaudhry, B., Dreyer,
P., Greenberg, M. D., Meili, R. C., et al. (2009).
*Identify crisis: An examination of the costs and
benefits of a unique patient identifier for the
U.S. health care system.* Retrieved July 1, 2010,
from http://www.rand.org/pubs/monographs/
MG753/?ref=homepage&key=t_stethoscope_keyboard

Kaissi, A. A., & Parchman, M. (2009). Organizational factors
associated with self-management behaviors in diabetes primary care clinics. *The Diabetes Educator, 35*(5),
843–850.

Lauer, G. (2008, October 30). *Privacy advocates reject unique
patient identifier study.* Retrieved July 1, 2010, from
http://www.ihealthbeat.org/features/2008/privacy-advo-
cates-reject-unique-patient-identifier-study.aspx

Lecker, R., Armijo, D., Chin, S., Christensen, J., Desper, J.,
Hong, A., et al. (2007, January 5). *Review of the personal
health record (PHR) service provider market.* Retrieved
November 25, 2010, from http://www.hhs.gov/healthit/
ahic/materials/01_07/ce/PrivacyReview.pdf

Liederman, E. M., Lee, J. C., Baquero, V. H., & Seites, P. G.
(2005). The impact of patient–physician web messaging
on provider productivity. *Journal of Healthcare Information
Management, 19*(2), 81–86.

Markle Foundation, & Westin, A. F. (2008, June). *Americans
overwhelmingly believe electronic personal records could
improve their health.* Retrieved June 29, 2010, from
http://www.connectingforhealth.org/resources/
ResearchBrief-200806.pdf

McDonald, K., & California Healthcare Foundation. (2003,
November 18). *Online patient–provider communication tools: An overview.* Retrieved August 17, 2011,
from http://www.chcf.org/publications/2003/11/
online-patientprovider-communication-tools-an-overview

Miniwatts Marketing Group. (2010, June 31). *World Internet
stats: Usage and population statistics.* Retrieved November 16,
2010, from http://www.internetworldstats.com/stats.htm

Monegain, B. (2009, September 25). *NAHIT disbands after
seven years of advocacy. Healthcare IT News.* Retrieved
from http://www.healthcareitnews.com/news/
nahit-disbands-after-seven-years-advocacy

National Alliance for Health Information Technology.
(2008, April 8). *Defining key helath information technology terms.* Retrieved November 16, 2010, from http://
healthit.hhs.gov/portal/server.pt/gateway/PTA
RGS_0_10741_848133_0_0_18/10_2_hit_terms.pdf

Office of the National Coordinator for Health Information
Technology. (2009, December 4). *Health IT terms.*
Retrieved November 25, 2010, from http://
healthit.hhs.gov/portal/server.pt/community/
healthit_hhs_gov__glossary/1256

Ross, S. E., & Lin, C. (2003). The effects of promoting patient
access to medical records: A review [corrected]. *Journal of
the American Medical Informatics Association, 10*(2),
129–138. [Erratum: *Journal of the American Medical
Informatics Association* May–June 2003, *10*(3), 294.]

Roter, D. L., Larson, S., Sands, D. Z., Ford, D. E., & Houston,
T. (2008). Can e-mail messages between patients and
physicians be patient-centered? *Health Communation,
23*(1), 80–86.

Sands, D. Z. (2004). Help for physicians contemplating use
of e-mail with patients. *Journal of the American Medical
Informatics Association, 11*(4), 268–269.

Smart Card Alliance. (2006). *University of Pittsburgh Medical
Center.* Retrieved November 26, 2010, from http://
www.smartcardalliance.org/resources/pdf/University_of_
Pittsburgh_Medical_Center.pdf

Smart Card Alliance. (2009, February). *A healthcare CFO's
guide to smart card technology and applications.* Retrieved
November 26, 2010, from http://www.smartcardalliance.
org/resources/lib/Healthcare_CFO_Guide_to_Smart
_Cards_FINAL_012809.pdf

Tang, P. C., Ash, J. S., Bates, D. W., Overhage, J. M., & Sands,
D. Z. (2006). Personal health records: Definitions,
benefits, and strategies for overcoming barriers to
adoption. *Journal of the American Medical Association,
13*(2), 121–126.

U.S. Department of Health and Human Services. (2010a).
Health information privacy. Retrieved June 28, 2010, from
http://www.hhs.gov/ocr/privacy/hipaa/understanding/
consumers/medicalrecords.html

U.S. Department of Health and Human Services. (2010b).
Summary of the HIPAA privacy rule. Retrieved June 28,
2010, from http://www.hhs.gov/ocr/privacy/hipaa/under-
standing/summary/index.html

Wasson, J. H., Johnson, D. J., Benjamin, R., Phillips,
J., & MacKenzie, T. A. (2006). Patients report positive
impacts of collaborative care. *Journal of Ambulatory Care
Management, 29*(3), 199–206.

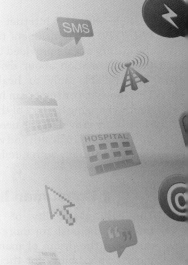

CHAPTER 14

The Empowered Consumer

Objectives

After studying this chapter you will be able to:

▶ Analyze the effect of consumer empowerment on healthcare.

▶ Describe approaches to guiding clients to high-quality web-based health information.

▶ Analyze the effects of health literacy and health numeracy on patient care and teaching.

▶ Demonstrate finding and evaluating a web-based support group for a client with a specific condition.

▶ Explore the potential for web-based health education.

Key Terms

Accessibility	HEDIS
Alt Tag	Image Map
Braille Reader	Navigation Bar
Broadband	NCQA
Consumer Informatics	Patient Portal
Decision Support	Plug-in
Dial-up Connection	Screen Reader
Extranet	Support Group
Flash Animation	URL
Health Literacy	Usability
Health Numeracy	

An imagined dialogue with Socrates, in Chapter 12 of the book *Consumer-Driven Healthcare,* asks why consumers who can intelligently purchase financial products, cars, and computers cannot do the same with healthcare (Hyde, 2004). The answer given was that they have never been allowed to do so. In the past, consumers did not have the knowledge that healthcare providers did, which resulted in a culture of paternalism. Patients were expected to accept what was prescribed disregarding cost and were labeled "noncompliant" if they did not. Additionally, there was an underlying assumption on the part of payers and consumers that all healthcare was equal; hence, there was no concern about quality or cost.

Spearheaded by many large corporations, who formed the Leapfrog Group to study how they could work together to have an influence on the quality and affordability of healthcare (Leapfrog Group, 2009a), the movement to give consumers more control over how to spend their healthcare dollar is increasing. Much of this progress has been made possible with the Internet and the World Wide Web (WWW). Consumers today can learn about the quality of care provided by many hospitals and find information about diseases that previously was available only to healthcare professionals. This move to consumerism in healthcare is permanently changing the face of the healthcare industry. Healthcare providers will need to evolve from being care providers to health and wellness brokers, a role that fits naturally with nursing.

Consumer Informatics

The easy availability of information on the Internet, the push for more cost-effective healthcare, and the desire of many consumers to take more responsibility for their health has resulted in the development of **consumer informatics**, a subspecialty in healthcare informatics. The goal is to improve the consumer decision-making processes and healthcare outcomes with electronic information and communication (American Medical Informatics Association, 2010). This field is an applied science using concepts from communication, education, behavioral science, and social networking (Houston & Ehrenberger, 2001). It is designed to provide healthcare information to consumers, allow consumers to make informed decisions, promote healthy behaviors and information exchange, and provide social support to clients. Practitioners analyze consumer needs and information use and develop ways to facilitate consumers in finding and using health information. They also evaluate the effectiveness of electronic health information and study how this affects public health and the consumer–healthcare provider relationship (Eysenbach, 2000; Lewis, 2007).

Consumer informatics is differentiated from healthcare informatics not by the technology, but by its focus on the consumer, rather than healthcare providers, as end user. The hope is that "intelligent informatics applications" will result in the healthcare information that reaches consumers, creating a healthy balance between self-reliance and professional help (Eysenbach, 2000). It is related to all of healthcare informatics because full realization of its potential depends on the features and breadth of information systems. Consumer informatics applications may include

interaction with healthcare providers; however, others may not. Examples include websites, information kiosks, blood pressure kiosks, and personal health records. Consumer informatics applications are part of the move to empower healthcare consumers.

Consumer Empowerment

The term "consumer empowerment" means that patients are provided with enough information so that they can make informed decisions. In other words, they can become consumers or clients, not patients. Patient empowerment got its start in a 1905 Illinois Court of Appeals decision that established that patients have the right to know in advance what surgery is going to be performed (*Pratt v. Davis*, 1905). The case resulted from a physician who performed a hysterectomy on an epileptic patient without her consent. According to the case, the physician obtained consent from the husband, instead of the wife, stating that the patient could not consent because of her mental condition, yet, he never established her incompetency. Scholendorff v. New York Hospital (1914) is the seminal case that supported informed consent and patient empowerment. A woman consented to surgery to diagnose a thyroid tumor as benign or malignant, but she did not give consent to remove the tumor. After determining that the tumor was malignant, the surgeon removed it against the patient's wishes. Justice Benjamin Cardoza noted:

> Every human of adult years and sound mind has a right to determine what shall be done with his own body; and a surgeon who performs an operation without his patient's consent commits an assault for which he is liable in damages. (Schloendorff v. New York Hospital, 1914)

Although the courts supported patient rights to consent for treatment, medicine was largely a paternalistic practice for many decades. Informed consent did not include the right to understand the personal medical condition, treatment options, risks associated with the options, or prognosis. That was finally changed in 1972, when the American Medical Association approved the Patient's Bill of Rights (Tung & Organ, 2000).

Further court cases in the 1970s affirmed the rights of patients to be given this information in plain English. Despite the slow beginning, today many consumers expect to receive understandable information about their health conditions and be full partners in their healthcare, not passive recipients. Consumers are also beginning to expect to be able to make intelligent decisions about healthcare based on cost and quality.

The Office of the National Coordinator (ONC) for Health Information Technology (IT) was established to coordinate programs established by the Health Information Technology for Economic and Clinical Health Act (Office of the National Coordinator for Health Information Technology, 2009). The ONC also facilitates the adoption of health IT programs in the United States. In 2004, Dr. Brailer, as national coordinator, outlined the strategic framework for the ONC. The report advocated for consumer empowerment, personalized care, and the consumers' ability to select healthcare based on their values and information. Consumer empowerment has the ability to affect the rising rate of health plan costs by incorporating economic consequences for low-quality care. It can also improve healthcare by providing consumers with data such as the cost and quality of healthcare services along with information for self-diagnosis and referral to appropriate providers. At the same time, it can preserve the best elements of our present system of clinical support for those who suffer from acute illnesses, injuries, or chronic conditions.

Accessing Quality of Care Information

In an attempt to control healthcare costs, the U.S. Department of Health & Human Services now requires hospitals to report quality indicators. Under the auspices of the Centers for Medicare & Medicaid Services and the Hospital Quality Alliance, this information, which is updated quarterly, is posted on a web page (U.S. Department of Health & Human Services, 2010a). Visitors can see how often a given hospital provides recommended care for heart attack, heart failure, pneumonia, or surgery. The Leapfrog Group also rates hospitals, but differently (Leapfrog Group, 2009b). It looks at high-risk treatments for such things as abdominal aortic aneurysm repair, pancreatic resection,

and bariatric surgery. It also rates intensive care units based on the use of intensivists, or healthcare providers who have special training in critical care, and the use of computerized provider order entry systems. Its site provides information and criteria to use in selecting a hospital as well as the dates that the information used for the rating was submitted. (On its page at http://www.leapfroggroup.org/cp, it may be necessary to scroll to the right to see the dates!)

The Healthcare Effectiveness Data and Information Set **HEDIS** provides information to consumers and employers that allows them to compare the performance of health plans with other plans and to national or regional benchmarks. HEDIS measures performance in quality of care, access to care, and member satisfaction with the health plan and doctors. HEDIS is used by more than 90% of the U.S. healthcare plans. CMS requires that health maintenance organizations (HMOs) submit data to HEDIS if they provide HMO services for Medicare enrollees. HEDIS was developed and is maintained by the National Committee for Quality Assurance **NCQA**, a private nonprofit corporation dedicated to improving health quality (National Committee for Quality Assurance, 2010).

Rating of hospitals is in the introductory stage. The benefits for use are not yet fully recognized. Werner, Bradlow, and Ash (2008) suggest that multiple assessment measures (structure, process, and outcomes) be used to assess performance. Hospitals should identify unmeasured factors that relate to better performance. Like any database, what is collected to calculate the ratings determines the results. Even if not perfect, if consumers are to make good decisions about healthcare, providing even this level of information is needed. Expect to see this situation improve as more factors affecting the quality of care are teased out. In any quality study, nurses need to learn what data are being collected and how much of it reflects actual nursing care.

In 1994, the American Nurses Association initiated the Safety and Quality Initiative. The initiative transformed into the National Database of Nursing Quality Indicators™ (American Nurses Association, 2010). The goal was to further the development of nursing knowledge about patient safety and quality improvement efforts by using comparative data on nursing care and the relationship to outcomes (National Database of Nursing Quality Indicators, n.d.). Participation is voluntary, but currently there are over 1,500 contributors. Results at this time are not available to consumers but only to participating agencies, but it is an excellent step toward helping nursing to further the quality of care.

Health Portals

A portal is by definition any website that offers a wide array of resources and services such as e-mail, forums, a search tool, and links to useful sites. It is the blending of many Internet tools into one useful service. Generally, a portal is targeted at a specific population such as professionals in a discipline, healthcare consumers with a specific medical condition, those looking for either general or specific health information, or shoppers for specific products such as baby products.

Health portals are common, and many are government sponsored. In Canada, the government sponsors the Health Canada site (http://www.hc-sc.gc.ca/index-eng.php), which has general health information as well as information specific to Canadians. The United Kingdom has several health portals, including a health screening portal (http://www.screening.nhs.uk/), health sites (http://www.healthsites.co.uk/), and health information sites (http://www.bbc.co.uk/health/). Similar sites are provided by the Australian government (http://www.healthinsite.gov.au/) and the New Zealand government (http://www.nzhis.govt.nz/). The U.S. government sponsors Healthcare.gov (http://www.healthcare.gov/) (see **Figure 14-1**), the National Library of Medicine (http://www.nlm.nih.gov/), Medline Plus (http://medlineplus.gov/), and PubMed Home (http://www.ncbi.nlm.nih.gov/pubmed). Other governments also provide online health information; some of these sites are integrated with general information about the government.

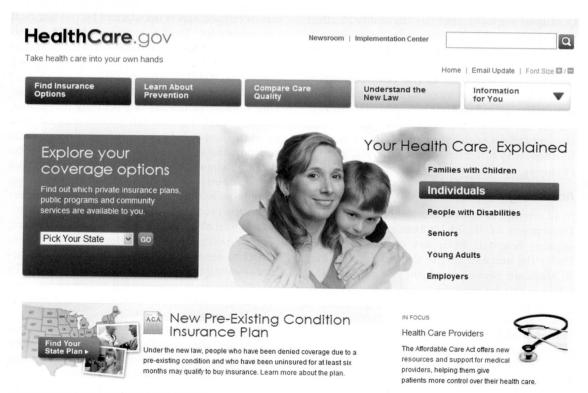

Figure 14-1 Healthcare.gov health portal.

Patient Portals

Patient portals take the portal concept one step further and individualize the portal by using clinical communication and, in some cases, the electronic patient health record. A patient portal may offer only one-way communication to a patient, but the information will be specific to that patient. Common communication functions include the ability to make routine appointments or renew prescriptions. Examples include sending diabetic patients reminders about making an appointment for a foot examination or alerting patients about abnormally high cholesterol results with a link to a video about cholesterol control (Gardner, 2010). Some portals allow patients to upload blood glucose results and then provide feedback on glucose control. Assisting diabetic patients to manage their chronic condition has the potential of saving healthcare dollars (Paylor, 2010) and improving their quality of life.

This type of personalization of information has been shown to be successful, especially in the care of patients with chronic diseases such as diabetes and heart disease. Most of these systems also contain some type of **decision support** using computerized prompts (Dorr et al., 2007). Some patient portals provide e-mail messaging features, and others provide patients access to their electronic medical record (EMR) (Gardner, 2010), which is similar to a personal health record (PHR), but without access to provider data outside the system. Using patient portals is one way of meeting the needs of clients who today expect attention that is more personal. They desire the same services that the financial industry provides,

namely, personalized information that is targeted for them.

In the United Kingdom, NHS Direct (http://www.nhsdirect.nhs.uk/) provides a patient portal that is not tied to a consumer's patient record. The portal provides answers to common questions, includes a health encyclopedia, and provides a self-help decision support guide. This site also allows consumers to send a health inquiry to the NHS team and find a local health service. To accommodate the sight impaired, NHS Direct provides a free **screen reader**. Eysenbach (2000) predicted that the professionals who staff this service might evolve to "cyber licensed professionals," or a healthcare provider who receives specialty education and whose practice is monitored for quality but whose practice is online. In the United States, specially trained nurses in hospitals provide some of these services.

Although the number and types of patient portals are growing, the usage as of 2010 is less than 10% (Harris Interactive, 2010). The percentage for use of patient portals is greater if the consumer has a health insurance plan that provides a patient portal. For example, 50% of patients who had Kaiser and 30% of patients who had United Healthcare reported that they had a PHR. What is interesting is that the 2010 Harris Interactive poll indicated that only 30% of the population believed that insurance companies should have access to their health information, although most believed that an electronic record would be valuable to track their health progress (see **Figure 14-2**).

Currently, there are many nongovernmental groups that sponsor healthcare portals; some are

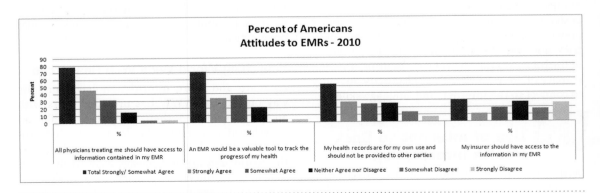

Figure 14-2 Consumer attitudes to EMRs 2010.

commercial, and some are nonprofit. Examples of free resources include Microsoft HealthVault (http://www.healthvault.com/), MyPHR by AHIMA (http://www.myphr.com/), and My Family Health Portrait sponsored by the U.S. Surgeon (https://familyhistory.hhs.gov/). Before recommending a site, or portal, to a client, it needs to be thoroughly evaluated. Because many portals depend on advertisements for support, special care needs to be taken to ensure that the information and links provided are bias free and complete.

The Digital Divide

One of the criticisms often leveled against the growing importance of the Internet and web as a means of dispersing information is that there is a "digital divide," a term that originated in the mid-1990s (van Dijk, 2006). It is often interpreted as the gap between those who have access to the Internet and those who do not. Before use of the term "digital divide," more general concepts such as information inequality, information gap, or knowledge gap were used. van Dijk states that this term has probably created more confusion than clarification. "Digital divide" suggests that there is a clear gap between two clearly defined groups that is difficult to bridge and that the condition is static. In reality, the gap is continually shifting.

The major accomplishment of the term "digital divide" seemed to be putting the topic of information inequality on the scholarly and political agenda. In the developed world, the problem is often a lack of knowledge of how to access the resources resulting from a lack of technical skills. It might also be a lack of knowledge about community resources such as a public library and/or perhaps, from motivation to take responsibility previously borne by others. In the developing countries, however, the ability to tap the rich resources of the Internet is still a problem resulting from the scarcity of computers, lack of electricity, inability to connect to the Internet, and language skills.

Use of Internet to Seek Health Information

With the transformation of the healthcare provider–client relationship from a paternalistic approach in which the healthcare providers

have all the knowledge to a more participatory approach in which clients take responsibility for their own care, the need for individuals to have more health-related information has increased 10-fold. The web has met this need. Searching for health information online has never been easier. A search for a condition such as diabetes using Google™ produces not only a list of sites but also allows the selection of sites specific to either professionals or consumers. If the consumer site is selected, clients can narrow their search by selecting from categories such as treatments, tests, or alternative medicine.

There is always concern about the quality of information on the web. Currently, the trend is not to criticize online resources but to guide users to evaluate the quality of online information. In looking at the behavior of consumers when finding health information on the web, a classic study found that although the searching technique may be suboptimal, consumers usually found the answers to their questions (Eysenbach & Kohler, 2002). They also usually selected the first few links that the search tool found. In assessing the quality, they looked at the source, the professional design, whether there was a scientific or official touch, the language, and ease of use. When their searching behavior was observed, it was found that participants never checked the About Us section, disclaimers, or disclosure statements. In interviews after searching, it was found that very few participants had even noticed or remembered from which websites they had retrieved information. Although there is certainly inaccurate information on the web, it can be argued that the accuracy of the information is comparable to many traditional sources such as pamphlets, acquaintances, and popular press articles.

Searching World Wide Web Resources

As more and more information has found its way online, the WWW has provided users with an encyclopedia in their computer. Unlike an encyclopedia, however, the documents that provide the needed information are located all over the world and are not always easy to discover. Additionally, the WWW provides an outlet to anyone who wishes to share personal views. Thus, the use of the WWW puts a burden on the user to become adept not only at finding sources but also at evaluating the sources. If we are going to help consumers to find and analyze web-based sources, it behooves us to develop some expertise first. Discovery of quality resources requires us to understand the different types of search engines, recognize what might be buried in the invisible web, and understand criteria to use to scrutinize the resources.

Types of Search Tools

There are many search tools available on the WWW. The search tools are automated or human-driven. The search tools can be classified into three general categories, crawler or spider, human-powered directories, or a combination. The popularity of specific search engines tends to fluctuate. Crawler or spider search engines visit each website, "read" each web page and the associated links, and then index or catalog the information in preparation for a search (European Commission, 2010). Currently, crawler or spider search engines, such as Google (http://www.google.com/), Yahoo! (http://www.

yahoo.com/), and Bing (http://www.bing.com/), have widespread use. Ask Jeeves (http://www.ask.com/) specializes in answering questions by using natural language. Dogpile (http://www.dogpile.com/) is a metasearch engine that searches all of the popular search engines.

There are fewer human-driven directories available than electronic crawlers. The Open Directory (http://www.dmoz.org) is an example. Other examples include the Google Directory (http://www.google.com/dirhp) and Yahoo! Directory (http://dir.yahoo.com/). The Yahoo! search engine is classified as a hybrid because it is both a crawler and a directory.

Many of the search engines are specialized. Although, there is a default search engine built into each web browser, you can change the search engine. To do so, go to the window where you enter a search term. Click on the search engine icon to obtain a dropdown menu with other choices (see **Figure 14-3**). Firefox web browser allows you to search for additional search engines to add to the dropdown menu. For example, eBay search

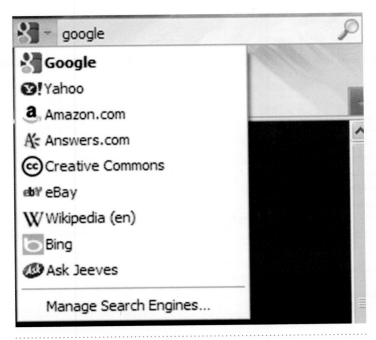

Figure 14-3 Change search engine in a web browser.

engine will look for sale items on the eBay website, Flickr will search for photos, and Internet Movie Database will search for movies. Find Articles will search print publications, including magazines and selected scholarly journals. The Combined Health Information Database (DHID) will search for medical topics.

The Invisible Web

Only a portion of the offerings on the web can be searched by using a search tool. Some pages and links cannot be located by search engines, and some are excluded by the policy of the specific search tool. These pages are called the invisible web. There are several reasons for documents to be invisible; one is that not all pages are static or permanent. Some are dynamic, that is, created on the fly in response to a question. An example would be a schedule of flights required by a user or a list of resources in response to a question. Some sites require a password or login that keeps spiders, which cannot type, out.

Sometimes, the type of page prohibits it from being found by the search tool. For example, some sites use the Acrobat Reader format instead of html for their pages. Other types of files that may not be found with a standard search engine are images, sound files, and streaming video files. Some search engines are programmed to avoid any page with a question mark in the **URL**. A question mark indicates that there is a script in the web page. Although, there are many legitimate reasons for including a script, a script can also be a trap, designed to bog a spider down in an infinite loop. Lacking any human judgment, most spiders just back off and ignore the URLs.

Although thousands of online resources are invisible to standard searches, a little user ingenuity can make them discoverable. Any of the specialized search engines noted above should identify sites that may not be visible with standard search engines. Even if the standard search engine did make the discovery, you may not know it because of the thousands of returns. If you want a particular type of file format, use the advanced search feature in the search engine (see **Figure 14-4**). As an example, advanced searches will allow you to look for only.xls spreadsheet files or .ppt PowerPoint files. To discover the latest information about revealing the invisible web, conduct your own search by using the search terms "invisible web search engines." Like any search of the literature, finding

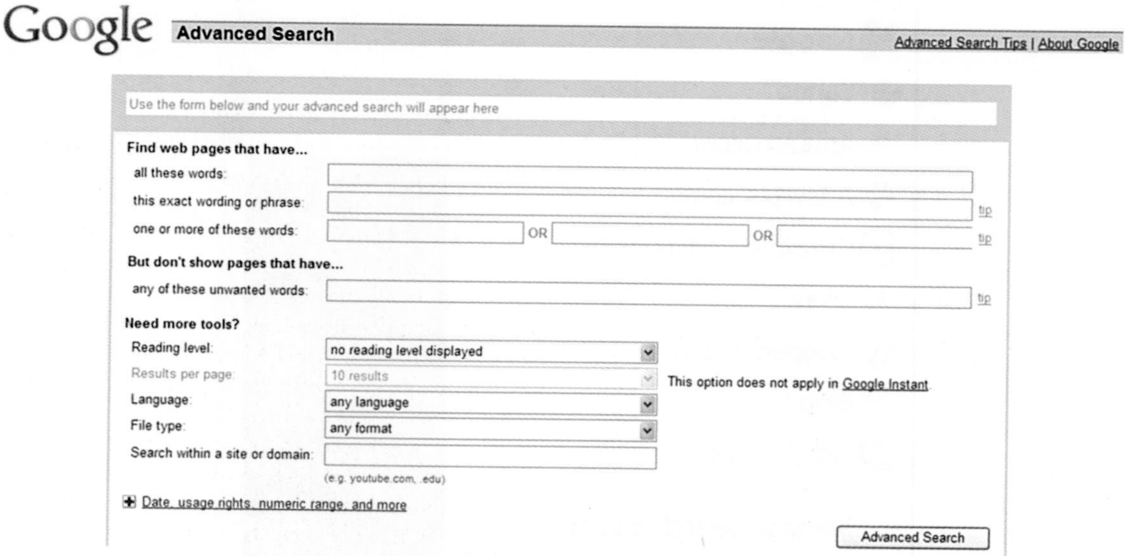

Figure 14-4 Advanced search feature in Google.

documents that are useful depends on the search strategy employed. For simple topics, using a one-word search may be helpful, but locating all of the pertinent information on many topics requires a good preplan, just like digital library searches.

Evaluating Web Resources

The freedom of publication on the Internet allows an airing of ideas, many of which are not in the mainstream. The authenticity that we count on in the print world with the reputations of various newspapers is not yet available on the WWW. Although we may long for the security of a library in which all material is vetted to a degree, the fact that yesterday's "far out idea" may become today's newest knowledge would make this undesirable. Additionally, as hard as we can, evaluation is never 100% objective. There is always the value of the evaluator involved.

The great variety of types of information on the web means that using only one set of yes/no criteria for web document evaluation is not valid. Use of an evaluation rubric that addresses the authority of the site, quality, currency, ease of use, privacy, and other resources provides a way to evaluate websites. The Medical Library Association has an online user's guide for finding and evaluating healthcare websites at http://www.mlanet.org/resources/userguide.html (Medical Library Association, 2009). The site includes a link designed specifically for healthcare consumers.

Certification from an authority, such as the Health on the Net Foundation, an international nonprofit organization, mitigates the need for personal evaluation of the site. Certification from the Foundation is signified with the HONcode icon. Health on the Net Foundation provides an evaluation tool online at https://www.hon.ch/cgi-bin/HONcode/Inscription/site_evaluation.pl?language=en&userCategory=individuals (Health on the Net Foundation, 2009). The Foundation also provides a downloadable search toolbar to assist users to find certified health information websites.

Teaching Clients How to Find and Evaluate Web-Based Information

You can guide clients to many trusted websites for web-based health information. Government sites are trustworthy, as are many organizational sites.

When working with clients, be sure to emphasize the importance of looking closely at the last letters in the name of the computer hosting the site. For example, the site http://www.cancer.com belongs to Ortho Biotech Products, L.P., the site http://www.cancer.org belongs to the American Cancer Society, and the site http://www.cancer.gov/ belongs to the National Cancer Institute. Links to some sites for locating quality health information are on the web page for the book at http://dlthede.net/Informatics/Informatics.html.

A 2008 study conducted by Keselman, Browne, and Kaufman indicated that the healthcare consumer's misconceptions about a healthcare condition are often a factor when using the web for information seeking. The consumer might have good search skills but search sites to support their mistaken understanding of the condition (Keselman et al., 2008). As a result of the study, the authors recommended the use of patient portals and websites analyzed and recommended by healthcare professionals. Nurses should guide clients to ask for assistance when searching the web for healthcare information. Consumers should be advised to look at information such as About Us, the last update date, qualifications of any listed authors, and the source of the page. It is very possible today to find credible health information on the web, but it is, and always will be, a "buyers beware" situation.

When Clients Come With Health Information From the Web

Given the plethora of new knowledge that research is constantly creating, it has become almost impossible for healthcare providers to stay abreast of recent developments. Additionally, most web-savvy clients will search the web for information about any condition they suspect they have, or that has been diagnosed. Unfortunately, less than half the people who find health information on the web will discuss the information with their healthcare provider (Harris Interactive, 2008). Those who do want to discuss this information will often arrive for an office visit or hospitalization with information printouts. This information, which may or may not be accurate, may be the one that the healthcare provider is unaware of. Conflicts may arise as the client questions the provider and second-guesses treatment, with the result of a lack of trust in the provider.

When the information a client brings is suspect, or new to you, several avenues are open. If the information is not from a respected peer and a computer is near, you may want to access the site, the URL (universal resource locator – web address) of which should be on the printout. If this is a personal account of a disease, the information may or may not be accurate, and may or may not be helpful to the client. If the information is posted by an organization, check out their About Us section. If the information has cited references that can be accessed, check them to see if they are accurately cited. Be wary of a list of references that are not cited in the text. Also watch for a pitch for a product. If the printout has no URL, ask the client how he or she found the site and see if you can duplicate the search. Even if you are unsuccessful, you have demonstrated to the client that you respect him or her and are interested in his or her well-being.

Always keep in mind that even though the information the client brings is new to you, or even refutes current practices or strongly held theories, it may be correct. For example, most hospitals and surgical centers still prescribe nothing by mouth after midnight before surgery, with no regard to the scheduled time of surgery. A search of the web for preoperative fasting will reveal, however, that this is not necessarily the best practice (Brady, Kinn, Stuart, & Ness, 2003; Maltby, 2006; McLeod, Fitzgerald, & Sarr, 2005).

Whatever your decision about the information, you will need to discuss it further with the client. If the information is from a reliable source and contradicts what you "know," you will need to acknowledge this. This may lead to you discovering that the client has unanswered questions, is scared, needs more understanding of the underlying disease, or just needs more information. In many cases, especially if the information is suspect, working with this client will take a great deal of patience and tact, but it is vitally important in providing care. More troubling can be the clients who have accessed information about their condition, do not discuss it with their healthcare provider, but use it in decisions regarding their treatment. Asking if a client has accessed information about his or her condition on the web may start a conversation that

leads to better understanding on both yours and the client's part.

Cyberchondriacs

The searching by consumers for health information on the web has led to a new term "cyberchondriac." The term is a combination of the terms "cyber" and "hypochondria" to coin a word that tends to appear pejorative, or implying that a person is obsessive about illness. Researchers at Harris Interactive (2002) say that the term is not pejorative, but indicates a person who has concerns about health and searches for health information on the web. They believe that this behavior is a positive sign. Although many worry that as the public gets more information from the web, the healthcare provider–patient relationship will erode, these researchers believe just the opposite. The 2002-posted survey reported that 30% of the U.S. online population, 23% in France, 33% in Germany, and 17% in Japan found that online information influenced the discussions they had with their healthcare provider in a positive manner. The researchers also found that this information affected people's understanding of any health problems they had and improved their health management.

Unfortunately, there are many who imply that cyberchondriacs are those who think they have a given disease because their symptoms match those on an Internet health site (Cohen, 2008). Although this is possible, it is no more likely that people who use the web for health information will develop imaginary diseases than those who read about conditions in the popular literature or see health information on television. As a nurse, you can influence how patients are affected by any information they have found (from any source) by answering clients' questions about this information and clarifying any misunderstandings. In these discussions, always remember that a client may be accurate in self-diagnosis. More than one person has accurately diagnosed himself or herself from web information.

Internet Pharmacies

Lawful online pharmacies require a prescription for any medication. Most well-known chain pharmacies in the United States have a pharmacy portal that allows healthcare consumers to order and renew prescriptions. The portals also provide patient education information about drugs. Other services include sending an e-mail or text message when a prescription is ready. Examples of legitimate online pharmacies include CVS (http://www.CVS.com), Walgreens (http://www.walgreens.com/pharmacy/), and Rite Aid (http://www.riteaid.com/).

Unfortunately, the high cost of drugs has forced many people to search for less expensive alternatives on the web. Unlawful Internet pharmacies allow consumers to purchase medications without prescriptions or consultation with a healthcare provider. Additionally, because their only interest is in making a sale, they may sell counterfeit or out-of-date medications, provide the wrong dosage, or sell medications that can create drug reactions. Furthermore, they do not warn purchasers of side effects or the appropriate method of taking a drug. In 2010, the search engines Google, Bing, and Yahoo all agreed to a policy to allow only Verified Internet Pharmacy Practice Sites (National Association of Boards of Pharmacy, 2011) to advertise on the search engine web pages. Despite the policy, unverified pharmacies have been known to show up on web searches (Hogans, 2010). To help your clients avoid the pitfalls of these suspect pharmacies, you should assess their sources for drugs and assist them to find a legitimate online pharmacy (see **Box 14-1**). Warn your clients that any online site that does not require a prescription operates outside the law and may send questionable drugs. The U.S. Department of Justice Drug Enforcement Administration maintains a website that allows the public to report unlawful Internet pharmacies at https://www.deadiversion.usdoj.gov/webforms/jsp/umpire/umpireForm.jsp.

Health Literacy

The benefit that consumers will gain from all the information available today depends not only on its quality and availability but also on the ability of the consumer to understand it. Referred to as **health literacy**, it is "the degree to which individuals have the capacity to obtain, process, and understand basic health information and services needed to make appropriate health decisions." It includes the ability to understand instructions on prescription drug bottles, appointment slips, medical education brochures, doctor's directions, consent forms, and the ability to negotiate complex healthcare systems. Health literacy is not simply the ability to read. It is "the degree to which individuals have the capacity to obtain, process, and understand basic health information and services needed to make appropriate decisions" (U.S. Department of Health & Human Services, 2000).

Health literacy is not static; it varies with context and setting. Health literacy is not necessarily

BOX 14-1 When Considering Buying Health-Related Items Online

- Be wary of extravagant claims about performance or treatment potential. Get all promises in writing and review them carefully before making a payment or signing a contract.
- Read the fine print and all relevant Internet links. Fraudulent promoters sometimes bury the disclosures that they are wary of sharing by putting them in very small, fine print or in a location where you are unlikely to find them.
- Look for a privacy policy. If you do not see one or if you do not understand it, you should seriously consider taking your interests elsewhere.
- Be skeptical of any company or organization that does not state its name, street address, and telephone number. Websites should have some form of feedback or contact information available. Check the site out with the local Better Business Bureau or consumer protection office.
- Always consult a healthcare professional before altering any current treatment regimen or buying a "cure all" product that claims to treat a wide range of ailments or offers quick cures and easy solutions to serious illnesses.

Reproduced from HIMSS from Marconi, J. (2002). *E-Health: Navigating the Internet for health information (advocacy white paper)*. Retrieved November 16, 2010, from http://www.himss.org/content/files/whitepapers/e-health.pdf, with permission.

correlated with years of education or general reading ability. Today, especially in the developed world, health literacy is more important in determining health than the digital divide. The correlation between health literacy and poor health was first reported in a 1999 report by *Journal of the American Medical Association* (Report of the Council on Scientific Affairs, 1999). It was reported to be a greater predictor of health than age, income, employment status, level of education, or race. When working with clients, face to face, either by phone, or by computer, or when designing educational materials, it is necessary to assess their health literacy (see **Box 14-2**).

Health Numeracy

Health numeracy is the ability of a consumer to interpret and act on all numerical information, such as graphical and probabilistic information needed to make effective health decisions (Rothman, Montori, Cherrington, & Pignone, 2008). Similar to health literacy, health numeracy is not correlated necessarily with educational level or the ability to read. Although much of the information that we provide to clients is quantitative, for example, laboratory values and medication schedules, a growing body of knowledge demonstrates that clients are not able to fully comprehend or use this information (Ancker & Kaufman, 2007).

Understanding a treatment, complying with a medication regime, or making decisions about a dosage of insulin based on a glucosometer require not only health literacy but also the ability to understand numbers in healthcare directions or information. It involves the skills necessary to understand quantitative data, the ability to do basic calculations, make sense of numerical information, and enough statistical knowledge to compare knowledge presented with different scales, for example, probability, proportion, and percent, and the ability to interpret graphs. Health numeracy is an essential skill for reading food labels and refilling prescriptions and interpreting the meaning of laboratory values, such as potassium or cholesterol.

Even deciding the timing of medication dosages can be difficult without health numeracy skills,

---

BOX 14-2 Skills Needed for Health Literacy

Patients are often faced with complex information and treatment decisions. Some of the specific tasks patients are required to carry out may include

- evaluating information for credibility and quality,
- analyzing relative risks and benefits,
- calculating dosages,
- interpreting test results, or
- locating health information.
  In order to accomplish these tasks, individuals may need to be
- visually literate (able to understand graphs or other visual information),
- computer literate (able to operate a computer),
- information literate (able to obtain and apply relevant information), and
- numerically or computationally literate (able to calculate or reason numerically).

Oral language skills are important as well. Patients need to articulate their health concerns and describe their symptoms accurately. They need to ask pertinent questions, and they need to understand spoken medical advice or treatment directions. In an age of shared responsibility between physician and patient for healthcare, patients need strong decision-making skills. With the development of the Internet as a source of health information, health literacy may also include the ability to search the Internet and evaluate websites.

more so when several medications with different time schedules are involved. Lack of numeracy has been associated with poor outcomes in anticoagulation control and history of hospitalization in asthma (Ancker, Senathirajah, Kukafka, & Starren, 2006). This lack can also create difficulties when consumers have to calculate dosages as well as make it difficult for consumers to use quantitative information effectively to make health decisions and guide health behaviors. Studies have found that many consumers lack basic probability skills, making it difficult to decide the numerical probability of heads or tails in a coin toss, or to convert between percentages and whole numbers. Even determining which the larger risk is, 1%, 5%, or 10%, can be difficult. This lack will create difficulty in making informed healthcare decisions or in granting permission to be in a research study.

The ability to comprehend numerical information is greatly influenced by the presentation, whether in a questionnaire, document, graphic, or medical device (Ancker et al., 2006). Some of these difficulties can be surmounted with a systematic design of information that considers these factors. For example, using stick figures to demonstrate 1 in 10 is usually clearer than using percentages or a graph. Although graphs appear to be an appealing alternative to using numbers, interpreting them often requires more effort and cognitive skills.

Helping Consumers to Use Computers

In your career, unless you work in an undeveloped country through the Peace Corp or missionary work, you will eventually find yourself both assisting consumers to find healthcare information and evaluating this information. Given that telemonitoring and computer support or education is becoming an accepted care protocol, you may be called on to help a client install or learn to use such a device. **Box 14-3** lists some of the steps that are needed to accomplish this.

Internet Support Groups

Even in the earliest days of the Internet, clients sought online support, information, and decision support. The idea of **support groups** is not new; they date back to the early 1900s as a method of working with persons suffering from psychological disorders (Klemm et al., 2003). Today, much of this support has migrated to the Internet. As of 2009, an estimated 20% of healthcare consumers had used the Internet and online support groups for help (Shapiro, 2009). Support groups may be

---

BOX 14-3 Installing a Technology Device in a Client's Home

- Evaluate the technical skills of the new user.
- Assess whether the physical skills needed to use the device are present.
- Before visiting describe the physical needs of the device and ask the patient to select a location in the home.
- Rehearse the installation steps so that you are thoroughly comfortable with the skills.
- Use a checklist to ensure a 100% installation.
- Use everyday terms when teaching how to use the device. Explain any terms such as login, password, and so forth before using them.
- Explain how the device functions and describe any idiosyncrasies.
- If there is a lag time between starting the device and it becoming functional, prepare the client.
- If there are sounds such as one would find with a dial-up connection, describe and demonstrate.
- Thoroughly teach the consumer how to use the device, including several return demonstrations.
- Provide written instructions. As you teach you may want to revise these or highlight those where difficulties occur.
- Have technical support available for follow-up instructions.

Adapted from Dauz, E., Moore, J., Smith, C. E., Puno, F., & Schaag, H. (2004). Installing computers in older adults' homes and teaching them to access a patient education Web site. *Computers, Informatics, Nursing: CIN, 22*(5), 266–272.

a combination of the patient portals discussed above, a message board, e-mail list, chat room, or any combination of these. Help given is similar to that in face-to-face groups.

There are hundreds of online support groups. Support group sites with the HONcode include Daily Strength.org (http://www.dailystrength.org/) and Mayo Clinic (http://www.mayoclinic.com/health/support-groups/MH00002). CaringBridge (http://www.caringbridge.org/) is an online support group that allows those with "significant health challenges" to stay in touch with their loved ones. PatientsLikeMe.com is especially popular for individuals with neuromuscular disorders. The site also bears the HONcode. To learn more, view a YouTube video at http://www.youtube.com/watch?v=nqm-3nHJdGw&feature=related. A survey of 1323 patients by Wicks et al. (2010) revealed that 74% of the participants felt that the PatientsLikeMe.com site was moderately or very helpful. Participants also noted that sharing with others helped them when starting a new medication or changing a treatment plan. The GriefNet Support (http://www.griefnet.org/) offers support to persons suffering the loss of a loved one. The GriefNet Support discussion groups are varied and are oriented to the type of loss. They include, but are not limited to, support groups for those affected by terrorist attacks, widows or widowers, parents who have lost children, children who have suffered a loss, and those who are grieving the loss of a pet. Trained counselors moderate many of their lists.

Support groups vary in sponsorship and the quality of the information. Healthcare providers who will answer questions sponsor some. Others are moderated; that is, nothing is posted that is not first vetted by the moderator. In groups sponsored by laypersons or organizations, the moderator may or may not be healthcare providers. Most groups allow open discussion and permit members to answer each other's questions just as they do with listservs. Although there may be erroneous information posted, especially in non-moderated groups, other members often quickly correct the misinformation.

For those groups that allow open discussion, membership is usually free and the discussion open for anyone to read, but one must join to post questions or replies. As a nurse, you may want to find one or two such groups in your specialty so that you can refer your patients to them. Before referring a patient, assess the group carefully. If referring a client to a group that is moderated, check the qualifications of the moderator. If the group is not moderated, look at the archives, and follow the list for a while before recommending it. You may even wish to join the group. A search by a web search tool for the name of the disease or condition followed by "forum" or "support group" will yield many groups for that condition. For all support groups you should remind clients that the information they receive may be only an opinion; it may be an informed opinion, or it may not be. If information posted is a new treatment, the client needs to do further research by using qualified medical sites such as those sponsored by the government, or formal organizations whose reputation in the field is known. Just as with web information, it may be necessary to teach clients how to evaluate the information they find in these groups. Additionally, unless users are very familiar with the reputation of the site sponsor and the provider, they should be careful about giving their names, e-mail addresses, and especially their credit card numbers.

Message Content Analyses

Message content from support groups has been an object of study for several researchers. Coulson, Buchanan, and Aubeeluck (2007) studied messages posted to a Huntington Disease support forum. They found that informational and emotional supports were the most frequent messages. Messages also often included teaching or referral to experts. Messages containing esteem support and tangible assistance, although not uncommon, were the least frequently posted. Reminders that the group was available for support were also a common topic. Klemm (2008) analyzed messages from support groups for long-term cancer survivors and categorized them as focusing on information exchange, symptomatology, or frustration with healthcare providers. Case et al. (2009) noted that since bulletin boards are generally blind to factors such as race, gender, age, and similar characteristics, bulletin board use has the potential of minimizing health disparities.

Advantages for Online Support Groups

There are many advantages to online groups over face-to-face groups. They are asynchronous, members can participate at any time of day or night, and membership is not restricted by time, geography, or space (Coulson et al., 2007). Messages to the group can be carefully thought out and edited before posting, which relieves participants from having to think on their feet, or having one or two people monopolize the conversation. Furthermore, members come from diverse perspectives, which provide varied experiences, opinions, and information sources. Lastly, the provision of being anonymous, which many groups are, is helpful in discussing sensitive or potentially embarrassing situations. A drawback may be that the individual may be spending too much time online alone when the company of others is needed.

Provider-Sponsored Groups

Healthcare providers, particularly hospitals or healthcare organizations, may provide online support for those for whom they provide care. These sites generally require passwords to enter, and sometimes require specialized software. One of the earliest groups of this type was the ComputerLink project (Brennan & Moore, 1994; Brennan & Smyth, 1994). This service provided support to caregivers of those with Alzheimer's disease. Users could access the service at a time convenient to them and select from a variety of services. It was designed to link these individuals to each other and to a nurse moderator. Services were provided in three areas – communication, information, and decision support. Communication involved private e-mail, a forum where members could post and read messages, and a question-and-answer session. The information module provided an electronic encyclopedia and over 200 indexed screens about selected illnesses, home care, and social services. In decision support, users were guided through an analysis process using their own words and preferences to making choices consistent with their values (Brennan, 1996).

Another example, although much different in scope, is the Comprehensive Health Enhancement Support System (CHESS) (https://chess.wisc.edu/chess/home/home.aspx). Instead of being designed for just one group, this service is a

vendor-supported service, developed at the University of Wisconsin-Madison's Center for Health Systems Research and Analysis and provided to member organizations. Several major health organizations in the United States and Canada are using it. This product is provided to member healthcare agencies that can either use it as is or tailor it for their use. Using both computer-based and human support, the service is designed to help individuals cope with a health crisis or medical concern (Mayer et al., 2010). Currently, CHESS has several initiatives, including improving the quality of addiction and mental health services, oncology treatment and support, and emergency medical services for children (The Center for Health Enhancement Systems Studies, 2010). It also provides social support and decision-making and problem-solving tools. The service includes discussion groups, which are monitored by a nurse who is provided by the member agency (A.L. Salner, personal communication, October 1, 2007, CHESS). The nurse can provide expert advice or contact a physician for more help if needed. Participants must download and install the specialized software; then they use it in the privacy of their own home. Potential users without a computer may receive a loaned computer for a year. Research has demonstrated that CHESS has improved participants' quality of life, reduced demands on physician time, and sometimes, the cost of care. It has also been found that it can be used equally, although in different ways, by all people regardless of gender, income, age, or education. (See **Box 14-4** for a description by a nurse of her experience with CHESS.)

Providing Web-Based Patient Information

Most healthcare agencies have websites. The exact contents vary but generally, they provide information about the organization, a map and directions to the agency, a list of the services offered, and other organizational information aimed at marketing. Some hospitals with obstetric services feature a web page that posts pictures of newborns that can be accessed by those whom the new parents specify. Still others will post healthcare information related to their specialty.

BOX 14-4 One Nurse's Experience with Chess

CHESS, for our breast cancer patients, was absolutely my best informatics experience. Our program was implemented in the early 1990s, and many thought the older women would not participate because of the technology. They were wrong! We had age 40 to age 85 burning up the wires, which filled an obvious need. Any newly diagnosed breast cancer patient was eligible to join at no charge. We held fundraisers to defray costs of the technology and were able to purchase refurbished computers from local vendors at very low cost. The biggest problem then was to find space for the computer in patient homes.

The stories they shared were great and intimate. We all got laughs when one woman, sunning herself after mastectomy, shared that she forgot she was bare chested (sans breast) and answered the door to the UPS guy who nearly fainted. I don't know how much of it was really true – but we all belly-laughed.

It was interesting that a lot of the activity occurred very late at night (I assume when their spouses and family were taken care of and asleep). Many developed intense support structures with the other patients as well as our designated CHESS nurse. At our annual "Celebrate Life" survivor event – many of them came to meet each other under the big tent in the cancer center parking lot.

I highly recommend programs such as this that provide reliable information, support from those in the same situation, and access to healthcare providers when needed.

D. Deborah Ariosto, MS, RN, October 2007.

Healthcare agencies may even develop a site specific to a given condition that functions more like an **extranet** where access is restricted to only their clients; however, the site is not tied to an EHR. Healthcare agencies should have written guidelines for use of the information provided on agency-developed web health sites. Agency guidelines are pertinent for extranets that deliver information designed for specific patients. Privacy and security issues should be addressed, as do the rights and responsibilities of the users and providers. If the site permits patient input and it will become a permanent part of its healthcare record, the patient must be informed of this practice.

Creating a Web Page

Although you may not need to learn how to prepare a page to be posted on your agencies' website, your expertise may be needed to either create or evaluate the information that will be posted. Just as when writing, you need to think carefully about who the audience will be. If your topic lends itself to illustration, choose carefully the illustration; remember that a simple schematic drawing is often more instructive than a complex one in which a learner must cognitively pull out the parts needed to understand the topic. If you want to use objects such as **Flash® animation**, ask yourselves what percentage of your audience is using **broadband** Internet access. In rural areas, **dial-up connections** are common. Additionally, be very concerned with readability.

General Design Principles

There are two approaches to designing a web page. The first uses an artistic approach in which artistic sensibilities are primary. These are often designed by those schooled in print graphics who wish to emulate this style on the web. In the other, the web designer sees the page as a way to assist a user to solve a problem. Although a pleasing design is helpful, sites that wish to compete for viewers successfully will need to focus on users and their needs (see **Box 14-5**). Web users are an impatient lot; force them to cope with myriad of decisions and much trial and error to find what they want and they will leave. Several

BOX 14-5 Thoughts on Designing a Web Page for Health

A Web Page Is an Agency's Front Door to the World. Make it Helpful.

1. Write down some answers to the following questions:
   a. What is the purpose of the site?
   b. Who is the intended audience?
   c. What information should be shared? Is it copyrighted?
   d. From a user viewpoint, what is the most intuitive organizational plan for the site?
   e. Will it provide interactivity? If so:
      i. Who will respond? When?
      ii. What features will be supported?
   f. How will the site be publicized?
2. Use established web conventions that are intuitive to users, such as blue underlined text for links to avoid making the user think about the interface.
3. The information.
   a. Who will provide it?
   b. Who will approve it?
   c. Evaluate carefully for grammatical and spelling errors.
   d. Match the readability level to the audience.
4. Designing the page.
   a. Use proportional fonts rather than specifying the size; this allows users to set their own preferences.
   b. Be 100% consistent in navigation aids.
   c. Use a similar page design for pages of a similar type. This can be achieved with the use of style sheets.
   d. Keep information in small manageable chunks.
   e. Use clear and concise language.
   f. If using audio or movie clips, provide a text transcript.

5. Consider download time. Not everyone has unlimited Internet access.
   a. Use a graphic only if it is small and/or contributes information necessary for understanding.
   b. If graphics are used, check to see how the page looks without them. Not all browsers have graphics capabilities; some users turn them off to shorten download time.
   c. Keep file size as small as possible.
6. Think carefully before designing pages that require a user to have special **plug-ins**.
   a. Is it necessary to make the content clear?
   b. Is the user apt to have it?
7. Consider maintenance of the site.
   a. Who will maintain the site? Links are here today and gone tomorrow, necessitating constant checking.
   b. Who is responsible for updating what content?

Additional Tasks

Design a prototype and have outsiders test it without any input from anyone connected with designing the site to see whether it is intuitive to use. Revise.

If your site necessitates the use of a browser plug-in, include the URL that leads directly to a place for downloading the plug-in. Don't use the front page of the organization and leave users to hunt for it – they won't.

Include the date each page was created, and all update dates.

Include a disclaimer in the form of user agreements to limit liability.

---

methods can be used to create a web page ranging from coding to use of an application program. **Table 14-1** compares three methods of creating a web page.

Accessibility *Factors in Web Design*

Whether you are creating a web page or evaluating one for use with clients, you need to consider that the visitors will include not only fully physically functioning individuals but also those with disabilities. It is imperative, therefore, that all healthcare websites are designed so that they are accessible. A 2008–2009 survey lists over 27 million (11.4%) U.S. citizens with one or more disabilities (Center for Personal Assistance Service, 2010). It is likely that the percentage of those who are disabled is

Table 14-1 Comparison of Some Methods of Web Page Creation

Method	Advantage	Disadvantage
Office application program	Minimal knowledge required beyond use of the program itself.	Creates "dirty code" that is difficult to maintain outside the application program used to create it. Often creates a very large file. May not provide needed flexibility.
WSYWIG authoring tool	Has many features such as methods to ensure that page designs are identical, spell check, and creating forms.	Some use nonstandard code that requires special software on the server.
HTML editor	Provides good flexibility	Steep learning curve
Coding HTML	Provides good flexibility	Very steep learning curve

even higher in the population of those who access healthcare websites.

Screen Readers. The possibility that visitors will use a screen reader needs to be provided for in the design. Although elementary screen readers are bundled with operating systems, for example, Microsoft Windows™ comes with Narrator, the Apple Mac™ with VoiceOver™, full-function screen readers are best for those who are visually limited. The bundled screen readers, however, can help a visually challenged person install a screen reader. Besides translating text to speech, some screen readers can send information to a **Braille reader**, a device that is placed near or under the keyboard. Users then use their fingers to "read" the information.

Screen readers have vastly improved from earlier times when they could not interpret tables; however, considerations for alternatives to using the mouse, such as keyboard commands for navigation, are still necessary. Because screen readers cannot "read" a graphic, when graphics are used text alternatives (called **Alt tags**) should be used. The tag should provide either textual information that can be used by a screen reader in place of the illustration or a link to a site that explains the illustration in text. If there are clickable spots on a graphic (known as an **image map**), make provisions for finding these links using a screen reader. **Navigation bars** or graphical bars across the top of a page that provide multiple choices also need alternative methods of access. Some sites provide this with a list of links for all these choices on the bottom of the page. Because this print is not intended for humans to read, it can be in a small font.

Color Blindness. Color blindness, which affects 12% of males of European descent and about 0.5% of females, can interfere with reading a web page, while the hearing disabled will miss any audio. Seizures can be caused in people with photosensitive epilepsy by blinking items on a web page or quick changes from dark to light (BC Epilepsy Society, 2008).

Usability

When health websites were evaluated by both **usability** experts and older adults, they agreed on many problem areas such as difficulty finding drop-down menus, too much information on the screen, too small a font size, lack of instructions for playing video, and navigation problems (Nahm, Preece, Resnick, & Mills, 2004). To prevent these difficulties, it is imperative that a healthcare website be evaluated by a sampling of the intended audience. Although healthcare providers can evaluate the web content, it requires members of the intended audience to do thorough usability testing. The National Institute on Aging and the National Institutes of Health have published guidelines on how to make a website senior friendly (National Institutes of Health, 2009). Furthermore, the U.S. Department of Health and Human Services has a website dedicated to assist web designers to address usability issues (U.S. Department of Health & Human Services, 2010b).

Some suggestions for making websites easier to understand are the use of adequate contrast between text and background, intuitive navigation, the avoidance of distracting features, and the inclusion of users in the design phase. Designers should also gauge the health literacy and health numeracy skills of the intended audience. Additionally, content should be written clearly and simply in a language the user will understand. For example, medical terminology is appropriate when the audience is healthcare providers, but not with laypeople.

Summary

The field of consumer informatics has developed along with the empowerment of the healthcare consumer. Consumers now have access to information that was previously unavailable such as the quality of care provided by hospitals and disease conditions. As consumers use the web more and more to find information, their relationship with healthcare providers will change. As this continues, greater attention will be paid to how health literacy and health numeracy affect the teaching of clients. Nurses will find themselves directing clients to high-quality websites and providing guidance in selecting support groups as another way to improve healthcare. By using patient portals healthcare agencies will provide more consumer education, some of it restricted to and individualized for their clients. These portals will also serve as a marketing device. Whether you ever design a website or part of a patient portal, you can still use the design principles as well as those in health literacy and health numeracy in evaluating the appropriateness of websites for clients and other educational materials. Helping clients to use computers, whether this involves installing a computer, referring clients to places where they can be taught basic computer skills, or providing help in finding and installing items to assist the physically challenged to use a computer, will become more frequent nursing interventions.

APPLICATIONS AND COMPETENCIES

1. The fact that only slightly more than half the people who have found health information on the web have discussed the information with their healthcare provider is somewhat disturbing (Cline & Haynes, 2001). Discuss the following statements.

   a. Patients are leery of discussing information with their healthcare providers versus just listening to advice.

   b. Patients are afraid to take a more participatory approach to their healthcare.

   c. Reluctance to discuss information found on the web affects an individual's decision to follow the provider's treatment plan.

2. You are the nurse in a surgical center. A patient arrives with a printout of the complications of the surgery for which he or she is scheduled. Additionally, the information advocates alternative treatments. Discuss how you can work with this patient.

3. Find a high-quality web-based support group for a client with a condition of your choice and outline how you would teach the client about this site.

4. You are a nurse practitioner. The clinic where you are working wants to institute providing an online support group. What things would you want to consider?

5. Evaluate a web-based health site.

REFERENCES

American Medical Informatics Association. (2010). *Consumer health informatics.* Retrieved August 21, 2011, from http://www.amia.org/applications-informatics/consumer-health-informatics

American Nurses Association. (2010). *NDNQI.* Retrieved July 8, 2010, from http://www.nursingworld.org/MainMenuCategories/ThePracticeofProfessionalNursing/PatientSafetyQuality/Research-Measurement/The-National-Database.aspx

Ancker, J. S., & Kaufman, D. (2007). Rethinking health numeracy: A multidisciplinary literature review. *Journal of the American Medical Informatics Association, 14*(6), 713–721.

Ancker, J. S., Senathirajah, Y., Kukafka, R., & Starren, J. B. (2006). Design features of graphs in health risk communication: A systematic review. *Journal of the American Medical Informatics Association, 13*(6), 608–618.

BC Epilepsy Society. (2008). *Epilepsy fact sheet.* Retrieved July 31, 2010, from http://www.bcepilepsy.com/files/PDF/Epilepsy_Fact_Sheet.pdf

Brady, M., Kinn, S., Stuart, P., & Ness, V. (2003). Preoperative fasting for adults to prevent perioperative complications. *Cochrane Database of Systematic Reviews* (4). doi: 10.1002/14651858.CD004423

Brennan, P. F. (1996). The future of clinical communication in an electronic environment. *Holistic Nursing Practice, 11*(1), 97–104.

Brennan, P. F., & Moore, S. M. (1994). Networks for home care support: The ComputerLink project. *Caring, 13*(8), 64–66, 68–70.

Brennan, P. F., & Smyth, K. (1994). Elders' attitudes and behavior regarding ComputerLink. *Proceedings from the Annual Symposium Computer Applications in Medical Care,* 1011.

Case, S., Jernigan, V., Gardner, A., Ritter, P., Heaney, C. A., & Lorig, K. R. (2009). Content and frequency of writing on diabetes bulletin boards: Does race make a difference? *Journal of Medical Internet Research, 11*(2), e22.

Center for Personal Assistance Service. (2010). *Disability prevalence data from the current population survey (2008–2009).* Retrieved July 31, 2010, from http://www.pascenter.org/state_based_stats/disability_prevalence.php?state=us&project=

Cline, R. J., & Haynes, K. M. (2001). Consumer health information seeking on the Internet: The state of the art. *Health Education Research, 16*(6), 671–692.

Cohen, E. (2008). *Are you a 'cyberchondriac'?* Retrieved July 30, 2010, from http://www.cnn.com/2007/HEALTH/12/20/ep.cyberchondriacs/index.html

Coulson, N. S., Buchanan, H., & Aubeeluck, A. (2007). Social support in cyberspace: A content analysis of communication within a Huntington's disease online support group. *Patient Education and Counseling, 68*(2), 173–178.

Dorr, D., Bonner, L. M., Cohen, A. N., Shoai, R. S., Perrin, R., Chaney, E., et al. (2007). Informatics systems to promote improved care for chronic illness: A literature review. *Journal of the American Medical Informatics Association, 14*(2), 156–163.

Pratt v. Davis, 118 Ill., App. 161 (Ill. Ct. App., Chicago, First District 1905).

European Commission. (2010). *How search engines work.* Retrieved July 29, 2010, from http://ec.europa.eu/ipg/go_live/search_engine/index_en.htm

Eysenbach, G. (2000). Consumer health informatics. *British Medical Journal, 320*(7251), 1713–1716.

Eysenbach, G., & Kohler, C. (2002). How do consumers search for and appraise health information on the world wide web? Qualitative study using focus groups, usability tests, and in-depth interviews. *British Medical Journal, 324*(7337), 573–577.

Gardner, E. (2010). Will patient portals open the door to better care? *Health Data Management, 18*(3), 58.

Harris Interactive. (2002). 4-Country survey finds most cyberchondriacs believe online health care information is trustworthy, easy to find and understand. *Healthcare News, 2*(12). Retrieved from http://www.harrisinteractive.com/news/newsletters/healthnews/HI_HealthCareNews2002Vol2_Iss12.pdf

Harris Interactive. (2008). *Number of "cyberchondriacs" – adults going online for health information – has plateaued or declined.* Retrieved July 10, 2010, from http://www.harrisinteractive.com/vault/HI_HealthCareNews2008Vol8_Iss08.pdf

Harris Interactive. (2010). *Few Americans using 'e' medical records.* Retrieved June 29, 2010, from http://www.harrisinteractive.com/NewsRoom/HarrisPolls/tabid/447/mid/1508/articleId/414/ctl/ReadCustom%20Default/Default.aspx

Health on the Net Foundation. (2009, August 9). *HONcode site evaluation form.* Retrieved August 30, 2010, from https://www.hon.ch/cgi-bin/HONcode/Inscription/site_evaluation.pl?language=en&userCategory=individuals

Hogans, A. (2010, July 28). *Unverified pharmacies easy to search online.* Retrieved July 30, 2010, from http://www.cbsnews.com/8301-31727_162-20011928-10391695.html

Houston, T. K., & Ehrenberger, H. E. (2001). The potential of consumer health informatics. *Seminars in Oncology Nursing, 17*(1), 41–47.

Hyde, S. S. (2004). Dialogues with Socrates. In R. E. Herzlinger (Ed.), *Consumer-driven healthcare* (pp. 262–269). San Francisco: Jossey-Bass.

Keselman, A., Browne, A. C., & Kaufman, D. R. (2008). Consumer health information seeking as hypothesis testing. *Journal of the American Medical Informatics Association, 15*(4), 484–495.

Klemm, P. (2008). Late effects of treatment for long-term cancer survivors: Qualitative analysis of an online support group. *CIN: Computers Informatics Nursing, 26*(1), 49–58.

Klemm, P., Bunnell, D., Cullen, M., Soneji, R., Gibbons, P., & Holecek, A. (2003). Online cancer support groups: A review of the research literature. *CIN: Computers Informatics Nursing, 21*(3), 136–142.

Leapfrog Group. (2009a). *About us.* Retrieved June 10, 2010, from http://www.leapfroggroup.org/about_us

Leapfrog Group. (2009b). *Leapfrog quality hospital ratings.* Retrieved July 6, 2010, from http://www.leapfroggroup.org/cp

Lewis, D. (2007). Evolution of consumer health informatics. *CIN: Computers Informatics Nursing, 25*(6), 316.

Maltby, J. R. (2006). Preoperative fasting guidelines. *Canadian Journal of Surgery, 49*(2), 138–139; author reply 139.

Mary, E. Schloendorff, v. The Society of New York Hospital, 211 N.Y. 105 N.E. (1914).

Mayer, D. K., Ratichek, S., Berhe, H., Stewart, S., McTavish, F., Gustafson, D., et al. (2010). Development of a health-related website for parents of children receiving hematopoietic stem cell transplant: HSCT-CHESS. *Journal of Cancer Survivorship: Research and Practice, 4*(1), 67–73.

McLeod, R., Fitzgerald, W., & Sarr, M. (2005). Canadian Association of General Surgeons and American College of Surgeons evidence-based reviews in surgery. 14: Preoperative fasting for adults to prevent perioperative complications. *Canadian Journal of Surgery, 48*(5), 409–411.

Medical Library Association. (2009, August 20). *A user's guide to finding and evaluating health information on the web.* Retrieved July 30, 2010, from http://www.mlanet.org/resources/userguide.html

Nahm, E. S., Preece, J., Resnick, B., & Mills, M. E. (2004). Usability of health web sites for older adults: A preliminary study. *CIN: Computers Informatics Nursing, 22*(6), 326–334; quiz 335–326.

National Association of Boards of Pharmacy. (2011, August 21). *Verified Internet pharmacy practice sites (VIPPS).* Retrieved August 21, 2011, from http://vipps.nabp.net/

National Committee for Quality Assurance. (2010). *About NCQA.* Retrieved July 8, 2010, from http://www.ncqa.org/tabid/675/default.aspx

National Database of Nursing Quality Indicators. (2011). *Transforming data into quality care.* Retrieved August 21, 2011, from https://www.nursingquality.org/

National Institutes of Health. (2009). *Making your website senior friendly: Tips from the National Institute on Aging and the National Library of Medicine.* Retrieved July 31, 2010, from http://www.nia.nih.gov/HealthInformation/Publications/website.htm

Office of the National Coordinator for Health Information Technology. (2009, March 3). *Summary of strategic framework (TAB)*. Retrieved July 8, 2010, from http://healthit.hhs.gov/portal/server.pt?open=512&mode=2&cached=true&objID=1249&PageID=15652

Paylor, M. (2010). Patient portals and health records in diabetes care. *British Journal of Healthcare Management, 16*(3), 142–145.

Report of the Council on Scientific Affairs. (1999). Health literacy. *Journal of the American Medical Association, 281*, 552–557.

Rothman, R. L., Montori, V. M., Cherrington, A., & Pignone, M. P. (2008). Perspective: The role of numeracy in health care. *Journal of Health Communication, 13*(6), 583–595.

Shapiro, J. (2009, November 16). *Patients turn to online community for help healing*. Retrieved July 30, 2010, from http://www.npr.org/templates/story/story.php?storyId=120381580

The Center for Health Enhancement Systems Studies. (2010, July). *Current studies and projects*. Retrieved July 30, 2010, from https://chess.wisc.edu/chess/projects/current_studies_and_projects.aspx

Tung, T., & Organ, C. H., Jr. (2000). Ethics in surgery: Historical perspective. *Archives of Surgery, 135*(1), 10–13. Retrieved from http://archsurg.ama-assn.org/cgi/content/full/135/1/10.

U.S. Department of Health & Human Services. (2000). *Health People 2010 – Health literacy (Vol. I)*. Retrieved from http://www.healthypeople.gov/document/html/volume1/11healthcom.htm

U.S. Department of Health & Human Services. (2010a, May 25). *Hospital compare*. Retrieved July 8, 2010, from http://www.hospitalcompare.hhs.gov/

U.S. Department of Health & Human Services. (2010b). *Usability.gov home*. Retrieved July 31, 2010, from http://www.usability.gov/

van Dijk, J. A. G. M. (2006). Digital divide research, achievements and shortcomings. *Poetics, 34*(4–5), 221–235.

Werner, R. M., Bradlow, E. T., & Asch, D. A. (2008). Does hospital performance on process measures directly measure high quality care or is it a marker of unmeasured care? *Health Services Research, 43*(5, Part 1), 1464–1484.

Wicks, P., Massagli, M., Frost, J., Brownstein, C., Okun, S., Vaughan, T., et al. (2010). Sharing health data for better outcomes on Patients Like Me. *Journal of Medical Internet Research, 12*(2), e19.

CHAPTER 15

Interoperability at the International and the National Level

Objectives

After studying this chapter you will be able to:

▶ *Define the three types of interoperability: technical, semantic, and process.*

▶ *Describe a general pattern for developing standards.*

▶ *Explain the need for standards.*

▶ *Interpret the effects on nursing of standards at all levels of healthcare.*

▶ *Identify organizations involved in setting standards at the international and the national level.*

Key Terms

Clinical Decision Support (CDS)	Mapping
Electronic Health Record (EHR)	Nationwide Health Information Network (NHIN)
Electronic Medical Record (EMR)	Process Interoperability
Granular	Protocol
Health Information Exchange (HIE)	Reference Terminology
Health Information Exchange Organization	Reference Terminology Model
Interoperability	Semantic Interoperability
	Standards
	Technical Interoperability
	Unified Medical Language System (UMLS)

An individual who is unknowingly infected with a very contagious stage of a new type of flu walks into the international airport in Houston on his way to Seattle. While standing in the baggage check line, he starts up a conversation with the woman behind him, who will be in New Delhi in 24 hours. After checking his bag, he goes to the security line and there strikes up a conversation with a man who will be in San Diego in 4 hours. He is early for his plane, so he goes into one of the airport bars and starts talking to a woman who will be in Tokyo in 8 hours and then in Shanghai in 48 hours.

This is the world in which we live today. Jet travel makes all points on the globe vulnerable to any communicable disease. Thus, health is an international concern. To protect ourselves, it is necessary that countries be able to exchange information pertaining to contagious diseases with other countries and within their own frontiers. This demands that healthcare systems be interoperable between communities, regionally and internationally. To achieve this goal, data transfer and reception must be interoperable.

Interoperability

Simply stated, **interoperability** is the ability of two or more systems to pass information and to use the exchanged information. In healthcare, interoperability means that healthcare information systems can transmit and receive information within and across organizational boundaries to provide the delivery of optimum healthcare to individuals and communities (Healthcare Information and Management Systems Society, 2005). This can be achieved either by adhering to accepted interface and terminology **standards** or by using a third system that seamlessly integrates the two systems. An example of the first option is the **protocols** that made the Internet possible, plus the use of a standardized terminology. The use of an "rtf" file to "translate" a file from one word processor to another is similar to the second option.

There are three different types of interoperability: technical (sometimes referred to as functional), semantic, and process. **Technical interoperability** refers to the transmission and reception of information so that it is useful (Gibbons et al., 2007). When systems are technically interoperable, they are able to receive usable data from a different system and send it to that system. This type of functionality enables data from a laboratory system to be exchanged with the pharmacy system. It also enables data from one healthcare provider to be exchanged with another.

Semantic interoperability takes this one step further. In semantic interoperability, not only is the information transmitted so that it is understandable, but, at its highest level, the messages exchanged by two computers can be automatically interpreted and acted on by the computers without human intervention. How effective semantic interoperability depends on the interaction between algorithms, the data used in the message, and the terminology used to designate that data.

Process interoperability is a rather new concept that is intended to coordinate work processes. It has been referred to as workflow management and is related to integrating computer systems into work settings. It includes such considerations as a user-friendly system and effectiveness in actual use. Those who have had experience with healthcare systems that did not have interoperability are aware of the extra work and difficulties that this creates such as duplicate data entry and having to remember login and password for different systems.

Standards

Interoperability is not possible without standards. Imagine a situation in which each community sets its own time. In one city it would be 1:00 p.m., whereas in another 30 miles east it would be 1:30 p.m. and in still another 40 miles northwest it would be 12:30 p.m. This is more or less the situation that existed until the mid-19th century. Of course, then the time was not so important and the population was not as mobile. When the railroads arrived, it became necessary to standardize the time. In the United States, the railroads set the first time zones, which were eventually adopted by state governments. As the industrial revolution progressed, it became necessary to have more and more standards if the economy was to prosper. Some may remember the Beta *v.* VHS videotape standards conflicts. A more recent standard conflict involved DVD formats – the Blu-ray disc *v.* HD DVD. These standards, of course, were decided in the market place. However, in healthcare, leaving standard setting to the marketplace has resulted in great inefficiencies.

A standard is an agreement to use a given protocol, term, or other criterion that has been formally approved by a nationally or internationally recognized professional trade association or governmental body. Standards are vital to communication as well as in other areas. Even in casual communication, differences in language can result in miscommunication. For example, the word "stroller" has several meanings depending on one's cultural background. Two meanings that it can have are a type of baby carriage or walking slowly. Hence, a sign reading "No strollers" in a museum could be understood by some that one should not meander through the museum and by others that baby carriages are not allowed – a situation that has happened. Although the results in casual life are not serious, in healthcare they can be. Not only can they lead to serious communication errors, but they can also result in no communication when electronic records are involved.

Standards impact nursing. They affect the equipment we use and affect how we document in **electronic healthcare records (EHRs)**. Decisions are being made today about the healthcare data that will be recorded, how it will be recorded, the terminology that will be used, and what data will be reported to what organizations. Because nursing is affected by these decisions, it is imperative that nurses have some understanding not only of the process but also of the groups involved in setting standards. Some of the groups involved in setting standards, along with their acronyms, are seen in **Box 15-1**. You could probably play a game of Scrabble by using just these acronyms.

BOX 15-1 Acronyms for Standards

ABCs – Alternative Billing Coding Set
AHIC – American Health Information Community
AMA – American Medical Association
ANA – American Nurses Association
ANSI – American National Standards Institute
APR-DRG – All Patient Refined – DRG
ASTM International – American Society for Testing and Materials
CAP – College of American Pathologists
CDC – Centers for Disease Control and Prevention
CDS – Clinical Decision Support
CEN – Comité Européen de Normalisation (or European Committee for Standardization)
CMS – Centers for Medicare and Medicaid Services
CPT® – Current Procedural Terminology
DHHS – Department of Health and Human Services
DICOM – Digital Imaging and Communications in Medicine
DRG – Diagnosis-Related Group
EHR – Electronic Health Record
EMR – Electronic Medical Record
EPR – Electronic Patient Record
FHA – Federal Health Architecture
HCFA – Health Care Financing Administration (now CMS)
HCPCS – Healthcare Common Procedure Coding System
HHS –Health and Human Services
HIE – Health Information Exchange
HIMSS – Healthcare Information and Management Systems Society
HIO – Health Information Exchange Organization
HIPAA – Health Insurance Portability and Accountability Act
HISPC – Health Information Security and Privacy Collaboration
HIT – Health Information Technology
HITECH – Health Information Technology for Economic and Clinical Health
HITSP – Health Information Technology Standards Panel
HL7 – Health Level Seven
ICD-# – International Classification of Disease Version #
ICD-#-CM – ICD "number" Clinical Modifications

(continued)

BOX 15-1 Acronyms for Standards *(continued)*

ICD-#-PCS – ICD "number" Procedural Codes
ICF – International Classification of Functioning, Disability and Health
IEC – International Electro-technical Commission
IHTSDO – International Health Terminology Standards Development Organisation
ISI – International Statistical Institute
ISO – International Organization for Standardization (a name, not an acronym)
NCVHS – National Committee on Vital and Health Statistics
NEDSS – National Electronic Disease Surveillance System
NEMA – National Electrical Manufacturers Association
NHIN – Nationwide Health Information Network
NHS – National Health Service (UK)
NIST – National Institute of Standards and Technology
NLM – National Library of Medicine
OASIS-C – Outcome and Assessment Information Set
OBQI – Outcome-based Quality Improvement
OMB – U.S. Office of Management and Budget
ONC or ONCHIT – Office of the National Coordinator for Health Information Technology
OSI – Open Systems Interconnect
PHIN – Public Health Information Network
PHR – Personal Health Record
SNOMED CT – Systematized Nomenclature of Medicine – Clinical Terms
TC 215 – ISO Technical Committee 215 (the group that set the nursing reference terminology model
UHDDS – Uniform Hospital Discharge Data Set
UMLS – Universal Medical Language System
WHO – World Health Organization

International Standards

Many organizations are involved in developing the standards demanded by the global nature of today's commerce. The two international groups that oversee much of the work involved in developing standards are the International Organization for Standardization (ISO) and the International Electrotechnical Commission (IEC, 2010). As may be suspected, the IEC is concerned with electrical standards. It sets the standards for the equipment used in hospitals. The ISO sets standards in all other areas including health. An international group is made up of member national groups that also perform work at the national level. There is often collaboration between these groups, as well as crossovers. For example, the U.S. National Committee of the IEC is an integral member of the American National Standards Institute (ANSI), which is the US member of the ISO.

International Organization for Standardization

The ISO is a nonprofit group, established in 1947, that oversees many international standardization efforts. It has member national groups from more than 150 countries. There is a Central Secretariat in Geneva, Switzerland, that coordinates the system (ISO, 2010). Some of its member institutions are part of the governmental structure of their countries, whereas others are from the private sector. Their purpose is to expedite standardization to facilitate international commerce and to promote cooperation in intellectual, technological, scientific, and economic activity.

ISO has technical committees in many fields. The committee for health informatics is technical committee number 215 (TC 215). Each technical committee has working groups within it whose work is done by volunteers. Under TC 215, a working group of volunteers from many nations established a nursing **reference terminology** model. Known as ISO 18104:2003, some of the potential uses for this standard include facilitating the documentation of nursing problems (diagnosis) and actions (interventions) in electronic information systems and the creation of nursing terminologies in a form that will make **mapping** (a form of matching concepts from one standardized terminology with those having similar meaning from another) among them easier.

International Electrical Commission

The IEC creates and publishes international standards for all electrical-related technologies (IEC, 2010). These standards serve as the basis for national standards in international contracts. The objectives include efficiently meeting the goals of a global market, assessing and improving the quality of products covered by its standards and contributing to the improvement of human health and safety. In the healthcare field, their standards include medical electrical equipment and magnetically induced currents in the human body.

ASTM International

Although ASTM International was originally created in 1898 as the American Society for Testing and Materials for the purpose of addressing the frequent rail breaks in the ever-growing railroad industry, it has become international (ASTM International, 2010). However, it still exerts a dominant influence among standards developers in the United States. Membership is by request, not by appointment or invitation, and anyone interested in its activities may join. Although there is no enforcement policy, in 1995 the United States passed the National Technology Transfer and Advancement Act, which requires the federal government to comply with privately developed standards when possible. Other governments – both local and worldwide – as well as corporations

doing international business also reference ASTM standards.

 ## International Healthcare Standardization

Both the modern world with jet airplanes, which created a need for the quick dissemination of health data concerning disease outbreaks, and a new focus on healthcare outcomes have made the need for the collection of healthcare data more visible. Healthcare data collection is not new; the first healthcare data collections occurred in the 16th century in England. Known as the London Bills of Mortality, parish clerics recorded and published weekly the number of burials. These were used as an early warning system against the Bubonic Plague epidemics that decimated the European population several times in the 16th and 17th centuries. In 1570, baptisms were added to the statistics. Because the data were found to be valuable, in 1629 the London government took over responsibility for collecting these data. In the last half of the 17th century, John Gaunt used these data to make some insightful observations on the patterns of mortality (Chute, 2000; WHO, 2010a). These efforts led to the modern concepts of epidemic and endemic disease patterns and the beginning of the disciplines of population-based epidemiology and the modern study of data terminologies and classifications.

International Classification of Disease

Developing the standards needed to implement data terminologies and classifications, however, was slow. It was 1900 before there was any agreement in medicine on standardizing even the causes of death. The first international classification of disease standardization was the Bertillion Classification List of the Causes of Death. In 1998, the American Public Health Association recommended the use of the Bertillion Classification by Canada, the United States, and Mexico at a meeting in Ottawa, Canada (WHO, 2010a). It was accepted in 1900 and became the International Classification of Disease Version 1 (ICD-1). At that time it was recommended that the classification be revised every 10 years to ensure that the system remained current with medical practice advances. The Mixed Commission, a group composed of representatives from the International Statistical Institute and the Health Organization of the League of Nations, had responsibility for the updates through ICD-6, a version that added morbidity and mortality conditions. The World Health Organization (WHO) took on this responsibility in 1948 and has published revisions ever since.

The ICD classification of codes, whose full name is the International Statistical Classification of Diseases and Related Health Problems, is a detailed listing of known diseases and injuries (WHO, 2010a). It is used worldwide for mortality and morbidity statistics. Every known disease (or a group of related diseases) is described, classified, and assigned a unique code. In the United States, the ICD codes are part of the standards required for use by the Health Insurance Portability and Accountability Act.

The ICD-10 version was adopted for international use in 1990. Almost immediately, WHO began discussions and initiated the workgroup to address development of ICD-11. The United States, however, continued to use ICD-9 despite the fact that most of the rest of the world uses ICD-10 (CDC, 2011b). The National Committee on Vital and Health Statistics (NCVHS) forwarded several recommendations to the Office of the Secretary of Health and Human Services (HHS) to move to ICD-10. In August 2008, HHS had proposed that the United States adopt ICD-10 by October 1, 2011. WHO projected the use of ICD-11 to be in place by May 2014 (WHO, 2010b). The ICD codes, which are now used worldwide for morbidity and mortality statistics and in the United States for billing, were the first efforts to standardize healthcare data for both national and international use. Unless you are a nurse practitioner or certified nurse midwife, it is unlikely that you will be asked to code a diagnosis, yet you need to be aware of these classifications. ICD codes are used in nursing quality improvement efforts to identify aggregate groups of patients by disease type. Although useful for statistical purposes, the ICD codes are not **granular** enough, that is, they do not capture enough data, to be used to document patient care in either **electronic medical records (EMRs)** or EHRs (Centers for Disease Control and Prevention [CDC], 2010a; Centers for Medicare & Medicaid Services [CMS], 2010a).

International Classification of Functioning, Disability and Health

The International Classification of Functioning, Disability and Health (ICF) falls under the auspices of the WHO. The ICF codes are used to measure health and disability for both individuals and populations (WHO, 2010c). These codes focus on the impact of disease on the human experience including social and environmental factors (see **Figure 15-1**). They are relatively new, having been officially endorsed only at the Fifty-Fourth World Health Assembly in 2001. The ICF classification acts to complement ICD-10 to provide information regarding functional status. These codes are organized around body structure, functions, activities of living, and participation in life situations. They also contain information on severity and environmental factors. Although not intended as a measurement tool, these codes place emphasis on function rather than disease. They were designed to be relevant across all cultures, age groups, and genders, making them useful with heterogeneous populations.

Health Level Seven

Although the Health Level Seven (HL7) organization is based in Ann Arbor, MI and is accredited by ANSI, it is an international community of healthcare subject matter experts and information scientists (Health Level 7, n.d.-b). Founded in 1987, it is an all-volunteer, not-for-profit organization that sets standards for functional and semantic interoperability for electronic healthcare data. Its mission is to provide a "comprehensive framework and related standards for the exchange, integration, sharing, and retrieval of electronic healthcare information" (Health Level 7, n.d.-b).

The term HL7 is derived from the position of these standards in the seven-level Open Systems Interconnect model. This model is a seven-layer model for implementing protocols that pass control from the bottom layer up the hierarchy to the top level (Health Level 7, n.d.-a). The number seven in the name means that the standards being set are at the seventh, or the highest, messaging level of this model. At this level, the standards include those that address the terminology used; and at the functional level, identification of participants, electronic data exchange negotiations,

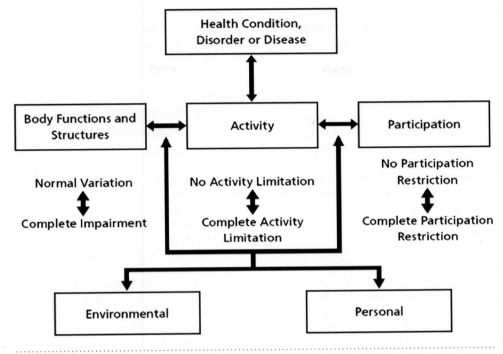

Figure 15-1 ICF codes.

and data exchange structuring. The lower six levels focus on the physical and logical connections between machines, systems, and applications. In very basic terms, HL7 standards are concerned with what data will be transmitted, for example, vital signs and demographic information, and what terminology and protocols will be used to transmit the data. There are many HL7 standards, each addressing a different portion of this process. The HL7 organization is very involved in setting standards for the EHR; several nurses are involved in these efforts.

Digital Imaging and Communications in Medicine

Another standards development group that has ties to both national (National Electrical Manufacturers Association) and international groups (IEC) is the Digital Imaging and Communications in Medicine (DICOM) organization. DICOM sets and maintains standards that allow electrical transmission of digital images (DICOM, 2010). Their work makes it possible to exchange medical digital images worldwide. Thus, if you have an magnetic resonance imaging done in London, England, and your doctor is in Chicago, IL, using the DICOM standards, it is possible for him or her to see the image in Chicago just as if it had been done in his or her radiology department.

Comité Européen de Normalisation

The European Committee for Standardization, or Comité Européen de Normalisation (CEN), is a collaboration of standards bodies in Europe. CEN has strong ties to the European Union politics, and common European legislation makes approved CEN standards the national standards (CEN, 2010). The standardization of healthcare informatics is the province of the CEN/Technical Committee 251. Several standards that are relevant to nursing have been developed including the PrENV 14032, health informatics systems of concepts for nursing. This standard focuses on the application of nursing terminology within electronic messages and healthcare information systems.

International Health Terminology Standards Development Organisation

The International Health Terminology Standards Development Organisation (IHTSDO), a standards development organization created in 2007, is the outgrowth of the joint development of the Systematized Nomenclature of Medicine – Clinical Terms between the National Health Service in the United Kingdom and the College of American Pathologists in the United States (IHTSDO, 2011). Working with representatives of countries worldwide, this organization was created to promote more rapid development and worldwide adoption of standard clinical terminology for EHRs.

Developing Standards

The work of the above standard setting organization groups is done by small groups of volunteers within the organization. Group members are experts in their field who become members of a working or technical group of an organization, which has been delegated to set a specific standard. Anyone (including you) who is an expert in an area and has the time to devote to this endeavor can be a member of a working or technical standard setting group.

There are four main steps for developing standards. The first step in setting a standard is identification of a need. In the second step, the group, which has been designated to define the standard, must state in operational terms what the standard will accomplish and how it will do this. The third step is the longest, and one that will be returned to more than once. Standards development involves a lengthy period of discussion, study of the literature, communication with those outside the group who will be affected by the standard, and possibly even research. Eventually, terms or specifications will be defined, which will be tested in the fourth step.

If the number of parties who will be affected by the new standard is large, the proposed standard will be opened for public comment. If the comments indicate problems, the group will return to the third step to refine the standard. If the changes from the original are many, the new proposal will again be submitted for public comment. Eventually, members of the group will vote on the standard. If they vote in favor, it is submitted to the parent organization for endorsement.

If accepted by the parent organization, it then becomes a standard with a prefix indicating the group that set the standard and a number specific to that standard. When updates are needed, steps three and four are repeated.

Billing Terminology Standardization

In the United States, there is an agreement that administrative or healthcare costs are too high. The National Health Expenditures Accounts reported that the administrative costs for 2008 were about 160 billion dollars (American Medical Association [AMA], 2010). Healthcare providers are hopeful that the Patient Protection and Affordable Care Act that went into effect in 2010 will address the cost concerns. Efforts to standardize government payments for hospital care were initiated in the 1980s with the diagnosis-related groups and modifications to the ICD codes. Following the lead of the government, many private insurers have also adopted them. Efforts to standardize billing for alternative healthcare, such as nurse practitioners, have led to the Alternative Billing Coding (ABC) Set.

International Classification of Disease – Clinical Modification

The ICD codes discussed above, although useful for certain statistical and billing purposes, present a one-dimensional view of disease because they focus only on etiology. To make the codes useful in billing, modifications were added. Clinical modification (CM) codes were developed to capture morbidity data from inpatient and outpatient records, physician office records, and National Center for Health Statistics surveys (CDC, 2010a). Currently in the United States, ICD-9-CM codes are used for billing purposes. ICD-10-CM is scheduled for use beginning October 1, 2013. The ICD-10-PCS for procedure codes is also used for billing purposes (CMS, 2010a).

Diagnosis-Related Groups

The diagnosis-related groups, sometimes referred to as the "daily rate guide," or simply DRGs, is a standardized patient classification system developed in the early 1980s under the auspices of the former Health Care Financing Administration, now called the CMS. Originally intended as a review of the use of hospital resources, they have since become a system for prospective payment. Under this system, patients are categorized into groups for which studies have determined the average hospital resources patients in those groups consume. Hospitals are then paid based on the category into which a patient is classified. The criteria used for assigning categories include medical diagnosis, surgery, complications, and usually age (Sermeus, Weber, Chu, Fischer, & Hunstein, 2006).

Every patient is assigned a single DRG, a process that is done by a computer program called a "grouper," based on information from the Uniform Hospital Discharge Data Set. More than one DRG system is in use beyond the main one used by CMS for Medicare patients. For example, the All Patient Refined–DRG (APR-DRG) is used to represent non-Medicare patients. Other countries, such as Australia, Belgium, Germany, France, the Netherlands, and Austria, have developed their own DRG system based on the US system. In some countries with nationalized health systems, these codes are used to determine hospital funding.

Although nursing is resource intensive, the DRGs do not do well in capturing this information. They tend to determine costs predominantly based on medical diagnoses and medical services consumption. It has been shown that adding nursing data to the DRG data can improve the DRG cost analysis by about 80%. One attempt to fix this was a project at Yale University (Doble, Curley, Hession-Laband, Marino, & Shaw, 2000). Using the APR-DRG, which has subclass ratings for severity of illness from 1 as minor to 4 as extreme, they sorted the DRGs into categories of high and not-high users of nursing resources. The DRG categories were used with the AACN Synergy Model, which matches nurse competencies to the needs and characteristics of a patient, unit, or system (American Association of Critical Care Nurses, 2010). They used patient characteristics such as stability and complexity and added nursing competencies required to care for patients with a given DRG such as clinical judgment, collaboration, and systems. They then designated that DRG on a scale of 1 (low) to 6 (high) for nursing care requirements.

This created a system that allowed nursing care to be articulated to payers in meaningful terms.

The Healthcare Common Procedure Coding System

The Healthcare Common Procedure Coding System, established in 1978, "is a standardized coding system that is used primarily to identify products, supplies, and services not included in the Current Procedural Terminology (CPT) codes, such as ambulance services and durable medical equipment, prosthetics, orthotics, and supplies" (CMS, 2010b). It is intended to supplement the CPT® codes that were developed by the AMA and updated annually.

Alternative Billing Coding Set

The ABC Set or ABCs supports electronic and paper claims processing for providers, healthcare payers, managed care organizations, and affiliated organizations. The system is intended for use in coding and support documentation for reimbursement by third parties for alternative medicine, nursing, and other nonmedical healthcare interventions (ABC Coding Solutions, 2010). The codes are designed to fit into existing standard claim forms, software applications, and information management systems. These codes permit accurate reimbursement for clinical nurse specialists, nurse midwives, nurse practitioners, licensed practical nurses, registered midwives, registered nurses, and other healthcare specialists. Although not the typical terminology that the American Nurses Association (ANA) recognizes, these codes are one of the standardized terminologies recognized by the ANA because they support nursing practice by providing a standardized method of billing for nurse practitioners.

Outcome and Assessment Information Set

The DRGs are not the only government actions to try and contain healthcare costs. Medicare-certified home care agencies must submit Outcome and Assessment Information Set data set to CMS as a part of the reimbursement procedure. OASIS is a group of data elements that represent a comprehensive assessment for an adult home care patient and the basis for measuring outcomes for Outcome-Based Quality Improvement (Department of Health and Human Services [DHHS], 2010e). Federal regulations require home healthcare agencies to collect, code, and transmit these data to their state center, which uploads them to CMS. OASIS standardizes what items are collected, and, by the use of a checklist, the terms used.

CMS provides the home health agencies feedback reports based upon the OASIS data. Currently, four reports are generated: (1) Agency Patient-Related Characteristics Report, (2) Potentially Avoidable Event Report, (3) Outcome-based Quality Improvement Report, and (4) Process Quality Measurement Report. The items in OASIS were derived from a study to develop a system of home care outcome measures. The development was co-funded by the Robert Wood Johnson Foundation and CMS (CMS, 2011). The items include sociodemographic and environmental data, support systems, health status, and functional status attributes of adult (nonmaternity) patients. OASIS data are also used by individual agencies for care planning, demographics, and case mix reports of such patient characteristics as health and functional status at the start of care.

US Efforts Toward an Interoperable Electronic Health Record

The Institute of Medicine's report "To Err is Human" resulted in the open realization that efforts toward improving the delivery of healthcare in the United States were needed. Creating EHRs has become one of the pillars of these endeavors.

Office of the National Coordinator for Health Information Technology

In May 2004, President Bush called for an EHR for Americans by 2014. To further this aim, he established the position of National Coordinator for Health Information Technology who heads the Office of the National Coordinator for Health Information Technology (ONC). The ONC advises the Secretary of the US Department of HHS on issues pertaining to the use of health information technology (ONC, 2010). It also coordinates the health information technology policies and programs for HHS. Together with other executive branches, the ONC is responsible for developing, maintaining, and directing the implementation of the strategies for health information technology in both public and private healthcare sectors and for providing advice to the Office of Management and Budget about specific federal health information technology programs.

The Health Information Technology for Economic and Clinical Health (HITECH) Act, passed in 2009, provided funding opportunities to advance health information technology. The ONC established five initiatives to assure the success of HITECH and to achieve IT adoption (DHHS, 2010d).

- State-level health initiatives
- Nationwide Health Information Network (NHIN)
- Federal health architecture (FHA)
- Health IT adoption surveys
- **Clinical decision support (CDS)**

State-Level Health Initiatives

The complexity of the effort to achieve interoperable IT adoption cannot be overstated. There are a number of state-level initiatives in place (DHHS, 2010f). There is a State Health Policy Consortium that is working on policy issues to allow for **health information exchanges (HIEs)** across state lines. The State Alliance, created by the National Governors Association, provides an executive body to assist state governments to identify best practices and solutions that allow inter- and intrastate HIE. The Health Information Security and Privacy Collaboration is composed of multistate work groups to address privacy and security practices, policies, and laws. Finally, the State-Level Health Information Exchange Consensus Project is working to assure that there is alignment of HIE throughout the United States.

Nationwide Health Information Network

The NHIN consists of standards, policies, and services necessary to allow for secure HIE (DHHS, 2010c) (**Box 15-2**). The work is conducted by federal agencies and state-level, regional, and local **health information exchange organizations**, as well as integrated delivery networks (formerly known as NHIN Cooperative). Direct Project is an example of outcomes of the information network.

BOX 15-2 Benefits of NHIN

- Standards-based, secure data exchange nationally.
- Improvements in the coordination of care information among hospitals, laboratories, physicians' offices, pharmacies, and other providers.
- The availability of appropriate information at the time and place of care.
- Secure and confidential consumers' health information.
- Consumers able to manage and control their personal health records and have access to their health information from EHRs and other sources.
- The reduction of risks from medical errors and the delivery of appropriate, evidence-based medical care.
- Lower healthcare costs resulting from correcting inefficiencies, preventing medical errors, and providing complete patient information at the point of care.
- A more effective marketplace, greater competition, and increased choice through accessibility to accurate information on healthcare costs, quality, and outcomes.

Based on HHS. Nationwide Health Information Network (NHIN). *Background*. Retrieved November 11, 2010, from http://www.hhs.gov/healthit/healthnetwork/background/

Direct Project workgroups are developing standards and procedures to allow for secure information exchange at the local level so that a primary provider can electronically exchange information with another provider.

Federal Health Architecture

The FHA is responsible for coordinating health IT activities for the federal agencies that provide healthcare and health services to citizens (DHHS, 2010b). It supports federal efforts for disseminating health IT standards. It also makes sure that there are seamless health IT exchanges within federal agencies and between state, local, and tribal governments and with private sector.

Health IT Adoption Surveys

The ONC conducts health IT adoption surveys of physician offices and hospitals in order to monitor the outcomes of the use of electronic HIE efforts. The surveys, conducted annually, monitor basic and full levels of use for the EHR. See **Table 15-1** for an example of comparison of basic and full levels of HIE for physician offices.

Clinical Decision Support

CDS support provides the "just in time" prompts to assist users to use health information systems effectively. The users include nurses, other healthcare providers, and patients. There are three important benefits of CDS use. CDS can improve care quality and outcomes. It can also prevent errors and adverse events. Finally, it can improve "efficiency, cost-benefit, and provider and patient satisfaction" (DHHS, 2010a).

Table 15-1 Comparison of Basic and Full Levels of HIE for Physician Offices

	Basic	Full
Health information and data		
Patient demographics	X	X
Problem list	X	X
Current medications	X	X
Clinical notes	X	X
Medical history (hx) and follow-up		X
Order entry management		
Rx (treatment) orders	X	X
Laboratory orders		X
Radiology orders		X
Rx sent electronically		X
Orders sent electronically		X
Results management		
View laboratory results	X	X
View imaging results	X	X
Images returned		X
Clinical decision support		
Drug warnings		X
Out of range levels highlighted		X
Clinical reminders		X

From DHHS. (2010, March 30). *Health IT adoption – Survey tables*. Retrieved November 11, 2010, from http://healthit.hhs.gov/portal/server.pt?open=512&objID=1152&&PageID=17154&mode=2&in_hi_userid=11113&cached=true#P

National Committee on Vital and Health Statistics

The NCVHS was established by Congress in 1949 to advise the DHHS on "health data, statistics, and national health information policy" (NCVHS, 2006). The NCVHS fosters collaboration for consensus on data standards and privacy issues. Historically, the committee has been involved with disease classification, health surveys, uniform data sets, state and community data sets, and health information privacy.

US Public Health Information Network

Although not part of the EHR efforts, the Public Health Information Network (PHIN) will benefit from it. The PHIN is a part of the CDC, which is a national effort to increase the ability of public health agencies to electronically use and exchange information by promoting the use of standards (CDC, 2010b). The National Electronic Disease Surveillance System (NEDSS) is a major component of these efforts (CDC, 2011a). The objective of the NEDSS is to develop and support integrated surveillance systems that can transfer appropriate public health, laboratory, and clinical data efficiently and securely over the Internet to allow quick identification and tracking of disease outbreaks, whether natural or from bioterrorism.

Unified Medical Language System

As you have seen, there are many different standardized efforts and terminologies. Although some of these express concepts particular to a specific discipline (those for nursing will be examined in the next chapter), there are many that are interdisciplinary. It is essential, however, for users to be able to find all the information related to a given concept in all machine-readable sources such as clinical records, databases, biomedical literature, and various directories of information sources. "The UMLS integrates and distributes key terminology, classification and coding standards, and associated resources to promote creation of more effective interoperable biomedical information services, including electronic health records" (National Library of Medicine, 2010).

The **Unified Medical Language System (UMLS)** consists of three different, but related, types of information: the Metathesaurus, Semantic Network, and the SPECIALIST Lexicon and Lexical Programs. The Metathesaurus is a large vocabulary database with information about health-related concepts, their names, and the linkages between them. The semantic network provides consistent categorization of the Metathesaurus concepts, including the categories that may be assigned to the concepts, and defines relationships between the semantic types. The SPECIALIST Lexicon provides information needed for the SPECIALIST Natural Language Processing (NLP) System. It contains many biomedical terms along with the information needed by the SPECIALIST NLP System. The future of the UMLS is envisioned to link information from EHRs with the biomedical literature.

Effect on Nursing and Patient Care

The decisions from the different HIT initiatives and the standards they set will affect nursing. These standards will be used for HIE and will determine what and how nurses document patient care. These decisions will determine the information that secondary analysis of the data will provide, which will determine national healthcare policy. Without nursing participation, the data will be unlikely to represent the contribution of nursing to patient care or provide national healthcare policy that is in the best interest of the patient and client.

Summary

Standards make commerce possible. From the light bulb you buy to the railroads, there are standards both nationally and internationally. The technology that is used to care for patients has also met standards. In information standards, healthcare is still in its infancy, particularly in electronic information standards. Currently, there are many systems that are not interoperable with other systems. This situation prevents early identification of epidemics and serious drug side effects as well as contribution to errors in patient care.

Data input into computers will become the healthcare records of the future; if these data are to be useful, it must meet standards. Professional organizations at the international and the national level as well as governments have recognized this problem and are working to overcome it. Healthcare, however, is very complex and composed of many different stakeholders and disciplines, which further complicates this problem. The standards that are developed and adopted will determine what is viewed as important in healthcare and will have a great effect on nursing and healthcare policy.

The epidemic in the beginning of this chapter was avoided. Cooperation of the international community allowed data on the various outbreaks of flu to be collected at the time and place of origin and preventative measures be undertaken.

The information in a chapter of this sort, because it is tied to the politics of healthcare, is changeable. Every effort has been made to make this chapter current at the time of its going to press.

APPLICATIONS AND COMPETENCIES

1. In your own words, describe interoperability and its three subtypes.

2. Working with two or three others, arrive at some standards for something simple such as entering a classroom or opening a book that could be interpreted by a computer.

3. Interview, in person or by e-mail, a local person who is involved in a regional, national, or international standards setting group.

4. using the web, investigate further the activities of one of the standards setting groups. Employ the principles of evaluating websites for use seen in Chapter 10.

5. By using a digital library, find an article that extends your understanding about interoperability and HIE. Make a list of "talking points" noted from the article to share with others.

6. Describe the function of the UMLS.

REFERENCES

ABC Coding Solutions. (2010). *ABC Codes explained*. Retrieved November 11, 2010, from http://www.abccodes.com/ali/abc_codes/

American Association of Critical Care Nurses. (2010). *The AACN Synergy Model for patient care*. Retrieved November 11, 2010, from http://www.aacn.org/WD/Certifications/Docs/SynergyModelforPatientCare.pdf

American Medical Association. (2010, October 8). *Getting the most for our health care dollars: Administrative costs of health care coverage*. Retrieved November 10, 2010, from http://www.ama-assn.org/ama1/pub/upload/mm/health-care-costs/administrative-costs.pdf

ASTM International. (2010). *The history of ASTM International – 1898–1998: A century of progress. Chapter one: A broader view*. Retrieved November 9, 2010, from http://www.astm.org/HISTORY/hist_chapter1.html

Centers for Disease Control and Prevention. (2010a, January 4). *Classification of diseases, functioning, and disability*. Retrieved November 10, 2010, from http://www.cdc.gov/nchs/icd.htm

Centers for Disease Control and Prevention. (2010b, May 17). *Public Health Information Network – About PHIN*. Retrieved October 29, 2010, from http://www.cdc.gov/phin/about.html

Centers for Disease Control and Prevention. (2011a, February 7). *National electronic disease surveillance system*. Retrieved October 28, 2010, from http://www.cdc.gov/nedss/

Centers for Disease Control and Prevention. (2011b, June 10). Classification of diseases, functioning, and disability. Retrieved August 21, 2011, from http://www.nationmaster.com/encyclopedia/International-Statistical-Classification-of-Diseases-and-Related-Health-Problems

Centers for Medicare & Medicaid Services. (2010a, October 5). *2011 ICD-10-PCS ICD-10*. Retrieved November 10, 2010, from https://www.cms.gov/ICD10/11b_2011_ICD10PCS.asp

Centers for Medicare & Medicaid Services. (2010b, June 15). *Healthcare common procedure coding system (PCPCS) Health Level II coding procedures*. Retrieved November 11, 2010, from https://www.cms.gov/MedHCPCSGenInfo/Downloads/LevelIICodingProcedures.pdf

Centers for Medicare & Medicaid Services. (2011, May 13). *OASIS Overview*. Retrieved August 21, 2011, from https://www.cms.gov/oasis/

Chute, C. G. (2000). Clinical classification and terminology: Some history and current observations. *Journal of the American Medical Informatics Association, 7*(3), 298–303. Retrieved from http://www.ncbi.nlm.nih.gov/pmc/articles/PMC61433/?tool=pubmed

Comité Européen de Normalisation. (2010). *European Committee for Standardization*. Retrieved November 10, 2010, from http://www.cen.eu/cen/pages/default.aspx

Department of Health and Human Services. (2010a, October 8). *Clinical decision support*. Retrieved November 11, 2010, from http://healthit.hhs.gov/portal/server.pt?open=512&objID=1218&parentname=CommunityPage&parentid=30&mode=2&in_hi_userid=11113&cached=true

Department of Health and Human Services. (2010b, July 16). *Federal Health Architecture*. Retrieved November 11, 2010, from http://healthit.hhs.gov/portal/server.pt?open=512&objID=1181&parentname=CommunityPage&parentid=26&mode=2&in_hi_userid=11113&cached=true

Department of Health and Human Services. (2010c, September 3). *Nationwide Health Information Network*. Retrieved November 11, 2010, from http://healthit.hhs.gov/portal/server.pt?open=512&objID=1142&parentname=CommunityPage&parentid=25&mode=2&in_hi_userid=11113&cached=true

Department of Health and Human Services. (2010d). *ONC initiatives*. Retrieved from http://healthit.hhs.gov/portal/server.pt/community/healthit_hhs_gov__onc_initiatives/1497

Department of Health and Human Services. (2010e, August). *Outcome-based Quality Improvement (OBQI) Manual*. Retrieved November 11, 2010, from https://www.cms.gov/HomeHealthQualityInits/Downloads/HHQIOBQIManual.pdf

Department of Health and Human Services. (2010f, August 13). *State level initiatives*. Retrieved November 11, 2010, from http://healthit.hhs.gov/portal/server.pt?open=512&objID=1154&parentname=CommunityPage&parentid=20&mode=2&in_hi_userid=11113&cached=true

Digital Imaging and Communications in Medicine. (2010, October 8). *DICOM homepage*. Retrieved November 10, 2010, from http://medical.nema.org/

Doble, R. K., Curley, M. A., Hession-Laband, E., Marino, B. L., & Shaw, S. M. (2000). Using the synergy model to link nursing care to diagnosis-related groups. *Critical Care Nurse, 20*(3), 86–92.

Gibbons, P., Arzt, N., Burke-Beebe, S., Chute, C., Dickinson, G., Jepsen, T., et al. (2007, February 7). *Coming to terms: Scoping interoperability for health care*. Retrieved November 9, 2010, from http://www.hln.com/assets/pdf/Coming-to-Terms-February-2007.pdf

Health Level 7. (n.d.-a). *HL7 FAQs*. Retrieved November 10, 2010, from http://www.hl7.org/about/FAQs/index.cfm?ref=nav

Health Level 7. (n.d.-b). *What is HL7?* Retrieved November 10, 2010, from http://www.hl7.org/about/

Healthcare Information and Management Systems Society. (2005, June 9). *Interoperability definition and background*. Retrieved November 9, 2010, from http://www.himss.org/content/files/interoperability_definition_background_060905.pdf

International Electrotechnical Commission. (2010). *About the IEC: Mission and objectives*. Retrieved November 9, 2010, from http://www.iec.ch/about/mission-e.htm

International Health Terminology Standards Development Organisation. (2011). *IHTSCO: International health terminology standards development organisation*. Retrieved November 10, 2010, from http://www.ihtsdo.org/

International Organization for Standardization. (2010). *ISO – About ISO Retrieved*. November 9, 2010, from http://www.iso.org/iso/about

National Committee Vital Health Statistics. (2006, March 13). *Introduction to the NCVHS: Information for Health*. Retrieved November 11, 2010, from http://www.ncvhs.hhs.gov/intro.htm

National Library of Medicine. (2010, November 2). *UMLS*. Retrieved November 11, 2010, from http://www.nlm.nih.gov/research/umls/

Sermeus, W., Weber, P., Chu, S., Fischer, W., & Hunstein, D. (2006). The DRG imperative: Overview and nursing impact. In C. Weaver, C. W. Delaney, P. Weber & R. L. Carr (Eds.), *Nursing and informatics for the 21st century: An international look at practice trends and the future* (pp. 231–245). Chicago, IL: Healthcare Information and Management Systems Society.

The Office of the National Coordinator for Health Information Technology. (2010, August 13). *The Office of the National Coordinator for health Information Technology (ONC)*. Retrieved November 11, 2010, from http://healthit.hhs.gov/portal/server.pt/community/healthit_hhs_gov__onc/1200

World Health Organization. (2010a). *History of the development of the ICD*. Retrieved November 9, 2010, from http://www.who.int/classifications/icd/en/

World Health Organization. (2010b). *ICD revision project plan: Version 2.0*. Retrieved November 10, 2010, from http://www.who.int/classifications/icd/ICDRevisionProjectPlan_March2010.pdf

World Health Organization. (2010c). *International classification of functioning, disability and health (ICF)*. Retrieved November 10, 2010, from http://www.who.int/classifications/icf/en/

CHAPTER 16

Nursing Documentation in the Age of the Electronic Health Record

Objectives

After studying this chapter, you will be able to:

▶ Compare the focus of documentation of patient care in an agency with the ways patient care data are used.

▶ Define standardized nursing terminologies and the associated concepts.

▶ Interpret how electronic documentation using standardized terminologies can inform evidence-based care.

▶ Differentiate between the nursing minimum data set and nursing focused terminologies.

Key Terms

Artificial Intelligence Classification
Clinical Care Classification (CCC)
De-identified Data
Granularity
Interface Terminology
International Classification of Nursing Practice (ICNP)
Logical Observation Identifiers Names Codes (LOINC®)
Mapping
NANDA, NIC, and NOC (NNN)
Natural Language Processing (NLP)
Nomenclature
North American Nursing Diagnosis Association (NANDA)
Nursing Information and Data Set Evaluation Center (NIDSEC)

Nursing Interventions Classification (NIC)
Nursing Management Minimum Data Set (NMMDS)
Nursing Minimum Data Set (NMDS)
Nursing Outcomes Classification (NOC)
Omaha System
Ontology
Outcomes Potentially Sensitive to Nursing (OPSN)
Perioperative Nursing Data Set (PNDS)
Reference Terminology
Secondary data use
Standardized terminology
Systematized Nomenclature of Medical – Clinical Terms (SNOMED CT)
Taxonomy

while attending a special meeting of the ICN in Paris, I was naturally at once struck by the fact that the methods and the ways of regarding nursing problems were ... as foreign to the various delegations as were the actual languages, and the thought occurred to me that ... sooner or later we must put ourselves upon a common basis and work out what may be termed a "nursing Esperanto" which would in the course of time give us a universal nursing language. (Hampton Robb, 1909)

Healthcare is undergoing a transformation worldwide. In the United States, fee-for-service is giving way to a demand for reimbursement for outcomes, not procedures. Evidence to prove positive outcomes of care is required for full reimbursement of service rendered. The evidence requires the use of documented data. The United States is one of the many countries in the world that supports the use of electronic clinical records (Boyd, Funk, Schwartz, Kaplan, & Keenan, 2010). If clinical nursing is to provide evidence that nursing care has an effect on outcomes, a readily identifiable and measurable documentation must be captured in the electronic record. This chapter focuses on the issues and challenges associated with capturing of nursing documentation and evaluating the effectiveness of nursing care. The development of standardized nursing terminologies is discussed by using an historical perspective.

Nursing and Documentation

Healthcare documentation has been done for over 100 years. Prior to documentation, healthcare was delivered by the family physician who knew the patient, the family, and all their maladies. Given the relative simplicity of healthcare before the 20th century, detailed records were not viewed as necessary. In the current healthcare system, care is often delivered by relative strangers. Care is often provided by a multidisciplinary team of healthcare professionals. Moreover, the cost of care has skyrocketed. As a result, the need to document and communicate among providers has become essential to the delivery of safe and effective care. Documentation of care is also tethered to the complex billing and reimbursement systems.

Today, an individual person may have health records with no shared data among many providers. The silo method of care results in minimal communication between the care providers treating the person. Care data that are stagnated in data silos cannot be collected, aggregated, and analyzed to improve care outcomes. This issue hopefully will be resolved as the United States and other countries worldwide move to an electronic health record (EHR), which uses standardized terminologies.

Invisibility of Nursing Data

In the absence of nursing data, nursing was often measured by negative qualities, such as adverse events (Ozbolt, 2000). For example, the US government used **outcomes potentially sensitive to nursing (OPSN)** to study outcomes and their relationship to the nurse–patient ratio (Needleman, Buerhaus, Mattke, Stewart, & Zelevinsky, 2001). An OPSN is a medical diagnosis that is thought to measure the contributions of nurses in providing inpatient care. Some OPSNs are urinary tract infections, skin pressure ulcers, pneumonia, shock, upper gastrointestinal bleeding, and length of stay. Using OPSNs, a study done by the Department of Health and Human Services, employing data from more than 5 million patient discharges from 799 hospitals in 11 states, found that the more the registered nurses, the fewer the adverse outcomes; that is, these complications did not occur as often. Additional studies have also demonstrated this as well as the fact that failure to rescue episodes increase as nurse staffing decreases beyond a certain level (Aiken, Clarke, Sloane, Sochalski, & Silber, 2002; Medical News Today, 2007; Needleman, Buerhaus, Mattke, Stewart, & Zelevinsky, 2002).

Although these studies identify that there is a relationship between nursing care and medically oriented outcomes, we are just beginning to understand what nurses do to prevent bad outcomes. What is it that nurses do to prevent infections, for example, catheter-associated bloodstream infections, catheter-associated urinary tract infections, or sepsis? The lack of nursing data that demonstrate what it is that a registered nurse does that prevents adverse outcomes makes it impossible to determine the true value of nursing.

The root of this problem lies in the "invisibility of nursing," a phenomenon identified in 1990 in an editorial in the *Journal of the American Medical Association* (Friedman, 1990). The editorial noted that although nursing is critical to patient care, it has a low profile. Even administrators have trouble identifying nursing's contribution to patient care. Hansten and Washburn (1998) wrote about a chief executive officer in a hospital who commented to his chief financial officer:

> To tell you the truth, George, I don't know what RNs do. Every time I've been on walking rounds in this hospital and asked nurses what they've done recently for our hospital's survival, some tell me I should already know, others struggle to come up with an answer, but can't explain. I know we need some RNs here, but I'm not sure why? (p. 42).

As nurses, we may not understand that what we do is not clear through the lens of others when they read our documentation. The absence of coded standardized nursing data that are incorporated into electronic databases contributes to the invisibility of nursing. As an example, a state public health group found that there was a "mystique" about nursing's contribution to public health; the care was invisible to partners and stakeholders (Correll & Martin, 2009). The nursing documentation did not clearly demonstrate nursing's value and was not easily accessible or measurable. Hannah, White, Nagle, & Pringle (2009) reported that when the focus in EHRs is on physicians, there is no visibility for "... nurses' clinical judgments and decision making that are within the scope of nursing practice" (p. 524).

In many settings, even those that use an electronic medical record, nursing documentation for secondary use research to improve care is about the same as it was in the 1920s. In 2010, the *American Journal of Nursing* reran an article about a research from 1927 (Marvin, 2010). According to the article, a new method of discovering and applying medical knowledge was identified in 1854. The method involved demonstrating effects versus blindly accepting practice. In 1927, nurses used the same thermometer on multiple patients. The thermometers were believed to be cleaned from soaking in a solution thought to disinfect them. One hospital decided to verify that the disinfecting procedure was effective. They discovered that the thermometers were contaminated with streptococcus and pneumococcus. Yet, use of the soaking procedure for decontamination was common practice in many settings until the 1960s.

There were other procedures that were used without supporting evidence. For example, how, how long, and when to scrub hands, the need for sterile towels when draping for catheterization, and the preparation and care of the surgical dressing cart lacked supporting research-based evidence. Each healthcare agency made decisions based on "what we have always done." The article ended with the thought that "... scientific research would mean that the art of nursing the patient would be more nearly perfected in a shorter time than it could possibly be by slow accumulation of knowledge gained though casual experiences" (Marvin, 2010, p. 69, in reprint). Evidence-based nursing exploration continues to be arduous when the record is in narrative form or the electronic documentation system does not allow nursing data to be visible for extraction.

Nursing has made much progress since 1927 and many healthcare settings today have made use of evidence-based procedures since 1927. However, many variations in procedures may exist according to the agency. Some procedures may be based on "how we have always done it" and casual experiences. Moreover, expert opinions may vary about nursing care. In the late 1980s, the developers of the **Nursing Interventions Classification (NIC)** found that interventions listed for given conditions varied by textbook (Dochterman, Bulechek, & Iowa Intervention Project, 1992). Different terminologies were used for the same interventions. More revealing, interventions were often traditionally versus empirically based.

Revealing Nursing Data

Nurses have always been respected healthcare providers, but the value of nursing documentation was not always seen as important. As difficult as it may be to believe, nursing data were purged from the medical record for several decades prior to the 1970s. In a 1972 book on medical record management, Edna Huffman, asserted that the purpose of nurses' notes was to serve as a means for nurses and physicians to communicate during a patient's hospitalization. When discussing medical record retention, she stated:

> ... in order to reduce the bulk and made records less cumbersome to handle, many hospitals remove the nurses' notes when the medical record personnel assemble and check the medical record after patient discharge .... The nurses' notes are then filed in chronological order in some place less accessible than the current files until the statute of limitations has expired. Then they are destroyed. (Huffman, Price, & American Medical Record Association, 1972, p. 203).

It was clear that the healthcare community at large did not recognize the importance of nursing data. Fortunately, nursing notes are no longer purged and destroyed today. A number of visionary nurse leaders were responsible for the significant progress in valuing nurses' documentation. A historical perspective on the work to develop standardized nursing languages should provide a framework to understand the journey to reveal nursing data. The realization about the importance of emerging computer and nursing information systems served as an impetus to speed up the process for naming and structuring nursing data.

Initial emphasis on research and data collection is attributed to Florence Nightingale, who kept careful statistics on diseases and mortality during the Crimean War (Nightingale, 1860; Nightingale & Goldie, 1997). Nightingale was well educated and excelled in mathematics (School of Mathematics and Statistics, St. Andrews University Scotland, 2003). She used the analysis of data to make recommendations about environmental hygiene and hospital design. She documented her findings in several books. Unfortunately, nursing did not embrace the importance of data collection and analysis to improve care outcomes for almost another century.

The concept of a prescribing nursing care is credited to Bertha Harmer, a Canadian nurse, who went on to be a nursing professor at Yale and McGill universities and author of several nursing textbooks. When discussing nursing assignments and a scientific method of study, Harmer stated: "*We* [nurses] are held responsible for the nursing care – should we not prescribe nursing care for each patient as doctors prescribe medical care?" (Harmer, 1926, pp. 111–112). She went on to note that physicians had acknowledged that "[a patient's] life will depend upon the nursing care he receives" (p. 112). When discussing nursing documentation, she noted the importance of aggregating data embedded in nursing documentation to "formulate principles, to organize knowledge – the process of making knowledge, which is science" (p. 116). Harmer had a clear vision about the value of documenting and aggregating nursing data to improve nursing care and patients' outcomes.

In order to capture the complexity of nursing for communication, research, and documentation, groups of nursing scientists have worked to identify standard language that reflects nursing diagnoses, interventions, outcomes, and other essential elements related to the care experience. The American Nurses Association (ANA) Committee for Nursing Practice Information Infrastructure) has recognized standardized terminologies that have met definitive criteria. **Table 16-1** summarizes the ANA standardization efforts pertinent to nursing.

In 1995, the **Nursing Information and Data Set Evaluation Center (NIDSEC)** was established by the ANA to evaluate vendor implementation of the ANA standardized terminologies in nursing information systems. The evaluation criteria included clinical content, a clinical data repository (how data are stored and retrieved), and general system characteristics. The ANA encourages nursing system developers to have their systems evaluated against the NIDSEC standards.

North American Nursing Diagnosis Association

Almost 50 years later, nurses took action on diagnosing and prescribing nursing care. Discussion about the need to reveal nursing data formalized in 1973, when Kristine Gebbie and Mary Ann Levin initiated a task force to name and classify nursing diagnoses. The first set of nursing diagnoses was established from their set of collective experiences. Nine years later, in 1982, **North American Nursing Diagnosis Association (NANDA)** was

Table 16-1 ANA Recognized Standardization Efforts Pertinent to Nursing

Name	Elements	Year Recognized by ANA	Relationships/ Maps To:	Description/Comments
		Nursing Minimum Data Sets		
USA Nursing Minimum Data Set (NMDS) http://www.nursing.umn.edu/ICNP/USANMDS/	Nursing care Patient/demographic Service	1999	CCC, ICNP, NANDA, NIC, NOC, OMAHA, PNDS, ABC	Delineates and defines categories of data needed to describe clinical nursing practice. Useful for nursing education, health information systems design, and clinical research.
Nursing Management Minimum Data Set (NMMDS) http://www.nursing.umn.edu/ICNP/USANMMDS/	Environment Nursing care Financial resources	1988	LOINC	Designed for nursing managers and administrators. Contains some terms as well as the categories. Permits nursing managers to have more and better information about their nursing services as well as provide comparable data for benchmarking with other organizations.
		Interface Terminologies Specific to Nursing (Alphabetically listed)		
Clinical Care Classification (CCC) http://www.sabacare.com/	Nursing diagnoses and outcomes Nursing interventions and actions/care components	1992	NMDS, ICNP, ABC. SNOMED-CT, LOINC, HL7	An interface terminology. Until 2003 was called HHCC. Originated to assess and classify home health patients for Medicare to predict resources. Expanded for all settings. Use by permission, no license fee. Maintained by Sabacare, Inc.
North American Nursing Diagnosis Association - International (NANDA-I) http://www.nanda.org/	Nursing diagnoses	1992	NMDS, NIC, NOC, PNDS, SNOMED-CT, UMLS, ICNP, HL7	Categorizes and defines nursing problems for documentation for all settings. Serves as a basis for most nursing terminologies' nursing problems. Requires license fee to use. Maintained by NANDA International. An interface terminology.
Nursing Interventions Classification (NIC) http://www.nursing.uiowa.edu//excellence/nursing_knowledge/clinical_effectiveness/nic.htm	Nursing interventions	1992	NMDS, NANDA, NOC, ABC, SNOMED-CT, UMLS, ICNP, HL7	Categorizes and defines nursing interventions for documentation in all settings. Requires license fee to use. Developed and maintained by the University of Iowa Center for Nursing Classification & Clinical Effectiveness. An interface terminology.
Nursing Outcome Classification (NOC) http://www.nursing.uiowa.edu/excellence/nursing_knowledge/clinical_effectiveness/noc.htm	Nursing outcomes	1997	NMDS, NANDA, NIC, ABC, SNOMED-CT, UMLS, HL7	Categorizes and defines nursing outcomes for documentation. Requires license fee to use. Developed and maintained by the University of Iowa Center for Nursing Classification & Clinical Effectiveness. An interface terminology.
Omaha Home Health Care System http://www.omahasystem.org/	Nursing problems Nursing interventions Problem rating scale for actions	1992	NMDS, SNOMED-CT, UMLS, ICNP, HL7, LOINC, ABC	Allows users to collect, classify, document, and analyze data for patients, families and communities in home care, public health, and community nursing. Used with permission, no fee. Developed by the Omaha Visiting Nurse Association in conjunction with seven other community health agencies. Maintained by the Omaha System Organization. An interface terminology.

Notes in Description/Comments column (aligned to Nursing Minimum Data Sets row): NANDA-I, NIC, and NOC are intended to be used together. Requires three separate licenses. When referencing all three, often named NNN.

(continued)

Table 16-1 ANA Recognized Standardization Efforts Pertinent to Nursing *(continued)*

Name	Elements	Year Recognized by ANA	Relationships/ Maps To:	Description/Comments
Patient Care Data Set (Retired) http://www.ncvhs.hhs.gov/990518t3.pdf	Nursing problems Nursing interventions Nursing outcomes	1998		Originally developed for acute care setting. Contained terms for Nursing Problems, Interventions, and Outcomes. Intended for nurses and non-physician healthcare providers. Retired in 2006.
Perioperative Nursing Data Set (PNDS) http://www.aorn.org/PracticeResources/PNDSAndStandardizedPerioperativeRecord/PNDSModel/	Nursing diagnoses Nursing interventions Nurse-sensitive patient outcomes	1999	NMDS, ICNP, SNOMED-CT, UMLS, HL7	Provides data around the complete peri-operative experience from pre-admission to discharge. Developed as a means to validate nursing in an operative setting. Development and maintained by the American Operating Room Nurses Association. Requires license fee to use. An interface terminology.
Reference Terminology Specific to Nursing				
International Classification of Nursing Practice (ICNP) http://www.icn.ch/pillarsprograms/international-classification-for-nursing-practice/	Nursing diagnoses Nursing actions Nursing outcomes	2000("Education listserv.")	UMLS. Harmonization with SNOMED-CT ongoing.	Based on a 7-axis model: focus, judgment, time, location, means, action, and client. Basically a reference terminology, it is compositional, terms selected from axes for nursing diagnoses and actions. "Subsets," or a pre-coordinated list of terms, are being developed for use as an interface terminology. Developed and maintained by the International Council of Nursing (ICN). With SNOMED is part of the International Health Terminology Standards Development Organisation (IHTSDO). Requires license fee to use.
Reference and Interdisciplinary Terminologies for Nursing and Other Healthcare Disciplines				
Logical Observation Identifiers Names & Codes (LOINC) http://loinc.org/	Assessment	2002	UMLS	Originally focused on standardization of names of laboratory tests. Now includes assessment measures for vital signs, obstetric measurements, and some clinical assessment scales. Has some interface properties. Developed by the Regenstrief Institute. Free to all users.
Systematized Nomenclature of Medicine (SNOMED-CT) http://www.ihtsdo.org/snomed-ct/	General terminology for the EHR	1999	CCC, NANDA, NIC, NOC, OMAHA, PNDS, LOINC, UMLS	Most comprehensive, multilingual, clinical healthcare terminology. Basically a reference terminology. Free to all US users through the National Library of Medicine. Originally developed by the American College of Pathology, now owned and maintained by the International Health Terminology Standards Development Organization (IHTSDO).
Billing Code for Nurse Practitioners				
Alternative Billing Codes (ABC) http://www.alternativelink.com/ali/home/	Services Remedies and/or supplies Practitioner type	2000	NMDS, CCC, NIC, UMLS	Supports electronic and paper billing claims processing for providers, healthcare payers, managed care organizations, and affiliated agencies. Provides a standardized method of billing for nurse practitioners and other alternative healthcare practitioners. Developed and maintained by ABC Coding Solutions (formerly Alternative Link).

EHR, Electronic health record;
HHCC, Home Health Care Classification;
HL7, Health Level 7, a standardization for exchanging messages between different computer systems to achieve interoperability;
NDNQI, National Database of Nursing Quality Indicator;
NQF, National Quality Forum;
UMLS, Unified Medical Language Systems.

Source: Education listserv. Retrieved July 29, 2003, from http://library.lib.binghamton.edu/subjects/education/listserv.html

established as an association. The ANA recognized NANDA in 1992. In 2002, NANDA name was changed to NANDA-I to reflect its international presence. NANDA-I is the most familiar standardized nursing terminology in the United States (Thede & Schwiran, 2011). It provides the basis for nursing problems in most of the other ANA-recognized nursing-focused terminologies. NANDA defined nursing diagnosis as "... a clinical judgment about individual, family, or community experiences and responses to actual or potential health problems and life processes" (NANDA, 2011).

Nursing Minimal Data Set

Harriet Werley first recognized the need for the ability to gather, store, and retrieve nursing data to use in research as a member of the ANA Committee on Nursing Research and Studies in 1962 (Werley & Lang, 1988). Werley acknowledged the importance of research on communication and decision making in nursing. She also understood the need to have a structured standardized vocabulary long before the widespread use of computers in the healthcare setting.

The concept of a **nursing minimum data set (NMDS)** was discussed at a Nursing Information Systems Conference at the University of Illinois in 1977. However, the concept was not formalized until 1984, when she and Norma Lang received a grant for an NMDS conference. Today, Werley and Lang are credited for the development of the NMDS, now known as USA-NMDS (Center for Nursing Minimum Data Set Knowledge, 2009). The NMDS was recognized by the ANA in 1999. The data set includes "essential, common, and core data elements to be collected for all patients/clients receiving nursing care" (Saba & McCormick, 2006, p. 249). A number of similar data sets were developed in Australia, Canada, Belgium, Ireland, the Netherlands, Iceland, Switzerland, and Thailand after the global nursing community recognized the value. Currently, i-NMDS is a term used to identify the international nursing minimal data set sponsored by the International Council of Nurses (2010). The i-NMDS is based on the collective work of individual countries. **Table 16-2** shows a comparison of the USA-NMDS and i-NMDS. Note that there are some distinct differences. For

Table 16-2 Comparison of the USA-NMDS with the i-NMDS

Data Categories	USA-NMDS	i-NMDS
Setting	• Unique facility or service agency number[a] • Unique health record number or patient or client[a] • Unique number of principal registered nurse provider • Episode admission or encounter date[a] • Discharge or termination date[a] • Disposition of patient or client[a] • Expected payer for most of the bill (anticipated financial guarantor for services rendered)[a]	• Agency location • Ownership of facility • Country system of payment • Clinical service type • Care personnel (number, gender, training and education) • Full-time equivalent for types of personnel • Ratio of patients to personnel
Patient/client demographics	• Personal identification[a] • Date of birth[a] • Sex[a] • Race and ethnicity[a] • Residence[a]	• Care episode start and stop dates • Country of residence • Clinical service type • Discharge status • Year of birth • Gender • Reason for admission
Nursing care	• Nursing diagnosis • Nursing interventions • Patient outcomes • Intensity of care	• Nursing diagnoses • Nursing interventions • Patient outcomes • Intensity of care

[a]Uniform hospital discharge data set (UHDDS) elements.

Center for Nursing Minimum Data Set Knowledge. (2009). *USA NMDS*. Retrieved February 11, 2011, from http://www.nursing.umn.edu/ICNP/USANMDS/; International Council of Nurses. (2010). *International Nursing Minimal Data Set (i-NDMS)*. Retrieved February 12, 2011, from http://www.icn.ch/pillarsprograms/international-nursing-minimum-data-set-i-nmdsseptember-2007/

example, the i-NMDS includes data elements relating to number, gender, training and education, and reason for admission, but those elements are not included in the USA-NMDS.

All but six items in the USA-NMDS are included in the UHDDS (Uniform Hospital Data Discharge Set), after which it was modeled. The NMDS was originally conceptualized as a way to support nursing research. It delineates and defines the categories of information needed to describe the care elements of patients and the patient's family experiences in a nursing care system (Westra et al., 2010). With the exception of intensity of nursing care, the nursing care elements in the NMDS have become the basis for the three categories in standardized nursing terminologies: problem or diagnosis, intervention, and outcome.

Nursing Management Minimum Data Set

The **Nursing Management Minimum Data Set (NMMDS)** was designed to capture data useful to nurse managers, administrators, and health care executives and complements the NMDS developed by Werley and Lang. It was developed by coresearchers, Huber and Delaney, from the University of Iowa in partnership with the American Association of Nurse Executives (Center for Nursing Minimum Data Set Knowledge, 2010; Huber, Schumacher, & Delaney, 1997; Simpson, 1997). The research on the data set began in 1989. The NMMDS allows administrators to pull together information that otherwise resides in different places, such as human resources, scheduling, and billing. By providing uniform names, definitions, and coding specifications, the NMMDS allows data to be collected and analyzed to provide information about nursing services at the local, regional, national, and international levels. Its data elements are mapped into the **Logical Observation Identifiers Names and Codes (LOINC®)** (Center for Nursing Minimum Data Set Knowledge, 2010) The NMMDS was recognized by the ANA in 1998.

Nursing Interventions Classification

The Nursing Interventions Classification System was developed by researchers at the University of Iowa in order to identify the activities (known then as treatments) nurses do in their daily work. The language system was developed to name what

nurses do in response to human needs in order to examine outcomes (McCloskey & Bulechek, 1994). The researchers developed the language system in anticipation of the widespread use of computerized patient records in healthcare, although the widespread use of EHRs was in its infancy. Computer clustering was used to identify the **classifications** (Gordon, 1998). The classification system includes physiological and psychosocial interventions, which may be independent or collaborative. While most of the interventions address the individual patient/client, interventions for use with families and communities are also included (Center for Nursing Classification & Clinical Effectiveness, n.d.-a). The fifth edition of NIC includes 542 interventions that are grouped into 30 classes and 7 domains. Its data elements are mapped to the Nursing Outcomes Classification, NANDA, and the **Omaha System**. NIC was recognized by the ANA in 1992.

Nursing Outcomes Classification

The **Nursing Outcomes Classification (NOC)** was also developed by researchers at the University of Iowa. The outcome classifications evaluate the effects of interventions and are designed to complement the NIC standardized language (Center for Nursing Classification & Clinical Effectiveness, n.d.-b). The third edition of the classification system included 330 outcomes. Each outcome includes a definition, indicators that can be used to evaluate the related patient/client status, a target outcome rating, data source, and a Likert scale to identify the patient status. NOC like NIC can be used with individuals, families, and communities. NOC is mapped to NIC, NANDA, and **Systemized Nomenclature of Medicine – Clinical Terminology (SNOWMED CT)**. NOC was recognized by the ANA in 1997.

Clinical Care Classification

The **Clinical Care Classification** (CCC) was developed by Virginia Saba and is designed for all care settings. It was originally designed for home health care and was called the Home Health Care Classification System. The CCC is a comprehensive nursing terminology system that includes nursing diagnoses, interventions, and outcomes that can be used in all settings (Saba, 2011). The classification system is designed to determine care costs. It includes 21 care components. The CCC is mapped to SNOMED CT. CCC has some unique characteristics including no licensing fee and an open architecture. The CCC was recognized by the ANA in 1992.

Omaha System

The Omaha System is a research-based **taxonomy** developed by Karen Martin, principal investigator, and fellow researchers. It is a comprehensive nursing terminology system that includes nursing problems, interventions, and an outcome problem rating scale (The Omaha System, 2010). Like similar taxonomies, it allows for aggregation and analysis of clinical data. It also links clinical data to "demographic, financial, administrative, and staffing data" (The Omaha System, 2010). The Omaha System is mapped to ABC Codes, LOINC®, and SNOWMED CT. It is currently being mapped to INCP. The Omaha System was recognized by the ANA in 1992.

Perioperative Nursing Data Set

The **Perioperative Nursing Data Set (PNDS)** was developed by the Association of periOperating Room Nurses (AORN) to standardize the terminology associated with the perioperative experience. The development began in 1993. The goal was to make the patient problems that perioperative nurses manage visible to administrators, financial officers, and healthcare policy makers (Baker, 2005). The system encompasses the entire perioperative experience from preadmission to discharge by using standardized elements for nursing diagnoses, interventions, and outcomes (AORN, 2011). It covers four domains: behavioral responses – knowledge, rights, and ethics; patient safety; physiological system; and the health system. It provides a framework for documentation for perioperative nurses (Kleinbeck, 2002). The PNDS is mapped to NANDA and SNOWMED CT (American Nurses Association, 2007). The PNDS was recognized by the ANA in 1999.

Systematized Nomenclature of Medicine – Clinical Terms

SNOWMED CT was developed by the National Health Service in England and the College of American Pathologists. It was initiated in 1965 as a standardized language for pathology and known as Systemized Nomenclature of Pathology and later expanded to address the needs of medicine and healthcare, in general (International Health Terminology Standards Development Organisation, n.d.). In 2003, SNOMED CT was licensed by the National Library of Medicine for use without charge in accordance to the regulations set for by the International Health Terminology Standards Development Organization (U.S. National Library of Medicine, 2010). It maps to most of the nursing terminologies recognized by the ANA. SNOWMED CT was recognized by the ANA in 1999.

Because of its comprehensiveness, ability to capture data from all healthcare professionals, and availability, SNOMED CT is fast becoming an important standard in the EHR. It has been approved as a standard for nursing documentation. There are, however, difficulties with, depending on SNOMED CT, capturing nursing documentation without the use of one or more of the seven nursing-oriented terminologies as the **interface terminology**. Given the nature of SNOMED CT, unless an application is specifically designed by a vendor or agency to link nursing problems, interventions, and outcomes and allow this information to be retrieved as nursing data, these data can be easily lost for purposes of determining best practices.

International Classification for Nursing Practice

The International Classification for Nursing Practice (ICNP) is a standardized terminology developed by the International Council of Nurses. It includes nursing diagnoses, interventions, and outcomes (International Council of Nursing, 2009). The ICNP serves as an international standard that assists with the aggregation and analysis of nursing practice. It serves to represent international nursing practice specialties, languages, and cultures. The INCP was recognized by the ANA in 2000.

ABC Codes

The ABC Codes were discussed in Chapter 15. It was designed especially for billing and insurance claims. The ABC Codes were recognized by the ANA in 2000.

Logical Observation Identifiers Names and Codes

LOINC® in its original form standardized the names and reporting of laboratory tests. It was created by, is maintained by, and is distributed free by the Regenstrief Institute (2011). Since its beginnings, LOINC® has expanded to include terms useful in assessment as well as clinical care, outcomes management, and research. Parts of the CCC and Omaha System are integrated into LOINC. It has been recognized as a standard for laboratory test names by the National Committee for Vital and Health Statistics. Although basically a **reference terminology**, there are places that use LOINC® as an interface terminology. In these cases, instead of displaying all the choices, the data requested is only what makes sense in the situation (S. Matney, October 25, 2010, personal communication). LOINC® was recognized by the ANA in 2002.

Standardizing Clinical Documentation Terminology

Electronic clinical records allow for nursing documentation terminology to be structured and standardized. Data retrieved for multiple patients by using the same criteria provide the ability to determine the effect on many patients, not just one. Clinical information systems are databases that allow for data to be grouped and analyzed according to nursing diagnoses, age groups, or any other criterion present in the documentation. The data analysis can provide useful information about the effectiveness of nursing interventions. It can also be used to demonstrate how nursing care contributes to outcomes in a way that is measurable (see **Box 16-1**).

The reuse of nursing data to analyze the effectiveness of nursing care, known as **secondary**

BOX 16-1 Using a Standardized Terminology

In our public health nursing agency, we use the Omaha System, one of the ANA-recognized standardized nursing terminologies. Use of this standardized terminology has been very valuable from my perspective as both a field nurse and an informatics consultant. The Omaha System has improved my ability to articulate the essence and the details of nursing care in both my roles. Although it has taken patience and commitment for me to become proficient in "speaking the language," the results, in terms of strengthened patient care, have been well worth the effort. The learning task is made easier because the grammatical rules, syntax, concepts, and content are those of the nursing process: assessment, planning, intervention, and evaluation.

The terminology is fully integrated into my agency's computerized nursing information system (CNIS). On the basis of the terminology's foundation, powerful care plans have been created and are easily accessible at the point of care. They help me plan care and allow my charting to be more efficient and complete at the point of care. The care plans are easily customizable, allow me to address

the unique needs of my patients, and reflect the organization's policies and procedures. Because we are using a standardized terminology, we can engage in electronic exchange of information across the state. This has created opportunities to learn from and collaborate with my nursing colleagues in the delivery of highly diverse public health nursing services, from tuberculosis control to the prevention of childhood lead poisoning.

The standardized data generated by the terminology and stored in the CNIS enable quality assurance and improvement activities to be based on actual patient care data rather than data extracted from charting. The data are sufficiently atomic to generate meaningful information that enables me to describe to public health payers and partners the needs of patients, outcomes of nursing care, and the unique services that nurses provide in meeting the public's health needs.

Pamela Correll, RN, BSN, Nursing Informatics Consultant, Public Health Nursing Program, Maine Center for Disease Control and Prevention

data use, depends on data entry using words (terms) that are the same for each given problem, intervention, and outcome. Computers use rules for data analysis. A semicolon and a colon are as different to a computer as the sun and a building. Although the terms heart attack and myocardial infarction (MI) convey (Westra et al., 2010) the same meaning to nurses, the computer regards them as two different entities. You may have had a similar experience when using search terms in an Internet search engine or when searching a bibliographic index in a digital library database.

The secondary data use that is becoming mandatory for reimbursement and reporting requires use of **standardized terminology**. Standardized terminology uses terms with agreed-upon definitions. The standardized terms allow information systems to record and exchange data (Westra, Delaney, Konicek, & Keenan, 2008). Standardized terms allow interoperability among different information systems. Keenan (1999) described nursing standardized terminology as a description of nursing care that uses a common language, which is readily understood by all nurses. Information represented by a standardized term can be measured (Rutherford, 2008).

Standardizing terminology in healthcare is not new. As noted in Chapter 15, during the early 20th century standardized terminology describing patient mortality and morbidity was adopted. The standardization was formalized in the International Classification of Disease. Other standards used in healthcare were discussed in Chapter 15 on interoperability.

Nursing has used standardized terms with shared meanings for a long time. For example, nurses document a potential or actual pressure ulcer using staging numbers based on definitions that have been agreed upon and promulgated. Charting a stage 3 pressure ulcer communicates the same information to other nurses and healthcare providers. The Glasgow Coma Scale is another standard that permits accurate, quick communication about neurological status between professionals. The APGAR measurement of a newborn infant is still another standard that improves communication and promotes the appropriate treatment. Nursing, however, encompasses much more than pressure ulcer staging, the Glasgow Coma Scale, and the APGAR. To bridge the gap, standardized nursing terminology was developed.

Prior to the use of standardized nursing diagnoses, traditional nursing focused on documentation around medical diagnoses. Today, nurses independently diagnose and treat nursing problems. As an example, a patient's mother shared a situation when her daughter was on the ventilator and unable to speak. Her nurses took the time, in a very stressful environment, to recognize her need to communicate. They provided the patient with paper and pencil and the time to write her needs. The mother commented that this intervention "... met needs related to impaired communication and it went a long way toward easing discomfort, because that was the only way she could direct them to position her for any degree of discomfort whatever" (P. Schwirian, October 22, 2010, personal communication). Enough has been written about the effect of discomfort on healing to realize the value of this intervention. If the nursing diagnoses, interventions and, outcomes provided by the nurses were documented by using standardized phrases, the outcomes could be compared to patients who did not have the intervention, as well with the level of required pain medication.

Table 16-3 Comparison of Medicine and Nursing Focus

	Medical Data and Focus	**Nursing Data and Focus Added to Care**
Diagnosis	Osteoporosis, mild	Physical injury, potentially due to: throw rugs on hardwood floor, bathtub without hand grips, and inadequate lighting in bedroom
Treatment/intervention	Calcium 500 mg 3× a day Calcitonin – 200 U intranasally in alternate nostrils daily	Remove rugs, install hand grips in shower, use higher wattage bulb in ceiling fixture
Outcome	Fall, fractured hip	Freedom from falls

The goal for the development of standardized nursing terminologies was to describe nursing clinical judgments for problems that nurses are educated and licensed to treat. Nursing problems are not identified in medical language systems (Gordon, 1998). Medicine and nursing have different, but complementary foci. **Table 16-3** shows a comparison of a medical diagnosis, treatment, and outcome with the complementary nursing diagnosis, interventions, and outcome. The efforts to develop different terminologies specific to nursing began in the early 1970s. Nursing visionaries recognized the importance of outcomes from improved communication.

Concepts for Understanding Standardized Terminologies

There are several recognized standardized terminologies used in healthcare that use the same concepts. Definitions of nine concepts should be helpful for understanding standardized terminologies. The vocabulary and definitions for the concepts are summarized in **Table 16-4**.

Granularity describes the detail that is captured by a term or phrase; the greater the granularity, the greater the detail or specificity of the term or phrase. Different levels of granularity are needed for different purposes. At the clinical level, very

granular data are usually needed. Billing and secondary data uses often require less granular data.

Some terminologies use coordinated terms selected from various lists. To describe a nursing problem with the **International Classification of Nursing Practice** (**ICNP**), you would select one term from an axis, such as "focus," and add it to terms from other axes. For example, selecting "pain" from the focus category and "extreme" from the judgment category creates the nursing diagnosis "Extreme pain." See **Table 16-5** to visualize the different levels of granularity that can be applied by using coordinated terms.

Mapping, in simple terms, refers to matching a concept in one standardized terminology with a concept in another standardized terminology. For example, the NANDA nursing diagnosis, "ineffective airway clearance," could be mapped with the CCC nursing diagnosis, "airway clearance impairment."

Organization refers to how the terms are structured for usefulness. There are several terms that are used to describe the structure for standardized terminology. **Nomenclature** and **ontology** describe the levels of classification. Classification is a grouping of related ideas into a taxonomy based on one perspective.

Nomenclature (names of words) is the lowest level of classification. Words in a dictionary are

Table 16-4 Vocabulary for Standardized Terminologies	
Term	**Definition**
Granularity	The detail that is captured by a term or phrase
Mapping	Matching of terms in one standardized terminology to concepts in a higher-order terminology
Post-coordinated term	A term used in documentation that has been created "on the fly" by selecting parts of the term from various categories
Pre-coordinated term	A term that is presented to the user that has been created by selecting parts of the term from various other lists
Nomenclatures	A list of terms from which users choose a term for documentation, often a "pick list," or lists of terms that can be picked for a given category of documentation
Classifications	A nomenclature that has been organized into taxonomical hierarchies. The term can still be used as if it were a nomenclature; analysis can be performed at a level in the domain above the term. For example, the term "acute pain" can be part of an analysis that includes all pain
Ontology	A sophisticated classification that allows terms to be a part of more than one hierarchy and that specifies relationships
Interface terminology	One that is used by clinical personnel for documentation. Usually at the nomenclature level
Reference terminology	One that is organized at the ontology level, which accepts terms from an interface terminology and maps them to the appropriate concept

Table 16-5 Creation of Post-coordinated Nursing Diagnoses From the Axes of the ICNP

From Axes	Term Selected
Focus of nursing practice	Pain
Judgment	Extreme (to a very high degree)
Frequency	Intermittent
Topology	Right
Body site	Foot
Nursing diagnoses	
Extreme pain	
Extreme, intermittent pain	
Extreme, intermittent pain in the foot	
Extreme, intermittent pain in the right foot	
From Axes:	**Term Selected**
Focus of nursing practice	Food supply
Judgment	Deficiency
Likelihood	High risk
Bearer	Community
Nursing diagnoses	
Food supply deficiency	
High risk for food supply deficiency	
High risk for food supply deficiency in the community	

examples of a list organized alphabetically for ease of use. A pick list in computer documentation is another example of nomenclature. Nomenclature has been described as follows:

- Lists of ideas with no inherent structure (Levy, 2004)
- Enumerative classification using an alphabetized list of subject headings (Hardiker, 2009)
- Lists of words from which to name or describe a phenomena within a language or knowledge base (Lang et al., 1995)

Ontology is the highest level of organization of classification. By definition, ontology refers to "relation of being" (Free Merriam-Webster Dictionary, 2011). Ontology is complex and powerful, providing the ability for terms to be represented and linked to multiple concepts.

Classifications and ontologies are useful in data analysis and comparisons, while nomenclatures are used for documentation. The terms interface terminology and reference terminology describe how a terminology is used. An interface terminology is intended for use by clinicians documenting actual care. With the exception of the ICNP, nursing-specific standardized terminologies are interface terminologies. A reference terminology is used behind the scene to transform the input from interface terminology and translate it or map it to concepts at a higher level of classification. Clinical terminology at a higher level allows for broader analysis. Most of the interdisciplinary terminologies used by all healthcare professions are reference terminologies.

Natural Language Processing

Although narrative text is the most expressive form of communication, and one with which most nurses are familiar and comfortable, it can lead to incomplete documentation when a busy nurse tries to remember every detail that needs documentation for many patients. Further, data in narrative text are difficult to extract for comparisons or to coordinate the effect of interventions on outcomes. Electronic healthcare records today vary in the amount of free text versus structured data that are used. One school of thought believes that the information that needs to be recorded in patient care will never be captured in a structured manner. The other school believes that if the information is needed, a way to capture it electronically can be devised. There is truth in both perspectives.

Those in the first school hope that **natural language processing (NLP)** can be used with free text to capture needed data. NLP is a computer process, part of **artificial intelligence**, that identifies and understands words or phrases in text entered into a computer in English or another spoken language and makes them available for use in a structured format. Hoehn (2009) reports that when a large percentage of clinical electronic documentation is in free text, agencies find it next to impossible to go back and mine data for quality and safety information. Also, although easier to get initial buy-in, it is much more difficult to move practitioners to using the structured data that are needed for data mining. Interestingly, when in Korea free text was analyzed to see if it could be structured, they found the most frequent statement was "Slept well" (Park, 2007).

There have been, however, some successes with NLP. Hyun, Johnson, and Bakken (2009) studied the use of an NLP system in retrieving concepts in oncology nursing process notes. They found that although they were able to retrieve many concepts, many additional terms needed to be added to the product that they used. Ware, Mullett, and Jagannathan (2009) fairly successfully used NLP to extract information about obesity from physician discharge summaries.

The general consensus about NLP is that the performance of NLP for automated coding and classification is relative to the complexity of the task (Stanfill, Williams, Fenton, Jenders, & Hersh, 2010). Although NLP is an appealing idea and has worked in some instances, it is not feasible with nursing notes given the variability of documentation from nurse to nurse as well as institution to institution. Another study by Chapman and Haug, cited by Stanfill et al. (2010), found that for every task a new set of regular expressions, or terminology used to express an idea, must be found. To cover all of nursing would require a tremendous amount of work, so for at least the next decade, if not longer, NLP is not feasible.

Issues in Standardized Terminologies

The numerous nursing terminologies available for nursing are a mixed gift. Whether nursing needs one or many terminologies brings to mind similar disciplinary debates about nursing theory and research methodology (McCormick & Jones, 1998). If there is one terminology, the assumption is that everyone will understand, accept, and use it. One terminology would eliminate confusion about the terms and meaning. However, no single medical language exists for healthcare (Levy, 2004) and the same can be said for nursing. In a national healthcare environment that supports many types of delivery, reflecting the entire scope of nursing practice is difficult.

The idea of one terminology, however, is appealing. Although that goal has not yet been attained, the ICNP is working toward this aim (Rutherford, 2008) by attempting to establish a common language for nursing practice. Many of the ANA-recognized nursing-focused terminologies have been mapped to the ICNP.

Today, with the exception of a few medical centers where one or more standardized nursing terminology is used, most nurses do not have a background in using standardized terminologies. Many completed their formal education before the nursing terminologies were readily available. As a result, there is a lack of understanding of what a standardized terminology is and a lack of recognition of its importance in improving nursing care (Kripps, 2008). In this climate, even when it is taught to students, they soon discover that it is not actually used in practice and indeed is often derided.

The task of trying to implement standardized terminologies faces the additional challenges of some nurses who do not see the value of standardization and regard it as a waste of time (Kripps, 2008). Furthermore, there is an insufficient number of nursing informaticists who realize the importance of standardized terminologies; hence, their use is not yet demanded in electronic documentation systems.

Given this background, when standardized terminologies are implemented the nursing staff needs much education and retraining in it uses (Correll & Martin, 2009; Hendrix, 2009; Klehr, Hafner, Spelz, Steen, & Weaver, 2009; Kripps, 2008). Energy is also required to sustain the documentation once it is implemented. Constant attention needs to be paid to the accuracy of the data entered. There is evidence that nurses' interpretation of data differs (Lunney, 2008) with the result that some of the interpretations represent low accuracy and incorrect nursing diagnoses. "This is serious because low diagnostic accuracy contributes to harm to patients through: wasted time and energy, implementing ineffective interventions, absence of positive outcomes, and patient and family dissatisfaction" (Lunney, 2008). However, the problem of inaccurate diagnoses of nursing problems exists whether standardized terminology is used or not. With standardized terminology, it becomes easier to identify and rectify.

Despite difficulties, if nursing is to gain visibility, there is no choice but to move forward with using standardized terminologies. Standardized terminologies are not a panacea and do not obviate the need for critical thinking and creative work (Hardiker, 2009); they merely supports the documentation of nursing's role, both in interventions and cognitively. They are a means to an end, the end being the improvement of patient care by using knowledge hidden in our documentation and identifying care that under too many circumstances is never recorded, and hence, not valued.

Summary

Using standardized nursing terminologies for nursing care involves changes in traditional thinking about documentation. There is much knowledge that is currently concealed in nursing data that could be uncovered with the use of standardized terminologies. As with other healthcare disciplines, there are many gaps in what is needed for documentation with standardized terminologies. Creating and using standardized terminology is a relatively new phenomenon. Its importance was brought about by the use of electronic records. Standardized nursing terminologies provide data that can be used in linking assessments, interventions, and outcomes, as well as linkages to the literature. Documentation data uncovered with nursing research will make nursing's contributions to healthcare visible.

One impediment for implementing nursing terminology is not outside forces, but the culture of nursing. Nursing history as well as the fact that nursing has been primarily a feminine occupation has contributed to our not voicing opinions or making our contributions known. Old customs of communicating to physicians with comments such as "The patient appears to be bleeding" instead of stating it as a fact have also been a contributing factor. Fortunately, this type of communication is no longer prevalent, but the mind set behind it lingers along with our historical legacies. If we are to truly become valued for our healthcare contributions, we will need to take over responsibility for our nursing actions, visibly label them, and support one another in using the terminologies. Only we as nurses can accomplish this.

APPLICATIONS AND COMPETENCIES

1. List the uses of patient documentation in health planning. Compare these purposes with the documentation format used in a clinical area with which you arefamiliar. What conclusions can be drawn?

2. Match the data that you collect from a patient with potential uses beyond the care of an individual patient. Which of these data could be used to document?

3. Think of some cases in which nursing interventions are not electronically documented, yet can affect outcomes. What solutions would you recommend?

4. Discuss the concept of the invisibility of nursing.
   a. How prevalent do you see it as being?
   b. What actions can change this?

5. Why is it necessary for nursing documentation to contain comparable data?

6. Describe the differences between interface mode and reference mode terminologies.

7. The use of the ICNP in Korea keeps free text to a minimum; however, when free text is audited, the most frequent item found is "Slept well." What would be the most common phrase if your narrative documentation were analyzed?

8. How would you compromise between the need for free text in nursing documentation and the need for structured documentation?

9. How do you see the thinking about documentation and nursing changing with the use of standardized terminologies?

10. List some benefits of using standardized terminologies in your work setting.

REFERENCES

Aiken, L. H., Clarke, S. P., Sloane, D. M., Sochalski, J., & Silber, J. H. (2002). Hospital nurse staffing and patient mortality, nurse burnout, and job dissatisfaction. *Journal of the American Medical Association, 288*, 1987–1993.

American Nurses Association. (2007, June 5). *Relationships among ANA recognized data element sets and terminologies.* Retrieved February 16, 2011, from http://www.nursing-world.org/npii/relationship.htm

Association of periOperating Room Nurses. (2011). *The PNDS model.* Retrieved February 11, 2011, from http://www.aorn.org/PracticeResources/PNDSAndStandardizedPerioperativeRecord/PNDSModel/

Baker, J. D. (2005). Specialty nomenclature: A worthwhile challenge. *Gastroenterol Nursing, 28*(1), 52–55.

Boyd, A. D., Funk, E. A., Schwartz, S. M., Kaplan, B., & Keenan, G. M. (2010). Top EHR challenges in light of the stimulus: Enabling effective interdisciplinary, intradisciplinary and cross-setting communication. *Journal of Healthcare Information Management, 24*(1), 18–24.

Center for Nursing Classification & Clinical Effectiveness. (n.d.-a). *Nursing Interventions Classification (NIC).* Retrieved February 13, 2011, from http://www.nursing.uiowa.edu/excellence/nursing_knowledge/clinical_effectiveness/nicoverview.htm

Center for Nursing Classification & Clinical Effectiveness. (n.d.-b). *Nursing Outcomes Classification (NOC).* Retrieved February 11, 2011, from http://www.nursing.uiowa.edu/excellence/nursing_knowledge/clinical_effectiveness/nocoverview.htm

Center for Nursing Minimum Data Set Knowledge. (2009, May 26). *USA NMDS.* Retrieved February 11, 2011, from http://www.nursing.umn.edu/ICNP/USANMDS/

Center for Nursing Minimum Data Set Knowledge. (2010, January 7). *USA NMMDS.* Retrieved February, 2011, from http://www.nursing.umn.edu/ICNP/USANMMDS/

Correll, P. J., & Martin, K. S. (2009). The Omaha System helps a public health nursing organization find its voice. *CIN: Computers, Informatics, Nursing, 27*(1), 12–16.

Dochterman, J. M., Bulechek, G. M., & Iowa Intervention Project. (1992). *Nursing interventions classification (NIC): Iowa Intervention Project.* St. Louis, MO: Mosby Year Book.

Free Merriam-Webster Dictionary. (2011). *Ontology.* Retrieved February 10, 2011, from http://www.merriam-webster.com/dictionary/ontology

Friedman, E. (1990). Troubled past of "invisible" profession. *Journal of the American Medical Association, 264*(22), 2851–2855, 2858.

Gordon, M. (1998). Nursing nomenclature and classification system development. *Online Journal of Issues in Nursing, 3*(2). Retrieved from http://www.nursingworld.org/MainMenuCategories/ANAMarketplace/ANAPeriodicals/OJIN/TableofContents/Vol31998/No2Sept1998/NomenclatureandClassification.aspx

Hampton Robb, I. (1909). *Report of the third regular meeting of the International Council of Nurses.* Geneva: ICN.

Hannah, K. J., White, P. A., Nagle, L. M., & Pringle, D. M. (2009). Standardizing nursing information in Canada for inclusion in electronic health records: C-HOBIC. [Research Support, Non-U.S. Gov't]. *Journal of the American Medical Informatics Association, 16*(4), 524–530. Doi: 10.1197/jamia.M2974

Hansten, R., & Washburn, M. J. (1998). Professional practice: Facts and impact. *American Journal of Nursing, 98*(3), 42–45.

Hardiker, N. (2009). Developing standardized terminologies in nursing. In D. McConigle & K. Mastrian (Eds.), *Nursing informatics and the foundation of knowledge* (pp. 97–105). Sudbury, MA: Jones & Bartlett.

Harmer, B. (1926). *Methods and principles of teaching the principles and practice of nursing.* New York, NY: Macmillan.

Hendrix, S. E. (2009). An experience with implementation of NIC and NOC in a clinical information system. *CIN: Computers, Informatics, Nursing, 27*(1), 7–11.

Hoehn, B. J. (2009). The pen is the tongue of the mind: developing a strategy for computerizing provider documentation. *Journal of Healthcare Information Management, 23*(3), 10–11.

Huber, D., Schumacher, L., & Delaney, C. (1997). Nursing Management Minimum Data Set (NMMDS). *Journal of Nursing Administration, 27*(4), 42–48.

Huffman, E. K., Price, E., & American Medical Record Association. (1972). *Medical record management* (6th ed.). Berwyn, IL: Physicians' Record Co.

Hyun, S., Johnson, S. B., & Bakken, S. (2009). Exploring the ability of natural language processing to extract data from nursing narratives. *CIN: Computers, Informatics, Nursing, 27*(4), 215–223; quiz 224–215.

International Council of Nursing. (2009). *Nursing matters: International Classification for Nursing Practice.* Retrieved February 16, 2011, from http://www.icn.ch/images/stories/documents/publications/fact_sheets/3a_FS-ICNP.pdf

International Council of Nurses. (2010). *International Nursing Minimal Data Set (i-NDMS).* Retrieved February 12, 2011, from http://www.icn.ch/pillarsprograms/international-nursing-minimum-data-set-i-nmdsseptember-2007/

International Health Terminology Standards Development Organisation. (n.d.). *History of SNOWMED CT.* Retrieved February 16, 2011, from http://www.ihtsdo.org/snomed-ct/history0/

Keenan, G. M. (1999). Use of standardized nursing language will make nursing visible. *Michigan Nurse, 72*(2), 12–13.

Klehr, J., Hafner, J., Spelz, L. M., Steen, S., & Weaver, K. (2009). Implementation of standardized nomenclature in the electronic medical record. *International Journal of Nursing Terminologies and Classifications, 20*(4), 169–180.

Kleinbeck, S. V. (2002). Revising the perioperative nursing data set. *AORN Journal, 75*(3), 602, 605–610.

Kripps, B. J. (2008). Toward standardized nursing terminology: The next steps. *Caring Newsletter, 23*(3), 4–8. Retrieved from http://www.thefreelibrary.com/oward+standardized+nursing+terminology%3A+the+next+steps.-a0187327610

Lang, N., Saba, V. K., Hudgings, C. J., Stenvig, T. E., Jacox, A., & Zielstorff, R. D. (1995). Toward a national database for nursing practice. In N. Lang (Ed.), *Emerging Framework: Data System Advances for Clinical Nursing Practice* (pp. 7–17). Washington, DC: American Nurses Publishing.

Levy, B. (2004). Evolving to clinical terminology. *Journal of Healthcare Information Management, 18*(3), 37–43.

Lunney, M. (2008). Critical need to address accuracy of nurses' diagnoses. *Online Journal of Issues in Nursing, 13*(1). Retrieved from http://www.nursingworld.org/MainMenuCategories/ANAMarketplace/ANAPeriodicals/OJIN/TableofContents/vol132008/No1Jan08/ArticlePreviousTopic/AccuracyofNursesDiagnoses.aspx

Martin, K. S., Monsen, K. A., & Riemer, J. G. (2010, September 17). *The Omaha System*. Retrieved February 11, 2011, from http://www.omahasystem.org/

Marvin, M. M. (2010). Research in nursing. 1927. *American Journal of Nursing, 110*(10), 65–69.

McCloskey, J. C., & Bulechek, G. M. (1994). Standardizing the language for nursing treatments: An overview of the issues. *Nursing Outlook, 42*(2), 56–63.

McCormick, K., & Jones, C. (1998). Is one taxonomy needed for health care vocabularies and classifications? *Online Journal of Issues in Nursing, 3*(2). Retrieved from http://www.nursingworld.org/MainMenuCategories/ANAMarketplace/ANAPeriodicals/OJIN/TableofContents/Vol31998/No2Sept1998/Isonetaxonomyneeded.aspx

Medical News Today. (2007, January 15). Hospital death rate study reveals wide variations and stresses importance of registered nurses. *Medical News Today*. Retrieved February 8, 2011, from http://www.medicalnewstoday.com/articles/60785.php

North American Nursing Diagnosis Association. (2011). *Nursing diagnosis frequently asked questions*. Retrieved February 13, 2011, from http://www.nanda.org/NursingDiagnosisFAQ.aspx#NDxBasics

Needleman, J., Buerhaus, P. I., Mattke, S., Stewart, M., & Zelevinsky, K. (2001). *Nurse staffing and patient outcomes in hospitals (2001): Executive summary*. Retrieved February 8, 2011, from ftp://ftp.hrsa.gov/bhpr/nursing/staffstudy/staffexecsum.pdf

Needleman, J., Buerhaus, P., Mattke, S., Stewart, M., & Zelevinsky, K. (2002). Nurse-staffing levels and the quality of care in hospitals. *The New England Journal of Medicine, 346*(22), 1715–1722.

Nightingale, F. (1860). *Notes on nursing: What it is and what it is not* (1st American ed.). New York, NY: D. Appleton.

Nightingale, F., & Goldie, S. M. (1997). Letters from the Crimea, 1854–1856. Retrieved from http://preview.tinyurl.com/2auahra

Ozbolt, J. G. (2000). Terminology Standards for nursing: Collaboration at the summit [electronic version]. *Journal of the American Medical Informatics Association, 7*(6), 517–522.

Park, H.-A. (2007). *International perspectives on nursing terminology and data standards*. Paper presented at the Summer Institute in Nursing Informatics, Baltimore, MD.

Regenstrief Institute. (2011). *Logical Observation Identifiers Names and Codes (LOINC®)*. Retrieved February 16, 2011, from http://loinc.org/

Rutherford, M. (2008). Standardized nursing language: What does it mean for nursing practice? *Online Journal of Issues in Nursing, 13*(1). Retrieved from http://www.nursingworld.org/MainMenuCategories/ANAMarketplace/ANAPeriodicals/OJIN/TableofContents/vol132008/No1Jan08/ArticlePreviousTopic/StandardizedNursingLanguage.aspx

Saba, V. K. (2011). *Clinical Care Classification System™*. Retrieved February 11, 2011, from http://www.sabacare.com/

Saba, V. K., & McCormick, K. A. (2006). *Essentials of nursing informatics* (4th ed.). New York, NY: McGraw-Hill.

School of Mathematics and Statistics, St. Andrews University Scotland. (2003). *Florence Nightingale*. Retrieved July 31, 2010, from http://www-history.mcs.st-andrews.ac.uk/Biographies/Nightingale.html

Simpson, R. L. (1997). Technology: Nursing the system. The Nursing Management Minimum Data Set initiative needs you! *Nursing Management, 28*(6), 20–21.

Stanfill, M. H., Williams, M., Fenton, S. H., Jenders, R. A., & Hersh, W. R. (2010). A systematic literature review of automated clinical coding and classification systems. *Journal of the American Medical Informatics Association, 17*(6), 646–651.

Thede, L., & Schwiran, P. (2011). Informatics: The standardized nursing terminologies: A national survey of nurses' experiences and attitudes. *OJIN: The Online Journal of Issues in Nursing. 16*(2). DOI: 10.3912/OJIN.Vol16No02InfoCol01. Retrieved August 31, 2011, from http://www.nursingworld.org/MainMenuCategories/ANAMarketplace/ANAPeriodicals/OJIN/TableofContents/Vol-16-2011/No2-May-2011/Standardized-Nursing-Terminologies.aspx

U.S. National Library of Medicine. (2010). *SNOWMED Clinical Terms®*. Retrieved February 16, 2011, from http://www.nlm.nih.gov/research/umls/Snomed/snomed_main.html

Ware, H., Mullett, C. J., & Jagannathan, V. (2009). Natural language processing framework to assess clinical conditions. *Journal of the American Medical Informatics Association, 16*(4), 585–589.

Werley, H. H., & Lang, N. M. (Eds.). (1988). *Identification of the nursing minimum data set*. New York, NY: Springer.

Westra, B. L., Delaney, C. W., Konicek, D., & Keenan, G. (2008). Nursing standards to support the electronic health record. *Nursing Outlook, 56*(5), 258–266, e251.

Westra, B. L., Goosen, W., Choromanski, L. M., Collins, B. J., Hart, C. M., & Delaney, C. (2010). Application of iNMDS using ICNP. In C. Weaver, C. Delaney, P. Weber, & R. L. Carr (Eds.), *Nursing and informatics for the 21st century: An international look at practice, education, and EHR trends* (2nd ed., pp. 262–268). Chicago, IL: Healthcare Information and Management Systems Society.

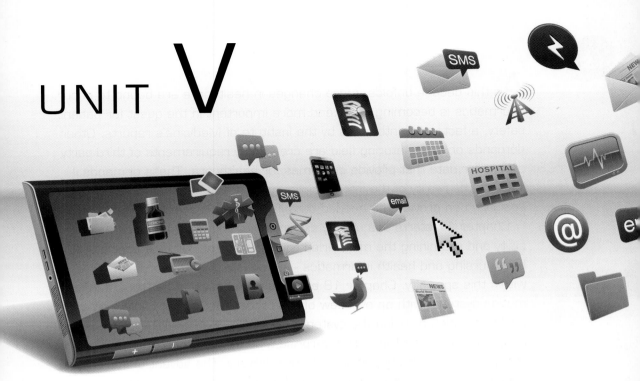

UNIT V

Healthcare Informatics

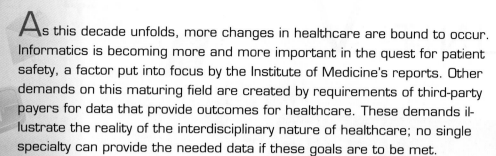

As this decade unfolds, more changes in healthcare are bound to occur. Informatics is becoming more and more important in the quest for patient safety, a factor put into focus by the Institute of Medicine's reports. Other demands on this maturing field are created by requirements of third-party payers for data that provide outcomes for healthcare. These demands illustrate the reality of the interdisciplinary nature of healthcare; no single specialty can provide the needed data if these goals are to be met.

Chapter 17 starts this unit by exploring nursing informatics as a specialty and examining the multivaried roles in this specialty – a specialty in both nursing and health informatics – as well as the standards for roles within this specialty. Chapter 18 examines the basics of healthcare information systems with an overview of the process for system selection and implementation by using the systems' life cycle. Chapter 19 explores healthcare information systems as enterprise-wide systems designed to improve the quality and efficiency of patient care delivery. The advent of informatics opportunities is associated with new challenges. Chapter 20 discusses some of the unresolved issues associated with clinical information systems. Finally, Chapter 21 discusses some of the cutting-edge telehealth developments in which care is provided or monitored by healthcare professionals in another location.

CHAPTER 17

The Informatics Discipline

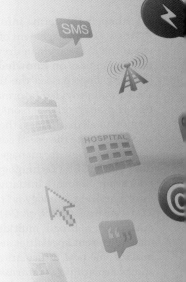

Objectives

After studying this chapter you will be able to:

- ▶ *Describe seven theories on which informatics relies.*

- ▶ *Differentiate between the roles of informatics nurses and nursing informatics specialists.*

- ▶ *Evaluate whether a specific nursing informatics educational program is appropriate for your career goals.*

- ▶ *Analyze nursing informatics roles for all nurses.*

- ▶ *Identify professional health informatics groups.*

Key Terms

Alliance for Nursing
   Informatics (ANI)
ANIA-CARING (American
   Nursing Informatics
   Association – Capital Area
   Roundtable on Informatics
   in Nursing)
American Health Information
   Management Association
   (AHIMA)
American Medical
   Informatics Association
   (AMIA)
British Computer Society (BCS)
Data
Driving Force
Early Adopter
Early Majority
European Federation for
   Medical Informatics (EFMI)
Healthcare Informatics
Healthcare Information
   Management Systems
   Society (HIMSS)

Informatics Nurse
Informatics Nurse Specialist
Information
Informatics Theory
Innovator
Input
International Medical
   Informatics Association
   (IMIA)
Knowledge
Laggard
Late Majority
Moving
Nursing Informatics
Nursing Informatics Working
   Group (NIWG)
Output
Refreezing
Restraining Force
Social Informatics
Sociotechnical Theory
Throughput
Unfreezing
Wisdom

Although the term "informatics"[1] is relatively new, the management of **information** started when the first caveman drew pictures to communicate and pass on **knowledge**. Society, however, has long since passed the time when pictures on a cave wall provided information. While information is managed by persons and in a coordinated fashion in all disciplines, the term informatics has come to denote the use of computers and information technology to manage healthcare information. The TIGER (Technology Informatics Guiding Education Reform) Initiative Report states that information technology is "the stethoscope of the 21st century" (2009, p. 24). **Healthcare informatics** is a broad multidisciplinary field with many different specialties such as **nursing informatics**, medical informatics, dental informatics, and pharmaceutical informatics. Generally, those who practice in their discipline's subspecialty are also licensed in their own profession such as nursing or dentistry. Health informatics is also broad enough to include subspecialties that are multidisciplinary, for example, social and consumer informatics. Despite all the subspecialties in healthcare informatics, a primary goal is interdisciplinary data management that facilitates holistic health and community health.

Nursing Informatics as a Specialty

Nursing is a subspecialty in informatics, with roles and tasks in both disciplines. The focus of **informatics nurses** varies with their job and specialty in healthcare, but the focus of nursing informatics is in one of the following seven areas (NCNR Priority Expert Panel on Nursing Informatics, 1993):

1. using **data**, information, and knowledge for patient care
2. defining data in patient care
3. acquiring and delivering patient care knowledge
4. creating new tools for patient care from new technologies
5. applying ergonomics to nurse–computer interfaces

6. integrating systems
7. evaluating the effects of nursing systems.

Practice in each of these areas requires different knowledge and skills on the part of the **informatics nurse specialist**. These areas can be matched with Warner's five categories of what people in medical informatics do: "(1) signal processing, (2) database design, (3) decision making, (4) modeling and simulation, and (5) optimizing the interface between the human and the machine" (Warner, 1995, p. 207). These areas are compared in **Table 17-1**.

Ozbolt, Nahm, and Roberts (2007) state that those who enter the nursing informatics field with on-the-job training are informatics nurses and those with either a degree in nursing informatics or a postgraduate training are informatics nurse specialists. Some would probably say that the first informatics nurse specialist was Florence Nightingale, despite her lack of a formal educational program, given that the fundamental building block in informatics is data. Recognizing the value of data in effecting healthcare, she collected data and systematized record-keeping practices in Crimea (Nightingale & Goldie, 1997). Using these data, she developed the first version of the pie graph known as a "polar area diagram" or "coxcombs" to dramatize the need for reform to stop the needless deaths caused by the unsanitary conditions in military hospitals (School of Mathematics and Statistics, St. Andrews University Scotland, 2003). With the advent of the computer, the use of data has become far easier and more widespread than it was in Ms. Nightingale's time.

When decisions are based on the data available, collection and analysis of nursing data become very important. Without nursing data, the value of nursing will continue to be hidden to those in policy-making positions. Through nursing informatics, the healthcare information systems that are being developed can include the nursing data needed to improve patient care and show the value that nurses add to healthcare.

One of the main objectives of nursing informatics in the clinical area is to integrate data from all areas pertinent to nursing care and present it in a manner that enables the clinical nurse to provide quality care. Many sources of information

---

1 Definitions of informatics are in Chapter 1.

Table 17-1 Categories of Informatics Tasks

Task	Warner's Description of Task	Nursing Informatics Areas of Focus from Pillar and Golumbic
Obtaining and processing	Data must be obtained from diverse	Acquiring patient care knowledge
Data	Sources including, but not limited to, clinician input, diagnostic device, patient registration, insurance information, research, systematic reviews, practice guidelines	Integration of systems
Database design	Identification and definition of data needed and designing data storage so that it can be retrieved by others	Identifying and defining of data needed in patient care
Decision making	Restructuring of data and its presentation in a manner that facilitates decision making	Using data, information, and knowledge for patient care. Creating patient care knowledge
Modeling and simulation	Building of structural models that provide insight into the data. Purpose is to increase knowledge from the data	Creating new tools for patient care from new technologies Evaluating the effects of nursing systems
Optimizing the human interface	Improving the method that humans use to gain meaning from the output. Involves not only screen design and navigation, but also how the data is structured. Educating users	Applying ergonomics to nurse–computer interfaces

Adapted from Warner, H. (1995). Medical informatics: A real discipline? *Journal of the American Medical Informatics Association,* 2(4), 207–214; Pillar, B., & Golumbic, N. (Eds.). (1993). *Nursing informatics: Enhancing patient care.* Bethesda, MD: National Center for Nursing Research, U.S. Department of Health and Human Services.

are needed for patient care. These were broadly classified into four areas by Corcoran-Perry and Graves (1990), who studied the information needs of practicing cardiovascular nurses as outlined in **Table 17-2**. The overall goal in nursing informatics is to optimize information management and

communication to improve individual healthcare and the health of populations (American Nurses Association [ANA], 2008).

In 1992, the ANA recognized nursing informatics as a specialty with the first certification examination held in 1995. The prerequisites for

Table 17-2 Information Sources for Patient Care

Information about the patient	Documentation. History and physical, medications and laboratory reports, demographic information, and information about the patient's support system
Institutional information	Data of immediate concern such as tracking a piece of equipment or an individual as well as agency policies for admission criteria, release of information, and confidentiality of patient data. Information needed for external bodies, such as that needed for reporting to third-party payers, regulatory agencies, and policy-making bodies
Domain knowledge	Nursing knowledge as well as knowledge from related disciplines, literature, and clinical experiences
Procedural knowledge	Focuses on the procedures for performing tasks such as starting an intravenous line

Adapted from Corcoran-Perry, S., & Graves, J. R. (1990). Supplemental-information-seeking behavior of cardiovascular nurses. *Research in Nursing & Health, 13*(2), 119–127.

writing the examination for certification include a bachelor's degree, an active registered nurse (RN) license, 2 years of practice as an RN, and 30 hours of continuing education in informatics within the last 3 years. The applicant must also meet *one* of the following three practice requirements (American Nurses Credentialing Center, 2010):

1. 2,000 hours in informatics nursing within the last 3 years
2. A minimum of 1,000 hours in informatics nursing in the last 3 years plus completion of a minimum of 12 hours of academic credit in informatics courses as part of a graduate level informatics nursing program
3. Completion of a graduate program in nursing informatics containing a minimum of 200 hours of a faculty-supervised practicum in informatics

Passing the examination provides certification for 5 years at which time the certification can be renewed if specified educational and practice requirements are fulfilled.

The third edition of the *ANA Nursing Informatics: The Scope and Standards Practice* is now available. The publication outlines the characteristics of the specialty, defines the specialty, and describes how it differs from other health and nursing specialties (ANA, 2008). It also explains in detail the basic theories behind nursing informatics, presents a discussion of the sciences that provide a foundation for informatics, and discusses standardized nursing terminologies and the importance of interoperability. The publication is a necessary basic reference for anyone interested in the field.

Theories That Lend Support to Informatics

Although information has been managed in one way or another since the beginning of time, in the early 1900s as society became more complex, theories about managing information developed. Information theory itself is a mathematical theory about communication, with the goal of finding the limits on reliably compressing, storing, and communicating data, and is a branch of applied probability theory (Gray,

2009; Schneider, 2010). **Informatics theory** builds not just on information theory, but uses concepts from change theories, systems theory, chaos theory, cognitive theory, and **sociotechnical theory**.

Nursing Informatics Theory

Nursing informatics theory is concerned with the representation of nursing data, information, and knowledge to facilitate the management and communication of nursing information within the healthcare milieu. It focuses on nursing phenomena and provides a nursing perspective, clarifies nursing values and beliefs, produces new knowledge, and develops standardized nursing terminology for use in electronic records. Graves and Corcoran (1989), in their seminal article on nursing informatics, devised an information model for nursing informatics based on Bloom's taxonomy. This model identified data, information, and knowledge as the key components of nursing informatics. **Wisdom** was first added to this structure by Nelson and Joos (as cited in Joos, Whitman, Smith, & Nelson, 1992) shortly thereafter, but it was the 2008 ANA *Nursing Informatics: Scope and Standards of Practice* that officially made this a part of the nursing informatics model.

Data

Data are discrete, objective facts that have not been interpreted (Clark, 2009) or are out of context; they are at the atomic level. Data are described objectively without interpretation. They are the building blocks of meaning but lack context, and hence are meaningless.

Information

Information is data that have some type of interpretation or structure; that is, it has a context. It is derived from combining different pieces of data (Clark, 2009). A set of data, such as vital signs, when interpreted over a period of time is information.

Knowledge

Knowledge is a synthesis of information with relationships identified and formalized. It changes something or somebody by creating the setting for formulating possible effective actions, evaluating their effects, and deciding on the required action (Clark, 2009). For example, interpreting a set of vital signs over a period of time and deciding on an action based on this information combined with nursing knowledge and experience is an example of knowledge.

Wisdom

Wisdom is achieved through evaluating knowledge with reflection. It involves seeing patterns and metapatterns and using them in different ways (Clark, 2009) and knowing when and how to apply knowledge to a situation (ANA, 2008). For example, wisdom would be interpreting vital signs in a postsurgical patient as indicative of an infection and taking the appropriate action.

The Continuum

The above concepts are constructs, not absolutes, and are a continuum or an analog process. The examples given are very simplified and are used to help you grasp the process of converting data into wisdom. Where something falls on the continuum depends on the person or situation. A nurse with 10 years of experience may possess a great deal of tacit knowledge. This is the knowledge that has been earned with experience and reflection, but the knowledge is so ingrained that it is difficult for the nurse to verbalize or acknowledge. Nonetheless, this tacit knowledge provides a higher level of wisdom than that possessed by a new graduate. For a

less experienced nurse, wisdom may be identical to knowledge in an experienced nurse.

The general idea of informatics theory is that the move from data to knowledge is a progressive process that follows a given path. As one moves up the continuum, each level becomes more complex and requires intellect that is more human. In practice, one finds the lines between each of these entities are blurred and that the process is iterative. The processes of converting data into knowledge include capturing, sorting, organizing, storing, retrieving, and presenting the data to give it meaning and produce information.

Figure 17-1 is a simplification of this continuum, one that might apply to a nursing student or a new graduate. In this figure, data are combined to produce information, and information is combined to produce knowledge. As another example, the number 37 is a piece of datum. It is the smallest unit that can be processed. If we combine the number 37 with the datum that this is a Celsius temperature for a person, we now have some information. Combining this still further with the information that this is the normal body temperature, we have a small piece of knowledge. The individual adds wisdom by deciding on the action, if any, to take because of this knowledge.

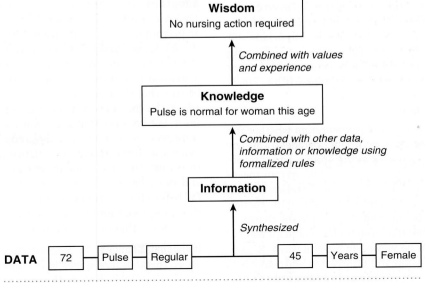

Figure 17-1 Progression of data to wisdom.

Sociotechnical Theory and Social Informatics

Sociotechnical theory developed in the middle of the last century when it became evident that not all implementations of technology were increasing productivity. The overall focus is the impact of technology's implementation on an organization. To this end, it focuses on the interactions of an organization between information management tools and techniques and the knowledge, skills, attitudes, values, and needs of its employees as well as the rewards and authority structures of the employer (Wade & Schneberger, 2005). Its precepts can increase the understanding of how information systems should be developed (Berg, Aarts, & van der Lei, 2003).

Introducing an information system is a social process that deeply affects an organization. Research based on sociotechnical theory is aimed at maximizing performance by designing or redesigning systems that fit the organizational system into which they are implanted. The sociotechnical point of view, which is the basis of **social informatics**, holds that a good design is based on an understanding of how people work and the context of the work, not just technologic considerations (Sawyer & Rosenbaum, 2000). The importance of social informatics is well evidenced by the failure of many information systems including the much publicized shutdown by Cedars-Lebanon Hospital in Los Angeles in early 2003 of their multimillion dollar computerized physician order entry. This system created a change that was seen as too radical by the physicians who believed that their interests were not sufficiently represented, the system was jammed down their throats, and that it was poorly designed (Chin, 2003).

Change Theories

Instituting a change in documentation whether it is relatively simple such as a minor upgrade to a system or major one such as **moving** from a paper record to a completely paperless electronic system means change. "What will this mean to me?" is always uppermost in everyone's mind when faced with change. Whether affected individuals perceive the change as minor or major differs from individual to individual.

Change can be viewed in several ways. Rogers' theory of diffusion and innovation addresses how change occurs in a society and in an individual.

Lewin's Field Theory talks about stages in moving people and enterprises from a comfortable state before the change, through the discomfort of change, and finally back to a comfort with the change. Ignoring the psychosocial nature of changing information management is too often a one-way ticket to failure of the system.

Rogers' Diffusion of Innovation Theory

Rogers' theory, the diffusion of innovations, was first published in his book of the same name in 1962. This theory examines the pattern of acceptance that innovations follow as they spread across the population and the process of decision making that occurs in individuals when deciding whether to adopt an innovation. It was based on depression era rural research that studied how Midwestern farmers adopted hardier corn (Rogers, 2003). This theory is still timely in North America and other parts of the world.

Societal Changes. Rogers divides people into five categories to view how innovations are accepted by the general population (Rogers, 2003). **Innovators**, the first category, readily adopt the innovation. They constitute a very small percentage, about 2.5% of the population. These persons are often seen as disruptive by those who are averse to risk taking, and are not able to sell others on the innovation. This job is left to the next category, **early adopters**, who comprise 13.5% of the population. They are respectable opinion leaders who function as promoters of an innovation. The next group is the **early majority** (34%) who is averse to risks, but will make safe investments. The **late majority**, who make up another 34% of the adopters, need to be sure that the innovation is beneficial. They may adopt the innovation not because they see a use for it, but because of peer pressure. The last group, comprising 16%, is termed **laggards**. They are suspicious of innovations and change and are quite resistant. They see their resistance as a rationale and must be certain that the innovation will not fail before they can adopt it. Instead of discounting this group, we should be listening. They may grasp weaknesses that others fail to see.

Individual Changes. In Rogers' theory, individuals go through five stages in deciding to adopt an innovation. Like all stage theories, progress is not uniform, and adopters can show behaviors from more than one stage at a time or revert completely to an earlier stage. The first stage is knowledge of an innovation in which the potential adopter gains an understanding of how the innovation operates (Rogers, 2003). This can occur passively, either through education or advertisements, or actively in response to a felt need or incentives. The second stage, persuasion, is based on the perception of the relative advantage of the innovation, compatibility with existing norms, and its observability. At this stage, an individual forms an opinion about the innovation, negative, neutral, or positive. In the third stage, the individual uses his opinions to make a decision. A potential adopter may try the innovation or base an opinion on the experience and opinion of a respected peer who has tried the innovation. The individual then decides to either adopt or reject the innovation. If the decision is positive, the fourth stage, or implementation, follows. At this stage, the adopter wants knowledge, such as how to use the innovation and how to overcome problems with its use. Confirmation, or the fifth stage, may occur when reinforcement of the decision is sought. Conflicting information about the innovation may cause the adopter to reverse a decision.

Lewin's Field Theory

Rogers' theory identified the stages that individuals go through in making a change, whereas Lewin's field theory provides a guide to helping individuals achieve a positive decision in relation to an innovation. This theory holds that human behavior is related to both personal characteristics and the social milieu in which the individual exists (Smith, 2009). It focuses on the variables that need to be recognized and observed in a situation of change and uses these variables to create a model of the stages that occur during change. Lewin divides these changes into three stages or force fields: **unfreezing**, moving, and **refreezing**. Ways of moving a group from the first to the last stage need to be part of a plan for implementation of a system.

Unfreezing. This stage is based on the idea that a balance of driving and **restraining forces** that creates equilibrium supports human behavior. To institute change, the driving and restraining forces that are part of the maintenance of equilibrium in the organizational culture and individual have to be changed. To unfreeze, one must identify and change the balance so that the **driving forces** are stronger than the restraining forces. Driving forces can be involvement in the process, respect of one's opinion, and continuous communication during the process. Unfortunately, restraining forces are harder to identify and treat because they are often personal psychologic defenses or group norms embedded in the organizational or community culture (see **Figure 17-2**).

Moving. In this stage, the planned change is implemented. Its success depends on how situations were

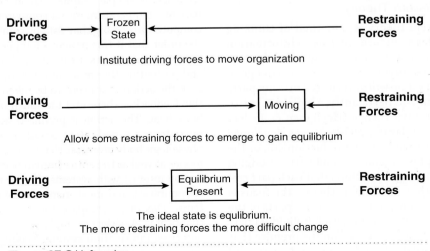

Figure 17-2 Unfreezing.

handled in the first stage. This is not a comfortable period. Anxieties are high, and if they are not successfully dealt with, the change may be unsuccessful. Additionally, it is important to recognize that in this stage, movement may occur in the wrong direction. This is especially likely to happen if the new system has many problems, if it is not supported by administration, or if it has had no end-user involvement. Thus, it is important to have the support of administration in the planning process, involve users so that the system serves them instead of creating more work, thoroughly test the system before implementation for both bugs and usability, provide adequate training, and deal with any implementation problems immediately. In the Cedars-Lebanon case, the system created more work and resulted in a movement in the wrong direction despite a decree that all people must use the system (Bass, 2003). Decrees do not "move" people.

Refreezing. In this stage, equilibrium returns as the planned change becomes the norm and it is surrounded by the usual driving and restraining forces. For this state to occur, individuals need to feel confident with the change and feel in control of the procedures involved in the new methods. A well-designed help system that can provide answers to frequent procedures as well as those that a user may use only occasionally will assist in this process, as will recognition by the organization of new skills. If too strongly reinforced, this stage can become a problem for the next change.

General System Theory

General system theory is a method of thinking about complex structures such as an information system or an organization. A simplified description of systems theory holds that any change in one part of a system will be reflected in other parts of the system. Von Bertalanffy, a biologist, introduced the original theory (Heylighen & Joslyn, 1992; von Bertalanffy, 1973). It was developed in part as a reaction against reductionism, or the reducing of phenomena to small parts, studying each, and ignoring the actions that each part creates in the other. In systems theory, the focus is on the interaction among the various parts of the system instead of regarding each individual part as standing alone. It is based on the premise that the whole is greater than the sum of its parts and is the basis for holistic nursing.

To be part of a system, a phenomenon must be able to be isolated from its surrounding area for analysis, yet be part of the functioning of the whole system. Systems are described as being either open or closed. An open system continually exchanges information with the environment outside the system, while a closed system receives no **input** from the outside. This classification is more of a continuum than an absolute. Few, if any systems, are 100% closed or 100% open.

The objective of any system is to be in equilibrium, which is maintained by the correction forces from a feedback loop. Negative feedback results when there is a lack of something. The action it produces is to add the missing item to restore a variable to its state of equilibrium. Positive feedback results when there is too much of something. The action in positive feedback is to take away the excess. These two concepts can be confusing until one remembers that positive feedback results when the system finds too much of something and negative feedback when it finds something missing. Whether feedback is positive or negative is based on what the system finds, not its action.

The feedback loop operates using input, **throughput**, and **output**. Input involves adding information or matter to a system. Throughput is the processing, or evaluation of the input, that the system performs using the input information; output is the information or action that results from what the processing finds. This output may produce no action, or the action needed from either negative or positive feedback. A simple example would be inputting a patient's temperature into a computer system, the computer processing that data by combining it with the order that if this patient's temperature is more than 101°F, a specific medication should be given, and presenting the information to the nurse along with the action that needs to be taken. This is positive feedback – there was too much of something, body heat. The action it produced was to tell the nurse to give a medication. Another example is the physiologic body processes that are governed by hormones as well as the entire human body.

You interact with systems all your life. Families, communities, and most inanimate objects are systems. The more complex the system, the more chaotic it is. A perfect example of a system is a computerized information system. Making a change in one area invariably affects other sections in ways that were never envisioned, which explains why it is often not a simple matter to make desired changes in systems. Adding an information system to a health-care agency produces an even more complicated system. Systems theory provides a way of studying both the information system itself and its interaction with the environment. These interactions are also the focus of sociotechnical theory, but that theory would frame the problem in a different way.

Chaos Theory

Chaos theory was first encountered by a meteorologist, Edward Lorenz, in 1963 (Holden, 2005) when attempting to predict the weather with a set of 12 equations. This theory is often associated with the so-called "butterfly effect," or the result on world-wide atmospheric conditions caused by the flapping of one butterfly's wings in the Amazon jungle (Kauffman, 1991). Yet, chaos theory has a true mathematical basis. The analogy comes from the small differences in the starting points of a butterfly flapping its wings, which produce different effects and which over time produce changes. Chaos theory deals with the differences in outcomes depending on conditions at the starting point. For example, the conditions where an information system is first envisioned will affect the overall design.

Chaos theory, such as general systems theory, addresses an entire structure without reducing it to the elemental parts. This makes it useful with complex systems such as information systems. The idea behind this theory is that what may appear to be chaotic actually has an order. It is based on the recognized fact that events and phenomena depend on initial conditions. Chaos theory is nonlinear. It allows us to question assumptions that we normally might reach using linear thought (Vincenzi, 1997). Seeing things reframed as a whole can stimulate new thinking and new approaches.

Cognitive Science

Cognitive science is gaining more importance in informatics. It is the study of the mind and intelligence (Thagard, 2010) and how this information can be applied. It is interdisciplinary, includes philosophy, psychology, artificial intelligence, neuroscience, linguistics, and anthropology, and is a part of social informatics. It adds to informatics concepts that focus on how the brain perceives and interprets a screen (Turley, 1996). These factors are important in all aspects of information systems. When designing input screens, the screen locations where information is entered must be organized to facilitate data entry.

Cognitive science is also a factor when presenting information; for example, characteristics such as color, font, and screen display affect clinical judgment because they are processed along with onscreen text and data. Additionally, cognitive science addresses the amount of information that an individual can absorb and use constructively. Principles from these theories provide a guide to developing systems that allow users to concentrate on the task, rather than requiring cognitive tasks to deal with the computer interface. Cognitive theory can also aid an informatics nurse specialist in understanding the information processing done by a nurse in decision making, thus facilitating the design of tools to support these processes (Staggers & Thompson, 2002).

Usability

Although usability has been a problem long before computers, the topic has become more visible with the advent of computer systems and the web and it is an integral part of informatics. It represents a multidimensional concept and involves users' evaluation of several measures, each one representative of their effectiveness in performing a task. It involves the ease of use, users' satisfaction that they have achieved their goals, and the aesthetics of the technology. It uses information from both the cognitive science and sociotechnical theories (see **Box 17-1**).

BOX 17-1 The Five Goals of Usability

1. It is easy for users to accomplish basic tasks the first time they use the product.
2. Once learned, the design permits users to quickly and easily perform the needed tasks.
3. If it is not used for a period of time, it is easy to reestablish one's proficiency in using the product.
4. Users make very few errors, but any that they do make are easily remedied.
5. The design is pleasant to use.

From Peters, L. A. (2004, August). *Web site usability*. Retrieved March 26, 2008, from http://www.da.ks.gov/itab/was/usability.htm

Table 17-3 Contributions of Theories to Informatics

Theory	Contributions to Informatics
Nursing informatics	Convert data into information and information to knowledge. Nurse adds wisdom
Sociotechnical theory and social informatics	Improve interaction between an information system and the organizational culture
Change	Increase the chance of success in implementing a system by attending to the reactions to the change
General systems	Contribute to the understanding of the complexity of an information system
Chaos	Improve the design of an information system
Cognitive science	Improve the ability of user to gain knowledge from an information system
Usability	Improve ease of use and satisfaction with an information system
Learning theory	Teach use of a system and design or select computer-aided instruction

Learning Theories

Learning theories are important in informatics as well as in all nursing endeavors. Users must be taught to use a system, and use of these theories can decrease the time for training as well as the time for learning.[2] See **Table 17-3** for a summary of what the various theories contribute to informatics.

Roles for Informatics Nurse Specialists

As can be seen from the broad areas that informatics and its subspecialty nursing encompass, as well as the evolving nature of nursing informatics, the roles and areas in which informatics nurses work are many. Although the role they play may differ depending on the area, there is much overlap. You may find informatics nurses with only on-the-job training in many roles, but with the increase in complexity and expectations for systems, many of these roles are becoming limited to nursing informatics specialists. Informatics nurses may be systems educators, an information technology advocate, superuser, system specialist, or clinical systems coordinator. Positions such as project director, director of clinical informatics, researcher, product developer, policy developer, or entrepreneur are more apt to be filled by a nursing informatics specialist

(see **Table 17-4**). Although job descriptions may vary from agency to agency, understanding the role of the informatics nurses in your area will help you to work with them to improve clinical systems.

Part of the job for all informatics nurses, regardless of their role or area of practice, is to interact with a variety of individuals at many different organizational levels, from anyone who uses the system to the chief executive officer. These interactions are important in gaining collaboration with clinicians, making decisions about how to interpret data, and obtaining administrative support for new practices. They also permit the informatics nurse to identify how information flows through an organization, assess for real and potential communication problems, and, when necessary, devise alternative methods of communication. These are all areas where it is important for clinicians to provide information to the staff and administrators, who are, in effect, clients.

User liaison is an important role performed by informatics nurses. In this role, the nurse is the communications link between nurses and others involved in computer-related matters. Other job functions can be managing nursing applications or chairing the nursing computer coordinating committee. Informatics nurses may also act as data systems managers for a specialty such as oncology.

Nursing informatics specialists working for either a healthcare agency or a vendor may be a project director for the installation of an information system. They may also be involved in product management or product definition. In this position, the nurse may also be responsible for seeing that the product is updated. This involves being aware of

---

2 Learning theories are addressed in Chapter 22 about educational informatics.

Table 17-4 Some Roles for Informatics Nurses

Roles	Responsibilities
Systems educator	Plans, coordinates, and facilitates education for all computer applications and computer software for all user groups. Develops and trains all user groups on clinical computer applications and online documentation processes. If employed by a vendor, systems educator may be responsible for documenting a new system and providing "train the trainer" education to healthcare agency personnel
Information technology nursing advocate	Assesses the needs and opportunities for nurses with the technology. Looks at both the functional and operational needs of clinical users when using the system and translates these needs into information technology–specific solutions
Super user	Supports the system in a given unit. Assists users with functionality, procedural issues, and basic troubleshooting. Often holds a clinical position in the assigned unit
System specialist	May work at many different levels from the unit to the full agency. Acts as a link between nursing and information services and is both a nursing resource and a representative
Clinical systems coordinator/analyst	Responsible for coordinating aspects of planning, design, development, implementation, maintenance, and evaluation of the clinical information system. Troubleshoots issues with systems. Supports a clinical system
The following roles are more apt to be filled by an informatics nurse specialist	
Project manager	Plans and implements an informatics project. Must be able to communicate effectively with all levels of management, users, and system developers. Must also be cognizant of all factors involved in the project including, but not limited to, managing change, assessing the need for the new project, and planning for its implementation
Consultant	Provides expert advice, opinions, and recommendations from consultant's area of expertise. Must be able to analyze what the client wants, as well as what is needed, and integrate these to create what is possible, technologically and politically. May be employed within an organization, by a vendor, or self-employed
Director of clinical informatics	Facilitates the development, implementation, and integration for an agency information system. Assists in developing the strategic and tactical plans of the system. Develops plans for implementation and gaining acceptance of systems
Researcher	Uses informatics to create new knowledge. Encompasses research in any area of nursing informatics. May be involved in basic research on the symbolic representation of nursing phenomena, clinical decision making, or applied research of information systems. Could be involved in developing decision support tools for nursing or models of representation for nursing phenomena
Product developer	Participates in the development of new information systems including designing, developing, and marketing of informatics solutions for nursing problems. Must understand the needs of both business and nursing
Policy developer	Contributes to health policy development by identifying nursing data, its availability, structure, and content, which are used to determine health policy. These policies encompass not only information management but also health infrastructure development and economics
Entrepreneur	Analyzes nursing information needs in clinical areas, education, administration, and research; develops and markets solutions

new developments in the field as well as the current and future needs of clients.[3] Some nurse informatics specialists who work for vendors are involved in marketing. For marketing, skills in listening and

anticipating needs, as well as the ability to identify the real decision maker, are necessary.

Some nursing informatics specialists act as consultants, either working independently or working for an organization. Consulting is a high-pressure field in which individuals often must make instant decisions based on personal knowledge and an analysis of only the known facts. This involves the

3 When working in a role that involves working with system users, a client is not necessarily a person outside the agency, but an individual who needs the services that an informatics person can provide.

role of a liaison and an expert. Many consulting jobs involve a heavy travel schedule. Nurses in academia who are involved in nursing informatics are usually involved in teaching nursing informatics, research, or both (see **Box 17-2**).

Educational Preparation

Both the National League for Nursing and the American Association of Colleges for Nursing, which are accrediting bodies for nursing programs, have made recommendations for including informatics in nursing education preparation (American Association of Colleges of Nursing, 2008; National League for Nursing, 2008). Basic informatics knowledge is essential for safe and effective nursing practice at the generalist level and all advanced practice levels. Understanding the possibilities and limitations of information management and technology assists the nurse to have realistic expectations of information systems.

The overall discipline of informatics has a core curriculum that is supplemented by informatics principles and knowledge specific to each

healthcare discipline, plus knowledge from one or more of the five categories described in **Table 17-1**, which is appropriate for the focus of the learner. Although formal educational programs provide an excellent foundation for jobs in informatics, as with all healthcare providers, there must be a commitment to lifelong learning.

Today many of the nurses who are practicing in the field of nursing informatics have gained their knowledge through self-learning and continuing education; nevertheless, there is a move toward requiring advanced formal academic preparation in the field, especially for the high-end jobs. Before commencing on a career in informatics, it is helpful to have a thorough, in-depth, understanding of clinical practice in one's discipline, which can only be gained through 3–5 years of experience in the field. Computer competency alone, although helpful, is insufficient for a career in informatics. Computers are only a tool in informatics; information management is the focus. This knowledge requires clinical experience.

To be a nursing informatics, a specialist requires a formal academic degree at the master's or doctoral level or a formal postmaster's

---

BOX 17-2 An Informatics Nurse Speaks

My mother introduces me these days as "my daughter who used to be a nurse." But that's not true – I am and always will be a nurse. I'm just practicing in a different area. Advances in technology have improved our ability to care for patients. What nurses (or others, such as my mother) don't often think about is that these technologic advances also include computer systems. All nurses need to have the skills to be able to use a PC, a monitor, or other piece of equipment, just like they need the skills to be able to do a physical assessment. You cannot keep up with the information or reports needed in today's world unless you have some system (besides paper) to help you.

I got into the field of nursing informatics several years ago when I was manager of a hospital ambulatory services department.

Being responsible for the business aspects of the department as well as the clinical, I was on the project team for implementation of the new computer systems. I found that my innate curiosity and need to always ask "Why" proved very helpful in this endeavor. I also discovered that computers are only a tool; it takes humans to analyze information needs and to plan how to best meet them – a discovery that led me to the field of nursing informatics.

I have never regretted the move! Just as in clinical nursing, you never know what to expect. Although you anticipate what you need to do each day, anything can happen to interrupt those plans and change your priorities. The next thing you know, it's 5:30 p.m. and you haven't been able to do one thing on your to-do list.

BOX 17-2 An Informatics Nurse Speaks *(continued)*

I start out each day by turning on my PC. Then I open my e-mail system. I read my new messages and respond when necessary. This usually takes an hour or two. Sometimes an e-mail I receive will require a telephone contact for follow-up, or users may contact me by telephone. Much of the time in my office spent either answering a question, providing clarification, explaining how a function works, or troubleshooting. When I am troubleshooting, I often access the software system with which the caller is having difficulty. This allows me to try to do what the user has done or attempted to do, so I can assess whether the caller is using the right function or routine and using it correctly. If the function is being used appropriately, I try to recreate what the user has done to see if I can elicit the same response or responses that she or he did. This method gives me a better picture of the difficulty and allows me either to solve the problem or to pinpoint a software problem. One day, I logged 6 hours 45 minutes of telephone time; the majority of which was nonstop.

Sometimes I need to contact one of the vendors to get a problem resolved. Talking with vendors may also include discussing product enhancements, a new product or feature that they are developing and releasing to clients or an upcoming class or meeting. Software testing is another function of the job. New features or updates may be released that need to be tested. This process involves creating different scenarios in which you enter data and print reports to make sure the software does what it's supposed to do. This can take hours, days, or even weeks to complete.

Reports are the end result of information processing. When you buy software, you sometimes get standard reports (those that the majority of all users need) but you usually have to write custom reports. Users give me requests for reports that they would like to have. To create them I may be able to modify an existing report, or I may need to create a

new one. This involves determining which file or files the information resides in, how the output of the report should look, what fields the report needs to include, what to name it so that the users will know which report to run, and perhaps which menu to put it on. Writing reports can take anywhere from a few minutes to several days, depending on the complexity, as well as the amount of time you can devote. (Remember all those interruptions!) Testing a report is also part of modifying or creating one. As the creator, I need to test it to be certain that it produces what the user wants. Then I need to have the user test it to see if the data and design meet his or her needs.

Another role of the informatics nurse is one of teacher. I develop the lesson plans and teaching materials to train the staff on the use of the computer systems. Training is done formally or informally, depending on the situation, and can take a few minutes to several days. In addition, I attend meetings, both in my department and with other departments. Many times, I am the leader of the meeting, which also involves putting together the agenda and handouts, and doing minutes. There are also user group and informatics organizations to which I belong.

A key element in this role is communication. When you are working in nursing informatics, you are providing help and support to end users: staff, managers, directors, and vice presidents, as well as the programmers/developers. (Very often, the programmer or developer is at your vendor's location and not in-house.) Nursing informatics is extremely dynamic, and I love the challenge. It offers me the opportunity to work with many different people, do many different things, and be creative. This role is never boring!

Judith Hornback, RN, BSN, MHSA,
Informatics Nurse Specialist,
Senior Consultant, RHI, Inc.,
Highland, Indiana

or postdoctoral degree program leading to a certificate. All informatics careers require continuing education that is often obtained at professional conferences. The **American Medical Informatics Association (AMIA)**, **Healthcare Information Management Systems Society (HIMSS)** , and **American Health Information Management Association (AHIMA)** have large educational and research meetings including tutorials for novice practitioners. Additionally, some universities sponsor 1- or 2-week intensive informatics courses. Three annual conferences, one sponsored by Rutgers College of Nursing, a second one by the University of Maryland School of Nursing, and a third by **ANIA-CARING** (American Nursing Informatics Association – Capital Area Roundtable on Informatics in Nursing) are all excellent places for continuing education.

Nursing informatics education can be classified into four categories: (1) online courses, (2) graduate programs with a specialty in nursing informatics, (3) graduate and undergraduate programs with minors or majors in nursing informatics, and (4) individual courses in nursing informatics within graduate/undergraduate programs. Online courses may be stand-alones that just provide continuing education, be part of a program that leads to a certificate in nursing informatics, or belong to a formal degree-granting program that may or may not be 100% online.

Many educational institutions have informatics programs. Given the many foci of informatics, it follows that each educational program will have a different focus. Some concentrate on applied informatics, others on informatics research. At present, there are no accrediting bodies that examine informatics education. Thus, there are many questions that prospective students need to ask of any program. Questions specific to an informatics program are listed in **Box 17-3**.

Informatics Missions for All Nurses

Informatics nurse specialists cannot work in a vacuum. The best systems are developed by collaboration between informatics nurse specialists and practicing clinicians. This avoids one of the common reasons for system failure: neglecting the expertise and needs of end users. To make this a productive relationship, practicing clinicians need to have a basic understanding of informatics (see **Box 17-4**). If a system is to assist the clinician in providing quality care, it is imperative that there be an understanding of the role of data in not only providing but also tracking and trending individual patient care. As data are synthesized and converted to information and knowledge, all nurses need to use this

---

BOX 17-3 Questions Specific to an Informatics Program

(In addition to those normally asked of any educational program)

1. What is the focus of the informatics program? For example:
   a. Clinical systems
   b. Knowledge generation/research
   c. Decision support
   d. Healthcare specialty
2. What types of jobs do graduates of the program obtain?
3. Who are the faculty in informatics?
   a. What is their informatics experience?

   b. What are their qualifications to teach informatics?
   c. What are there interests in informatics?
4. Is there a preceptorship or internship?
   a. If so, for how long?
   b. How are these assignments found?
5. How long has the program been operating?
6. What courses are currently available versus those being planned, but not yet offered?
7. If the program is online, how much on-campus time is required?

> **BOX 17-4** Some Informatics Facts for All Nurses
>
> **Data should be entered only once.**
> - One piece of data can be presented in many different ways and contexts.
> - Data from monitors of physiologic processes can be integrated into an electronic record.
> - Computers can transform data by calculating either numbers or words.
> - Computers require standardization of data if they are to permit learning from aggregated data.
> - Decision support can be part of an informatics system.
> - Output is only as good as input.
> - Only a clinician understands how information flows through the clinical area, it is imperative that this information be communicated to informatics personnel.
> - An information system will not solve organizational problems.
> - Aggregated, unidentified data about patient care can, and should, be available to all practicing clinicians for the purpose of improving patient care.

information/knowledge wisely. Everyone needs to realize that a computer can only work with the data that it has. The principle "garbage in, garbage out" should have a corollary "data lacking, output defective". When evaluating output, whether research or from a computer, examine the data categories (fields) on which it was based.

There is often an unrealistic expectation that a new information system will solve all problems, some of which may be organizational problems. An information system is apt to magnify organizational problems such as poor communication between departments, lack of accountability, and lack of administration support for the planned information system. It is important to be able to separate organizational problems from informational system problems and solve the former before the new system is implemented.

 Informatics Organizations

Health and healthcare concerns are worldwide, as is the interest in the use of informatics to improve healthcare.

Multidisciplinary Groups

Given the interdisciplinary nature of informatics, many of the formal organizations involve practitioners from all areas.

International Medical Informatics Association

The largest informatics group is the **International Medical Informatics Association (IMIA)** , which was established in 1967 as TC4, a Technical Committee within the International Federation for Information Processing. This group soon was renamed IMIA. IMIA is a nonpolitical, international, scientific organization whose goals include promoting informatics in healthcare, promoting biomedical research, advancing international cooperation, stimulating informatics research and education, and exchanging information.

Many countries belong to IMIA through national organizations such as the AMIA, which represents the United States and the **European Federation for Medical Informatics (EFMI)**, which represents Europe. The members have national meetings to focus on issues pertaining to their nation, which allow members to establish a national network where ideas can be shared, and provide a place to gain information for specific national problems. These organizations also provide journals and are a source of up-to-date information for their country. The members of IMIA also take part in MedINFO, a feature of IMIA, which is held every 3 years. A list of member countries' organizations is present on the IMIA web page (http://www.imia.org/).

Healthcare Information and Management Systems Society

Another international organization is HIMSS, which was founded in 1961, with offices in Chicago, Washington, DC, Brussels, and other locations across the United States and Europe. HIMSS is a not-for-profit organization dedicated to promoting a better understanding of healthcare information and management systems. At present, HIMSS represents more than 30,000 individual healthcare professionals and more than 470 corporate members (HIMSS, 2010). In 2003, HIMSS formed a Nursing Informatics Community to provide support to the nursing role in informatics. HIMSS meets annually and publishes a quarterly journal and several guides to the field. They offer accreditation as a Certified Professional in Healthcare Information and Management Systems.

American Health Information Management Association

The American College of Surgeons formed AHIMA in 1928. This is mostly a North American group whose goal is the improvement of clinical records (AHIMA, 2010). Originally named the Association of Record Librarians of North America, the organization has had several name changes. Currently named AHIMA, this name was adopted to reflect today's situation in which clinical data has expanded beyond either a single hospital or a provider. They offer credentialing programs in health information management, coding, and healthcare privacy and security.

Nursing Informatics Groups

The multidisciplinary groups sometimes have smaller working groups, some of which are nursing focused. The IMIA Nursing Working Group has sponsored an International Nursing Informatics Conference every 3 years since 1982. The themes of these conferences provide a look into how the concerns of nursing informatics have broadened from a concern in 1982 with computers in nursing through integrating caring and technology in nursing, a realization of the impact of informatics on nursing knowledge, to the recognition of the importance of the consumer or human in healthcare (**Table 17-5**).

Nursing Working Groups of Larger Organizations

AMIA and EFMI both have nursing working groups. AMIA's nursing working group, the **Nursing Informatics Working Group (NIWG)**, is responsible for promoting the integration of nursing informatics into the broader context of healthcare. NIWG also works to influence US policy makers regarding the use of nursing information. EFMI's nursing working group was formed to support European nurses and nursing informatics as well as to build informatics contact networks (EFMI, 2007).

British Computer Society Nursing Specialist Group. Other professional informatics organizations are primarily for nurses. A very active group is the **British Computer Society (BCS)** Health Nursing Group. One of its aims is to disseminate information about current nursing informatics applications and to encourage the publication of research and development material in this area (BCS, 2010). This is accomplished by interacting with other groups such as the Royal College of Nursing, the Clinical Professions and Health Visitor's Association (CPHVA/Amicus), and the NHS Connecting for Health's National Advisory Group for the National Programme.

Alliance for Nursing Informatics. In 2004, the **Alliance for Nursing Informatics (ANI)** was formed to unite many of the local, smaller, nursing informatics groups. The organization is sponsored by AMIA and HIMSS. Membership is through membership in a nursing-focused informatics group, either a nursing working group or a local or national group. These groups retain their dues, programs, publications, and organizational structures, but they are united through ANI to create a unified voice for nursing informatics. Representatives of each of the organizational groups make up the governing directors group that guides the strategic goals and activities of ANI (2010). Their website (http://www.allianceni.org/) features link to all the member groups. ANI membership includes the nursing working groups

Table 17-5 Themes and Locations of International Congress on Nursing Informatics Conferences

Year	Title	Location
1982	The Impact of Computers on Nursing	London, United Kingdom
1985	Building Bridges to the Future	Calgary, Alberta; California, United States
1988	Where Caring and Technology Meet	Dublin, Ireland
1991	Nurses Managing Information in Health Care	Melbourne, Victoria, Australia
1994	An International Overview of Nursing in a Technological Era	San Antonio, Texas, United States
1997	The Impact of Nursing Knowledge on Healthcare Informatics	Stockholm, Sweden
2000	One Step Beyond: The Evolution of Technology and Nursing	Auckland, New Zealand
2003	E-health for All: Designing a Nursing Agenda for the Future	Rio de Janeiro, Brazil
2006	Consumer-Centered, Computer-Supported Care for Healthy People	Seoul, Korea
2009	Nursing Informatics – Connecting Health and Humans	Helsinki, Finland
2012	Advancing Global Health Through Informatics	Montreal, Canada

of AMIA, HIMSS, and ANIA-CARING, another large nursing informatics organization.

Summary

Nursing informatics is a subspecialty in both nursing and health informatics and is a relatively new field. Nursing informatics focuses on helping clinicians acquire and integrate patient care data from many sources. Concerns in this field have moved from hardware and healthcare applications to perspectives that embrace sociotechnical, change, general systems, cognitive science, usability, and chaos theories.

Within nursing informatics, there are many different areas of concentration and roles including project manager, systems manager, and independent contractor. Nursing informatics, however, is not solely the province of nursing informatics specialists; all nurses must be involved if successful information systems are to be developed and implemented. There are many areas where informatics nurses work, as well as many different job foci.

Many of the nurses working in informatics have learned on the job, but the trend today is for a more formal education in the field. Many different types of programs exist for those who wish to specialize in nursing informatics. They range from programs granting graduate degrees to continuing education offerings. There is no accrediting body for education in this specialty yet, and the wise prospective student should investigate any academic program before enrolling.

Health informatics organizations at the international and national level are mostly multidisciplinary. Besides nursing working groups in the multidisciplinary groups, there are organizations that focus only on nursing informatics interests.

APPLICATIONS AND COMPETENCIES

1. Using one episode in a recent clinical experience, describe how you mentally move data through information and knowledge to wisdom. Keep it small, such as giving a medication or assessing a patient for lung congestion.

a. How did you evaluate and combine the different pieces of data?

b. What was the outcome of this process?

c. Reflect on how an information system could assist this process.

2. The theories supporting informatics come from many different areas.

a. By using the sociotechnical theory, make a plan to assess the readiness of an organization for either a new information system or an update to the current plan.

b. In adopting a spreadsheet, in which category of Rogers' diffusion theory would you place yourself?

c. Think of planning a change for an organization with which you are familiar. What are some of the restraining forces and the driving forces? How would you proceed?

d. Think of some of the various organizations with which you are familiar. Where would you classify them on the open–closed continuum of systems theory?

e. Relate the cognitive theory to the design of a web page.

3. Interview an informatics nurse to discover her or his responsibilities. Into which of the role(s) discussed in this chapter would you place this individual?

4. Conduct an Internet search to identify two formal educational programs in nursing informatics that would most interest you. Identify three key factors about the programs that you found to be most interesting and explain why.

5. Investigate the activities of one of the informatics professional organizations. Some methods for accomplishing this include checking their home page, attending a meeting, or interviewing a member/officer in one of the groups.

REFERENCES

Alliance for Nursing Informatics. (2010). *About ANI*. Retrieved August 3, 2010, from http://www.allianceni.org/about.asp

American Association of Colleges of Nursing. (2008). *The essentials of baccalaureate education for professional nursing practice*. Retrieved August 3, 2010, from http://www.aacn.nche.edu/Education/pdf/BaccEssentials08.pdf

American Health Information Management Association. (2010). *AHIMA facts*. Retrieved August 3, 2010, from http://www.ahima.org/about/facts.aspx

American Nurses Association. (2008). *Nursing informatics: Scope and standards of practice* (No. 1-55810-166-7). Washington, DC: American Nurses Publishing.

American Nurses Credentialing Center. (2010). *Informatics nursing certification eligibility*. Retrieved August 1, 2010, from http://www.nursecredentialing.org/Eligibility/InformaticsNurseEligibility.aspx

Bass, A. (2003, June 1). *Health-care IT: A big rollout bust. CIO*. Retrieved August 22, 2011, from http://www.cio.com/article/29736/Health_Care_IT_A_Big_Rollout_Bust

Berg, M., Aarts, J., & van der Lei, J. (2003). ICT in health care: Sociotechnical approaches. *Methods of Information in Medicine, 42*(4), 297–301.

British Computer Society. (2010). *About BCS – The Chartered Institute for IT*. Retrieved August 3, 2010, from http://www.bcs.org/server.php?show=nav.5651

Chin, T. (2003, February 17). Doctors pull plug on paperless system. *American Medical News*. Retrieved August 22, 2011, from http://www.ama-assn.org/amednews/2003/02/17/bil20217.htm

Clark, D. (2009, May 6). *Understanding and performance*. Retrieved August 1, 2010, from http://www.nwlink.com/~donclark/performance/understanding.html

Corcoran-Perry, S., & Graves, J. (1990). Supplemental-information-seeking behavior of cardiovascular nurses. *Research in Nursing and Health, 13*(2), 119–127.

European Federation for Medical Informatics. (2007). *EFMI WG NURSIE nursing informatics in Europe*. Retrieved August 3, 2010, from http://www.helmholtz-muenchen.de/ibmi/efmi/index.php?option=com_content&task=view&id=25&Itemid=121

Graves, J. R., & Cocoran, S. (1989). The study of nursing informatics. *Image: Journal of Nursing Scholarship, 21*, 227–231.

Gray, R. M. (2009). *Entropy and information theory*. New York, NY: Springer Verlag. Retrieved August 22, 2011, from http://ee.stanford.edu/~gray/it.pdf

Healthcare Information and Management Systems Society. (2010). *About HIMSS*. Retrieved August 3, 2010, from http://www.himss.org/ASP/aboutHimssHome.asp

Heylighen, F., & Joslyn, C. (1992, November 1). What is systems theory? In F. Heylighen, C. Joslyn, & V. Turchin (Eds.), *Principia Cybernetica Web (Principia Cybernetica, Brussels)*. Brussels: Principia Cybernetica. Retrieved August 22, 2011, from http://pespmc1.vub.ac.be/SYSTHEOR.html

Holden, L. M. (2005). Complex adaptive systems: Concept analysis. *Journal of Advanced Nursing, 52*(6), 651–657.

Joos, I., Whitman, N. I., Smith, M. J., & Nelson, R. (1992). *Computer in small bytes*. New York, NY: National League for Nursing Press.

Kauffman, S. A. (1991). Antichaos and adaptation. *Scientific American, 265*(2), 78–84. Retrieved August 22, 2011, from http://www.itee.uq.edu.au/~comp4006/CxSys%20Readings/Antichaos/Antichaos%20and%20Adaptation.htm

National League for Nursing. (2008, May 29). *NLN Board of Governors urges better preparation of nursing workforce to practice in 21st century, technology-rich health care environment*. Retrieved August 3, 2010, from http://www.nln.org/newsreleases/informatics_release_052908.htm

NCNR Priority Expert Panel on Nursing Informatics. (1993). *Nursing informatics. Enhancing patient care: A report of the NCNR priority expert panel on nursing informatics*. Bethesda, MD: U.S. Department of Health and Human Services,

U.S. Public Health Service, National Institutes of Health, National Center for Nursing Research.

Nightingale, F., & Goldie, S. M. (1997). *Letters from the Crimea, 1854–1856*. Retrieved August 22, 2011, from http://preview.tinyurl.com/2auahra

Ozbolt, J., Nahm, E.-S., & Roberts, D. (2007). How about a career in nursing informatics. *American Nurse Today, 2*(9), 34–36.

Rogers, E. M. (2003). *Diffusion of innovations* (5th ed.). New York, NY: Free Press.

Sawyer, S., & Rosenbaum, H. (2000). Social informatics in the information sciences: Current activities and emerging directions. *Informing Science, 3*(2), 89–95. Retrieved August 22, 2011, from http://inform.nu/Articles/Vol3/v3n2p89-96r.pdf

Schneider, T. D. (2010, January 8). *Information theory primer*. Retrieved August 1, 2010, from http://www.ccrnp.ncifcrf.gov/~toms/paper/primer/primer.pdf

School of Mathematics and Statistics, St. Andrews University Scotland. (2003). *Florence Nightingale*. Retrieved July 31, 2010, from http://www-history.mcs.st-andrews.ac.uk/Biographies/Nightingale.html

Smith, M. K. (2009, November 4). *Kurt Lewin: Groups, experiential learning and action research*. Retrieved August 1, 2010, from http://www.infed.org/thinkers/et-lewin.htm

Staggers, N., & Thompson, C. B. (2002). The evolution of definitions for nursing informatics: A critical analysis and revised definition. *Journal of the American Medical Association, 9*(3), 255–261.

Technology Informatics Guiding Education Reform. (2009). *The TIGER initiative: Collaborating to integrate evidence and informatics into nursing practice and education: An executive summary*. Retrieved January 24, 2011, from http://www.tigersummit.com/uploads/TIGER_Collaborative_Exec_Summary_040509.pdf

Thagard, P. (2010, June 9). *Cognitive science – The Stanford encyclopedia of philosophy*. Retrieved August 22, 2011, from http://plato.stanford.edu/entries/cognitive-science/

Turley, J. (1996). Toward a model for nursing informatics. *Image: Journal of Nursing Scholarship, 28*(4), 309–313.

Vincenzi, A. E. (1997). Using chaos theory: The implications for nursing. *Journal of Advanced Nursing, 37*(5), 462–469.

von Bertalanffy, L. (1973). *General system theory: Foundations, development, applications*. Harmondsworth: Penguin.

Wade, M., & Schneberger, S. (2005, October 13). *Theories used in research: Socio-technical theory*. Retrieved August 1, 2010, from http://www.istheory.yorku.ca/sociotechnicaltheory.htm

Warner, H. R. (1995). Medical informatics: A real discipline? *Journal of the American Medical Association, 2*(4), 207–214.

CHAPTER 18

Basic Electronic Healthcare Information Systems

Objectives

After studying this chapter you will be able to:

► *Compare and contrast the electronic medical record with the electronic health record and the electronic personal health record.*

► *Discuss the importance of the clinical nurse's role in the selection of a clinical information system process.*

► *Discuss the concept of workflow analysis as it relates to nursing care.*

► *Compare the systems life cycle with the nursing process.*

► *Discuss the role of the superuser in the systems life cycle.*

► *Display adherence to HIPAA regulations when working with health information.*

► *Discuss how a business continuity plan mitigates risk.*

Key Terms

American Recovery and
   Reinvestment Act (ARRA)
Big-Bang Conversion
Bugs
Business Continuity Plan
Clinical Document
   Architecture (CDA)
Context-Sensitive Help
Contingency Plan
Continuity of Care Document
   (CCD)
Cost Benefit
Debugging
Disaster Recovery
Electronic Health Record
   (EHR)
Electronic Medical Record
   (EMR)
Go-Live
Health Level 7 (HL7)
HIPAA (Health Insurance
   Portability and
   Accountability Act)

Health Information
   Technology for Economic
   and Clinical Health
   (HITECH) Act
Initiating
Intranet
Meaningful Use
Needs Assessment
Phased Conversion
Pilot Conversion
Project Goal
Project Scope
Regression Testing
Request for Information (RFI)
Request for Proposal (RFP)
Return on Investment (ROI)
Rollback
Rollout
Scope Creep
Superuser
Systems Life Cycle
Test Scripts
Vanilla Product
Vaporware

Healthcare information systems (HIS) are a composite made up of all the information management systems that serve an organization's needs. The complexity of HIS is largely independent of the size of the organization because healthcare provides a common core of patient care services. At the very minimum, most healthcare providers have electronic systems for billing patient care services. Facilities using advanced technologies have numerous systems that manage every service provided to the patient. This chapter focuses on a few basic components and processes common to HIS that are essential for all nurses to understand.

Every nurse needs to appreciate her individual role as it relates to HIS. As nurses, we need to understand what systems can "do" to help us efficiently manage information that relates to patient care. We must recognize how electronic documentation underpins the discovery of evidence-based practice for improved patient outcomes. We should expect HIS to support the nursing care delivery process and the documentation of care; HIS should not negatively impact our practice. That being said, we should not expect a technology solution to mimic the paper chart world. Adaption to electronic documentation requires a change in processes and workflow design. To manage the change process effectively, nursing leadership (Simpson, 2006, 2007) and clinical nurses must acquire technologic competence and take an active role in the selection process and design for new systems. When participating in the system selection process, we should be able to talk with information technology (IT) specialists and vendor representatives by using the appropriate terminology. Additionally, we must understand the **systems life cycle**, the process for health information technology (HIT) system selection and implementation.

EMR, EHR, ePHR, and Their Relationships to Emerging Clinical Information Systems

The patient's health information is the forefront of clinical information systems. A brief review of the different types of patient records should help set the scene for emerging clinical information systems. The EMR (**electronic medical record**), EHR (**electronic health record**), and ePHR (electronic personal health record) are now being

integrated into the design of clinical information systems.

As noted in Chapter 13, the EMR is an electronic version of the traditional record used by the healthcare provider. It is a legal record that describes the care that a patient received during an encounter with the healthcare agency. The EMR is an electronic clinical data repository that uses a controlled healthcare vocabulary (Garets & Davis, 2005). The EMR comprises order entry, computerized provider order entry (CPOE), pharmacy, and other applications for clinical documentation. Instead of hospital visit information being located in one or more manila folders in medical records, the EMR is a searchable database. For example, providers could search for all admissions for treatment of congestive heart failure or all surgeries. A patient can have many EMRs: one at the health department for immunizations; one at each hospital where care has been provided; and one at each healthcare provider's office.

The value of EMRs has been challenged because there is no standard for recording data, which leads to data redundancy (repeated entries of the same information) and subsequent entry discrepancies. As an example, the hospital where the care was originally provided may have accurate dates for the admission or surgery; however, on readmission when asked about previous surgeries, the patient's memory of those dates or types of surgeries may vary from the actual information. Although the information belongs to the patient, the healthcare provider owns the data in the EMR. Except for a few very large healthcare organizations, the EMR data reside in virtual silos among all the providers.

The EHR is a transportable subset of the EMR designed for use by healthcare organizations and physician practices and other providers (Garets & Davis, 2005). It provides a bridge connecting the EMR and the ePHR. "The EHR is a longitudinal record of patient health information generated by one or more encounters in any care delivery setting" (Health Information and Management Systems Society [HIMSS], 2010). The patient owns the data (Rowley, 2009). The EHR uses **Clinical Document Architecture (CDA)** data standards. CDA for common clinical document types was devised by **Health Level 7 (HL7)** to provide a common structure for clinical documents. The structure has three levels and provides the ability to send documents that have sufficient "code" in them to be machine-readable and yet are easily interpretable as a document by a human. This can be achieved by the use of extensible markup language tags that designate what a piece of text is. For example, a first name will be tagged just like in HTML, as will other required fields. The tagged items can be automatically placed as data into an electronic record, while humans can read the document. This format is intended for use by any type of clinical document such as demographics, vital signs, medications, progress notes, history and physical, consults, nursing documents, laboratory and radiology reports, and discharge summaries.

The **Continuity of Care Document (CCD)** uses the CDA architecture to provide a "snapshot" of a patient's health information, including insurance information, medical diagnoses and problems, medications, and allergies (Kibbe, 2010), which is to be integrated with EHRs to provide the sharing of data with multiple providers. It is a result of the harmonization of the CCD developed jointly by the American Society for Testing and Materials (ASTM) International, Massachusetts Medical Society, HIMSS, American Academy of Family Physicians, and the American Academy of Pediatrics ASTM's with HL7's CDA specifications (Healthcare IT News Staff, 2007). The CCD has defined what data are shared, and the CDA defines how data are shared with the EHR. In this manner, the CDA is used for other clinical documents that need sharing.

The terminology for an electronic record can be confusing because the terms EMR and EHR may be used as if the meanings are identical. Not only can healthcare providers extract pertinent information from electronic records that enhance the effectiveness of care, but the information also has the potential for use in quality and evidence-based care knowledge management. Both the EMR and EHR electronic clinical databases allow healthcare providers to review and analyze changes over time. Liang (2007) forecasted five (see **Box 18-1**) potential solutions that the EHR can provide to fill gaps in knowledge between evidence and practice.

In the effort to improve patient care outcomes, there has been somewhat of a chaotic effort for healthcare providers to transition from a paper

BOX 18-1 Ways the EHR Can Address the Gaps in Clinical Knowledge

The EHR can address the gaps in knowledge in evidence and clinical practice by the following ways:

- Detecting information and knowledge from current records that can efficiently affect clinical outcomes
- Shortening the time from knowledge discovery to implementation
- Monitoring quality improvement outcomes that result from knowledge-driven changes in providers' practices
- Empowering the patient to become a partner in care with the healthcare provider(s)
- Providing real-world knowledge versus controlled clinical trials about treatment effectiveness and outcomes

Adapted from Liang, L. (2007). The gap between evidence and practice. *Health Affairs, 26*(2), w119–w121.

record to an electronic record. Without any "mental models" about how information can be extracted from electronic systems, the adoption process is tainted by "paper chart thinking" (Baron, 2007). The process is under way to adopt and certify electronic records. There is still inconsistent communication between those who are involved in the universal design of the electronic record, those attempting to implement it, and those who are considering implementation. Agencies that are adopting or want to adopt electronic documentation may not understand the advantages of an interconnected record and the importance of interoperability for sharing information pertinent to improvement of patient outcomes. In the ideal world, the EHR summary data are owned by the patient, have patient input, and are used by multiple healthcare organizations. The vision for EHRs is that they will reside in Regional Health Information Organizations and will ultimately reside in the National Health Information Network in the United States (Garets & Davis, 2005).

Meaningful Use

There are a growing number of adopters for the use of the EHR. The **American Recovery and Reinvestment Act (ARRA)** (Recovery.gov, 2010), signed into law by President Obama on February 17, 2009, was a milestone in the history of HIT. **The Health Information Technology for Economic and Clinical Health (HITECH) Act** was a part of ARRA. The HITECH Act outlined four purposes:

- Define **meaningful use**
- Use incentives and grant programs to foster the adoption of EHRs
- Gain the trust of the public regarding the privacy and security of electronic healthcare data
- Promote IT innovation

The HITECH Act provided monetary incentives to hospitals and providers that met "meaningful use" requirements. The term "meaningful use" refers to the use of information from electronic health records to make improvements in the delivery of healthcare (Blumenthal & Tavenner, 2010). Meaningful use cannot be achieved unless the vast array of HIS is interoperable so that data can be exchanged. A full-text summary of the meaningful use objectives and measures is online in a *New England Journal of Medicine* article, "The 'Meaningful Use' Regulation for Electronic Health Records" (http://www.nejm.org/doi/full/10.1056/NEJMp1006114).

According to a research done by Health Affairs in 2009, only 11.9% of hospitals had adopted the EHR (Mayer, 2010). Smaller and rural hospitals have been slower to adopt than do larger, private, and urban hospitals. The meaningful use definition, finalized in July 2010, allowed hospitals and provider to qualify for incentive payments beginning in 2011. It provided a two-tiered implementation plan (see **Table 18-1**). The percentage of EHR adopters was anticipated to increase in the beginning of 2011.

The HITECH Act provided $27 billion in incentives for healthcare agencies and providers to adopt

Table 18-1 Meaningful Use Components, Purpose, and Examples

Meaningful Use Components	Purpose	Examples
Tier 1: Basic core functions	Enable EHRs to support healthcare	• Patient: Electronic record of • Vital signs • Demographics • Allergies • Medications • Diagnoses • Smoking status • Provider: • Use of decision support tools • Enter clinical orders, including prescriptions • Provide patients with electronic versions of their health information • Use systems that protect the privacy and security of EHR patient data
Tier 2: Support activities	Provide flexibility for hospitals and providers to choose five applicable support activities for implementation during the first 2 years	• Conduct drug formulary checks • Include clinical laboratory test results as structured data • Record advance directions for patient 65 years and older • Send patient reminders for preventive and follow-up care
Reporting	Report performance on three core quality measures to inform providers and the public	• Quality measures • Blood pressure • Tobacco status • Weight screening

From Blumenthal, D., & Tavenner, M. (2010). The "meaningful use" regulation for electronic health records. *New England Journal of Medicine, 363*(6), 501–504. Retrieved from http://www.nejm.org/doi/abs/10.1056/NEJMp1006114. doi:10.1056/NEJMp1006114

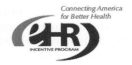

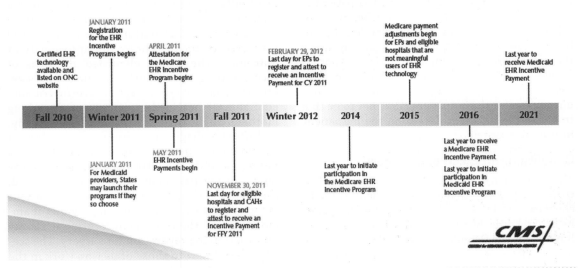

Figure 18-1 EHR incentive program timeline.

EHRs over 10 years. CMS (Centers for Medicare and Medicaid) was responsible for distribution of the incentive payments for providers. The first round of incentives began in 2011 and was scheduled to end by 2014 (see **Figure 18-1**). Comprehensive information about the HITECH Act is available online at http://healthit.hhs.gov/. Information about the CMS incentive programs is available online at http://www.cms.gov/ehrincentiveprograms/.

Need for Interoperability

In healthcare, it is common for one or two services or departments to adopt a HIT solution long ahead of others. As an example, laboratory systems and admission departments have used HIT for several decades. HIT problems do not begin to surface until the systems "bump into each other" because they cannot talk to one another; they are not interoperable. Interoperability[1] can be thought of as the ability to share data and, as noted above, is a goal of the HITECH Act for EHRs. Consider the following scenario posted to an informatics listserv and used with permission:

> The facility where I am currently employed is entertaining the idea of purchasing a new documentation system [Product A]. It is currently being used in outpatient areas, but inpatient is on [Product B] with both ER and Surgery on different systems as well. The systems are not interfaced, which is causing several problems throughout the inpatient world.

---

1 For a full discussion of interoperability, see Chapter 15.

Because inpatient and outpatient information needs are vastly different, it is still common for the systems not to "talk" with each other. As a result, nurses have had to use different passwords and learn to use two or more systems while also delivering complex patient care. When looking up patient visits, nurses may also have to query the systems independently. An example of a common problem is that the patient is seen in the emergency department (ED) and data are entered into the ED information system. When the patient is admitted to the hospital using a different clinical information system, the information has to be summarized or documented again by using the acute care documentation system. Another example is when the hospital-discharged patient is followed up in an outpatient clinic. It is not uncommon for the outpatient clinic not to be able to access the inpatient data from the outpatient information system.

Benefits of an Electronic Record

There are many benefits of the use of the electronic record in documenting patient care. In contrast, the inherent weaknesses of the paper health records were realized when Hurricane Katrina hit the US gulf coast in 2005. Thousands of Americans were affected when physicians' offices, healthcare agencies, and hospitals were underwater. Paper health records were destroyed, and the continuity of care was breached. In contrast, the Veteran's Administration (VA) patients experienced a relatively minor continuity of care issue because the VA uses EHRs. The VA patient care issues were associated with the initial isolation of patients, the lack of communication and electricity, and not the permanent loss of medical care information. Access to EHRs with a health information infrastructure, such as used by the VA, is just one of many benefits of an EHR.

Uses of the EMR, EHR, and ePHR all minimize the "decentralized and fragmented nature of the healthcare delivery system" that we were warned about in the Institute of Medicine (IOM) report *To err is human: Building a safer health system* (Kohn, Corrigan, & Donaldson, 2000, p. 3). The report was the first of several that followed, outlining the inherent weaknesses in our healthcare delivery

system. The report challenged us to make healthcare safe. The electronic record provides ways to make healthcare safer with the use of real-time documentation and instant communication with all providers who "need to know" wherever they are – in another department or in a remote office. In addition, decision support systems with just-in-time alerts can guide providers while delivering patient care.

The IOM report *Crossing the quality chasm: A new health system for the 21st century* (Committee on Quality of Health Care in America & Institute of Medicine, 2001) outlined the critical need for restructuring healthcare to improve patient outcomes. The report identified six areas of focus, stating that healthcare should be safe, effective, patient centered, timely, efficient, and equitable. It provided a scenario of a working mother's plight with healthcare before, during, and after her diagnosis of breast cancer. Many of the problems she experienced could have been mitigated with the EHR, beginning with the failure of her past mammograms to be mailed, the failure of the physician to notify the patient of an abnormal finding on a previous mammogram, and the time spent locating her x-ray information in preparation for surgery. The scenario is not new to those of us who work in the paper record world; we see it happening every single day.

Information privacy and security is a benefit of the EMR. The EMR includes an audit trail that details information about when the record was accessed, the origin point of access, what particular components were accessed, the date, and times. Access to the EMR is controlled by delineation of user privileges. In contrast, there is no means of knowing who picked up a paper chart or what information was reviewed.

The ability to search and extract information and to trend the information to create knowledge to inform practice is another benefit of the EMR. If the EMR is a well-designed database with a standardized healthcare vocabulary, it can be searched quickly and efficiently. For example, if a patient presented with a wound infection that was not responding to therapy, the patient's temperatures could be viewed in a graph output to visualize the patterns of temperature elevation spikes. Information from patients with chronic diseases, such as diabetes and heart failure readmission patterns, could be analyzed for proactive intervention.

Real-Time Information

The EMR provides the opportunity for real-time information that can be collected and communicated in an effective and efficient manner. As soon as a medication or vital sign is done, it can be entered into the record and viewed by other care providers who have access to the record. As another example, consider the patient who is referred from a provider's office to a facility for an outpatient test, such as a magnetic resonance imaging. If the referring office is connected to the same information system as the provider's office, the staff will be able to view the available appointments and schedule the test before the patient leaves the office. When the tests are completed, the test results can be communicated to the referring provider in an efficient manner and the test results can be added to the patient's record electronically.

Data entry can be automated by using synchronization with monitoring devices or the user can key it in. Multiple users can easily view and document on different parts of the EMR simultaneously, unlike the paper record. When providing care in the paper world, the chart is not usually with the patient, so the first step is to locate it. The paper chart may be in a stack of charts with doctor's orders, with a physician writing orders or progress notes, or being reviewed by another care provider.

The electronic record is simply a tool for the clinician to use when telling the story about patient care and making pertinent decisions. If we do not take advantage of the real-time documentation, we miss opportunities to share just-in-time information with other care providers. Real-time documentation provides a window of opportunity for early interventions and improved patient outcomes. Nurses must embrace the potential values of the electronic record, demonstrate real-time documentation that can facilitate communication, and use the record to extract information to improve patient outcomes. Real-time documentation requires a culture change for nurses who

practiced in a paper chart world. It also requires a workflow redesign, which includes ready access to computers for charting at the point of care.

Improved Quality

One of the most important benefits of the electronic record is improved patient care outcomes. In noncomputerized systems, test results can be easily lost or misplaced, requiring repeated testing. Ordered treatments can be overlooked or not documented. An electronic information system can improve the quality of care by preventing these all-too-common difficulties. When physicians enter orders into the system, transcription errors are eliminated. The electronic order can be compared with recommended dosages in the database, and the physician can be provided with information about the drug prescribed using clinical reminders (decision support system). When the order is integrated with the patient's information about the drugs that the patient is concurrently receiving, as well as drug allergies, drug mismatches can be better avoided. Clinical reminders can be generated to ensure that the patient is receiving the correct drug.

Healthcare Information Systems

Since the beginning of formalized healthcare, there have been HIS. As the complexity of healthcare has grown, so has the complexity of information. Patients see many providers and have records in many places. For several centuries, the paper record has proven its worth, but today's complex systems have outgrown the ability to be managed by paper.

Strengths of Paper Records

The wonderful thing about paper is that it is light and very transportable. The paper record can be used as soon as we find it and pick up a pen to write. We do not have to wait in line for a computer terminal, log in, click to drill down to menus, nor wait between window opening. The paper record requires no electricity, no maintenance, and no downtime. In the paper chart world, we can chart very quickly.

A nursing student completing her senior internship in a hospital that used the paper record system stated that documenting on paper "made her think." When asked what she meant, she said that she was used to a computer documentation system that provided checkboxes and data entry screen prompts, which, she felt, guided her in electronic documentation. She said that when there was a blank nursing progress note, she had to "think" about what to chart. It was clear that she realized that without those prompts her entries might be incomplete.

Weaknesses of Paper Records

Those of us who have used paper records can readily cite the inherent weaknesses. Unlike the electronic record, there is no backup system. Paper records can be easily damaged or destroyed. Parts of the paper record can be destroyed accidentally or, rarely, purposely. A part of the drudgery, particularly for night staff, includes stamping new forms and deleting duplicate updated patient information such as laboratory and x-ray reports. In the paper record world, it is very easy to stamp a chart form with the wrong stamp plate. Stamp machines are heavy and cumbersome and require maintenance. Filing copies of testing reports in paper records is very time-consuming and prone to human error, such as misfiling a report.

Legibility is another criticism of the paper record. It is often very difficult to read handwriting of others. Script versions of certain terms have led to serious and sometime fatal medical errors. As a result, the National Coordinating Council for Medication Error Reporting and Prevention (2010) and the Joint Commission (2010) made recommendations to stop using certain dangerous abbreviations. The Joint Commission issued a Sentinel Event Alert on the use of dangerous abbreviations in 2001, and healthcare agencies have worked fervently ever since to correct the problems. For example, the abbreviation for cubic centimeter (cc) was being misinterpreted as units, every day (q.d.) was being misinterpreted as four times per day (q.i.d.), and morphine sulfate (MSO_4) was being misinterpreted as magnesium sulfate ($MgSO_4$). The official "do not use" abbreviation list is available online at http://www.jointcommission.org/NR/rdonlyres/2329F8F5-6EC5-4E21-B932-54B2B7D53F00/0/dnu_list.pdf.

Trending data in the paper record world is tedious and prone to error. The user has to graph vital signs data and draw connecting lines to portray a trend on a vital signs flow sheet. Information such as intake and output (I&O) is initially charted on a clipboard in the patient's room and then transferred to the paper record at the end of the shift. If the patient got behind or ahead of his or her fluid volume needs, it usually is not discovered until the nurse charts the date – when it is too late to make an efficient correction. Totaling the I&O for complex care patients can be extremely time-consuming and prone to error. A calculator is often required to add and subtract numbers for an I&O total. All this is avoided with an EMR; the data can be entered as they are generated, and the total is automatically calculated. Further, it can provide an up-to-date record for the physician who wants this information before the end of the shift.

Paper records for patients who require a lengthy hospital stay can become very large, heavy, and difficult to store on a nursing unit. Retrieving old records for a new admission is often challenging. If the paper record is misfiled, there may be a significant time delay before the paper record is delivered to the nursing unit. Finding information for a patient with multiple readmissions is often overwhelming and may require searches through stacks of manila folders.

The Need for EHRs

Why is there a need for healthcare records to be electronic? As clearly outlined in the IOM reports, it is to make patient care safer (Committee on Quality of Health Care in America & Institute of Medicine, 2001; Page, A., & Institute of Medicine [U.S.]., 2004; Kohn et al., 2000). The paper record and the associated information silos are not good enough anymore. The need for an electronic record is recognized worldwide, not just in the United States.

Workflow Redesign

The need for workflow redesign when making a change from the paper record to an electronic documentation system cannot be emphasized enough. In contrast to the paper record environment where forms were often designed for the care providers, the electronic system focuses on the *patient* with collaborative information sharing patient data among the care providers. This means that workflow redesign has to consider the patient, the work done by all the care providers, and organizational needs, not just nursing needs. All participants in the design and implementation process must carefully listen to users' perceptions about the impact of a system implementation, recognize barriers to change, and identify strategies to work through the barriers (Lee, 2007). "Applying automation, even the newer, more sophisticated solutions, without focused, intentional process redesign can increase the very complexities intended to be streamlined" (Ball, Weaver, & Kiel, 2004, p. 454). One approach for workflow redesign is to use the same method as we do for patient problems: identify the purpose, goals, and expected outcomes (Schulman, Kuperman, Kharbanda, & Kaushal, 2007). The workflow redesign should be orchestrated by a multidisciplinary committee, which first identifies what an automated system is expected to accomplish. The committee should also establish broad goals and maintain compliance with standard setting organization requirements and rules and laws of regulatory agencies. The design of an efficient workflow process must include documentation of patient care, creation of reports, electronic prescribing of medications, and CPOE.

Workflow redesign is not for the faint-hearted. It requires a tremendous amount of work and collaboration between the various discipline members. Without that communication, the work could easily be compared to the Chinese parable about the blind men and the elephant. According to the parable, each blind man touched a different part of the elephant and came away believing that the part he touched represented the big picture. If the blind men had communicated what part of the elephant they were describing, they would have had a much richer picture of the true representation of an elephant. An example of a complex process in healthcare is the redesign of the paper medication administration record (MAR) to create the electronic version (eMAR).

In the paper record world, the MAR is used primarily by the nurse or medical secretary to record medication information and by the nurse when administering medications. In contrast, the eMAR is used by multiple disciplines. The physician uses it to order medications, the pharmacists use it to review/verify the orders and dispense the medications, and the nurses use it to organize their care for a group of patients and to document medication administration. Staggers, Kobus, and Brown (2007), in their study to identify critical online medication tasks for acute care, described some of the challenging issues associated with medication administration. For example, nurses often chart data associated with a medication, such as a pulse when administering digoxin and a blood sugar when administering insulin. In addition, nurses chart sites where injections were given. When carefully designed (see **Figure 18-2**), the eMAR can guide the nurse in organizing medication administration and facilitate documentation of this complex process.

Technologic Competencies

All users of computerized clinical information systems need to have effective technologic competencies. Examples of computer competencies for nurses include basic desktop software, documentation, and communication: the types of competencies discussed in this textbook. These competencies, computer literacy, and keyboarding skills should be addressed long before a system is implemented. Since it takes about 2 years to plan and install a system (Simpson, 2007), the staff should be expected to attend workshops and classes to gain the necessary skills during the planning period. Leadership should foster the skill-learning activities by encouraging the nursing units to develop **intranet** web pages and to use e-mail for communication.

Many healthcare agencies administer computer competency tests to assess learning needs of employees. The types of competency tests vary widely from self-assessments to timed, proctored quizzes. The 2009 TIGER (Technology Informatics Guiding Education Reform) report includes numerous informatics competencies educational resources (TIGER, 2009). June Kaminski maintains a nursing informatics website, Nursing-Informatics.com with links to a variety of tutorials and skills self-assessments. Because employees with low skill levels may feel intimidated by testing environments, it is very important to communicate that the purpose for the use of competency assessment tools is supportive rather than punitive. Computer games might be a strategy for the development of hand–eye motor skills necessary for using a mouse. See **Table 18-2**

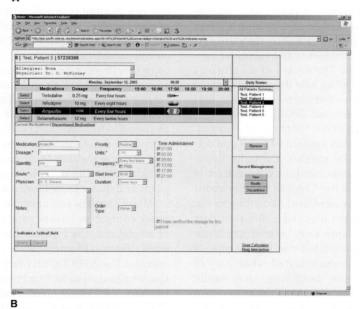

Figure 18-2 Sample eMAR screens. **A:** Medication administration time summary for all patients. **B:** Detailed medication information for a single patient. (From Staggers, N., Kobus, D., & Brown, C. (2007). Nurses' evaluations of a novel design for an electronic medication administration record. *CIN: Computers Informatics Nursing: CIN, 25*(2), 67–75, Figure 3, p. 71.)

for a listing of resources that can assist users to develop technology skills. There are free websites with online lessons that allow users to learn about computers and to gain competency with knowledge about how to use a computer and software, such as the operating system, e-mail, word processing,

Table 18-2 Resources for Technology Skills Development

Name	Where to Locate
Solitaire or Spider Solitaire	Microsoft Windows Operating System
Typing Game	http://www.freetypinggame.net/
GCFreeLearn	http://www.gcflearnfree.org/
HP Learning Center	http:// www.hp.com/go/learningcenter
Nursing-Informatics.com	http://www.nursing-informatics.com/
Others	Type "free typing practice" or "using mouse skills" into a search engine

and spreadsheets. GCFFreeLearn.org sponsored by Goodwill Community Foundation International includes online lessons that are enhanced with videos. HP Learning Center, sponsored by Hewlett-Packard, offers a wide assortment of online classes that range from office software, personal computer (PC) maintenance and security, business basics, graphics art, and digital photography. The HP Learning Center lessons include video tutorials, practice learning assignments, and quizzes. Both websites are free and require only for the user to register and create a user name and login.

The nursing staff should be strongly supported as they gain the computer competencies outlined for all nurses in the American Nurses Association publication *Nursing informatics: Scope and standards for practice* (American Nurses Association, 2008). Experienced nurses with little or no computer competencies may require significant support because they must revisit the role of a novice. Asking nurses to revisit the change theory concepts[2] may be a way to heal any feelings of inadequacy and discomfort. Although abuse of computer privileges is unlikely, if it occurs, it should be addressed the same way other performance issues such as time and attendance are addressed – with enforcement of policies and procedures and individual counseling.

Project Management and the Systems Life Cycle

Project management is an essential skill of the nursing informatics specialist. The term refers to the management of a project from start to finish. It requires excellent communication and team-building skills, organizational planning, and time and resource

management (Hunt, Sproat, & Kitzmiller, 2004). Project management database software, for example, Microsoft® Office Project and Project Kickstart™, are often used to chart the course of system development. Some healthcare agencies contract out or hire professional certified project managers to assure project success. The systems life cycle is the backbone for project management. The Project Management Institute (http://www.pmi.org) publishes the Project Management Body of Knowledge (PMBK®), an excellent resource for learning more about project management and the systems life cycle.

Systems Life Cycle

The term "systems life cycle" refers to the process that begins with the conception of a system until the system is implemented. The systems life cycle is analogous to the nursing process because it begins with assessment, has multiple places for iteration, and ends with evaluation (see **Figure 18-3**). Like the nursing process, it never really ends because changes can be made as a result of evaluation findings; thus, a new cycle begins. Unlike the nursing process, the wording and number of steps involved differ according to the agency or author (Hunt et al., 2004). To provide consistency in the use of terminology across an organization, healthcare agencies often provide glossaries and templates for users. One example is the Duke University Project Management website (http://www.oit.duke.edu/enterprise/project-mgt/) that includes a glossary, templates, and flow charts (Duke Office of Information Technology, n.d.).

Initiating

Every system begins with an idea. In the **initiating** phase, the **project goals** and needs (requirements) are identified and analyzed. This first phase is a critical step. Many system implementation failures

---

2 Change theory is examined in Chapter 17.

Systems Life Cycle

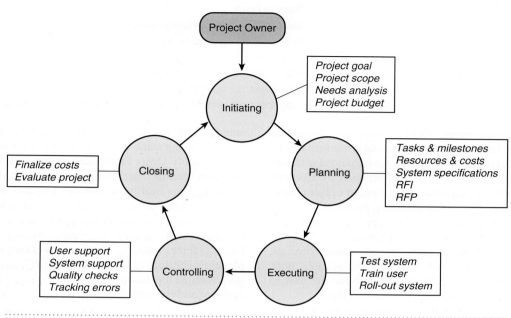

Figure 18-3 Systems life cycle.

can be attributed to a poor **needs assessment**. All system stakeholders must be a part of this process, not just the information systems personnel. A stakeholder is anyone who has something to gain or lose from a project. Examples of stakeholders include the healthcare agency's top executives, nursing executives, financial personnel, nursing clinicians, and any other personnel who may need to use the system.

Project Goals and Scope. The first task in initiating the process is to identify the project goal. The project goal is a succinct statement that describes the project. Goals should be specific and measurable. Instead of using the term project goal, some references use the term project definition (see **Box 18-2**).

The next task is to define the **project scope**, which refers to all the elements that are entailed in the project. For example, a project scope may address the implementation of an electronic documentation in the ED or it may entail deployment of electronic documentation throughout the entire hospital. **Scope creep** is a term that describes

BOX 18-2 Example of Project Goal Statements

- Implement computerized patient order entry CPOE by December 1, 2012.
- Implement computerized documentation in the ED by April 1, 2011.

unanticipated growth of the project. It can develop because of "we don't miss what we never had" situations. Once the users understand that a database or new system can manage information more effectively, they often specify new requirements, causing the scope of the project to creep (get larger). The problem with scope creep is that time and resources add up to money. Scope creep can cause project budget overruns.

Project Requirements. Every project involves risks; they should always be carefully explored and never be minimized. Risks are all those things that could interfere with the success of the project. They include personnel, finances, equipment, interoperability issues, training, security, and time issues.

The needs assessment is identification of the expectations or requirements of the system. In this part of the cycle, data and information pertinent to the project goal and scope are put together and translated to the needs for the system. The team identifies which features are essential to the new system and which features would be nice to have. At this point, a team member may go back to the clinicians and ask them to differentiate their needs from their wants. Some teams use a rating scale to determine the necessity of a feature, with patient safety features being given a higher priority.

The assessment is comparable to a brainstorming session. Questions that should be addressed include the following:

- Why do we want an information system?
- What do we want the system to do?
- Do we need to communicate with another department?
- Are generate alerts required?
- Do we record information in the patient record?
- Do we print reports?
- Of all the system "wants," which are essential needs and which are nice to have?

As a comparison, think about your needs assessment process when purchasing an automotive vehicle. Considerations for making a purchase would include the amount of money you have to spend. You also would want to consider the expected number of passengers and when and why you want to use the vehicle. Gas consumption may be another consideration – whether there is a **cost benefit** in purchasing a hybrid. Service should be important. You would want to consider the reputation and reliability of the service department, the cost of oil changes, and routine maintenance. In the process of making a purchase decision, the buyer usually reads news reports, compares auto manufacturers, vehicle types, and auto dealers.

Likewise, all the factors considered for the purchase of a vehicle should be taken into consideration when selecting an information system:

the reason for the purchase, what we want the system to accomplish, and the alternatives available. When reviewing the alternatives, decision makers must consider the alternatives that best meet their requirements, the experiences of other users, and the type and reliability of service. This detailed analysis is done to determine the **return on investment (ROI)** and cost-benefit analysis. ROI[3] is the cost savings that are realized. Cost-benefit analysis is an examination of the difference between the projected revenues and expenses (Investopedia, 2011).

The needs assessment for a HIS is similar to a vehicle purchase. All participants in the needs assessment process must do their homework. A list of possible vendor products should be determined. This is often done by using word of mouth, reading news reports, reading journal article reports, and listserv communication. A **request for information (RFI)** with a summary of the information is sent to vendors. Information from the return of the RFI is used to determine which vendors should be considered. Vendor products should be compared by using a tool such as a matrix. In doing so, participants need to learn the IT terminology. The time and quality of a needs assessment can make or break the success of system implementation. A **request for proposal (RFP)** is a detailed document sent to potential vendors asking them to submit information on how their product will meet the user's needs. The document should be a list that can be answered with using yes, yes with customization, yes with future releases, and no (Hunt et al., 2004). A well-written RFP will allow the users to compare products effectively. It has three parts – one that describes the method and deadline for responses; one that describes the organization; and one with a listing of details of expectations such as requirements, training, and support.

HIS project requirements refer to needs, such as

- schedule, design, and budget constraints;
- the number of system users;
- the department(s) that will use the system;
- the type of application, for example, desktop application or enterprise application;

---

3 ROI is discussed in greater detail in Chapter 20.

- where the software and data will reside;
- how and where the data are backed up;
- requirements for system redundancy (if one system fails, another system takes over seamlessly); and
- the type and availability of system support.

Planning

Planning is the second step in the systems life cycle. This critical phase requires a detailed assessment of the current processes including workflow analyses, timelines, and the implied changes of the new processes. Effective planning can breed trust and confidence among the users and team members (Hunt et al., 2004).

Analysis of Workflow. Workflow analyses are critical components of the planning phase. A workflow analysis analyzes and depicts how work is accomplished. Each nursing task has a distinct workflow. It is important to analyze workflow in the paper record system (or legacy electronic system) and then project work might best be accomplished using the new electronic system. As an example, consider the workflow that begins with

- a physician's medication order and ends with the medication administration of digoxin;
- administering intravenous Lasix and ends with the documentation of the drug; and
- checking a blood glucose level, subsequently administering a combination of NPH and regular insulin, and ends with the documentation of the procedures.

The process for "who" does what, when, and how differs for each example. The "it depends" has to be considered. In the first example, it depends on how the physician's order was written. Was it written by the physician or was it a verbal or phone order? If the order was written on the paper chart, did a medical secretary or a nurse transcribe the order?

An effective way to visualize what happens is to diagram the activity. Diagramming can be done by using drawing tools in any program that includes the use of drawing shapes such as OpenOffice.org Draw, MS PowerPoint®, or specialized software, such as MS Visio®. A process flow diagram uses special symbols to convey a certain meaning. As an

example, the oval shape is used to convey the start and stop processes, the rectangle shape indicates a process, and the diamond shape indicates a decision (see **Figure 18-4**).

Selecting a System. Selecting a system is one of the most daunting decisions for the stakeholder committee members. Healthcare organization enterprise solutions have the potential of improving or disrupting the complex care delivery process and are significant financial investments that range from thousands of dollars to millions of dollars. The risks of making a mistake can be mitigated with the use of a structured process, effective risk and needs analyses, and careful product investigation.

The selection member participants must educate themselves to be able to make an informed decision. Participants should investigate pertinent literature. Journals with comprehensive pertinent articles include *CIN: Computers Informatics Nursing*, *JAMIA: Journal of the American Medical Informatics Association*, *The Journal of Healthcare Information Management*, and the *International Journal of Medical Informatics*.

Nursing participants should consider membership in nursing informatics professional organization and stay abreast of common issues and concerns using informatics listservs. Nurses should network with other system users and attend professional informatics education sessions, such as HIMSS and American Medical Informatics Association. Listening to the experiences of others without a vendor present can uncover important issues, both good and bad.

It is important for the selection committee not to be overly dependent on the vendor's advice. Vendors are in the business of making money, and they are trained to market their product to make sales. They have been known to minimize system weaknesses. Be cautious about vendors' promises of upcoming new features or product releases. Broken promises of computer system products are known as **vaporware**. The selection committee members should also make site visits to interview others. Before selecting sites to visit, it is important to talk with several agencies and listen to both good and bad features. No system is perfect, and the success of a system may have as much

Flow Chart Symbols and Their Meaning Using the Systems Life Cycle

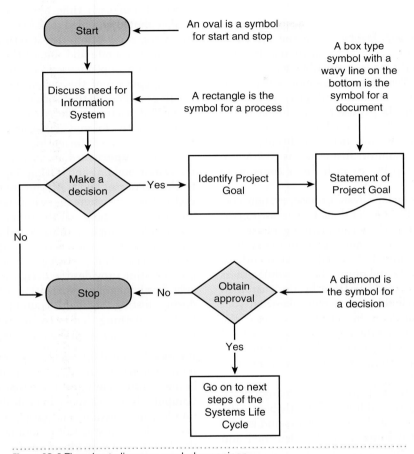

Figure 18-4 Flowchart diagram symbol meanings.

to do with the agency as the vendor. Although the vendors often arrange the visits, users should make sure that they candidly speak with other users without the vendor's presence. During a site visit, talking with clinical users as well as with information system personnel and those in leadership positions will provide the most knowledge.

The site visitation team should include several potential users, not just IT services or administrative personnel. Creating a list of questions that will be used for all visits will allow users to make comparisons between the different sites. Visitors should also be sure to see the system in operation.

The staff nurse may be a part of the visitation team or may be demonstrating the system from the host site. In either position, the selection team should be open-minded and both listen carefully to what is said and be attuned to what is not said. The nurse demonstrating the system at the host site should be honest and fair in discussing the system.

Executing

The third stage of the systems life cycle is executing the system. This phase involves customizing the system to meet the needs of the organization. The system is tested to make sure that it works as planned. Once there is agreement that the system meets the user requirements, the staff members are trained and the system is implemented (called a rollout).

System Design and Testing. Once the system is selected, the next step is to customize the system design so that it is compatible with the user requirements. Typically, the vendor will provide the user with a standard product, sometimes known as a **vanilla product**. It is similar to the standard desktop PC that the buyer can customize with additional features such as additional memory or an extra monitor. Just as in the customization of a desktop PC, extra features come at an additional fee.

During the system design phase, system documentation must be developed. It is an important feature started in the planning phase and continued with each change made in the system. Some vendors provide "canned" or standardized data entry objects and output boxes, while others allow unlimited customization by the customer. The decision to build-your-own or take-what-you-get should be made in the very early stages of the vendor selection and discovery process. The need for up-to-date and complete system documentation that flows with the user processes cannot be overemphasized.

The testing phase is just one of many critical phases that must be addressed intently before the system is implemented. System errors and issues, commonly called **bugs**, must be identified and addressed. The process of correcting the errors is called **debugging**. The testing of the new system is ongoing, during, and after the system build. The testing needs to include features and expected functionality of the system, hardware, backups, downtime, restarts, data capture and storage, and network communication. Application functionality is often referred to as **regression testing** and interfaces, and communication/network functionality is usually called integration testing. A set of situations commonly called scenarios or **test scripts** are devised to depict normal and abnormal events that could occur. Clinicians may be involved in devising the features and functionality scenarios and in the actual testing. Several test scripts should be written for each functional part of the software

and for the integration of data across interfaces to ensure consistent quality of output. A test script may not catch everything that does not work as expected, but each time a new issue is discovered, it should be added to the set of scripts. Over the years, a collection of test scripts can become extremely accurate and reduce the issues discovered during implementation. This will improve user acceptance of the system or changes to an existing system and the user's trust and confidence in the IT department. The trust and confidence for IT is imperative for moving the institution forward with an electronic information system.

System **superusers** are identified to assist in the system building and testing. Superusers should be clinical nurses and staff who are recruited from each of the areas where the system will be deployed. Superusers can help sell the other clinicians and assist in later implementation and training. They are invaluable to the success of the implementation phase. The participation of end users in initial testing provides the design team with valuable developmental information. Observer users during testing highlight training needs. Many times, something that is considered intuitive by the design team may prove confusing for the user.

Training. The need for basic computer training that is uncovered in the needs assessment phase should be met before training for the actual system occurs. Computer literacy issues can be dealt with in separate learning sessions and target only those who need to know instead of planning training with the lowest common denominator of learner in mind. User training is another essential step leading to a successful **go-live** or **rollout**. Both terms refer to the implementation of a new system. The training sessions should use effective pedagogical teaching/learning theory and methods.[4] Training should be done within a few weeks of the system implementation for "just-in-time" learning. If completed too early, without reinforcement, the learning will be forgotten.

Training should be done with the user needs in mind. Many facilities use superusers to assist with the training sessions. A needs assessment may be helpful to identify training resources. An

---

4 Information about teaching/learning theory is in Chapter 22.

analysis of needs can assist the training developers to create modules that meet the needs of novices to expert computer users. It can also be helpful to identify availability of the staff. Training should also include instructions on how to obtain help for the system. An ideal system will contain **context-sensitive help** or help that is modified based on where in the system help was accessed. Providing online tutorials and video clips on the computer can also assist clinicians to use the system successfully.

During training sessions, end users should take responsibility for learning to use the new system by asking questions and providing feedback on the functionality and features for the system to serve their needs best. Training activities should be viewed as multipurpose activities. The trainer not only teaches intended users how to use a system but also makes determinations about specific support that will be required during the rollout. During the training sessions, security and data accuracy must be addressed. By discussing these issues in the context of system use, the user responsibilities related to security become more meaningful.

A common training mistake is to simply show the user where system features are located and explain how they are used. A better approach is to develop several scenarios or simulation case studies that the clinician experiences on a daily basis so that the user can apply learning. After a brief introduction to the system, the user is allowed to work through the learning modules. Some agencies develop self-learning modules, place them on the nursing unit PCs, and use them in addition to classroom training.

Another mistake is to provide too much information in a single training period. Rather than planning a 4–5-hour class, it is better to break the training session down into shorter 1–2-hour classes. Learning to use a new computer system can be overwhelming to many. After a short period, the mind can become saturated, evident by restlessness and inattention of the learners.

Implementation. The implementation or go-live is a significant milestone. Many agencies build the momentum to that milestone with preparatory "count down the days …" presentations, memos, and posters. The implementation team may choose to order T-shirts – one color for the trainers and superusers and another for the staff. The celebration often includes a media release to the local newspapers. The implementation is yet another key phase in the systems life cycle. It needs to be carefully planned and implemented. If not done well, the users might be tempted to bypass essential features that were put in place to make patients safer.

Success of the go-live is dependent on the support system. Adequate system and user support are crucial. It may be necessary to schedule additional staff for the first few days or weeks, depending on the number of users affected and the workflow impact. Initially, 24-hour onsite support may be required, with later support provided from a help desk. Vendor support is important in the initial stages of implementation to troubleshoot unforeseen issues and to resolve any issues quickly. The goals should be to have as little disruption in patient care delivery as possible.

Each system implementation plan should have a **contingency plan** for a **rollback**. A rollback refers to backing out of the implementation – the cancellation of the system implementation. The contingency plan should be detailed and address risks of significant implementation problems. Clinicians should not be expected to use a clinical information system that jeopardizes patient care. If the system is carefully tested prior to implementation and the users are trained and ready, rollback issues are minimized.

There are three main approaches used to implement health information systems: the big-bang approach, **pilot conversion**, and **phased conversion**. There are strengths and weaknesses of each approach. All approaches involve change by very busy health practitioners, and change involving care of patients should never be considered lightly. To optimize the success of any new health information system, nursing leadership and clinical nurses should be involved in the selection, planning, training, and implementation planning processes.

Pilot Conversion. The pilot conversion is done to "test the waters" to see what issues might occur when making a transition to a new clinical information system. This approach enables the testing of a system on a smaller scale. For instance, a new documentation system or point-of-care device may be implemented on one care unit for a period of time for the purpose of evaluation. For the overall evaluation to be successful, specific evaluation criteria should be established. The pilot testing should be completed within a defined time period. The pilot conversion might be used when transitioning from the paper chart to an electronic charting system or when switching charting system vendors. Usually, pilot implementation is used to determine operational or training needs for future implementation of the system. It involves the least risk.

Phased Conversion. The phased conversion is used to bring up a new system gradually in a controlled environment. The phased conversion is done incrementally with several alternative approaches. One is to implement one component of the system to a group of departments throughout the organization. New systems can be phased in on one nursing unit or department at a time. The choice of the initial phased roll area is usually done with the staff members who are most likely to champion the system. The personnel who are implementing the system can learn from training sessions and go-lives and implement that learning in the next phase.

Parallel Conversion. The parallel conversion requires the operation and support of the new and the old system for a period of time. The implementation plan will normally address the specific operational needs and define the timing of the implementation. Specific departments or care units may be targeted with specific dates for a switchover to the new system. This method allows an organization to allocate resources in an efficient manner. It involves the least risks but increased workload for the users. Training can be done with just those who need to know.

Big-Bang Conversion. The **big-bang conversion** is used when switching from one computer system to another. The entire institution implements the system at the same time. This method can be most disruptive to the clinical setting. It is used most frequently when there is no initial system, the system in use is old, or there is a requirement for implementation on a specific date, such as the beginning of a new fiscal year. As a nonclinical example, many universities are switching from university-run old and failing e-mail systems to a free one provided by Microsoft® Windows Live or Google™ Mail. When making a switch, the universities use the big-bang approach and migrate all the e-mail accounts at one time. Likewise, healthcare agencies may use the approach when switching clinical information systems. The associated risk and required support for this major transition is dependent on the size of the agency.

Controlling (Maintenance and Evaluation)

Controlling (maintenance and evaluation) is the last critical phase of the systems life cycle. Even the best systems will have bugs and issues. System maintenance is an ongoing process. The information system staff members who work on the help desk are key personnel for keeping the system running smoothly. They need to have customer service communication skills and be able to talk using words that the user who is experiencing problems can understand, appreciate the complex role of the clinician, and be able to recognize potential patient safety issues. All issues should be documented, prioritized, and tracked by using a database.

Although evaluation should be a part of every phase of the systems life cycle, there should be a planned evaluation at least 6 months after implementation. Before that, improvements may be difficult to identify because of issues related to adjusting to new methods of working. If a preevaluation was done before implementation, comparisons can be made. Clinicians may find changes that would make the system easier to use. In such cases, clinicians should provide a thorough explanation of the needed change and the rationale behind it. In addition to clinician recommendations, issue tracking at the help desk about common problems will lead to the establishment of effective adjustments and system improvements. Established teams and analysts must continually evaluate and deal with identified issues.

 HIPAA Revisited

In the United States, the **Health Insurance Portability and Accountability Act (HIPAA)** of 1996 has had a tremendous impact on the policies and procedures for clinical information systems. The law initiated a new standard for protecting information for individuals who have health records that are stored or transferred by using clinical information systems. Under HIPAA, health information for individuals has federal protection. Although there is a tremendous amount of education and news about HIPAA and HIPAA breaches, the law is too often misunderstood. To complicate things, the law has been constantly amended. Moreover, HIPAA is frequently misspelled as HIPPA. The acronym is also misquoted as "health information," instead of "health insurance."

HIPAA law has two components: one is privacy and the other is security. The law reaches further than the origin of the clinical HIS and extends to consultants, agencies, and businesses that contract with the owner of the HIS. Nurses generally have an exceptional understanding of the privacy (confidentiality) part of the law. However, the data security part of the law may not be as clear to nurses and other healthcare providers. The Department of Health and Human Services (http://www.hhs.gov/ocr/privacy/hipaa/understanding/index.html) has easy to read information on HIPAA privacy and security.

Security of protected health information is more than logging in and out of the EMR or assuring that the computer screen is not viewed by those who do not have the need to know. It relates to transfer, removal, disposal, and reuse of the electronic information (Department of Health and Human Services, 2010). Every healthcare worker who works with patient information data must be familiar with the agency's policies and procedures for storage of data that are extracted from the EMR, such as for quality improvement studies. Storage of data pertains to remote shared agency servers, hard drives, flash drives, and any other optical media. The agency's HIPAA security officer is responsible for the policies and procedures that address data security issues.

Understanding the levels of security is important. When visiting certain websites, have you noticed whether the web address begins with "http" or "https"? The letter "s" in the "https" uniform resource locator (URL) indicates that the site is secure. If you are using a learning management system for school, the website is probably secure. For another example, it is a standard protocol for healthcare e-mail servers to send e-mail identified as "secure message delivery," where you have to click a button to view the e-mail. In addition to

the "View Email" button, there may be a web link to the e-mail content. Note that the web link URL will begin with "https." Secure e-mail stores the content of the message on a remote secure server. The e-mail may also include a note that the date when the e-mail can no longer be viewed. Secure is a level of e-mail encryption.

 ## Business Continuity Plan

Business continuity plan is the term use by IT for **disaster recovery**. Some resources differentiate the two terms indicating that business continuity refers to how to continue IT services in the case of a disruption (Public Safety Canada, 2009). The term "disaster recovery" may refer to the recovery of IT services after a disaster. It has significance as healthcare continues to adopt EHRs. If health information is stored electronically, what are the ramifications of a disaster, such as a tornado, fire, or hurricane destroying the HIS location? What are the ramifications of a pandemic where a significant number of the IT staff is ill and unable to work? What about major equipment failures?

IT, just like nursing services, must have a written plan, equipment, and services that outline actions to manage potential disasters. It includes precautions taken to minimize the loss of data due to a disaster. In the case of a major power outage, it might be use of the backup power supply. In the case of a fire, it might be an automated shutdown of the HIS system before the sprinklers turn on. Other precautions include mirroring the major servers to a remote site. The plan would include procedure to restore mission critical processes as quickly as possible. It would also include how to address data entry after the system is restored.

BCPWHO, Business Continuity Planning Workgroup for Healthcare Organizations (http://www.bcpwho.org/), is a nonprofit organization with comprehensive resources on business continuity management, emergency management, and disaster recovery (BCPWHO, 2010). Many of the resources are free. Examples include presentations, guides on how to develop a plan, and links to other resources that address IT management.

Summary

The original healthcare computer systems met financial and billing needs. As computerized systems moved into the clinical area, individual systems that focused on a department or a process became the norm. The most recent changes in clinical information systems focus on the patient and patient safety needs. Healthcare information should be stored in a data repository and used as a tool for quality assessments and uncovering evidence-based knowledge practices. Additionally, the information should serve the needs of healthcare planners, researchers, lawyers, and third-party payers.

To meet this need, healthcare agencies need a strategic plan to guide in selecting and implementing necessary information systems. The implementation process for information systems uses a process known as the systems life cycle, which parallels the nursing process. The involvement of end users, such as practicing nurses, in all stages of the systems life cycle is crucial to a successful system implementation. A well-planned and implemented system can provide many patient care benefits, including improved efficiency in both documentation and communication. Electronic information systems can also provide aggregated data for use in improving clinical practices. When standardized nursing languages[5] are included in the documentation system, nursing data will be available for unit, institution, and regional uses. Aggregated nursing data have the capacity to demonstrate the values that nursing brings to healthcare.

APPLICATIONS AND COMPETENCIES

1. Use a search engine such as Google Health to discover the most current EMR vendors. Compare and contrast two EMR vendors for ease of consumer use and interoperability with provider clinical information systems.

2. Do a literature search for the EHR. Summarize your findings for current development issues.

3. Interview a nurse informatics specialist to identify the specialist's role in the system selection and implementation process.

4. Use drawing word processing or presentation software to draw the process of medication administration beginning either with the physician's order in the paper record environment or with an electronic information system.

5. Compare the systems life cycle with the nursing process. How are they alike or different?

6. Discuss how the role of the nurse clinician superuser is helpful in the design and implementation of life cycles.

7. Create a lesson plan to use when implementing a clinical documentation system on a nursing unit. Be sure to incorporate concepts of change theory and teaching learning theories.

REFERENCES

American Nurses Association. (2008). *Nursing informatics: Scope and standards of practice* (No. 1-55810-166-7). Washington, DC: American Nurses Publishing.

Ball, M. J., Weaver, C., & Kiel, J. M. (Eds.). (2004). *Healthcare information management systems: Cases, strategies, and solutions* (3rd ed.). New York, NY: Springer-Verlag.

Baron, R. J. (2007). Improving patient care. Quality improvement with an electronic health record: Achievable, but not automatic. *Annals of Internal Medicine, 147*(8), 549–552.

Blumenthal, D., & Tavenner, M. (2010). The "meaningful use" regulation for electronic health records. *New England Journal of Medicine, 363*(6), 501–504. Retrieved from http://www.nejm.org/doi/abs/10.1056/NEJMp1006114. doi:10.1056/NEJMp1006114

Business Continuity Planning Workgroup for Healthcare Organizations. (2010). *About business continuity planning workgroup for healthcare organizations*. Retrieved September 18, 2010, from http://www.bcpwho.org/

Committee on Quality of Health Care in America & Institute of Medicine. (2001). *Crossing the quality chasm: A new health system for the 21st century*. Retrieved from http://books.nap.edu/catalog.php?record_id=10027#toc

Page, A., & Institute of Medicine (U.S.). Committee on the Work Environment for Nurses & Patient Safety. (2004). *Keeping patients safe: Transforming the work environment for nurses*. Washington, DC: National Academies Press. Retrieved August 22, 2011, from http://books.nap.edu/catalog/11151.html

Department of Health and Human Services. (2010). *Summary of the HIPAA security rule*. Retrieved September 18, 2010, from http://www.hhs.gov/ocr/privacy/hipaa/understanding/srsummary.html

Duke Office of Information Technology. (n.d.). *Project management*. Retrieved September 19, 2010, from http://www.oit.duke.edu/enterprise/project-mgt/

Garets, D., & Davis, M. (2005, October). *Electronic patient records: EMRs and EHRs*. Retrieved November 7, 2005, 2005, from http://www.healthcare-informatics.com/issues/2005/10_05/garets.htm

Healthcare IT News Staff. (2007, April 12). Continuity of care standards reach milestone. *Healthcare IT News.*

Retrieved from http://www.healthcareitnews.com/news/continuity-care-standards-reach-milestone

Health Information and Management Systems Society. (2010). *Electronic health record (EHR)*. Retrieved November 9, 2010, from http://www.himss.org/ASP/topics_ehr.asp

Hunt, E. C., Sproat, S. B., & Kitzmiller, R. R. (2004). *The nursing informatics implementation guide*. New York, NY: Springer.

Investopedia. (2011). *Cost–benefit analysis*. Retrieved August 22, 2011, from http://www.investopedia.com/terms/c/cost-benefitanalysis.asp

Kibbe, D. C. (2010). *Unofficial FAQs about the ASTM CCR standard*. Retrieved September 18, 2010, from http://www.centerforhit.org/online/chit/home/project-ctr/astm/unofficialfaq.html

Kohn, L. T., Corrigan, J. M. & Donaldson, M. S. (Eds.). (2000). *To err is human: Building a safer health system*. Retrieved August 24, 2011, from http://www.nap.edu/catalog/9728.html#toc

Lee, T. T. (2007). Nurses' experiences using a nursing information system: Early stage of technology implementation. *CIN: Computers Informatics Nursing, 25*(5), 294–300.

Liang, L. (2007). The gap between evidence and practice. *Health Affairs, 26*(2), w119–w121.

Mayer, H. (2010, August 27). Report: EHR adoption rates low. *DotMed News*. Retrieved from http://www.dotmed.com/news/story/14044

National Coordinating Council for Medication Error Reporting and Prevention. (2010). *National coordinating council for medication error reporting and prevention*. Retrieved September 18, 2010, from http://www.nccmerp.org/

Public Safety Canada. (2009, September 21). *A guide to business continuity planning*. Retrieved September 18, 2010, from http://www.publicsafety.gc.ca/prg/em/gds/bcp-eng.aspx

Recovery.gov. (2010). *The recovery act*. Retrieved September 20, 2010, from http://www.recovery.gov/

Rowley, R. (2009, April 30). *EHR bloggers: Who "owns" a patient's medical record?* Retrieved November 9, 2010, from http://www.ehrbloggers.com/2009/04/who-owns-patients-medical-record.html

Schulman, J., Kuperman, G. J., Kharbanda, A., & Kaushal, R. (2007). Discovering how to think about a hospital patient information system by struggling to evaluate it: A committee's journal. *Journal of the American Medical Informatics Association, 14*(5), 537–541.

Simpson, R. L. (2006). Evidence-based practice: How nursing administration makes IT happen. *Nursing Administration Quarterly, 30*(3), 291–294.

Simpson, R. L. (2007). The politics of information technology. *Nursing Administration Quarterly, 31*(4), 354–358.

Staggers, N., Kobus, D., & Brown, C. (2007). Nurses' evaluations of a novel design for an electronic medication administration record. *CIN: Computers Informatics Nursing, 25*(2), 67–75.

Technology Informatics Guiding Education Reform. (2009). *The TIGER initiative: Collaborating to integrate evidence and informatics into nursing practice and education. An executive summary*. Retrieved September 16, 2010, from http://www.tigersummit.com/uploads/TIGER_Collaborative_Exec_Summary_040509.pdf

The Joint Commission. (2010, June 17). *The official "do not use" list of abbreviations*. Retrieved September 18, 2010, from http://www.jointcommission.org/PatientSafety/DoNotUseList/

CHAPTER 19

Specialized Electronic Healthcare Information Systems

Objectives

After studying this chapter you will be able to:

▶ Discuss the potential impact of quality measures for the use of health information technology on patient care.

▶ Discuss the pros and cons for the use of best-of-breed versus integrated health information technology solutions.

▶ Identify two quality measures that would benefit the nurse who has a voice in the selection of an electronic clinical system.

▶ Describe the advantages for the integration of data from pharmacy, laboratory, and radiology information systems with the electronic patient record.

▶ Explain why the Leapfrog Group recommends the use of computerized provider order entry.

▶ Discuss the factors that impact the management of patient flow in hospitals.

▶ Identify at least three factors that would promote the adoption of clinical information systems by nurses.

Key Terms

Active RFID	Health Information
Aggregated Data	Technology (HIT)
Best of Breed	Progressive Disclosure
Certification Commission for	Integrated Interface
Healthcare Information	Mission Critical
Technology (CCHIT)	Passive RFID
Clinical Decision Support	Physician Quality Report
System (CDSS)	Initiative (PQRI)
Clinical Documentation	Picture Archiving and
Closed-Loop Safe Medication	Communication System
Administration	(PACS)
Electronic Medication	Positive Patient Identifier
Administration Record	(PPID)
(eMAR)	Radio Frequency Identifier
Enterprise	(RFID)

The healthcare industry uses a variety of information systems to support and communicate for the delivery of patient care and to manage business operations. Healthcare information systems (HISs) comprise applications that track patients and manage financial data associated with the staff payroll and billing for services rendered and patient care services including nursing, pharmacy, radiology, and laboratory services. In a well-designed system, there is an interface between systems to support the sharing of data so that the data do not have to be reentered. An interface allows for the sharing of data between systems. Two approaches are used when selecting a vendor system: **best-of-breed** or integrated solutions. The best-of-breed approach refers to the selection of systems that best meet the needs of particular services or departments from different vendors, and it requires building an **integrated interface** at the institutional level. The integrated approach refers to the selection of a collection of HISs that are already interfaced; however, the systems may not all be best of breed. An integrated **enterprise** system is an information system designed to meet the needs of the organization at large. The purpose of this chapter is to provide some background for quality initiatives and to explore some specific HIS applications.

Quality Measures for Health Information Technology

Several resources are available to healthcare organizations and care providers who make decisions to purchase **health information technology (HIT)**. Clinical nurses and nurse leaders should be familiar with nationally recognized quality measures for HIT. Nurses must also be knowledgeable about innovative reimbursement incentive efforts to reward quality care, such as the **Physician Quality Report Initiative (PQRI)** by the Centers for Medicare & Medicaid Services (CMS). Nurses, especially if involved in the system selection process, must also understand organizational efforts to address quality care and have the necessary knowledge to judge vendor systems. As an example, vendor system analysis reports might show software components for two different vendor systems to be very similar and equally robust, but the vendor support for planning and implementing the system differs. One vendor may have a better track record of successful implementation of computerized provider order entry (CPOE) than the other.

Physician Quality Report Initiative

The PQRI was authorized in December 2006 when the president signed the Tax Relief and Health Care Act of 2006 (Centers for Medicare & Medicaid Services, 2010). The purpose of the CMS initiative was to provide financial incentives to fee-for-service care providers for cost-effective high-quality care. The Act was designed to be renewed by the president on an annual basis. Information about PQRI is available online at http://www.cms.hhs.gov/pqri/.

Historically, our healthcare delivery system has paid for the number of patients served and the number of resources that were consumed. There have been no financial incentives to improve care – just moral and ethical ones. Hospitals that worked on decreasing patient care costs by decreasing the length of stay and reducing the number of unnecessary tests and medications lost revenue. In other words, the healthcare system rewarded poor care.

The PQRI is voluntary for all fee-for-service providers who bill Medicare, including nurse practitioners, clinical nurse specialists, and certified nurse midwives. As an incentive, qualified participants receive a bonus of approximately 2% (may vary by year) of the revenue, subject to a cap. The evidence-based quality measures used for reporting were identified through a collaborative effort of the Physician Consortium for Performance Improvement°, convened by the American Medical Association, the National Committee for Quality Assurance, and specialty medical associations. The quality measures address care classifications such as advanced care planning, perioperative care, medication reconciliation, imaging, and screening for fall risk. Participants are asked to include information on the use of electronic health records (EHRs) and electronic subscribing.

EHR Certification Organizations

The **Certification Commission for Healthcare Information Technology (CCHIT)**, an independent, private, nonprofit organization, pioneered the EHR certification process. CCHIT provides two certification programs to ensure EHR interoperability. One of the programs, developed independently by CCHIT, has been used to certify EHRs since 2006. The second program was developed specifically to meet the requirements of ONC-ATCB (The Office of the National Coordinator–Authorized Testing and Certification Bodies), set forth by the Health Information Technology for Economic and Clinical Health (HITECH) Act, supporting Meaningful Use Stage 1 (Certification Commission for Health Information Technology, 2010). The organization certifies the following types of EHRs:

- ambulatory EHRs for use by office-based clinicians,
- inpatient EHRs for use by hospitals and health systems,

- EHRs for health networks to allow sharing of EHR data with other health-related systems,
- specialty practice and special care EHRs, and
- electronic personal health record components.

CCHIT began certifying ambulatory EHRs and inpatient EHRs in 2007. The certification of health networks and specialty areas began in 2008.

New ONC-ATCB certification organizations are evolving to meet the needs of the HITECH Act's "meaningful use" requirements. As of January 2011, there were five additional certifying agencies (The Office of the National Coordinator for Health Information Technology, 2010). The number of certifying bodies is expected to grow to meet the needs of "meaningful use." The agencies were authorized to certify complete EHR and EHR modules.

Hit Research and Analysis Reports

Many companies specialize in researching HIT solutions to assist healthcare providers and institutions making purchase solutions. The research reports also serve to assist vendors make decisions for modifying their systems to meet market needs. Considering the millions of dollars involved in adopting new systems, the use of research findings to select a solution makes great sense. Examples of vendor research companies include HIMSS Analytics (http://www.himssanalytics.org/) and KLAS (http://klasresearch.com/). HIMSS Analytics,[1] a nonprofit organization associated with HIMSS, provides benchmarking reports based on provider information. KLAS provides reports based on information from providers who rate the systems. Both HIMSS Analytics and KLAS offer provider participants the results of their reports at no charge.

Healthcare Information Systems

Take a moment to think about all the different services that are necessary to deliver patient care. Even within the nursing department, there are various

services including nursing administration, intensive care units, surgery, and postanesthesia care. It is no different for any other discipline service in a hospital, such as the laboratory and radiology. Each of those smaller services has a specialized information need but most or all share two common needs: access to the patient electronic record and the ability to send charges to the financial management department. When healthcare providers select a system, they weigh the options for best-of-breed solutions, which serve as the best solution for a specialized service or they choose a vendor package that provides an integrated enterprise solution to meet the needs of many or all the services. This section addresses just a few of the many specialty HISs.

Admission, Discharge, and Transfer

The admission, discharge, and transfer (ADT) system was one of the first information systems used in healthcare. It is the backbone of the clinical and business portion of most hospital systems. In the early years, ADT systems were stand-alone best-of-breed systems with an interface to financial systems; however, ADT is now also a common part of integrated enterprise solutions. This application provides and tracks patient details, such as demographics and insurance information, medical record numbers, care providers, and next of kin. All patient interactions are tracked or linked to this basic information. Laboratory results find their way to the appropriate provider or care area based on the important information contained in this portion of the information system. It is important, therefore, that the data in this system should be updated and verified on a regular basis.

Financial Systems

Financial systems are another distinct application in the HIS. They are considered by some as the second backbone of the system because they track financial interactions and provide the fiscal reporting necessary to manage an institution. Financial systems are **mission critical**, which means that the services are vital to the existence of the organization. A few functions of financial systems are to ensure a higher collection rate from payers, to expedite payments for accounts receivable, to minimize third-party payer denials of care, and to prevent underpayment for care.

---

1 HIMSS Analytics is discussed in more detail in Chapter 21.

The problem that many healthcare organizations are facing today is how to get their legacy financial system to communicate with the clinical information system (CIS). Some of the systems in use date back several decades and are not able to meet the demands of regulators and consumers (Conn, 2007). To avoid building costly interfaces at the institutional level, some healthcare organizations choose to purchase enterprise systems that include financial systems, but it is an expensive proposition that costs in the hundreds of millions of dollars range. The integration of the two systems is necessary for efficient billing and to allow for process improvement analysis.

Healthcare agencies recognize the challenges of being able to stay in business and meeting the requirements of regulators and payers. Besides the billing and reimbursement from third-party payers, consumers want to know their out-of-pocket expenses prior to checking into the hospital. Hospitals want to be able to bill Medicare without being accused of fraud.

Unfortunately, fraud accusations–true or not– are in the news daily. As an example, a New Jersey physician received fraudulent reimbursement from Medicaid by billing personal services performed by three people with no medical licenses (Bowman, 2010). An Illinois cardiologist went to prison for fraud after receiving $13 million from Medicare and 30 other private and public insurance programs for services he never rendered (Yin, 2010). He accessed insurance information on patients without their knowledge and hired others to bill for fake services. To place the gravity of the fraud matter in perspective, the costs for Medicare and Medicaid in 2009 were $54 billion. In 2010, CMS initiated a program that uses auditors and high-tech computer software to scan Medicare and Medicaid records for bogus claims (Versel, 2010). The anticipated savings are 2 billion dollars over a 3-year period. The initiative is clearly only a dent in the rampant fraud problem.

Clinical Information Systems

CISs are a conglomerate of integrated and interoperable information systems and technologies that provide information about patient care. The core information systems are the ancillaries: laboratory, radiology, and pharmacy. The **clinical documentation** system is built by using data from the core ancillary systems. Other components of the CIS are the CPOE, the **electronic medication administration record (eMar)**, and **positive patient identifier (PPID)** systems, such as the bar-coded medication administration system.

CIS vendors, like other software companies, continuously work to improve the quality of their products. They make the improvements available as version releases and as major upgrades. Major upgrades are usually associated with a fee and may require equipment upgrades. Major software upgrades could also introduce new software bugs. For these reasons and others, healthcare institutions may choose not to make software changes. On the other hand, nurses who are critical of a certain CIS need to be aware that their concerns may be related to the version of software, not the manufacturer.

Ancillary Systems

The laboratory and radiology systems provide a means of storing and viewing clinical testing and diagnostic patient information. Laboratory systems, one of the earliest clinical systems, have been in use by small and large hospitals for several decades. Laboratory systems integrate data from all the standard laboratory departments including hematology, chemistry, microbiology, blood bank, and pathology. Radiology systems integrate data from patient diagnostic and therapeutic services, including the **picture archiving and communication system (PACS)**. The PACS allows for digital versions of all diagnostic images, such as x-rays and magnetic resonance images, to be stored in the electronic patient record. The pharmacy system provides a means for stocking and recording medications dispensed by the pharmacy. The three ancillary information systems provide a foundation for other clinical systems.

Clinical Documentation

Clinical documentation applications are available in various formats. A good documentation system, whether for nursing or another discipline, is part of the clinical workflow and supports the communication of real-time information. Clinical documentation software is designed by using rules so that when the assessment data with abnormal values, such as a pulse rate or blood pressure, are entered, the abnormal values stand out because they are displayed in a different color (see **Figure 19-1**). These systems remove the need to find the paper chart and allow all who use the electronic chart to access information whenever and wherever it is needed.

Screens can be designed to support assessment documentation by listing systems, or practitioners can be alerted by the system with a pop-up box to complete or verify essential information, such as allergies. Numerical laboratory data, such as a white blood count, hemoglobin, and platelet count, can be displayed in a graph format to visualize trends (see **Figure 19-2**). In a well-planned documentation system, there is little need for the entry of free text, although the ability to do so should be maintained for those occasions when there is no place to document the information and a comment is necessary. When these systems work well, it is because the healthcare professionals who use the system were involved in the planning, designing, implementation, and evaluation of the system.

Nursing information systems sometimes use the nursing process approach with nursing diagnoses as the organizing framework. When properly designed, data collection supports clinical workflow instead of being distracting. It should provide flexibility in both data entry and in viewing data necessary for patient care. Additionally, it should provide easy access to reference information such as policies and procedures as well as online literature.

Clinical documentation systems should provide for the retrieval of data used in long-range planning and research. The use of clinical data by practicing nurses can be facilitated by easy availability of **aggregated data**. Aggregated data are a collection of data that are useful in seeing the big picture. It can be useful in determining best practices and evidence-based care, and can form the basis for decision support systems.

Computerized Provider Order Entry

The CPOE system allows a clinician to place an order by simply selecting a patient and the needed service from a computer screen. The letter "P" in CPOE can mean physician; however, this textbook uses "P" to refer to all care providers who write orders, including physician's assistants and nurse practitioners. The use of CPOE is the number one recommendation made by the Leapfrog Group to improve patient safety and quality (Leapfrog Group, 2009). The advocacy group promotes the safety, quality, and affordability of healthcare. A Leapfrog Group research study indicates that CPOE has the potential benefit of averting approximately 3.1 million preventable adverse medication errors – an annual benefit of $9.2 billion dollars per year (Lwin & Shepard, 2008).

When a provider writes an order by using CPOE, the order is immediately sent to the appropriate department. This saves time, and it prevents transcription errors. Additionally, order entry systems facilitate the capture of financial information for restocking and billing purposes. The advantages attributed to CPOE are electronic prescribing (e-prescribing) and quality improvement (Agency for Healthcare Research Quality, 2008; Dixon & Zafar, 2009). The use of e-prescribing can reduce errors and improve the quality of care because the medication order is checked against a set of rules, such as allergies, drug dosage, administration routes, frequency of administration, and drug-to-drug interaction, by using **clinical decision support system (CDSS)** information. Decision support is a computer application that uses a complex system of rules to analyze data and presents information to support the decision-making process of the knowledge worker. That is, if a medication order is entered and the dosage exceeds normal limits for that medication, the provider will be given this information. The system should also provide information about any potential drug incompatibilities and patient allergies.

Medication Administration

The use of HIT for medication administration is a process that goes hand-in-hand with CPOE with the purpose of making patient care safer by reducing potential and actual errors. In the paper record world, the medication administration process resided in three record silos – the doctor's order, the pharmacist's verification/dispensing records, and the nurse's administration/paper

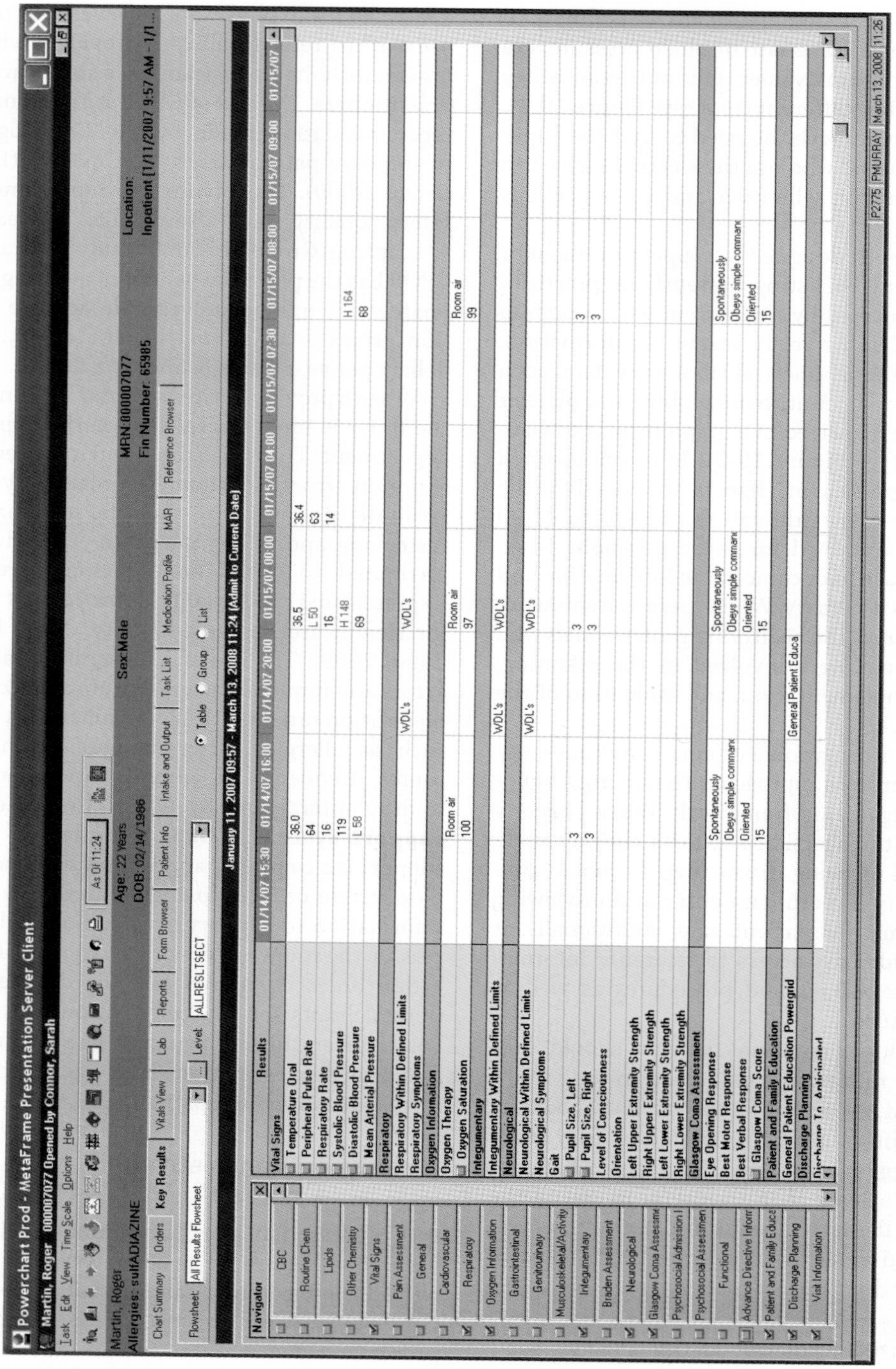

Figure 19-1 Clinical assessment data display with abnormal values. (Used with permission from Cerner Corporation.)

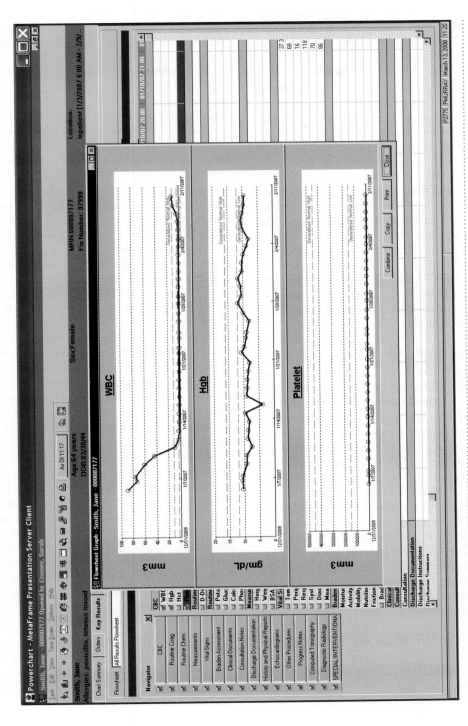

Figure 19-2 Laboratory values trended data display. (Used with permission from Cerner Corporation.)

documentation record. In reality, electronic medication administration is a medication-use process addressed with the use of the eMar.

eMar

The eMar discussed in Chapter 18 is a multidisciplinary record that communicates the complex process of medication use. The use of the eMar requires the implementation of CPOE and CDSS. The eMar guides the nurse to use the six rights when administering medications: the right drug, the right dose, the right time, the right route, the right patient, and the right documentation. If well designed, it includes all the pertinent documentation appropriate for the medication that is administered. Because the eMar can provide a view of information in the database, the nurse can query it to display scheduled medications and medications that are pending, past due, and/or previously administered. The eMar provides a mechanism for efficient nurse time utilization as well as facilitates the delivery of safe care.

Positive Patient Identifier

The PPID with bar-coded or **radio frequency identifier (RFID)**-tagged bracelets is used with the eMar for **closed-loop safe medication administration**. The term "closed loop" means that the right patient received the right medication, and it is an essential component of patient safety improvements. The Joint Commission first issued a recommendation for accurately identifying patients in 2003. The following year, the U.S. Food and Drug Administration recommended the use of barcodes on patient identification bracelets.

The medication administration procedures when using bar coding or **passive RFID** are similar. Both procedures require the use of a barcode or RFID scanner that is either handheld or built into a laptop or tablet computer. The nurses first scan their barcode or RFID tag on their ID badge to identify themselves in the system. Next, the nurses scan the barcode on the medication and finally scan the patient's armband prior to administering the medication. If the tag uses **active RFID**, which means that the RFID tag is battery powered and constantly transmitting signals, the use of a scanning device is not necessary, because the identifier will be recognized by the computer

(Sun, Wang, & Wu, 2008). The use of active RFID would allow PPIDs without disturbing the patient (e.g., when hanging an intravenous [IV] line while a patient is sleeping).

The outcomes of research on the use of PPID with the eMar are promising. A pilot study conducted at a 300-bed hospital after the implementation of barcode medication administration (BCMA) revealed an 80% error reduction (Foote & Coleman, 2008). A systematic review of 25 studies to analyze risk reduction after the implementation of CPOE revealed new insights. In 23 of the studies, there was a relative risk reduction of medication errors by 13%–99% (Ammenwerth, Schnell-Inderst, Machan, & Siebert, 2008). Two of the studies had negative results and revealed possible shortcomings in the design, implementation, and/or workflow analyses.

The complexity of the medication process cannot be overemphasized. CPOE and BCMA are not magic bullets. Examples of factors that facilitate or impede the safe administration of medications include the quality of the workflow analysis, physician verification of current medications, CPOE and BCMA hardware and software, the medication barcode, the barcode on the patient armband, and the process for medication administration. Nurses who find the BCMA impeding the ability to administer medications have been known to use workarounds in order to administer medications. However, they may not understand the possible negative consequences and threats to the patient's safety. The results of a study conducted in two large hospitals located in the Midwest and the East coast of the United States revealed 31 types of potential medication errors and 7 types of process workarounds (Kaplan, 2008; Koppel, Wetterneck, Telles, & Karsh, 2008). The classifications for potential errors were related to technology, tasks, organization, patients, and the environment. The types of workarounds were as follows:

- Scanning the medication without verifying the medication list, drug name, and dose.
- Physicians not verifying the eMar current medication list, resulting in additional medication given to the patient.
- Administering the medication without reviewing the parameters for administration.

- Bypassing the policy for a check by a second provider or the second nurse confirms without verifying the medication.
- Administering medications without reviewing new medication orders.
- Administering medications without scanning the patient barcode to confirm the patient's identification.
- Administering the medication without scanning the medication barcode to confirm the correct medication, dose, and time.

The researchers noted that when patient armband barcodes did not work, nurses often used nonstandard procedure and printed extra copies of the barcode (Kaplan, 2008). Consequently, information management services take efforts to thwart the nonstandard procedures. When workarounds are observed, there must also be an investigation and correction of the issues that impede the safe medication administration process.

Managing Patient Flow

Patient flow is a long-standing hospital issue that must be addressed to provide safe and efficient patient care. The problems associated with patient flow are multifactorial and are based on the principle of supply (hospital beds and resources) and demand (patients). Hospitals have to operate with nearly full bed capacity for economic efficiency purposes. Staffing, supplies, and resources are budgeted according to the average occupancy. Most hospital budgets have very little flexibility.

The demand for hospital care resources is affected by the aging population, many of whom have chronic diseases such as congestive heart failure, diabetics, and chronic renal disease. This medically fragile population often has acute episodic needs because of their disease processes. As a result, the population is negatively impacted during the annual flu season. Patients expect to be treated at the time of need. If they are unable to see a physician during office hours, they use emergency services where patient flow problems begin. Emergency beds fill quickly because of the lack of available hospital beds for patients who need to be admitted, causing a patient traffic jam.

The Joint Commission issued a new recommendation requiring hospitals to discover and minimize

barriers to well-organized patient flow in 2004 (McBeth, 2005). Scoring on the standard went into effect on January 1, 2005. The recommendation was the result of root cause analyses for sentinel events, which reported that emergency department (ED) overcapacity was a contributing factor in 31% of sentinel event cases (McBeth, 2005). Hospital leaders quickly recognized the difficulty in planning, tracking, and managing patient flow, and as a result, many, especially the large facilities, turned to informatics bed management systems. According to the American Hospital Association Quality Center (2007, p. 29), "The goal of bed management is to accurately place the patient in the right unit with the right level of staff and right level of care the first time."

Tracking Systems Solutions

A variety of informatics solutions are available that both track the processes involved with patient flow, such as bed availability, and provide documentation of time lapses, which is used in the analysis of data and planning. Radianse Reveal RTLS™, McKesson Horizon Enterprise Visibility, and the Versus® RTLS all use RFID tags to monitor patient locations (McKesson Corp, 2010; Radianse, 2009; Versus, 2010). Features common to many of the popular patient-tracking systems include the visual display of beds, which indicates the patient status (e.g., discharge, fall risk, methicillin-resistant Staphylococcus aureus [MRSA]), bed availability display, instant transport notification, and equipment (e.g., wheelchairs) locators.

Reports from a study conducted on a healthcare system at a hospital located in Delaware showed that information from patient flow management tools can be used to improve the care delivery system (ADVANCE, 2007). After the patient flow system was implemented, the time for the ED outpatients from triage to exit decreased by 14 minutes. For ED patients who were admitted to the hospital, the time from triage to exit decreased by 36 minutes. The percentage of patients who left the ED without being seen was decreased by 24%. The ED was able to accommodate a 7% volume increase in the number of patients seen.

Voice Communication Systems

Communication systems facilitate the exchange of information needed by the various healthcare disciplines. Examples include the use of e-mail, Internet, and intranet systems. Although these systems may not be integrated with clinical systems, they enhance information flow within the organization and work-flow patterns. They have an indirect impact on clinical practice. An example of a wireless communication system is Vocera™ Communications (Vocera Communications, Inc., San Jose, CA). The product uses a combination of technologies: a wireless local area network that is 802.11 compliant, speech recognition software, and voice over Internet protocol (VoIP) to allow mobile working to communicate interactively within the same building.

A study to determine the benefits of using Vocera technology was conducted at a 299-bed health-care organization located in Maryland (Breslin, Greskovich, & Turisco, 2004). The study design compared a traditional telephone and overhead paging system with the voice-activated communication device using two similar nursing units over a 4-day period. The researchers determined that communication with Vocera was five times quicker than traditional methods, and the time saved was equivalent to 3,477 hours per year or $74,000 per unit. A second study at the same healthcare organization was completed over 7.4 weeks during 2005 to study the time responses to a patient's request following the integration of Vocera technology with the nurse call system. The results of the study demonstrated a 51% reduction in response time for patient calls, which was equivalent to a potential savings of $37,700 (Kuruzovich, Angst, Faraj, & Agarwal, 2006).

Some suggest that VoIP is a technology of the past in the healthcare arena. Hospitals and healthcare providers are gravitating toward the use of smartphones for voice communication (Millard, 2010; Rawson, 2010; Voalté, 2010). Smartphones allow for voice communication, text messaging, and applications that facilitate the delivery of healthcare. It is clear that there is no "one size fits all" solution for healthcare providers (Blackberry, 2010). The promise is that the popularity of the smartphone with the benefits of multipurpose use will influence the adoption rate. By 2013, some suggest that there will be approximately 1 billion smartphones in the world and that smartphones will replace the traditional phone used in the past (Lyons, 2010; Rawson, 2010). Factors influencing the adoption include the ability to disinfect the device, data encryption and antitheft

prevention, and the ability to integrate with EMR (electronic medical record) and EHR. There is little certainty for the direction that voice communication systems will take in the future. However, we can anticipate that overhead paging systems and pagers will become extinct and that smartphones will be at least one component in future systems.

Critical Pathways

Information systems allow for the construction of critical pathways. Critical pathways provide a foundation for multidisciplinary documentation that focuses on the attainment of a specific clinical outcome within a defined length of time. The pathway identifies the patient-desired outcomes. The criteria required for their achievement are predetermined by representatives of the multidisciplinary groups involved in the care of patients with a particular diagnosis. The development of the critical path is based on a review of the literature and a synthesis of findings. The structure of the path allows for the documentation of assessment elements, interventions, patient response to interventions, and coordination of documentation by all disciplines.

Point-of-Care Systems

Clinical systems should be accessible at both the point of care and quiet places where the nurse is able to sit down and reflect on patient care events to chart accurately. Nurses' attitudes about the use of clinical systems are often shaped by the ease or difficulty in its use. For example, common complaints are about heavy carts that are difficult to get through doorways or into a patient's room. Any rolling device is subject to the same problems as those encountered with poles for IVs, such as wheels sticking because of spills on the floor from IV solutions or other solutions, wheels that "fall off" of moveable carts, or difficulty in pushing a cart because of the cart's weight or carpeting. To answer nurses' concerns, some facilities have chosen to use lightweight tablet computers with built-in scanning devices for barcode recognition. Others are using laptops on small rolling platforms. With every solution, new problems arise (e.g., problems with battery life, device failure, or theft of portable devices).

Summary

Today's complex healthcare delivery environment requires the use of numerous specialized electronic HISs. Nurses should be aware of the advantages and disadvantages of choosing best-of-breed systems versus integrated enterprise solutions. Quality initiatives such as the PQRI and CCHIT are driving forces for information technology adoption. CCHIT has an aggressive agenda for certifying vendor solutions for the electronic record, which includes ambulatory, inpatient, and specialty practice and specialty care EHRs. CCHIT is also certifying health networks that share data from the electronic record.

The two backbones for the clinical and business portion of most hospital systems are the ADT system and the financial system. Both have been in existence for several decades. Because many of the legacy systems have run their course, there is a growing trend to replace them by using integrated enterprise solutions to share data with the CIS.

The foundation for the CIS is made up of data from laboratory, radiology, and pharmacy information systems. Therapeutic and diagnostic data seamlessly interfaces with the clinical documentation system and allows the clinician visual alerts for abnormal values and data trends over time. CPOE is designed to reduce order errors and to expedite the delivery of safe patient care. Medication administration is a complex process involving the provider who orders the medication, the pharmacist who checks the order and dispenses the medication, and the nurse who administers the medication. The eMar provides real-time communication among all who are involved in the process. The PPID is verified by using bar coding or RFID-tagged armbands. It provides for a closed-loop medication administration in which the right patient receives the right medication correctly and on time.

The Joint Commission 2004 recommendation requiring hospitals to discover and minimize barriers to patient flow has spurred hospitals to look for informatics solutions. As a result, some hospitals have various electronic tracking systems for patient beds, personnel, and equipment such as wheelchairs.

Data from the tracking systems can be analyzed to improve patient flow from admission to discharge, thereby improving the efficiency of the use of scarce resources such as ED and telemetry beds.

The nurse plays a key role in the adoption and use of information technology. The access and use of CISs should be designed to assist the nurse in the delivery of efficient, safe care. Consideration must be made for the selection and placement of equipment such as desktop computers, laptops, tablets, scanners, and medication storage devices. Although the workflow using electronic systems is different from paper record systems, the focus on quality patient outcomes remains the same.

APPLICATIONS AND COMPETENCIES

1. Search the Internet for information about managing patient flow. Summarize your findings to explain how changing hospital processes can improve patient flow outcomes.

2. Review the PQRI website. Compare the incentive for a quality care concept with the traditional fee-for-service concept. Will the use of incentives impact the adoption of HIT on patient care? Why or why not?

3. Explore the use of best-of-breed versus integrated HIT solutions at a local hospital. Discuss the pros and cons for each approach.

4. Conduct an Internet search for HIS research and analysis services. On the basis of your findings, identify two quality measures that would benefit the nurse who has a voice in the selection of an electronic clinical system.

5. Describe the advantages for the integration of data with the electronic patient record for each of the ancillary information systems listed below.
   a. Pharmacy
   b. Laboratory
   c. Radiology

6. Review the Leapfrog Group website and then explain why the Leapfrog Group recommends the use of CPOE.

7. Review the Joint Commission website and at least one website for a company that provides informatics solutions to assist in the management of patient flow. Discuss the pertinent factors that leadership should plan to monitor to improve patient flow.

8. Does the healthcare agency where you work use a CIS? If so, do all the nurses support the use of technology? Why or why not? Explain at least three factors that would promote the adoption of clinical systems by nurses.

REFERENCES

ADVANCE. (2007). Using technology to protect patients. *ADVANCE for Health Information Executives, 11*, 29–32.

Agency for Healthcare Research Quality. (2008). *Health IT: Support for effective use of electronic prescribing* (No. 08-PFS015). Retrieved from http://portal.ahrq.gov/portal/server.pt/gateway/PTARGS_0_834454_0_0_18/08-PFS015_eRx.pdf

American Hospital Association. (2007). Improving patient flow patient satisfaction and patient safety. *Hospital & Health Networks, 81*(11), 28–29.

Ammenwerth, E., Schnell-Inderst, P., Machan, C., & Siebert, U. (2008). The effect of electronic prescribing on medication errors and adverse drug events: A systematic review. *Journal of the American Medical Informatics Association, 15*(5), 585–600.

Blackberry. (2010). *Six lessons learned as hospitals journey to smartphone utopia – Business exchange.* Retrieved November 6, 2010, from http://whitepapers.bx.businessweek.com/content9636

Bowman, D. (2010, September 10). 'Fake doctors' treated patients in Medicaid fraud scheme. *FierceHealthcare: Daily News for Healthcare Executives.* Retrieved from http://www.fiercehealthcare.com/story/fake-doctors-used-medicaid-fraud-scheme/2010-09-10

Breslin, S., Greskovich, W., & Turisco, F. (2004). Wireless technology improves nursing workflow and communications. *CIN: Computers, Informatics, Nursing, 22*(5), 275–281.

Centers for Medicare & Medicaid Services. (2010, September 16). *Overview physician quality reporting initiative.* Retrieved September 22, 2010, from http://www.cms.gov/pqri/

Certification Commission for Health Information Technology. (2010, September 14). *CCHIT certification update.* Retrieved September 22, 2010, from http://www.cchit.org/sites/all/files/CCHITCertificationOverview.pdf

Conn, J. (2007). Following the money. Financial data systems – which have long taken second billing to clinical IT – gain attention as focus turns to quality, consumerism. *Modern Healthcare, 37*(27), 28–30.

Dixon, B. E., & Zafar, A. (2009). *Inpatient computerized provider order entry (CPOE): Findings from the AHRQ portfolio.* Retrieved from http://portal.ahrq.gov/portal/server.pt/gateway/PTARGS_0_846328_0_0_18/09-0031-EF_cpoe.pdf

Foote, S. O., & Coleman, J. R. (2008). Medication administration: The implementation process of bar-coding for medication administration to enhance medication safety. *Nursing Economic$, 26*(3), 207–210.

Kaplan, M. (2008, July 2). *Barcoded technology to reduce medication administration has flaws.* Retrieved September 25, 2010, from http://www.medicalnewstoday.com/printerfriendlynews.php?newsid=113498

Koppel, R., Wetterneck, T., Telles, J. L., & Karsh, B. T. (2008). Workarounds to barcode medication administration systems: Their occurrences, causes, and threats to patient safety. *Journal of the American Medical Informatics Association, 15*(4), 408–423.

Kuruzovich, J., Angst, C. M., Faraj, S., & Agarwal, R. (2008). Wireless communication role in patient response time: A study of Vocera integration with a nurse call system. *CIN: Computers Informatics Nursing, 26*(3), 159–166. Doi: 10.1097/01.NCN.0000304780.27070.ee

Leapfrog Group. (2009). *The Leapfrog Group fact sheet.* Retrieved September 25, 2010, from http://www.leapfroggroup.org/about_us/leapfrog-factsheet

Lwin, A. K., & Shepard, D. S. (2008, September 23). *Estimating lives and dollars saved from universal adoption of the leapfrog safety and quality standards.* Retrieved September 25, 2010, from http://www.leapfroggroup.org/media/file/Lives_Saved_Leapfrog_Report_2008-Final_%282%29.pdf

Lyons, D. (2010, October 3). How Android is transforming mobile computing. *Newsweek.* Retrieved from http://www.newsweek.com/2010/10/03/how-android-is-transforming-mobile-computing.html

McBeth, S. (2005). Mitigate impediments to efficient patient flow. *Nursing Management, 36*(7), 16–17.

McKesson Corp. (2010). *Enterprise patient visibility and tracking software helps enhance patient flow and speed clinical decisions.* Retrieved September 25, 2010, from http://www.mckesson.com/en_us/McKesson.com/For%2BHealthcare%2BProviders/Hospitals/Interdisciplinary%2BCare%2BSolutions/Horizon%2BEnterprise%2BVisibility.html

Millard, M. (2010, May 10). Smartphones save money and stave off staffing shortages, study finds. *HealthIT News.* Retrieved from http://www.healthcareitnews.com/news/smartphones-save-money-and-stave-staffing-shortages-study-finds

Radianse. (2009). *The Radianse Reveal RTLS platform – How it works.* Retrieved September 25, 2010, from http://www.radianse.com/reveal-how-it-works.html

Rawson, M. (2010, October 20). From pagers to smartphones: Why hospitals are making the switch. *Healthview News.* Retrieved from http://healthviewnews.com/from-pagers-to-smartphones-why-hospitals-are-making-the-switch/

Sun, P. R., Wang, B. H., & Wu, F. (2008). A new method to guard inpatient medication safety by the implementation of RFID. *Journal of Medical Systems, 32*(4), 327–332.

The Office of the National Coordinator for Health Information Technology. (2010, December 28). *ONC-authorized testing and certification bodies.* Retrieved January 25, 2011, from http://healthit.hhs.gov/portal/server.pt?open=512&mode=2&objID=3120

Versel, N. (2010, March 29). CMS to fight Medicare, Medicaid fraud with high-texh 'bounty hunters'. *FierceHealthcare: Daily News for Healthcare Executives.* Retrieved from http://www.fiercehealthit.com/story/cms-fight-medicare-medicaid-fraud-high-tech-bounty-hunters/2010-03-29

Versus. (2010). *Versus IR RFID patient tracking, asset tracking, and hospital patient flow solutions.* Retrieved August 31, 2011, from http://www.versustech.com/

Voalté. (2010, May). *Smart hospitals embracing smartphones at the point of care.* Retrieved November 6, 2010, from http://www.voalte.com/uploads/docs/Smart%20Hospitals.pdf

Yin, S. (2010, August 12). Fraud: Cardiologist billed Medicare, other insurers $13M for untreated patients. *FierceHealthcare: Daily News for Healthcare Executives.* Retrieved from http://www.fiercehealthcare.com/story/fraud-cardiologist-billed-medicare-other-insurers-13m-untreated-patients/2010-08-12

CHAPTER 20

Electronic Healthcare System Issues

Objectives

After studying this chapter you will be able to:

Use the EMR Adoption model to analyze the level of adoption for a healthcare agency.

▶ Discuss the risks and opportunities for sharing clinical data.

▶ Discuss how the privacy and confidentiality of patient electronic information is currently being addressed in healthcare.

▶ Discuss how the issue of interoperability affects the sharing of patient health information.

▶ Provide an example that demonstrates the significance of workflow redesign as it relates to a clinical documentation system.

▶ Identify ways that healthcare is addressing the Joint Commission's patient safety goals with the use of health information technology.

▶ Provide at least two examples of strong passwords, with an explanation about why the password is strong.

Key Terms

Accuracy of Data	Return on Investment (ROI)
Authentication	Single Sign-On
Biometrics	Spear phishing
Clinical Decision Support System (CDSS)	Stark Rules
	Strategic Planning
Data Security	Tangibles
Intangibles	Unintended Consequences
Interoperability	Voice Recognition
Login	Workflow Redesign
Password	

The use of health information technology (HIT) is improving patient care outcomes. The rate of adoption of technology solutions is growing. All the issues associated with its use have not been resolved. The transition from a paper record world to an automated one is a huge endeavor. Healthcare practitioners are slow to adopt new solutions that they believe could jeopardize patient care while they are "unlearning" legacy processes and "learning" new approaches. This chapter focuses on a few of the issues associated with the adoption of HIT.

The Adoption Model for the Electronic Medical Record

Unraveling the complexity of healthcare delivery systems when planning the adoption of information technology can be a daunting process. HIMSS Analytics, a nonprofit subsidiary of Healthcare Information and Management Systems Society (HIMSS), has defined an adoption model, as seen in **Table 20-1**, for the electronic medical record (EMR). The model serves as a guide for healthcare providers

Table 20-1 EMR Adoption Model[sm]

Stage	Cumulative Capabilities
7	Complete EMR (electronic medical record); CCD (continuity of care document) transactions to share data; data warehousing; data continuity with ED (emergency department), ambulatory, OP (outpatient)
6	Physician documentation (structured templates), full CDSS (variance and compliance), full R-PACS (radiology – picture archiving and communication system)
5	Closed-loop medication administration
4	CPOE, CDSS (clinical protocols)
3	Nursing/clinical documentation (flow sheets), CDSS (error checking), PACS available outside radiology
2	CDR, controlled medical vocabulary, and CDSS may have document imaging; HIE–capable
1	Ancillaries – laboratory, radiology, pharmacy – all installed
0	All three ancillaries not installed

From HIMSS Analytics. (2008). *Healthcare providers: EMR Adoption model.* Retrieved November 23, 2008, from http://www. himssanalytics.org/hc_providers/index.asp)

who are transitioning from the paper record to the electronic record. It should be useful for multidisciplinary information technology implementation committees that are involved with system procurement and budget planning.

At stage 0, all the basic clinical systems (laboratory, pharmacy, or radiology) are not in place (HIMSS Analytics, 2009). At stage 1, all three of the basic clinical systems exist. At stage 2, there is physician access to obtain and view results from a clinical data repository (CDR) fed by the clinical systems. At this stage, there is also a "controlled medical vocabulary" (standardized healthcare vocabulary) and a **clinical decision support system (CDSS)** for conflict checking in place. At stage 2, the system is capable of health information exchange.

At stage 3, clinical documentation is integrated with the CDR with at least one other hospital service. There is error checking for order entry by using CDSS, and a picture archive and communication system available outside of radiology by using a secure network such as an intranet is in place. Clinical documentation is described as nurses' notes, the electronic administration record (eMAR), flow sheets, and care plans. At stage 4, computerized provider order entry (CPOE) and CDSS related to evidence-based care protocols are in place on at least one patient care area. This level is achieved with implementation on only one patient service.

At stage 5, the closed-loop medication administration is achieved by using the eMAR and a

method for auto-identifying the patient is integrated with the pharmacy system. At stage 6, physician patient documentation and the ability to view all radiology images is available on at least one patient care area. At the highest level of implementation, stage 7, clinical information can be shared electronically with authorized providers, payers, patients, and others through a regional health network, creating a true electronic health record (EHR), as defined in this book. The hospital does not use paper records to manage patient care. Furthermore, a clinical data warehouse is used to analyze clinical data patterns for the purpose of improving the quality of care.

The issues associated with the adoption of HIT become evident when viewing the percentage of adoption at each stage. According to HIMSS Analytics, as of 2008, 4.3% of 5,050 healthcare agencies were between stages 4 and 7 (HIMSS Analytics, 2008). By 2010, 19.2% of 5,281 healthcare agencies were between stages 4 and 7, with the highest level of adoption achieved by 1% of providers. The most current adoption data for the United States and Canada is on the HIMSS Analytics website at http://www.himssanalytics.org.

Adoption of the EHR places the patient as the first and foremost recipient of benefits. Providing the best possible patient care requires access to the data generated in patient care situations and systems, which can monitor for known problem areas and anticipate others (**Box 20-1**). Although

BOX 20-1 Some Benefits of a Fully Integrated Electronic Health Record

To clinicians	To patients	To researchers and policymakers
• Availability of information when and where it is needed. This information includes patient data and bibliographic resources.	• Knowledge of who has access to their data.	• Time savings in obtaining data.
		• Large databanks yielding more valid and precise research.
	• Individualized treatment anywhere the computer-based patient record is available.	
		• Ability to answer questions at local, state national, and possibly international levels.
• Decision support.	• Ability to check the accuracy of their record.	
• Organization of information specific to the discipline so that it can be easily located.	• One location for all healthcare data.	
	• Evidence-based healthcare.	
• Facilitation of the process of preparing reports for internals and external entities.		
• Ease of order entry.		
• Elimination of multiple entries of the same data.		

we are making headway, there is still much work ahead before this goal becomes an everyday reality.

Strategic Planning

Healthcare agency **strategic planning** lays the groundwork for the adoption of healthcare information technology; it is absolutely essential for successful system implementation. A strategic plan is a roadmap that guides the institution in meeting its mission. It is used to guide decision-making practices over a 3- or 5–10-year period. It also provides a guide for the acquisition of resources and for budget priorities. It should be a living and breathing document that allows for flexibility. As an example, it should provide the ability to incorporate the use of new evolving technologies. The costs associated with the use of an HIT solution, such as CPOE, are often in the thousands to millions of dollars range, depending on the size of the institution (Conrad & Gardner, 2005). As a result, the stakeholders must be able to see that the expenditures are offset by patient outcome benefits; they must see a **return on investment (ROI)**. If the use of information technology is not supported by the institution's strategic plan, it will probably not be funded (Hunt, Sproat, & Kitzmiller, 2004).

Return on Investment

The ROI is an important issue serving as a barrier to the adoption of electronic systems. "Chief financial officers toil to accurately present their financial counterparts with measures that capture the impact on items such as averting medication errors or reducing future cost outlays by catching illnesses in early stages" (Runy & Towne, 2005). Improving patient care outcomes and managing costs should align with the strategic plans for healthcare agencies. The process of ROI requires scrutiny regarding risks and the associated values. In other words, is risk offset by the potential value? If so, what data are available to support the value? Those persons involved in budget-making decisions must identify goals and methods for measuring achievement for both tangible and intangible values and risks. A 2006 study indicated that although there are increased expenses associated with the use of information technology, there is an ROI in the acute care setting (Menachemi, Burkhardt, Shewchuk, Burke, & Brooks, 2006).

Tangibles are those values that can be clearly measured, calculated, and quantified with numerical data (Runy & Towne, 2005). Examples of tangibles include a decrease in length of stay, a decrease in anti-infective medication costs, a decrease in the number of unnecessary medications and tests, and a decrease in charges per admission. The literature reports that after the implementation of CPOE for intensive care unit patients in one setting, the costs associated with anti-infective medications fell by 70% and total hospital costs for the patients decreased by 25% (Conrad & Gardner, 2005).

Intangibles are those values that are not easily calculated or in which the results cannot be directly attributed to the investment. Examples of intangibles include improved decision making, communication, and user satisfaction (Runy & Towne, 2005).

Intangibles may vary between healthcare settings as a result of the differences in factors such as organizational culture, physical environments, population served, and staffing.

Fortunately, the results of a number of studies (Agency for Healthcare Research and Quality, 2001; Birkmeyer & Dimick, 2004; Conrad & Gardner, 2005) have spurred efforts by individual healthcare organizations in larger geographical areas to initiate the adoption of CPOE to improve patient care outcomes. The results from the research studies have been used to benchmark data and to calculate ROIs.

Reimbursement

Reimbursement is a crucial issue for healthcare agencies, physicians, and other providers. The Centers for Medicare & Medicaid services passed the Physician Self-Referral Law in an effort to prevent Medicare fraud (Centers for Medicare & Medicaid Services, 2010c). The law is more commonly known as Stark Law or **Stark Rules** because Congressman Peter Stark introduced it. It has been criticized for interfering with collaborative innovations and limiting the ability of healthcare agencies and providers to design seamless solutions for sharing healthcare information using technology (Milstein, 2007). The law was relaxed in August 2006 to provide an incentive for physicians to adopt a certified EHR. The amended law allowed hospitals to donate "certified" interoperable systems to physicians (Kibbe & Mongiardo, 2010). On the other hand, the law has been criticized for swaying physicians to use the hospital's choice of clinical information system vendor.

Electronic Medical Record Versus Electronic Health Record

The terms EMR and EHR are often used interchangeably, but the differences are very important. The EMR belongs to the healthcare agency. Information associated with the EMR can be a composite of several different information systems that may or may not be intergrated. The

EHR includes certain information from healthcare agency EMRs as well as other healthcare providers (e.g., physicians, nurse practitioners, and pharmacies). The EHR allows health information to be shared with consumers, authorized providers, and public health personnel (National Committee Vital Health Statistics, 2001). Information embedded in the EHRs provides a strong foundation for new knowledge formation. Examples of information stored in the EHR include patient histories, medical tests, medications, and images (Health Information Technology, 2010).

There are five main issues associated with electronic health information: (1) **interoperability** standards, (2) user design, (3) **workflow redesign**, (4) quality measurement, and (5) **data security**. Theoretically, the certification requirement has resolved issues associated with the EHR. However, they still apply to commercial vendor EMR products.

Interoperability

The lack of interoperability standards interferes with the ability to share information by authorized users, including the patient. Interoperability is especially a significant issue as it relates to clinical information system and the EMR. Clinical information systems refer to a group of technology-enabled systems, which may or may not be originally designed to share data with one another. Purchasing from a single vendor does not assure the buyer that the system is seamlessly interoperable. Large well-known vendors commonly purchase smaller popular applications and then design interfaces with other vendor applications. The resulting lack of interoperability requires nurses to document the same data in more than one area or application because the data do not flow over to another application. Many times the deviations seem minor, but in reality the deviation from system standard can become a huge issue when attempting to standardize, update, and maintain data (Campbell, Sittig, Ash, Guappone, & Dykstra, 2006) or to integrate applications, develop interfaces, or aggregate data between systems. One of the significant rewards of a clinical information system is the ability to share data.

User Design

User design of data entry screens is an issue because many healthcare providers involved in the design process have no background knowledge of or skills with database design. As a result, providers approach user design by using paper-chart thinking (Baron, 2007). Until all healthcare providers have some kind of education on informatics and database design basics, the issue will not be resolved. Examples of screen-design issues include lack of use of uniform pain scales, pain documentation, pressure ulcer prevention programs, and falls prevention programs. These design issues impact the ability to analyze the data for evidence-based practice decisions. They also make documentation of care challenging for nurses who float to other units or who work for temporary assistance agencies. Finally, lack of uniformity introduces new opportunities for extending the time for documentation, user frustration, and documentation errors.

Workflow Redesign

Workflow redesign is one of the many difficult issues that healthcare providers face when planning and designing the application of electronic systems. As noted several times earlier, one of the problems is the lack of experience or lack of knowledge about other ways to accomplish work. Another problem relates to resistance to change. Workflow redesign also relates to the tedious processes involved in identifying how work is changed with a technology solution. It involves creating process flow diagrams that paint "before" and "after" pictures of workflow. Finally, redesign involves the nuts-and-bolts questions about the presence of computers. Common questions faced by nurses are as follows:

- How many computers are needed?
- Where should the computers be located?
- Should the computers be placed on wheeled stands (computer on wheels) so that they can be moved or should they be at the bedside?
- What are the fire marshal regulations for storing moveable or wall-mounted computers in patient unit hallways?
- If laptops or tablets are used, can these be prevented from being stolen?

- How can the patient or their visitors be prevented from using the computer?
- When documenting care in public places, can unauthorized eyes be prevented from viewing the data?

Quality Measurement

A CDR has the potential to allow us to measure quality. The goal for the use of HIT is improved patient outcomes and quality of care, not the use of HIT (Milstein, 2007). A quality measurement issue is that the data fields have to be designed in a way that allows users to query the data for answers. Clinical application vendors need to work with providers to identify quality measures and design data entry windows to capture the data so that the computer can analyze it.

Introduction of Unintended Consequences

The introduction of technology into a healthcare delivery system can result in unintended and unexpected consequences (Ash, Berg, & Coiera, 2004; Ash, Sittig, Campbell, Guappone, & Dykstra, 2007; Ash, Sittig, Poon, et al., 2007). An unintended consequence refers to an outcome, good or bad, that was not planned or deliberate. Researchers have reported on **unintended consequences** for the use of CPOE and CDSS. The findings from the research studies should assist nurses in avoiding these problems and recognizing the necessary compromises that must be made to ensure patient safety.

CPOE

Research investigating CPOE revealed nine types of unintended consequences (Ash, Sittig, Poon, et al., 2007; Campbell et al., 2006). Two of the consequences related to the way work (more and new work) and workflow changed after CPOE. For example, the providers were responsible for entering orders instead of the nurses or secretaries. At least initially, work tasks took a longer time as the users learned to adjust to a new ordering system.

System demands were the third consequence. The CPOE system required unintended system design, support, and maintenance that involved personnel, software, and hardware requirements. Communication and emotions were two other unintended consequences. Although patient information was readily available, some users used the computers to replace face-to-face communication when indeed communication never occurred; there was only the appearance of communication. The information was entered into the computer, but the person who needed it did not know. Computers should enhance, not replace, other types of communication.

Emotions ranged from love to hate. Personnel who were comfortable with automated systems acclimated to CPOE, but those who were uncomfortable experienced strong negative emotions. CPOE led to power shifts, and some believed the physician was perceived as losing power, but others felt that pharmacists lost power because the physician took responsibility for ordering medications. The dependence on technology was considered an unintended consequence of problems and productivity loss associated with computer downtimes.

The research on the effects of CPOE revealed new kinds of errors and problems with confusing user-screen designs, and order option presentations had the potential to result in new errors. Use of long drop-down menus had the potential for inadvertent selection of the wrong patient. Other potential errors were related to medication dosing errors and orders that overlapped.

Decision Support Systems

Another research study that investigated CDSS also revealed unintended consequences (Ash, Sittig, Campbell, et al., 2007). The research findings identified "patterns" of unintended consequences as (1) those related to content and (2) those related to the way information was presented on the computer screen. Consequences related to content included the possibility of continuing unnecessary daily orders, such as chest x-rays. Content also related to the way orders had to be entered, resulting in a lack of full information from other professionals. There were problems that related to difficulties in updating the clinical decision support rules and wrong or misleading alerts. There were also problems related to inadequate communication between systems, resulting in a lack of supplies or misinformation about the costs of laboratory testing. Consequences related to clinical decision support representation on the computer screen related to order information that was required but not available and alert fatigue from too many alerts.

As in the CPOE research, CDSS research revealed unintended potential errors. Examples include the accidental selection of an auto-complete word when typing and notifications that were delivered in an untimely manner. Finally, potential errors could occur when editing and correcting a clinical decision support rule.

Rules and Regulations: The Joint Commission

The Joint Commission has challenged the healthcare organizations it surveys with annual national safety goals (The Joint Commission, 2010). The patient safety goals can be viewed at http://www.patient safety.gov/TIPS/Docs/TIPS_JanFeb10Poster.pdf. Three of the top patient safety goals for years 2003–2008 can be augmented with the use of HIT. The first goal (2010) is to improve the accuracy of patient identification. Some agencies are using bars or armbands embedded with the radio frequency identification (RFID) chip code to meet the goal (stage 5 of the EMR Adoption model in **Table 20-1**).

The second safety goal is to improve communication. The communication goal 2.2 addresses standardization of abbreviations, acronyms, and symbols, and goal 2.3 addresses notification for critical test values. Goal 2.5 recommends the use of a standard approach to "hand-off" communications. These goals promote interdisciplinary healthcare team communication.

Healthcare agencies have begun to develop a standardized electronic hand-off report to supplement the verbal report. The electronic report would be used when the patient is transferred to the care of an on-call physician. For example, physicians at Columbia University reported that they developed a standardized unofficial electronic document, signout, to use when handing off a patient and between patient admissions. The researcher reported that the report was accessed frequently after the handoff of the patient. The researchers were able to quantify collaborative use of the document by using a clinical information system logging mining technique (Stein, Wrenn, Johnson, & Stetson, 2007).

The next safety goal is to improve medication safety. Goal 3.1 recommends an annual review of look-alike/sound-alike drug lists. Clinical decision support could be used to alert the provider to

double-check their order intent. Automatic dispensing machines should be of benefit in addressing the problem if they are stocked correctly and if the drug vials for different concentrations are different. The nation was alerted to the problem when the infant twins of a movie star couple received 1,000 times the recommended dose of heparin in November 2007 (Nudd & Lee, 2007). The Joint Commission clearly acknowledges the use of HIT for patient safety but, within clearly defined guidelines, still allows healthcare agencies to arrive at decisions that are the best fit for their patients and staff.

Disease Surveillance Systems and Disaster Planning

When all health records are electronic, aggregated data from the records could be trended to detect infectious disease outbreaks and bioterrorism. In 2010, the Centers for Disease Control realigned its divisions within the Public Health Information Network to form the Division of Preparedness and Emerging Infections (DPEI). The division incorporated the responsibilities of the former National Electronic Disease Surveillance System (NEDSS). The purpose of DPEI is to work with public partners to "prepare for, prevent, and respond to infectious diseases, including outbreaks, bioterrorism, and other public health emergencies, through cross-cutting and specialized programs, technical expertise, and public health leadership" (Centers for Disease Control, 2011). Early detection (or potential disease) or bioterrorism health problems can be accomplished by using syndromic surveillance systems.

Syndromic Surveillance

There are four models used for syndromic surveillance (Mandl et al., 2004). Syndromic surveillance was defined as the collection of health indicators from individuals and populations that present before diagnoses are made (Uscher-Pines et al., 2009). The models vary according to the scope of the population served.

One model is the Special Events Model. It was used during the 1999 World Trade Organization meeting in Seattle, the 2002 World Baseball Series in Phoenix, and the 2001 World Trade Center in New York City terrorist attacks in which the twin towers were destroyed (Moran & Talan, 2003; Centers for

Disease Control and Prevention, 2002). The Special Events Model refers to events involving large numbers of people who are monitored by public health teams that collect data from regional hospitals under the legal authority of local health departments.

The second model is one that could be developed by a given region (e.g., city, county, or state) that crosses the jurisdiction of local health authorities. The PHIN is yet a third model. The PHIN covers the entire United States with state data collected under the authority of state or local health departments. Data are exchanged through the use of interoperable information systems for both routine and emergency purposes (Centers for Disease Control and Prevention, n.d.-a). Finally, the military model covers a community with a large military presence or global military communities. This model is currently in place in Washington, DC, where the Department of Defense monitors military emergency department and primary care clinic patient diagnostic codes through the use of a centralized medical information systems database (Lewis et al., 2002).

The National Bioterrorism Syndromic Surveillance Demonstration Program (NDP) was designed to provide an alternative model to current CDC reporting methods (Lazarus, Yih, & Platt, 2006). The NDP model used no identifiable health information; instead, aggregated data counts stored on a secure server were proposed for use. Analysis would be done from the data located in a secure server. Afterward, alerts and reports from the data analysis would be forwarded to the pertinent local public health authorities for appropriate alert distribution and care interventions.

Disaster Response and Planning

Hurricane Katrina, the disastrous storm that struck the U.S. Gulf Coast in August 2005, served to inform HIT about disaster planning. After the storm, the KatrinaHealth website (http://www.katrinahealth.org) was almost immediately established in conjunction with local and state governments, Dr. David Brailer, the then National Coordinator for HIT, the Markle Foundation, and pharmaceutical companies (Markle Foundation, American Medical Association, & Gold Standard, 2006). The website served as a portal for authorized physicians

and pharmacists to obtain electronic prescription medical records for victims of the storm. Reflective analysis for KatrinaHealth is available online at http://katrinahealth.org/katrinahealth.final.pdf. The report includes seven recommendations that local, state, and national policy makers and governments must consider:

- Plan for disasters now.
- Use existing available resources such as the regional health information organizations (RHIOs).
- Create interoperable EHRs.
- Integrate emergency response systems into nonemergent systems.
- Establish systems that can be easily accessed.
- Establish effective communication channels.
- Overcome policy barriers.

Healthcare professionals, information technology specialists, and those in leadership positions continue to learn from disasters such as the 2010 Haiti earthquake, Hurricane Katrina, and the World Trade Center attacks. The efforts serve as catalysts for improved communication channels and the development of improved informatics solutions to improve the lives of future victims.

The Regional Coordinating Center for hurricane response (RCC) was established in October 2005 (Mack, Brantley, & Bell, 2007). The mission for RCC was to work through the use of HIT with the National Institute of Health's Centers of Excellence in Partnerships for Community Outreach, Research on Health Disparities and Training to assist with the renewing and rebuilding of the healthcare systems that were affected by hurricanes Katrina and Rita. The RCC embarked on building partnerships with local healthcare systems among the different Gulf Shore states to assist in the rebuilding process. The goals for this project included the use of EHRs, telepsychiatry, and screening and surveillance systems. Project leaders for RCC recognized that the reconstruction process was very complicated and that it would take time to accomplish.

RCCs are now under the direction of FEMA (Federal Emergency Management Agency) and organized into regions of the United States as

Regional Response Coordinating Centers (RRCC). RRCCs coordinate the immediate emergency response to a disaster or catastrophic event for the Federal government (FEMA, 2011).

Protection of Healthcare Data

Health Insurance Portability and Accountability Act

The 1996 Health Insurance Portability and Accountability Act (HIPAA) has affected the entire healthcare entity, including HIT. The law addressed several areas pertaining to healthcare information, including simplifying healthcare claims, providing standards for healthcare data transmission, and ensuring the security of healthcare information. The purpose of the law was to improve the effectiveness and efficiency of healthcare. It was also designed to prevent medical fraud by standardizing the electronic exchange of financial and administrative data. The HIPAA law applies only to (1) healthcare providers that "furnish, bill, or receive payment for healthcare in the normal business day" and who also transmit any transactions electronically; (2) healthcare clearinghouses; or (3) health plans (Centers for Medicare & Medicaid Services, 2010a).

The area that has generated the most public attention has been the privacy and security rules that address many of the privacy, confidentiality, and security issues already discussed in this chapter. There have been many areas of disagreement among the stakeholders about the rules, and legitimate concerns exist on both sides. One rule requires that in each agency, a specific person be assigned the responsibility for overseeing efforts to secure electronic data. As a result, each healthcare agency that has to abide by the rules has a person designated as the HIPAA officer. This person must be proficient in information technology, auditing, agency policies and practices, ethics, state and federal regulations, and consumer issues.

Although data privacy issues generate the most media attention, HIPAA also maintains "technology neutral" methods for the transmission of data among healthcare organizations. Technology neutral means that any computer system can import

and read the data.[1] To simplify and encourage electronic transfer of administrative and financial healthcare data among payers, plans, and providers, HIPAA requires the use of national code standards.

HIPAA also calls for the use of "national identifiers for providers, health plans, and employers" (Centers for Medicare & Medicaid Services, 2010b). Use of the national provider identifier went into effect in 2008 for Medicare fee-for-service providers. The original call for a unique patient identifier has been put on hold permanently because of privacy issues.

Privacy

Protecting patient privacy is an important professional responsibility. Being sick does not make intrusions into one's personal life justifiable. In some instances, people have been denied employment because of known medical conditions. This can make patients hesitant to share their health history when they know that it will be entered into a record for anyone with access to read. Patient privacy also needs to be considered when interviewing a patient. The environment should be such that the interview cannot be overheard. Additionally, information that is routinely asked of patients should be scrutinized to ensure that it is pertinent to the care that can be rendered in the agency. Another item to consider is the placement of computers on which charting is done. Ideally, the computer screen should not be visible to anyone except the person charting. The nurse must log off before leaving the computer; otherwise, anyone who approaches the computer will be able to access private information.

Confidentiality

Confidentiality is a constant balancing act. The more confidential we make a record, the more difficult it becomes to use it. Before computerized records, we gave minimal concern to confidentiality. We believed that the record was safe. Yet, in most institutions, anyone with a white coat and a name badge that reads "Doctor or Nurse X" could pick up a

---

1 This is similar to the rich text format (RTF) that permits most word processors to read documents created by other word processors.

record and read it. Additionally, when a patient was sent to another area, such as the operating room, the chart was tucked under a corner of the gurney from where anyone could easily remove it. Not only did this make it easy for the staff in another area to view the record, but it also raised questions about confidentiality that were seldom addressed.

Authentication

Computerized records have brought the issue of confidentiality to the forefront. Even with the flaws in paper records, it was difficult to obtain information from more than one or two records at a time. When records are computerized, if one gains entrance to the system, it is easy to access many records. Hence, the first line of protection is to defend against unauthorized access or entrance to the system. This is achieved with a **login** process that authenticates that the person using the system is permitted access. **Authentication** simply means verifying the identification of the person logging into the system. It can be accomplished by using **passwords**, smartcards, **biometrics**, or a combination of these.

Login Name and Passwords

Anyone who has ever used a network in a healthcare agency or a secure site on the World Wide Web has become familiar with login names (user ID) and passwords. Most systems today rely on a login name and a password for authentication. Various systems of designating login names are used, such as first initial and last name, most of which are easy to guess, and they generally remain the same as long as one is using the same network. Thus, the rules for passwords are much more stringent and vary from agency to agency.

The best passwords involve a combination of upper and lower case letters and numbers in a manner that will not form a word, (e.g., "Sec9uR7ity"). This prevents someone with an electronic dictionary from trying various passwords until the right one is found. Additionally, making passwords case sensitive (i.e., one must use lower and upper case letters in the same way each time the password is used) also makes them more difficult to guess.

Password Policies

Policies on how often to change passwords are based on the premise that after a given length of

time, one's password has been compromised, either purposely or accidentally. The system administrator determines the length of time. Additionally, most systems prohibit users from reusing a password. Forcing a change too frequently can result in users writing the password down and pasting it either near the computer or on the back of an ID badge. Not changing frequently enough leaves users open to having the security of their account breached. One of the problems faced by network administrators is providing logins and passwords to temporary users, such as temporary staff and nursing students. Because an unused account is an invitation to hackers, there must be a network policy for closing the accounts of both temporary users and workers who leave their positions in the company or institution.

Network administrators require password access to clinical information systems to protect the privacy and security of patient records. They also have to deal with regulatory pressure, security threats, and the cost of help desks. Password problems are among the top day-to-day issues encountered at information technology help desks.

Automatic Logout

Automatic logout is another function used to preserve data confidentiality. Knowing emergencies often arise that involve calling a nurse away from the computer, most systems will time out after a given length of time with no input activity. If the time interval is too short, this can be annoying to users who have to go through the entire login process again. If it is too long, it could allow someone else to perform unauthorized activities by using the original user's login. If the clinician is at the computer and involved in a phone call, simply moving the mouse may be interpreted as activity and keep the system from logging the user out.

Single Sign-On

Use of a **single sign-on** is an issue for the use of clinical information systems. Single sign-on allows the user to access multiple clinical applications with only one login/password for authentication. Use of logins for each and every clinical application is problematic. Having multiple passwords that expire on a regular basis creates the same problem as having passwords expire too frequently – the users creatively use methods to write down the passwords by which they can easily be discovered. Each login requires authentication and forces the busy professional to wait before completing a transaction. It is more efficient for users to have a single sign-on for the use of clinical information systems, which improves workflow and prevents accidental breaches of security and confidentiality.

Professional Responsibility to Protect Confidentiality

Confidentiality of private information located in computerized records starts with the users. Users need to understand the need for protecting their account; they must tailor behaviors to guarantee this protection. Users need to understand that between the times they log in and out, they are responsible for anything that is done from their account. If a nurse leaves a computer screen unattended with patient data exposed, the patient's confidentiality has been breached. To make matters worse, any other person who recognizes that the nurse is logged in has the opportunity to make entries into the system under the nurse's name. The computer would not be able to tell the difference. It is very important for nurses to learn to always log off the computer before leaving. It is a habit that can be learned as easily as locking the doors of the house or car.

Biometrics

The most secure method of authentication is biometrics – the use of physiological characteristics such as iris or retinal scan, fingerprint, or a voiceprint that is presumably unique to the particular person. Of these, the iris scan seems to hold the most promise and return the least number of false "no matches." There are more than 200 unique points on the iris that can be used for comparison (Daugman, 2007; Dunker, 2003). For authentication purposes, users stand approximately 4–6 inches away from the scanner (Schiphol, 2010). Verification takes only seconds. The retinal scan is very accurate, but it is less beneficial in the busy healthcare environment because the users must remove their glasses, place their eye against a device, and focus on a point. The entire process takes about 10–15 seconds (Biometric Newsportal.com, n.d.).

The rich whorls, ridges, and patterns of fingerprints are still useful for authentication. The users press their fingers against an optical or silicon surface reader for less than five seconds. The accuracy is improved with the use prints from more than one finger. One of the limitations of fingerprint biometrics is that the finger should be clean and not smudged with grease, dirt, or ink, such as newspaper print (Erdley, 2006). Because optical scanners require reflected light, they may fail to read fingerprints of people with dry skin; some people with dark skin; and those with fine print ridges, such as children. Improved accuracy in fingerprint authentication is achieved with ultrasound technology because it has less trouble reading a fingerprint with contaminants (Pierce, 2003). Ultrasonic print scanners are able to read fingerprints on dark skin and require no special lighting conditions. Fingerprint recognition is a common option used to authenticate access to personal digital assistants and laptops.

Voice recognition is another type of biometric used for security. Voice recognition creates voiceprints using a combination of two authentication factors: What is said and the way that it is said (Anderson, 2007). It can also be used at a distance with a telephone. Voice biometrics is more commonly used in the banking industry as much of banking business is done over telephone lines. Voice recognition has potential for increased use in healthcare because it is two to three times more accurate than fingerprinting and less expensive than some of the other biometric systems.

Radio Frequency Identification

RFID refers to smart labels or intelligent bar codes that can communicate with a network. RFID is designed to take the place of the Universal Product Code that we see on almost any product we purchase, whether it is a package of CD-ROMs at the office supply store or a box of cereal at the grocery store. We may have seen or used RFID on a pass card attached to a vehicle windshield for access to toll roads. Another nonmedical use is to tag pet dogs and cats for easy identification in case they are lost. In 2006, the United States began to embed RFID chips in passports (Gross, 2005).

RFID is of two types: passive and active (American Electronic Association, 2005). The passive tags are lighter, less expensive ($0.5 per tag) (RFID Journal, 2010), have read-only capability, and can be read at a distance of 1–10 feet. The passive, implantable (inserted under the skin) tag uses a U.S. Food and Drug Administration chip. The active tags are more expensive (several dollars), have read–write capability, and can be read at distances of 1–300 feet.

Currently, RFID is used in many healthcare agencies to track patients, including newborn babies. The "Hugs" Infant Protection System by Stanley Healthcare Solutions is an example of how RFID is used in healthcare. Each baby receives an ankle band with an embedded RFID chip. If there is an unauthorized removal of the baby, an alarm is sounded. An example of successful use was reported when a baby's abduction was thwarted from Presbyterian Hospital in Charlotte, North Carolina (Sullivan, 2005).

RFID is also used in healthcare agencies to track equipment such as wheelchairs and intravenous pumps and used to track the location of patients (Supply Insight Inc., 2006). Another use of this technology is to track hospital personnel, such as doctors and nurses (Activewave Inc., 2009). Although the use of the technology with patients and personnel has been controversial in some settings, decisions have been made in favor of improved care delivery systems and patient safety.

RFID solutions have been used to facilitate identification. A unique identifier number can be used to identify "at-risk" patients who may need emergency medical treament. These unique identifier numbers can also be used to locate patients with memory impairments who may wander away from their rooms or care-givers (Positive ID, n.d.). The RFID tag can be implanted under the patient's skin or worn as a bracelet. The only information contained in the chip is the patient's name, address, allergies, picture, and the unique identifier, which is used to obtain health record information. The healthcare provider uses a wall or handheld scanner to obtain the information.

Data Security

The third element of healthcare data protection is data security. The data security issues are the responsibility of the information systems team. Data security has three aspects. The first deals with ensuring the accuracy of the data; the second, with protection of the data from unauthorized eyes inside or outside the agency; and the third, with internal or external damage to the data.

Informatics nurses and clinical nurses are involved in building entry screens prior to a system implementation. Nurses as well as the technical staff need to understand the principles of data security. **Accuracy of data** can be improved with methods that check the data during input. For example, when a user chooses phrases for input from a list, the person needs to be sure that only recognized terms are entered. To check that the desired phrase was chosen before leaving the page, the user can be presented with a screen that shows the items that will be entered into the record. Another factor that must be considered is how to handle incorrect entries. Generally, provision is allowed for the entry to be corrected within a time period, but a record of all entries is kept in an audit trail. An audit trail provides a list of who accessed the system, the date, the time, and the activity.

Protection of the data from prying eyes involves the use of audit trails and making decisions about how much access individual users should have. Who has access to what information differs from agency to agency. For pure ease of use, all professional healthcare workers would have access to any patient record in the system. This is very helpful when patients are transferred from one department to another, and it is allowed in some institutions. Its use must be backed up by audit trails or by a record of which individual worker accessed which record at what time and where. Additionally, those audit trails must be routinely examined to determine if breaches of security are occurring. Audit trails are closely scrutinized after the admission of persons who are well known. Making decisions about how much access users have varies from one institution to the next. Most institutions provide access only to records of those patients on the unit where the healthcare worker is stationed, and they index them by job description. Limiting access too severely will prohibit holistic care and can put patients in jeopardy.

Accuracy of the original data is also the responsibility of users. There have been situations in which clinicians have entered anything into a mandatory field just to continue in the system. Not only does this put patient care at risk, but it also compromises the integrity of the database. This cavalier attitude can be attributed to a multitude of factors: lack of awareness of what is done with the data, an unwieldy system for entering data, time pressures, and inadequate training on using the system. That being said, system designers must understand nurse workflow and require only essential mandatory fields, not ones that may be impossible to complete. Regardless of the cause, attempts to bypass mandatory data entry fields must be addressed if data are to be valid.

Protection From System Intrusions

With the rise of the Internet and the actuality that most agencies are now connected to it, preventing outsiders from accessing institutional information has become a major responsibility of the information services department. One of the first lines of defense for protecting against unauthorized access is a firewall. A firewall operates in one of two ways. Either it examines all messages entering and leaving a system and blocks those that do not meet specific criteria or it allows or denies messages on the basis of whether the destination port is acceptable. Firewalls require constant maintenance. To ensure that the system is safe from prying eyes, some agencies hire white hat hackers to try and penetrate their systems. White hat hackers are persons who are ethically opposed to security abuse. Their job is to attempt to penetrate systems to identify security weaknesses. Protection is then devised for any security breaches that are found.

Systems also need to be protected from outsiders who gain physical entrance to the agency and from insiders who are intent on gaining unauthorized access. Security audits completed by independent consultants are used to identify potential system security vulnerabilities. The first line of defense against this type of breach includes staff education on the importance of data security. Staff should be encouraged to expect identification from unfamiliar persons and to refuse access to anyone without recognized authorization.

Phishing and Spear Phishing Security Breaches

The concept of phishing was discussed in Chapter 5 on e-mail, so you may be curious about why it is being discussed again in this chapter on healthcare system issues. To steal confidential patient information, criminal hackers use phishing e-mail tactics to lure the care provider into revealing private information. **Spear phishing** tactics use what appears to be legitimate business e-mail from a person well known to the e-mail recipient. It is a scam that lures an employee into revealing private login information (Microsoft, 2005; SearchSecurity.com, 2010). For example, in a healthcare agency, the employees might receive what appears to be a legitimate employee e-mail from within the agency, such as from human resources, nursing services, or information services. The scam is that the e-mail will ask the recipients to update their login and password information or to verify it. When the recipients respond, the perpetrator steals their login and password and then uses the information for criminal purposes by hacking into the hospital's information system. All phishing scams should be reported to the Antiphishing Working Group at http://www.antiphishing.org.

Protection From Data Loss

Computer data need to be protected from being lost as a result of either a system problem or disaster, natural or otherwise. This latter element took on new importance after the fall of the World Trade Center on September 11, 2001, and hurricanes Katrina and Rita in 2005. To provide this protection, data must be backed up routinely and stored off-site in a secure place. These backups should be periodically examined to make sure that they are accurate and can be easily reinstalled on the system. Additionally, a disaster recovery plan needs to be devised and tested. This plan should be made in conjunction with key people in the agency to ensure adequate protection. The objective in disaster recovery is to allow work to resume by using the same standards as before the disaster with the least amount of effort. One of the first tasks in planning for disaster recovery is to do a risk analysis. This analysis will determine vulnerabilities and appropriate control measures. Identification of system weaknesses can prevent the actual occurrence of a disaster. A disaster plan should be tested at least twice a year. Healthcare accrediting bodies have standards to assure protection from data loss.

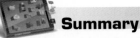

Summary

The issues associated with migration from a paper medical record to full implementation of the electronic record are extremely complex and arduous. The good news is that progress is being made one step at a time, and sometimes, one keystroke at a time. There is collaboration among the government, private and professional organizations, vendors, healthcare agencies, and healthcare professionals. The EMR Adoption model developed by HIMSS Analytics serves as a roadmap for those who have undertaken or plan to undertake the electronic journey.

The healthcare organization's strategic plan serves as a foundation for the successful implementation of a system. Selection decisions for health information system solutions don't come easily. In this day of financial scrutiny, stakeholders need to see an ROI. Risks and opportunities for tangible and intangible payoffs must be explored.

The HIT steering committee should be made up of a multidisciplinary team including the top leadership, clinicians, information technology personnel, and all others whose work might be influenced by the new system. The oversight committee must address hard issues such as interoperability standards, user design of data entry screens, workflow redesign, and quality measurement desired outcomes. All users must have a clear vision of the opportunities to improve nursing outcomes and save unnecessary, avoidable hospital costs while at the same time meet the Joint Commission's regulatory requirements. Everyone who is involved with the system design and implementation should be familiar with literature findings and research results to anticipate and avoid negative unintended consequences. No potential problem should be minimized; rather, it should be addressed proactively.

As the issues of interoperability and system integration are addressed, the United States will be able to take proactive interventions to recognize communicable disease outbreaks by using analysis of symptoms in a secure central database. Several initiatives addressing the creation of disease and syndromic surveillance systems can also be used for bioterrorism. As an example, the CDC NEDSS system is already in place. The EHR has the ability of expediting safe care and saving lives during a disaster if the data are stored in an RHIO's secure databases so that they are accessible wherever the victim receives care.

Issues regarding privacy, confidentiality, and data security still persist. Healthcare data privacy and security are of utmost importance to those who provide and receive care. The associated challenges are how to expedite the delivery of healthcare and communication among providers while at the same time protecting the health information system data. As new technology develops, new issues will surface. The more things change, the more they stay the same.

APPLICATIONS AND COMPETENCIES

1. Use the EMR Adoption model to analyze and describe the level of adoption for a local healthcare agency.

2. Discuss the opportunities for clinical data sharing in your city or region. Support the associated risks and opportunities with current literature.

3. Discuss the methods for ensuring privacy and confidentiality of patient electronic information in a local clinical setting. Identify the penalties the agency uses for employees that breach confidentiality and security policies.

4. Interview a leadership representative from information technology at a healthcare agency to assess interoperability issues within the different health information systems. Summarize the findings in a written report.

5. Create literature on workflow redesign, as it relates to a clinical documentation system. Afterward, interview a nurse on a unit that is using any method of HIT to assess any nurse workflow issues. Explain why workflow is or is not an issue for the nursing staff.

6. Analyze how a local healthcare agency is addressing the Joint Commission's patient safety goals. Is the agency using HIT to address the safety goals? Why or why not?

7. Search the web for tools that measure the strength of a password. Use the tool to assist you to create two examples of strong passwords. Provide an explanation for how you were able to create a strong password.

REFERENCES

Activewave Inc. (2009). *RFID solutions for hospitals*. Retrieved October 29, 2010, from http://www.activewaveinc.com/applications_hospitals.php

Agency for Healthcare Research and Quality. (2001). Reducing and preventing adverse drug events to decrease hospital costs. *Research in Action*, (1). Retrieved from http://www.ahrq.gov/qual/aderia/aderia.htm

American Electronic Association. (2005, December). RFID 101: Benefits of the next big little thing. *AeA Competitiveness Series*, 5, 1–4. Retrieved from http://www.techamerica.org/content/wp-content/uploads/2009/07/aea_cs_rfid_101.pdf

Anderson, N. (2007, May 13). *Voice biometrics: Coming to a security system near you*. Retrieved October 29, 2010, from http://arstechnica.com/security/news/2007/05/voice-biometrics-come-of-age.ars

Ash, J. S., Berg, M., & Coiera, E. (2004). Some unintended consequences of information technology in health care: The nature of patient care information system-related errors. *Journal of the American Medical Informatics Association*, 11(2), 104–112.

Ash, J. S., Sittig, D. F., Campbell, E. M., Guappone, K. P., & Dykstra, R. H. (2007). Some unintended consequences of clinical decision support systems. *AMIA Annual Symposium Proceedings*, 2007, 26–30.

Ash, J. S., Sittig, D. F., Poon, E. G., Guappone, K., Campbell, E., & Dykstra, R. H. (2007). The extent and importance of unintended consequences related to computerized provider order entry. *Journal of the American Medical Informatics Association*, 14(4), 415–423.

Biometric Newsportal.com. (n.d.). *Retina biometrics*. Retrieved October 29, 2010, from http://www.biometricnewsportal.com/retina_biometrics.asp

Birkmeyer, J. D., & Dimick, J. B. (2004). *The Leapfrog Group&APOS;S patient safety practices, 2003: The potential benefits of universal adoption*. Retrieved October 20, 2010, from http://www.leapfroggroup.org/media/file/Leapfrog-Birkmeyer.pdf

Campbell, E. M., Sittig, D. F., Ash, J. S., Guappone, K. P., & Dykstra, R. H. (2006). Types of unintended consequences related to computerized provider order entry. *Journal of the American Medical Association*, 13(5), 547–556.

Centers for Disease Control and Prevention. (2011, April 1). *Division of Preparedness and Emerging Infections (DPEI)*. Retrieved September 1, 2011, from http://www.cdc.gov/ncezid/dpei/

Centers for Disease Control and Prevention. (2002). Syndromic surveillance for bioterrorism following the attacks on the World Trade Center–New York City, 2001. *MMWR: Morbidity and Mortality Weekly Report*, 51 Spec No, 13–15.

Centers for Disease Control and Prevention. (n.d.-a). *Public Health Information Network – About PHIN*. Retrieved October 29, 2010, from http://www.cdc.gov/phin/about.html

Centers for Medicare & Medicaid Services. (2010a, July 19). *Overview HIPAA – General information*. Retrieved October 29, 2010, from http://www.cms.gov/HIPAAGenInfo/01_Overview.asp

Centers for Medicare & Medicaid Services. (2010b, August 31). *Overview national provider identifier standard*. Retrieved October 29, 2010, from http://www.cms.gov/NationalProvIdentStand/

Centers for Medicare & Medicaid Services. (2010c, September 9). *Physician self-referral*. Retrieved October 20, 2010, from http://www.cms.gov/PhysicianSelfReferral/

Conrad, D. A., & Gardner, M. (2005, May 2). *Updated economic implications of the Leapfrog Group patient safety standards: Final report to the Leapfrog Group*. Retrieved October 20, 2010, from http://www.leapfroggroup.org/media/file/Conrad_Updated_Economic_Implications_2_.pdf

Daugman, J. (2007). New methods in iris recognition. *IEEE Transactions Systems, Man, and Cybernetics, Part B*, 37(5), 1167–1175.

Dunker, M. (2003, November 20). *Don't blink: Iris recognition for biometric identification*. Retrieved October 29, 2010, from http://www.sans.org/reading_room/whitepapers/authentication/dont-blink-iris-recognition-biometric-identification_1341

Erdley, W. S. (2006). Personal digital assistants, wireless computing, smart cards, and biometrics: a hardware update for clinical practice. *Journal of Obstetric, Gynecologic, and Neonatal Nursing*, 35(1), 157–163.

Federal Emergency Management Agency (FEMA). (2011). *Disaster Response Division*. Retrieved September 1, 2011, from http://www.fema.gov/about/regions/regioni/operations.shtm

Gross, G. (2005, October 26). United States to require RFID chips in passports. *PC World*. Retrieved from http://www.pcworld.com/article/123246/united_states_to_require_rfid_chips_in_passports.html

Health Information Technology. (2010, October 7). *Frequently asked questions about electronic health records and health information networks*. Retrieved September 1, 2011, from http://healthit.hhs.gov/portal/server.pt/document/873991/cee_tool_press_faqs_doc

HIMSS Analytics. (2009). *U.S. EMR Adoption Model^sm trends*. Retrieved October 20, 2010, from http://www.himssanalytics.org/docs/HA_EMRAM_Overview_ENG.pdf

Hunt, E. C., Sproat, S. B., & Kitzmiller, R. R. (2004). *The nursing informatics implementation guide*. New York, NY: Springer.

Kibbe, D. C., & Mongiardo, D. (2010, October 7). *Health information security & privacy toolkit*. Retrieved October 20, 2010, from http://healthit.hhs.gov/portal/server.pt/document/872346/pet_1_tool_faq_script508_pdf

Lazarus, R., Yih, K., & Platt, R. (2006). Distributed data processing for public health surveillance. *BMC Public Health*, 6, 235.

Lewis, M. D., Pavlin, J. A., Mansfield, J. L., O'Brien, S., Boomsma, L. G., Elbert, Y., et al. (2002). Disease outbreak detection system using syndromic data in the greater Washington DC area. *American Journal of Preventative Medicine*, 23(3), 180–186.

Mack, D., Brantley, K. M., & Bell, K. G. (2007). Mitigating the health effects of disasters for medically underserved populations: Electronic health records, telemedicine, research, screening, and surveillance. *Journal of Health Care for the Poor and Underserved*, 18(2), 432–442.

Mandl, K. D., Overhage, J. M., Wagner, M. M., Lober, W. B., Sebastiani, P., Mostashari, F., et al. (2004). Implementing syndromic surveillance: A practical guide informed by the early experience. *Journal of the American Medical Informatics Association*, 11(2), 141–150.

Markle Foundation, American Medical Association, & Gold Standard. (2006, June 13). *Lessons from KatrinaHealth*.

Retrieved October 29, 2010, from http://katrinahealth. org/katrinahealth.final.pdf

Menachemi, N., Burkhardt, J., Shewchuk, R., Burke, D., & Brooks, R. G. (2006). Hospital information technology and positive financial performance: A different approach to finding an ROI. *Journal of Healthcare Management, 51*(1), 40–58; discussion 58–59.

Microsoft. (2005, December 9). *What is spear phishing?* Retrieved October 29, 2010, from http://www.microsoft. com/canada/athome/security/email/spear_phishing.mspx

Milstein, A. (2007). Health information technology is a vehicle, not a destination: A conversation with David J. Brailer. *Health Affairs, 26*(2), w236–w241.

Moran, G. J., & Talan, D. A. (2003). Update on emerging infections: News from the Centers for Disease Control and Prevention. Syndromic surveillance for bioterrorism following the attacks on the World Trade Center – New York City, 2001. *Annals of Emergency Medicine, 41*(3), 414–418.

National Committee Vital Health Statistics. (2001, November 15). A strategy for building the national health information infrastructure. *Information for Health*. Retrieved October 21, 2010, from http://ncvhs.hhs.gov/nhiilayo.pdf

Nudd, T., & Lee, K. (2007, December 4). Dennis & Kimberly Quaid sue drug company. *People*. Retrieved from http:// www.people.com/people/article/0,,20164211,00.html

Pierce, F. S. (2003). Biometric identification: Ultrasonic systems can succeed where optical systems may not. *Health Management Technology, 24*(5), 38–39.

Positive ID. (n.d.). *PositiveID – Identity theft, credit monitoring, implantable microchip, electronic health records*. Retrieved October 29, 2010, from http://www.positiveidcorp.com/ health-id.html

RFID Journal. (2010). *Frequently asked questions*. Retrieved October 29, 2010, from http://www.rfidjournal.com/faq/20

Runy, L. A., & Towne, J. (2005). Information technology ROI: A CEO's guide to measuring and evaluating IT's financial effectiveness. *H&HN: Hospitals & Health Networks, 79*(2), 45, 47–50, 52.

Schiphol. (2010). *Schiphol – FAQ*. Retrieved October 29, 2010, from http://www.schiphol.nl/Travellers/AtSchiphol/ PriviumIrisscan/FAQ.htm

SearchSecurity.com. (2010, September 10). *Spear phishing*. Retrieved October 29, 2010, from http://searchsecurity. techtarget.com/sDefinition/0,sid14_gci1134829,00.html

Stein, D. M., Wrenn, J. O., Johnson, S. B., & Stetson, P. D. (2007). Signout: A collaborative document with implications for the future of clinical information systems. *AMIA Annual Symposium Proceedings*, 2007, 696–700.

Sullivan, L. (2005, July 19). RFID system prevented a possible infant abduction. *Information Week*. Retrieved from http:// www.informationweek.com/news/mobility/RFID/show- Article.jhtml?articleID=166400496

Supply Insight Inc. (2006, April 20). *RFID in patient tracking*. Retrieved October 29, 2010, from http://www.supplyin- sight.com/RFID_in_Patient_Tracking.htm

The Joint Commission. (2010). *2010 Joint Commission national patient safety goals*. Retrieved October 28, 2010, from http://www.patientsafety.gov/TIPS/Docs/TIPS_ JanFeb10Poster.pdf

Uscher-Pines, L., Farrell, C. L., Babin, S. M., Cattani, J., Gaydos, C. A., Hsieh, Y. H., et al. (2009). Framework for the development of response protocols for public health syndromic surveillance systems: Case studies of 8 US states. *Disaster Medicine and Public Health Preparedness, 3*(2, Suppl), S29–S36.

CHAPTER 21

Carrying Healthcare to the Client

Objectives

After studying this chapter, you will be able to:

▶ *Define the two overall classifications of technology used in telehealth.*

▶ *Discuss some of the ways that telehealth can deliver healthcare.*

▶ *Illustrate the opportunities for autonomous nursing practice in telehealth.*

▶ *Discuss the main issues in implementing telehealth.*

▶ *Analyze the ways that telehealth could impact the present healthcare system.*

Key Terms

Biometric Garment	Telehomecare
E-Intensive Care	Telemedicine
Portable Monitoring Devices	Telemental health
Real-Time	Telenursing
Robotics	Telepresence
Store and Forward (S&F)	Teletrauma
Telehealth	

During the 1998 Around the World Alone sailboat race, one of the racers, while in the South Atlantic, developed an abscess on his elbow that could have caused him to lose his arm. Using a wireless computer and satellite technology, he was put in touch with a doctor in Boston who directed his treatment and saved the arm (Lynch, 1998). Not all **telehealth** applications are this dramatic, but the incident demonstrates the power of this emerging vehicle for delivering healthcare. Although much attention has been given to the aspect of telehealth that addresses the delivery of acute care or specialist consultations, telehealth has been shown to be far more versatile. Telehealth can be used to provide home **telenursing**, electronic referrals to specialists and hospitals, teleconsulting between specialists and general practitioners or nurse practitioners, minor injury consulting, and consulting through call centers.

Terms such as "telehealth" and "**telemedicine**" in the past have been used interchangeably to refer to health services delivered using electronic technology to patients at a distance. According to the American Telemedicine Association (ATA), telemedicine refers to the electronic exchange of patient information between two sites for improving the patient's health status, and telehealth, a broader term, extends beyond the delivery of clinical services (American Telemedicine Association, 2010). The International Council of Nursing defines *telenursing* as telecommunications technology in nursing to enhance patient care (International Council of Nurses, 2010). This chapter focuses on emerging developments and applications using the term telehealth unless specified otherwise in the references used to support the information.

Telehealth Basics

As the sailor in the Around the World Alone sailboat race proved, telemedicine technology does not have to be complex. Hopefully, most cases would not involve self-treatment. Generally, there are two uses of technology for delivering telehealth, either **store and forward (S&F)** or a two-way communication. The line between these two modes is becoming less and less distinct because many services use both types of communication. There is a wealth of information about telehealth on the Internet. A good place to begin is the Telemedicine Information Exchange at http://tie.telemed.org/links/specialties.asp.

Store and Forward Technology

In S&F technology, a digital camera, scanner, or technology (e.g., x-ray machine) that generates electronic images captures a still image electronically and then that image is sent to a specialist for interpretation later (American Telemedicine Association, n.d.). Radiology, dermatology, pathology, and wound care specialties lend themselves very well to this technique. S&F also includes asynchronous transmission of clinical data, such as the results of an electrocardiogram, magnetic resonance imaging, or blood glucose levels, between two sites. This type of communication is often between healthcare providers. S&F offers the only affordable way that medicine can be practiced in remote communities, such as those in Alaska. For example, S&F is used when an x-ray is read by a radiologist located at a different site from where it was done. This method is frequently used in healthcare.

Real-Time Telehealth

Real-time telehealth involves the patient and the provider interacting at the same time by using interactive video/television. Many telecommunications devices that permit two-way communication are used to provide real-time telehealth. The oldest of these is the telephone, but current telehealth technology generally includes videoconferencing using two-way video and audio. Although videoconferencing is possible with a modem and plain old telephone service, a higher quality of service is usually preferred. The required level of service depends on the type of services offered. Some services require at least a T1 line or a line on an integrated digital network, which must not only connect the sites but also extend to the rooms where both the patient and the distant consultant are located. Large satellite systems that have a global audience are also used in telehealth. In short, any two-way communication technology offering both audio and video has, or will find, a use in telehealth.

Real-time telehealth also makes use of special instruments that can transmit an image to a clinician at a different location. These include an ear–nose–throat scope, a camera that captures skin observations, and a special stethoscope. They can be used either in real-time or in S&F mode. In addition, by using a combination of **robotics** and virtual reality, a surgeon with special gloves and the appropriate audio and video technology is able to perform surgery by manipulating surgical instruments at the remote site. This procedure uses what is known as **telepresence**. It is still in development and requires a 100% reliable system and a very high bandwidth. Telepresence is the use of technology to provide the appearance of a person's presence, although he or she is located at a remote site (Federation of American Scientists, n.d.).

Telehealth Examples

As healthcare shifts away from the hospital and into the home and community, the therapeutic uses for telehealth increase. A much broader range of healthcare professionals such as nurse practitioners, nutritionists, social workers, and home healthcare aides will have a role in the provision of telehealth. One problem that has plagued the use of telehealth in the past is that payers have focused on acute medical care; however, reimbursement for telehealth services is slowly beginning to improve. Until the reimbursement issue is completely resolved, much of our population will remain underserved. As a result, illnesses, instead of being treated in the early stages, will progress to a stage where they are very costly to treat.

Telehomecare

A trend in modern healthcare is to focus on the patient instead of the provider or agency. **Telehomecare** refers to the monitoring and delivery of healthcare in the patient's home rather than the provider's work setting. The greatest use of telehomecare is that it allows the patient the comforts of his or her own home, improves quality of life, and avoids time-consuming costly visits to office appointments or hospital admissions. The ongoing monitoring allows potential problems to be identified before they become significant problems. Because telehomecare can eliminate unnecessary emergency room visits and hospital visits, it is cost-effective.

For patients with chronic diseases, telehealth can be a powerful self-management tool. Using telehomecare devices, patients can collect and transmit vital signs, cardiac rhythm, blood glucose, and weight (see **Box 21-1**). The data are sent by using a telephone line or broadband connection to the healthcare provider and are stored in the patient's electronic health record (EHR). The healthcare provider's central monitoring station can view data from all patients that they are monitoring and see any alerts indicating significant changes. The computer screen that the healthcare provider views looks very similar to the central monitoring station in an intensive care unit (ICU) or step-down unit. Various companies host home health monitoring services.

Portable Monitoring Devices

Portable monitoring devices, available from a number of vendors (see **Box 21-1**), have many similarities. For example, they include an input device and various peripheral monitoring equipments. Many of the input devices use a touch screen with text and audio to ask the patient health assessment questions. The patient can respond to questions by choosing answers such as true/false, none/better/worse, yes/no, and 0–10. Some of the devices can be programmed to include branching questions. Answers to some questions may result in the display of patient education information.

There are some differences for self-monitoring equipment. While most provide access to a central monitoring station using a telephone line, others allow access using high-speed and wireless connections. The peripheral monitoring accessories can vary among vendor products. Examples of monitoring accessories include a blood pressure cuff, electrocardiogram, blood glucose meter, weight scales, fluid status monitor, pulse oximeter, monitors for PT/INR, peak flow meter, and a spirometer.

What are the future trends for home monitoring devices? We can expect vendors to design the equipment so that the monitoring data will integrate with the EHR, where it can be shared with pertinent healthcare agencies and providers. For example, HOMMED® Health Monitoring System recently partnered with Procura, LLC, to integrate the patient monitoring data into an EHR (Business Wire, 2007). We can also expect the devices to provide patient decision support with context-sensitive health education information, reminders to take medication and doctor's appointments, feedback regarding vital sign monitoring results, and motivational messages. One example of a home monitoring system that uses a television monitor, Phillips Motiva remote care manager, is available at http://www.medical.philips.com/goto/motiva.

Pill Dispensers/Reminders

Automatic pill dispensers/reminders are another type of telehomecare device. The pill dispensers

---

BOX 21-1 Examples of Telehomecare Devices

Vendor
ViTelCare™ Health
RemoteNurse™ Patient Monitor by WebVMC
HOMMED® Health Monitoring System
Phillips Motiva remote care manager
MD.2 Medication dispensing system
VivoMetrics® Lifeshirt®
Heart Failure Management System

may include auditory reminders to prompt patients to take their medications even if the medication is not a pill. The reminders may remind the patient to take the medication with food or to take an insulin injection. If medications are not taken within a specified period of time, the caregiver is notified by telephone. If the caregiver does not answer the telephone, the device phones the support center. Compliance can be monitored remotely through a secure website. The systems are about the size of a coffee maker. One example of an automatic pill dispenser is the MD.2. A short video of the device can be viewed at http://www.epill.com/md2video.html.

Wearable Monitoring Garments

Our current healthcare system remains disease focused; we seek care after something has gone wrong. Emerging wearable **biometric garment** technology will allow for a proactive approach

where symptoms are identified early before problems develop. Early identification of symptoms has the potential for maintaining the patient's quality of life, reducing acute exacerbations of disease processes, and avoiding unnecessary medical costs. The concept of wearable garments with built-in physiological monitoring devices is fascinating.

Consider the concept of "smart underwear" where sensors printed on the waistband of underwear monitor biomarkers in sweat and tears (Kane, 2010; UC Health, 2010). The underwear sensors make "autonomous" diagnoses and dispense appropriate drugs. Researchers are developing smart underwear for use by warriors who might be injured in battle. Of course, they could also be used by others who have an altered health status.

A lightweight, washable biometric shirt can provide telehomecare noninvasive monitoring of temperature, cardiac rhythm, and pulmonary function (see **Figure 21-1**). Peripheral devices

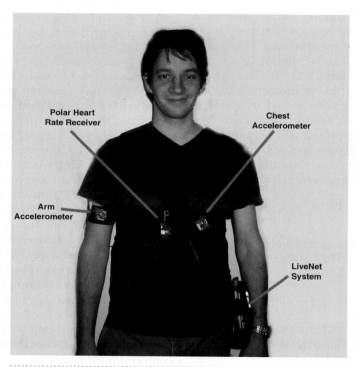

Figure 21-1 Livenet configured for noninvasive real-time soldier physiology monitoring. (From Sung, M., Marci, C., & Pentland, A. (2005). Wearable feedback systems for rehabilitation. *Journal of Neuroengineering and Rehabilitation, 2*, 17.)

for monitoring of the electroencephalogram, electrooculography, blood oxygen saturation, blood pressure, and cough can be used with the shirt. Research from the Massachusetts Institute of Technology (Sung, Marci, & Pentland, 2005) reported that wearable garments have potential uses for symptom detection and early treatment of

- hypothermia
- Parkinson's disease
- epilepsy seizures
- depression

Wearable biometric garments can also be designed for use with portable home monitoring devices (Villalba, Ottaviano, Arredondo, Martinez, & Guillen, 2006). Consider a shirt for cardiac and respiration monitoring in addition to a portable blood pressure cuff and weight scale with Bluetooth capabilities for data transfer. The grouping of devices is a part of the Heart Failure Management System. An example is available at http://www.cinc.org/Proceedings/2006/pdf/0237.pdf.

Telehomecare for Chronic Disease Management

Telehomecare used to manage the care of patients with chronic diseases such as heart failure (see **Figure 21-2**). Its use is associated with a decrease in hospitalization rates and more efficient uses of home care services. The Centers for Medicare & Medicaid Services have traditionally not reimbursed for telehomecare, so the studies reported in the literature are prototypes funded with grant money.

For example, home care agencies in New York began using telehomecare after receiving a York State Department of Health telemedicine grant (Wood, 2011). Home care service reported decreases in hospitalization rates ranging from 5% to 10% after implementing the service. A home care agency in Pennsylvania successfully reported a reduction of rehospitalization rates to 1.2% and improved resource utilization by decreasing the number of skilled nursing home care visits (Schneider, 2004; Schneider & Harris, 2003).

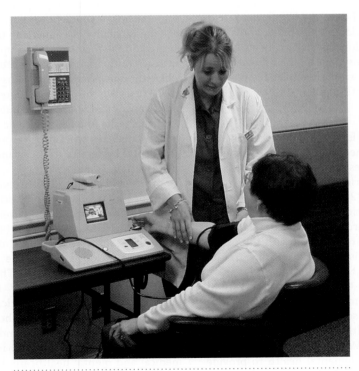

Figure 21-2 Nurse instructing patient on the use of home monitoring equipment.

Telehomecare is also in use by major medical centers worldwide. A large medical center located in Atlanta, GA, reported that telehomecare monitoring heart failure patient readmission rates were 75% lower than that for patients not in the program (Mattia, 2007). A hospital in Amsterdam reported monitoring over 100 patients with chronic heart failure at home with telehomecare monitoring equipment (Koninklijke Philips Electronics, 2007). Home monitoring was used to improve quality of life and to prevent hospital readmissions.

The Veterans Administration (VA) also uses telehomecare. The VA reported a study with two groups of veterans (Chumbler, Neugaard, Ryan, Qin, & Joo, 2005). One group, monitored weekly, photographed their wounds and mailed the photos to the care coordinator for evaluation and follow-up. The second group, using a telehomecare monitoring system, reported disease management data daily with a care coordinator. The group that was monitored with the telehomecare equipment had improved outcomes over the group that was monitored weekly. The telehomecare group had a 52% lower rate of hospital admissions for all causes, a 53% lower rate of hospital admissions related to diabetes, and a 55% lower rate for unscheduled primary care visits. The researchers reported a separate 4-year longitudinal study with 774 veterans with similar results (Jia, Chuang, Wu, Wang, & Chumbler, 2009).

Telemental Health

Telemental health is the use of telehealth to deliver psychiatric healthcare. The Telemental Health, a special interest group of the ATA, website at http://www.americantelemed.org/i4a/pages/index.cfm?pageID=3326 includes up-to-date educational presentations on current telemental health projects. Research on the use of telemental health reports that care provided with the use of telehealth technology is comparable to face-to-face care (Bensink, Hailey, & Wootton, 2006).

Telehealth is used to deliver care for various mental health problems. Its use is more prevalent in rural areas, prisons, and other areas where access to a mental health professional is difficult or impossible. Tschirch, Walker, and Calvacca (2006) reported the use of telemental health to provide care to victims of domestic violence in the medically underserved areas of East Texas. Telemental

care has been used to deliver patient care in areas of the world that are compromised by violence and war. For example, victims of violence that existed in the Gush Katif settlements of the Gaza Strip, Israel, received care to reduce the development of acute stress disorder and posttraumatic stress syndrome with the use of videoconferencing (Todder, Matar, & Kaplan, 2007). Military healthcare professionals have used videoconferencing to deliver care to soldiers involved in the Iraq war – again, to help treat mental health problems (Carmichael, 2005).

Clinic Visits

Other uses of telehealth are seen in rural areas where residents traditionally have few options for healthcare and few, if any, specialists. For example, Maine includes many barrier islands inhabited by residents, many of whom make their livelihood from lobster work. Travel to the mainland for these residents can be very inconvenient and result in loss of income. To address the healthcare delivery problem, Sunbeam Island Services provides clinic visits by using a ship staffed by nurses and equipped with two-way teleconferencing equipment (Daley, 2007). The ship has the capability of connecting to seven hub sites located on the mainland. The ship visits the islands twice a month. Island residents attend the ship clinic where the nurses make an initial assessment. Prior to the virtual visit, the nurses fax notes to the attending physician located at one of the hub sites. In addition to virtual visits, the floating clinic transports pediatricians, diabetes specialists, respiratory therapists, and dental hygienists to the island for face-to-face visits with the island residents.

Young and Ireson (2003) reported the use of telehealth at two elementary school health clinics. The study was conducted over a 2-year period. Of the 3,461 clinic visits, 150 (4.3%) resulted in telehealth consultations. Staff at the clinic telehealth site included a full-time nurse and part-time mental health therapist. The telehealth site was equipped with two-way teleconferencing using a telephone line. Pediatricians and pediatric nurse practitioners staffed the connecting hub site. Outcomes of the project indicated that telehealth was an effective means to improve access to medical and mental healthcare. Use of telehealth resulted in cost savings of $101–$224 per encounter for each of the children's families.

E-Intensive Care Units

Remote monitoring of critical care patients is not new. Hospitals, such as Stormont-Vail in Topeka, KS, were doing remote telemetry monitoring for patients in small outlying communities of Kansas in the 1970s. The current use of telepresence of ICU intensivists in critical care is redefining the meaning of critical care remote monitoring. According to the Leapfrog Group, the mortality rate of ICU patients is 10%–20%; however, the use of intensivists to manage or comanage patients can reduce hospital mortality by 30% and ICU mortality by 40% (Leapfrog Group, 2010). The Leapfrog Group recommends the use of ICU physician staffing and supports the use of telemedicine intensive services to meet that need. Telepresence in critical care is currently being delivered with the use of videoconferencing tools, such as eICU® (VISICU, Baltimore, MD), and robotics, such as RP-7 (InTouch Health, Santa Barbara, CA).

eICU

iCare Intensive Care at North Colorado Medical Center provides telepresence using a camera, microphone, and speaker in the patient rooms (Banner, 2010; Trenary, 2007). The bedside team activates the camera during patient rounds when there is a need for the off-site intensivists and the expertise of critical care nurses located at the iCare Command Center in Banner Desert Medical Center.

The Banner Health system includes 23 hospitals located across seven states: Alaska, Arizona, California, Colorado, Nebraska, Nevada, and Wyoming. The iCare Command Center, located in Mesa, AZ, monitored 126 critical care beds in 2007 with plans to extend the eICU for all of the Banner system ICU beds over a 2–3-year period (Banner, 2007). The command center staff has access to patient monitoring information, laboratory values, and x-rays. The cameras and microphones make it possible for the off-site experts to speak with the patients and on-site care providers by using HIPAA-compliant transmissions (Trenary, 2007). Patients receive information about the service upon admission to the hospital and are encouraged to ask questions or express concerns about the service. According to the Banner Health patient information, there is no additional charge for remote monitoring.

Research on the use of eICU provides promising results for the use of telehealth in critical care. Breslow et al. (2004) reported a 2-year study of 2,140 ICU patients cared for using eICU. They compared economic and clinical outcomes data collected during 6 months of remote monitoring with data collected before the eICU was implemented. Analysis of the data showed a decrease in patient mortality from 12.9% to 9.4%. The ICU length of stay decreased from 4.35 to 3.63 days.

Nurses agree that improved patient outcomes are extremely important, but implementing **e-intensive care** had implications for the entire ICU environment. The use of these tools and robots requires extensive planning and communications as well as workflow redesign. The most important factor is buy-in by all affected departments, including not only the ICU staff but also attending physicians, hospital leadership, information services, and respiratory therapy.

Robotics

Robotics is yet another way to provide telepresence of ICU intensivists. One example is the RP-7 robot; RP is short for remote presence (InTouch Health, n.d.-c). The robot is the height of a person who is 5 feet 6 inches and has a large flat screen monitor where a person's head would be; a small camera with tilt, pan, and zoom features; and a couple of antennas on top of the monitor (see **Figure 21-3**). The robot also has two-way audio that allows for conversations between the clinical site and the remote expert. It receives and sends data through a wireless network. It rolls about the floor on three spheres and has built-in infrared sensing devices to help guide it around obstacles.

The remote teleintensivist expert controls the robot using RP software and a joystick. The software can be used with either a laptop or a desktop computer. Dual monitors allow the physician to view a patient's electronic medical record on one monitor and to control the robot using the second monitor. The movement of the robot's camera tilt, pan, and zoom features allows the physician to examine the patient, read a chart, view x-rays mounted on a light board, or observe physiological monitor data. The robot's "head" (the monitor) is able to move 360 degrees, allowing it to "face" the ICU person. The robot's audio and video features allow for real-time

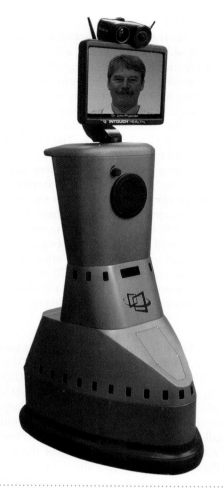

Figure 21-3 RP-7 robot. (Reprinted from InTouch Health, with permission.)

interaction between the physician at the remote site and the patient and care providers in the ICU.

The RP-7 robot is in use in a number of ICU settings. Children's Hospital Los Angeles was the first hospital in the United States to use robots to support the ICU physicians and staff in the pediatric ICUs (Children's Hospital Los Angeles, 2007). The University of California, Los Angeles reported using a robot named RONI (robot of the neuro ICU) in the neurological ICU (InTouch Health, n.d.-b). The Methodist Hospital in Houston, TX, reported using the RP-7 robot in the neurosurgical ICU and the stroke center (InTouch Health, n.d.-a). The Methodist Hospital staff members affectionately

named the robots MURDOC (mobile unit robot doctor) and ROHAS (remote-operated health assessment system). The common goal for use in each of the ICU settings was to improve the quality of patient care by supporting the ICU physicians and staff with a real-time expert opinion.

Research on the use of remote telepresence using robotics in critical care has demonstrated positive outcomes. Vespa et al. (2007) compared data for a period of time before and after using robot telepresence. They noted that the face-to-face response time for routine and urgent pages was reduced from 3.5 hours to less than 10 minutes. Because of the rapid response times, patient outcomes improved and the ICU length of stay was reduced. The researchers attributed a cost savings of $1.1 million to the use of robot telepresence.

Teletrauma Care

Rural hospitals have been able to use telehealth to augment trauma care (**teletrauma**) because they are able to obtain reimbursement for these services (Centers for Medicare & Medicaid Services, 2009). Teletrauma is used to obtain second opinions and advice from trauma care experts. Teletrauma care has also been used to deliver care in parts of the world torn by violence and war.

Rural hospitals in places like Northern California and Eastern Maine are using telehealth equipment to connect with trauma experts. The rural physicians and staff want to provide the best possible care to the patients while keeping the inconvenience of care, travel, and expense of care as low as possible. As of 2007, University of California, Davis (UC Davis), pediatric intensivists had completed over 200 videoconferencing consultations with remote hospital emergency departments and ICUs (UC Davis Medicine, 2007). Thirty percent of the consultations were related to trauma care for children. Eastern Maine Health System (EMHS, 2010) has reported the use of teleconferencing to improve emergency patient outcomes. The telemedicine hub site, located at Eastern Maine Medical Center, was designed to provide 24/7 support for the care of patients located in multiple rural care hospitals.

Research on the use of teletrauma care in rural settings has shown promising outcomes and significance for use in rural health settings. Duchesne et al. (2008) reported a 5-year study of 814 trauma patients, comparing the outcomes before and after the implementation of telemedicine in rural Mississippi settings. The trauma patients who experienced teletrauma care had a decrease in the length of stay at the local community hospital (1.5 hours vs. 47 hours) and a decrease in transfer time to trauma centers (1.7 hours vs. 13 hours). The hospital costs for the trauma patients decreased from $7,632,624 to $1,126,683.

Disaster Healthcare

Telehealth has been used successfully in providing healthcare in disasters (Block, 2010; Markle Foundation, American Medical Association, & Gold Standard, 2006). Almost immediately after Hurricane Katrina hit the Gulf Shore states in the United States, the KatrinaHealth website was established to facilitate communication and to assist victims to access their electronic prescription medication records. As a result, many nurses were able to distribute medications in temporary living communities established across the United States where victims had been transported. One example of such a community was the Rock Eagle 4-H camp in Georgia. The home economics building was converted into a clinic and was open 24 hours to serve 240–500 victims. Volunteer physicians and nurse practitioners staffed part of the clinic. Another part was staffed by volunteer nurses. The local health department nursing leadership coordinated all the care. Nurses used desktop computers with access to the Internet and secure logins to access information to assist the victims. With the assistance of the electronic prescribing, a local pharmacy was able to make daily deliveries of prescribed medication. The clinic volunteer nurses provided care in traditional ways, and the patient records were all on paper; however, access to the Internet played a major role in access to supplies and the provision of care.

Telenursing

Telenursing, as part of telehealth, is not new. The project mentioned in the previous section demonstrates the use of volunteer nurses in telehealth. Telenursing in nondisaster settings is a nursing specialty. Telenursing offers nurses a chance to create more collaborative and autonomous roles and at the same time reduce the overall cost of healthcare. One study compared the outcomes of 28 ostomy patients using only homehealth visits versus a combination of homehealth and telenursing visits (Bohnenkamp, McDonald, Lopez, Krupinski, & Blackett, 2004). The patients who experienced a combination of homehealth and telenursing visits had higher satisfaction, lower costs (although not statistically significant), and a lower cost (number) of ostomy pouches.

Today, telenurses work in various settings. An international study completed between 2004 and 2005 revealed that 37% of telenurses reported working in hospital and college settings (Grady & Schlachta-Fairchild, 2007). Telenursing was described as a nurse who works with telehealth technologies. The majority of the nurses indicated that they learned telenursing skills on the job. An interesting finding, given that majority of the nurses had no prior experience with telehealth before their telenursing positions, is that the majority (89.2%) of those surveyed indicated that telehealth should be included in basic nursing curriculum.

Education

Most telehealth projects have a built-in patient educational component. In some, education is delivered during the "visits" and in others through web pages. Telehealth is also useful in the educational needs of healthcare professionals, not only for continuing education but also for preparing practitioners. As an example, faculty from five University of Wisconsin nursing programs embarked upon an innovative curricular redesign that infused telenursing into learning (Gallagher-Lepack, Scheibel, & Gibson, 2009). Lead faculty members designed telenursing assignments for nursing theory, health assessment, community, research, and leadership/management courses. Students gained competencies with informatics and computers as outcomes. They also learned to appreciate the value of telenursing to complement face-to-face encounters with patients and families.

Issues

Telehealth in its many forms can provide many benefits such as enhanced patient care, reduced travel time, increased productivity, access to specialists, and enlarged educational opportunities for all. Many issues, however, surround this mode of healthcare delivery. Four main issues relate to (1) reimbursement, (2) medico-legal issues,[1] (3) technical issues, and (4) research.

Reimbursement

Reimbursement remains a large barrier to the widespread adoption of telehealth. Of the examples in this chapter, the majority was supported with grants. Despite successes, the telehealth projects were discontinued when the grants expired. Our healthcare system today is shaped by third-party payers, both government and private. Currently, there continues to be no uniformity for the reimbursement of telehealth/telemedicine services. According to the 2003 Telemedicine Reimbursement, "One of the barriers to telemedicine becoming completely integrated into the U.S. medical system is the absence of consistent, federal and state reimbursement policies" (Health Resources and Services Administration, 2003). For telemedicine to survive/thrive, reimbursement must be a joint effort between states, the federal government, and private payers. Reimbursement considerations must be made with the best interests of the patients' healthcare needs and outcomes in mind.

A 2006 study, a follow-up study on the ATA and AMD Telemedicine Study, showed progress in reimbursement for telehealth (Whitten, 2007). In 2008, the Centers for Medicare & Medicaid modified their reimbursement policy for telemedicine as a result of the 2006 Tax Relief and Healthcare Act (Naditz, 2008).

Technical

The safety of the patient is always a concern with developing uses of new technology. As stated earlier in the chapter, all the projects seen thus far have been of a very high quality, with no compromise in patient safety. In an endeavor to set standards in telenursing, the American Academy of Ambulatory Care Nursing (AAACN) established the telehealth nursing practice special interest group in 1995. The AAACN developed telehealth nursing practice administration and practice standards (American Academy of Ambulatory Care Nursing, 2007) that

address standards for telenursing, including staffing, competency, ethics, patient rights, and the use of the nursing process in telehealth. They followed this with the publication of the Telehealth Nursing Practice Essentials (Espensen & American Academy of Ambulatory Care Nursing, 2009). The organization also published the Telehealth Nursing Practice Resource Directory (American Academy of Ambulatory Care Nursing, 2008). The directory includes resources and information to assist nurses to "improve the quality, efficiency, and effectiveness" of their practice. The AAACN offers certification for telehealth nursing. The application can be downloaded from the AAACN website at http://www.aaacn.org/.

The ATA has adopted core standards for telemedicine operations, which address three types of standards: administrative, clinical, and technical. Administrative standards cover issues related to human resource management, HIPAA, research protocols, telehealth equipment use, and fiscal management. Clinical standards uphold the individual discipline standards of professional practice and standards of care as they relate to telehealth. Technical standards relate to requirements for safety and the function of telehealth equipment, the requirements for policies and procedures, and the need for redundant systems to ensure network connectivity.

Research

A Cochrane Library meta-analysis of research done in the early years of this century to examine the efficacy of telemedicine versus face-to-face patient care recommendations did not demonstrate strong evidence of clinical benefits (Currell, Urquhart, Wainwright, & Lewis, 2000, 2001). A main complaint was that the number of patients in the research studies was small. The meta-analysis did note that people were satisfied with home self-monitoring and video consultations. Technology and telehealth research have matured since then, and current literature has reported studies conducted over time with larger numbers of patients (Vespa et al., 2007); thus, the evidence for telehealth is now much stronger. Technology and telehealth research have matured since the meta-analysis of research was published. A meta-analysis of publications on telehealth published

---

1 Medico-legal issues are discussed in Chapter 25.

between 2001 and 2007 revealed a positive and significant effect on clinical outcomes (DelliFraine & Dansky, 2008). The outcomes for heart disease and psychiatric conditions were most significant.

Summary

As technology improves, the possibilities for telehealth are endless. Telehealth technologies can be classed as either S&F or real-time. S&F is an asynchronous method in which images are sent to a distant location and examined at the convenience of the specialist. Real-time telehealth, a synchronous mode, involves both the patient and the consultant interacting at the same time. Telepresence created with eICUs, two-way video teleconferencing, and robotics is being used to augment care delivered in ICUs and emergency departments. Telehomecare monitoring devices are empowering patients to live independently and to be proactive in the early detection of healthcare problems before they happen.

Telehealth offers many opportunities for nurses. Telehealth has also proved valuable in education, both professionally and for patient care and disaster care. As telehealth becomes more widespread, issues still need to be resolved. Medicare has finally begun to reimburse telehealth care in the United States; however, since Medicaid is controlled at the state level, variations in reimbursement still exist. The telecommunications infrastructure can also be a problem. As with many innovations, use of telehealth will change the way healthcare is delivered. These changes will create opportunities for many. Care that is more preventive reduces emergency room visits and hospital admissions. It has the potential to upset the financial base of the present acute care system.

APPLICATION AND COMPETENCIES

1. Define the two overall classifications of technology used in telehealth. Provide examples on how the classifications are used in your healthcare work setting.

2. Discuss some of the ways that telehealth can be applied to deliver healthcare.

3. Write two or three paragraphs illustrating the essential competencies for telenursing.

4. Select one of the issues in implementing telehealth and discuss the different approaches t&t; resolving the issue.

5. Analyze two research studies done with telehealth. Compare the findings for similarities and differences.

6. Explore the ways that telehealth could have ant; impact on the healthcare system in your country.

REFERENCES

American Academy of Ambulatory Care Nursing. (2007). *Telehealth nursing practice administration and practice standards* (4th ed.). Pitman, NJ: Author.

American Academy of Ambulatory Care Nursing. (2008). *Telehealth nursing practice resource directory* (3rd ed.). Pitman, NJ: Author.

American Telemedicine Association. (2010). *Telemedicine defined*. Retrieved October 29, 2010, from http://www.americantelemed.org/i4a/pages/index.cfm?pageid=3333

American Telemedicine Association. (n.d.). *Telemedicine/telehealth terminology*. Retrieved October 29, 2010, from http://www.americantelemed.org/files/public/abouttelemedicine/Terminology.pdf

Banner, H. (2007, May 11). *Banner health to add 50 new eICU beds in valley*. Retrieved February 14, 2008, from http://www.bannerhealth.com/About+Us/News+Center/Press+Releases/Banner+Health+adds+50+eICU+beds.htm

Banner, H. (2010). *iCare intensive care, utilizing eICU technology*. Retrieved October 30, 2010, from http://www.bannerhealth.com/Locations/Colorado/North+Colorado+Medical+Center/Programs+and+Services/iCare+Intensive+Care+Unit.htm

Bensink, M., Hailey, D., & Wootton, R. (2006). A systematic review of successes and failures in home telehealth: Preliminary results... 6th International Conference on Successes and Failures in Telehealth, SFT-6, Brisbane, Queensland, Australia, 24–24 August, 2006. *Journal of Telemedicine & Telecare, 12*(S3), 8–16.

Block, C. (2010, April 21). *UTMB responds to disasters*. Retrieved October 30, 2010, from http://telemedicinenews.blogspot.com/2010/04/utmb-responds-to-disasters.html

Bohnenkamp, S. K., McDonald, P., Lopez, A. M., Krupinski, E., & Blackett, A. (2004). Traditional versus telenursing outpatient management of patients with cancer with new ostomies. *Oncology Nursing Forum, 31*(5), 1005–1010.

Breslow, M. J., Rosenfeld, B. A., Doerfler, M., Burke, G., Yates, G., Stone, D. J., et al. (2004). Effect of a multiple-site intensive care unit telemedicine program on clinical and economic outcomes: An alternative paradigm for intensivist staffing. *Critical Care Medicine, 32*(1), 31–38.

Business Wire. (2007, December 11). *Honeywell HomMed partners with Procura to offer comprehensive telehealth solution*. Retrieved October 29, 2010, from http://www.allbusiness.com/technology/software-services-applications-information/5329380-1.html

Carmichael, M. (2005, March 1). *Combat stress teams and telemedicine: The new strategies for helping soldiers cope with war*. Retrieved February 15, 2008, from http://www.pbs.org/wgbh/pages/frontline/shows/heart/readings/telemedicine.html

Centers for Medicare & Medicaid Services. (2009, July). *Fact sheet: Telehealth services*. Retrieved October 30, 2010, from http://www.telemedicine.com/pdfs/TelehealthSrvcsfctsht.pdf

Children's Hospital Los Angeles. (2007). *Virtual robotic doctor' working with intensive care staff at Children's Hospital Los Angeles*. Retrieved October 30, 2010, from http://www.chla.org/site/apps/nlnet/content2.aspx?c=ipINKTOAJsG&b=3793521&ct=4909875

Chumbler, N. R., Neugaard, B., Ryan, P., Qin, H., & Joo, Y. (2005). An observational study of veterans with diabetes receiving weekly or daily home telehealth monitoring. *Journal of Telemedicine & Telecare, 11*(3), 150–156.

Currell, R., Urquhart, C., Wainwright, P., & Lewis, R. (2000). Telemedicine versus face to face patient care: Effects on professional practice and health care outcomes. *Cochrane Database Systems Review*, Issue 2, Art. No. CD002098.

Currell, R., Urquhart, C., Wainwright, P., & Lewis, R. (2001). Telemedicine versus face to face patient care: Effects on professional practice and health care outcomes. *Nursing Times, 97*(35), 35.

Daley, S. (2007). Riding the technological wave. *Health Management Technology, 28*(11), 18, 20.

DelliFraine, J. L., & Dansky, K. H. (2008). Home-based telehealth: A review and meta-analysis. *Journal of Telemedicine & Telecare, 14*(2), 62–66.

Duchesne, J. C., Kyle, A., Simmons, J., Islam, S., Schmieg, R. E., Jr., Olivier, J., et al. (2008). Impact of telemedicine upon rural trauma care. *The Journal of Trauma, 64*(1), 92–97; discussion 97–98.

EMHS. (2010). *EMHS telehealth: Improving access to healthcare in Maine's rural communities*. Retrieved October 30, 2010, from http://emh.com/dynamic.aspx?id=14710

Espensen, M., & American Academy of Ambulatory Care Nursing. (2009). *Telehealth nursing practice essentials*. Pitman, NJ: American Academy of Ambulatory Care Nursing.

Federation of American Scientists. (n.d.). *Glossary*. Retrieved October 29, 2010, from http://www.fas.org/spp/military/docops/usaf/2020/app-v.htm

Gallagher-Lepack, S., Scheibel, P., & Gibson, C. C. (2009). Integrating telehealth in nursing curricula: Can you hear me now? *Online Journal of Nursing Informatics, 13*(2), 16. Retrieved from http://ojni.org/13_2/GallagherLepak.pdf

Grady, J. L., & Schlachta-Fairchild, L. (2007). Report of the 2004–2005 International Telenursing Survey. *CIN: Computers, Informatics, Nursing, 25*(5), 266–272.

Health Resources and Services Administration. (2003, October). *Telemedicine reimbursement report*. Retrieved October 30, 2010, from http://www.hrsa.gov/telehealth/pubs/reimbursement.htm

International Council of Nurses. (2010). *Network history*. Retrieved October 29, 2010, from http://www.icn.ch/networks/tele-network-history/

InTouch Health. (n.d.-a). *24–7 coverage for patients at The Methodist Hospital in Houston*. Retrieved February 14, 2008, from http://www.intouchhealth.com/rpnews_081607-RP-7_Remote_Presence_Robots_help_provide_24-7_Coverage_for_Patients_at_The_Methodist_Hospital_in_Houston.html

InTouch Health. (n.d.-b). Increased neuro-ICU coverage in an academia setting. *UCLA Today*. Retrieved October 30, 2010, from http://www.intouchhealth.com/2UCLA-Neuro-ICU.pdf

InTouch Health.(n.d.-c). *Products: Overview*. Retrieved November 5, 2010, from http://www.intouchhealth.com/products.html

Jia, H., Chuang, H.-C., Wu, S. S., Wang, X., & Chumbler, N. R. (2009). Long-term effect of home telehealth services on preventable hospitalization use. *The Journal of Rehabilitation Research and Development, 46*(5), 557–562.

Kane, D. (2010, June 17). *NanoEngineers print and test chemical sensors on elastic waistbands of underwear*. Retrieved October 29, 2010, from http://ucsdnews.ucsd.edu/newsrel/science/06-17ElasticWaistbands.asp

Koninklijke Philips Electronics. (2007, November 1). *St. Lucas Andreas Hospital to start home monitoring of cardiac patients using Philips remote system*. Retrieved October 29, 2010, from http://www.newscenter.philips.com/main/standard/about/news/press/20071101_stlucas_andreas_hospital.wpd

Leapfrog Group. (2010, February 23). *ICU staffing*. Retrieved October 30, 2010, from http://www.leapfroggroup.org/media/file/FactSheet_IPS.pdf

Lynch, A. (1998). *Bleeding sailor performs self-surgery via e-mail/Boston doctor advises solo racer – SFGate*. Retrieved October 20, 2010, from http://articles.sfgate.com/1998-11-19/news/17737296_1_viktor-yazykov-sailor-e-mail

Markle Foundation, American Medical Association, & Gold Standard. (2006, June 13). *Lessons from KatrinaHealth*. Retrieved October 29, 2010, from http://katrinahealth.org/katrinahealth.final.pdf

Mattia, J. (2007, May 21). *How Piedmont Hospital cut heart failure patient readmissions by 75 percent*. Retrieved February 3, 2008, from http://www.healthleadersmedia.com/content/89750/topic/WS_HLM2_TEC/How-Piedmont-Hospital-Cut-Heart-Failure-Patient-Readmissions-by-75-Percent.html

Naditz, A. (2008). Medicare's and Medicaid's new reimbursement policies for telemedicine. *Telemedicine Journal & E- Health, 14*(1), 21–24.

Schneider, N., & Harris, D. K. (2003). Telemedicine success story. *Telemedicine Journal & E- Health, 9*(1), 115–116.

Schneider, N. M. (2004). Managing congestive heart failure using home telehealth. *Home Healthcare Nurse, 22*(10), 719–722.

Sung, M., Marci, C., & Pentland, A. (2005). Wearable feedback systems for rehabilitation. *Journal of Neuroengineering and Rehabilitation, 2*, 17.

Todder, D., Matar, M., & Kaplan, Z. (2007). Acute-phase trauma intervention using a videoconference link circumvents compromised access to expert trauma care. *Telemedicine Journal & E- Health, 13*(1), 65–67.

Trenary, K. (2007). Advances in technology affects nursing: iCare Intensive Care, Banner Health: Remote telepresence in the critical care setting. *Arizona Nurse, 60*(2), 6.

Tschirch, P., Walker, G., & Calvacca, L. T. (2006). Nursing in tele-mental health. *Journal of Psychosocial Nursing and Mental Health Services, 44*(5), 20–27.

UC Davis Medicine. (2007, Spring). *Telemedicine extends trauma care to rural areas*. Retrieved October 30, 2010, from http://www.ucdmc.ucdavis.edu/ucdavismedicine/issues/spring2007/features/3.html

UC Health. (2010). *Smart underwear*. Retrieved October 29, 2010, from http://universityofcalifornia.edu/sites/uchealth/2010/06/16/smart-underwear/

Vespa, P. M., Miller, C., Hu, X., Nenov, V., Buxey, F., & Martin, N. A. (2007). Intensive care unit robotic telepresence facilitates rapid physician response to unstable patients and decreased cost in neurointensive care. *Surgical Neurology, 67*(4), 331–337.

Villalba, E., Ottaviano, M., Arredondo, M. T., Martinez, A., & Guillen, S. (2006). Wearable monitoring system for heart failure assessment in a mobile environment. *Computers in Cardiology, 33*, 237–240. Retrieved from http://www.cinc.org/Proceedings/2006/pdf/0237.pdf

Whitten, P. (2007). Private payer reimbursement for telemedicine services in the United States. *Telemedicine Journal & E- Health, 13*(1). Retrieved from http://www.american-telemed.org/files/public/policy/Private_Payer_Report.pdf

Wood, D. (2011). *Telehealth successes in patient health management*. Retrieved August 31, 2011, from http://www.amnhealthcare.com/News/news-details.aspx?Id=35158

Young, T. L., & Ireson, C. (2003). Effectiveness of school-based telehealth care in urban and rural elementary schools. *Pediatrics, 112*(5), 1088–1094.

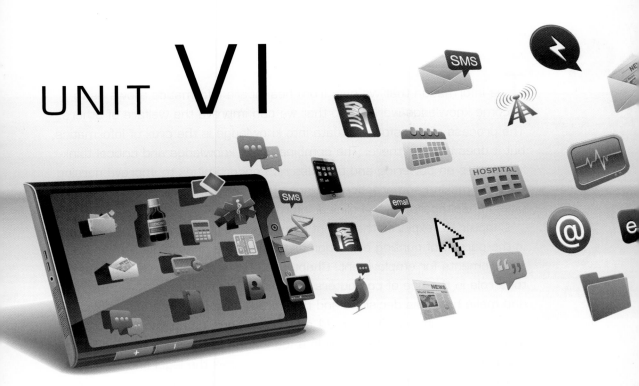

UNIT VI

Computer Uses in Healthcare Beyond Clinical Informatics

The information that we gain from healthcare informatics allows us to become knowledge workers so that we can improve the welfare of others. The process of transforming data into knowledge is the crux of informatics, but it does not end there. The combination of knowledge and critical thinking skills is empowering and provides rich opportunities to improve nursing decision making and practice settings. The theme for this unit is computer uses in healthcare beyond clinical informatics.

Chapter 22 explores the use of computers for online learning, whether in the pursuit of nursing education or to meet the ongoing clinical education requirements for employment. Chapter 23 looks at the nurse administrator's role in the use of computers and information systems to analyze data and make business decisions and the nurse's role as it relates to clinical information systems. Chapter 24 addresses basic competencies in data analysis and research that provide a foundation for decision making in nursing and healthcare. Finally, Chapter 25 addresses the legal and ethical responsibilities of the nurse as they relate to informatics. Topics that are discussed include the professional codes of ethics, Health Insurance Portability and Accountability Act of 1996 (HIPAA), Web 2.0, telehealth, the implantable patient identifier, and copyright issues.

CHAPTER 22

Educational Informatics: e-Learning

Objectives

After studying this chapter you will be able to:

▶ *Describe how different online teaching methodologies contribute to learning using Bloom's taxonomy of learning.*

▶ *Compare computerized quizzing and survey features with that of a print version.*

▶ *Describe how online databases of teaching/learning resources such as the MERLOT project benefit learners.*

▶ *Identify the strengths and weaknesses of e-learning.*

▶ *Interpret the factors affecting distance education outcomes.*

▶ *Discuss the role of the learner in distance education.*

▶ *Discuss three essential characteristics that contribute to success of learners who take courses online.*

Key Terms

Animation
Avatar
Bloom's Taxonomy of Learning
Computer-Aided Instruction (CAI)
Computer-Based Learning
Drill and Practice
E-Learning
Hybrid Courses
Instructional Games
Learning Assessment
Learning Content Management System (LCMS)
Learning Management System (LMS)
Learning Style
Multimedia
Simulation
Sharable Content Object Reference Model (SCORM®)
Simulation-Based Learning (SBL)
Streaming Video
Tutorial
Virtual Reality (VR)

You may have heard or read **e-learning** (electronic learning) advertisements – "Go to school in your pajamas" or "Earn a college degree without ever leaving your home." You may be taking courses that are offered completely online or with parts of the course online (**hybrid courses**). You may be earning an online degree. But then again, you may be taking classes at a traditional brick and mortar school where you have schoolwork that requires the use of a computer for learning activities and quizzing functions. If your learning falls into any of these situations, you have much personal experience on the topics presented in this chapter on e-learning.

Online educational activities are focused on increasing the knowledge level of learners. Resources for such activities appear in many formats, including lectures, reading, and self-learning computer activities. Education itself can be looked at as the mental manipulation of data, information, and knowledge by learners to increase their knowledge. Learning occurs only in the learner but can be facilitated by a teacher, whether face-to-face or mediated by learning resources ranging from paper to a DVD, an interactive **simulation**, or any combination of these. The job of an educator, whether a nurse providing patient education, a teacher in a formal class, a designer of educational aids, or a parent, is to facilitate this process. These functions can be called educational informatics, and they may or may not involve technology. Learning that is mediated by computer technology is termed "e-learning."

No matter what format is used for education, the primary focus must be on learning, not on the technology or lack of it. Informatics is about using the best methods to manage information, and e-learning focuses on the appropriate use of computerized technology to achieve educational aims. Factors such as learning goals, outcomes, and characteristics of the topic determine the best instructional methods needed. Simply moving a class or course to a computer format is not necessarily an improvement. Educators must pay attention to how the technology is used as well as to what it will add to the learning situation. Each technology method from simple computer-assisted learning to **virtual reality (VR)** possesses different attributes. An attribute such as color, movement, or music may or may not add to the learning process (Clark & Mayer, 2003).

E-Learning Basics

E-learning is another of the "e-words" that has crept into our language; it indicates a marriage between electronics – generally a computer – and educational software. It includes many different types of computerized instruction, from instruction using only the text portion of a computer to Internet-based distance learning using a **multimedia**-capable computer. The term "e-learning" places the emphasis on student learning and pedagogy. Older terms, such as computer-assisted instruction or **computer-aided instruction (CAI)** and **computer-based learning**, emphasized the technology.

Learning management is another concept that involves computer use in education. The term

learning management system (LMS) describes software that facilitates delivering course content electronically. Examples of commercial LMSs include Blackboard, ANGEL® Learning, and Desire 2 Learn. Free open-source solutions include Moodle, Sakai Project, and ATutor. **Figure 22-1** is a screenshot showing online course features in Sakai. The items on the menu are similar to commercial and other open source LMSs.

Today, the more sophisticated e-learning products are often a combination of LMS and **learning content management system (LCMS)** functions. LMS features can be as simple as delivering learning content, scoring computer-learning activities, and providing printable certificates of course completion. Other LMS features include e-mail, discussion forums, virtual student work areas, chat, wikis, and blogs. Sophisticated enterprise solutions synchronize with school student registration database systems so that when students register for courses, their names can automatically appear in the online grade book.

The purpose of LCMSs is to store and manage learning resources authored by faculty and content experts so that they can be reused by a variety of educators (Greenberg, 2002). The LCMS learning resources such as course content modules, slides, video clips, illustrations, and quiz questions can be assembled into course learning content by using infinitely changeable combinations according to the instructor's needs.

From the Learner's Perspective: Computer Technology and Learning

Although educational informatics involves all facets of education, this chapter focuses on computer technology and learning. Technology-enhanced instructional methodologies allow learners to take ownership for their learning. It provides mechanisms to allow the learner to interact with knowledge concepts and to practice and evaluate learning gains. E-learning provides a foundation for nurses who want to advance their education and obtain college degrees when time, work, family, or distance makes it difficult to attend school in the traditional brick building setting. E-learning is used in healthcare facilities

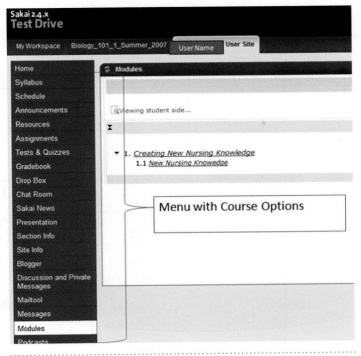

Figure 22-1 View of a sample course in Sakai.

to provide continuing education (CE) programs to nurses at times when they are mentally and physically able to learn, rather than after a busy 12-hour work shift. E-learning provides a means for nurses to obtain CE hours to acquire and maintain their specialty certifications. In spite of the pains of occasional technology glitches, nurses who truly embrace e-learning would rather fight than give it up.

How People Learn

Dale's Cone of Experience, based on the work of Edgar Dale in 1946 (see **Figure 22-2**), is often used to provide a visual about how people learn (Thalheimer, 2006). Dale's original model did not include any numbers. This particular model is concept based but not evidence-based and, as a result, remains very controversial. The model provides an intuitive explanation about the learning experience and helps to explain why student nurses learn best from clinical experiences with patients and families and from simulation laboratories. Interactive teaching methodologies using e-learning open up opportunities for

students to apply learning. How people learn is individualized. **Learning style** is the way people perceive, remember, express, and solve problems. Fortunately, learning style surveys are available online and provide excellent self-assessment tools. One example of an online survey is the index of learning styles questionnaire at http://www.engr.ncsu.edu/learningstyles/ilsweb.html.

Quality E-Learning

Seven principles of quality undergraduate education were identified in 1987, long before e-learning gained popularity (Chickering & Ehrmann, 1996). These classic principles apply to today's e-learning environment. The principles address (1) the importance of faculty–student contact in and out of class; (2) collaborative learning among students and faculty; (3) active learning techniques, which allow students to discuss, write reflectively, and incorporate learning into their lives; (4) opportunities for students to practice learning and receive just-in-time feedback; (5) learning strategies that help students to learn

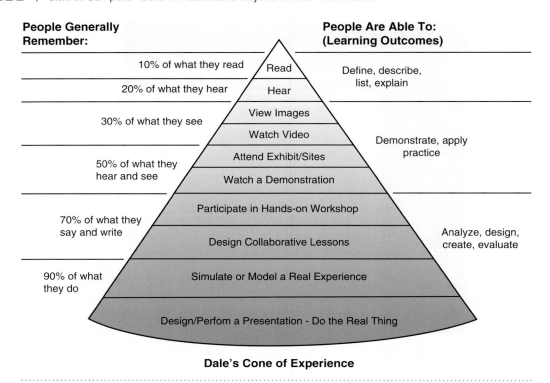

People Generally Remember:

- 10% of what they read
- 20% of what they hear
- 30% of what they see
- 50% of what they hear and see
- 70% of what they say and write
- 90% of what they do

People Are Able To: (Learning Outcomes)

- Read
- Hear
- View Images
- Watch Video
- Attend Exhibit/Sites
- Watch a Demonstration
- Participate in Hands-on Workshop
- Design Collaborative Lessons
- Simulate or Model a Real Experience
- Design/Perfom a Presentation - Do the Real Thing

- Define, describe, list, explain
- Demonstrate, apply practice
- Analyze, design, create, evaluate

Dale's Cone of Experience

Figure 22-2 Dale's cone of experience. (From Pastore, R. S. (2003). *Principles of teaching.* Retrieved November 5, 2010, from http://teacherworld.com/potdale.html.)

efficiently; (6) high faculty expectations for student learning; and (7) respect for various learning styles and individual student talents.

LMSs can supplement or replace face-to-face classes. LMSs provide a means for faculty/student interaction, collaborative learning, and prompt feedback on learning progress. The use of technology serves as a foundation for the design of a variety of interactive instructional methods. The methods can be combined in a number of ways like building blocks to provide learning content.

Bloom's Taxonomy and Learning Methods

According to **Bloom's Taxonomy of Learning** (Bloom, 1956), learning occurs at six levels: knowledge, comprehension, application, analysis, synthesis, and evaluation. E-learning can be designed to address one or more of the domains (see **Figure 22-3**). The taxonomy was later modified by Anderson and Krathwohl to make "creating" rather than "evaluating" the highest level of learning (Anderson, Krathwohl, & Bloom, 2001).

Knowledge, comprehension, and application are considered lower-order thinking skills. Knowledge indicates the ability to recite discrete facts. Flash cards, games, and quizzes are used to assist the learner to memorize terms. Comprehension indicates that the learner can explain the concept. Simulations, **animations**, and **tutorials** are used to assist the learner to visualize and describe complex concepts. Application indicates that the learner can understand the concepts well enough to apply it to a new situation. Interactive tutorials, simulations, **instructional games**, and case studies assist the learner to apply learning.

Analysis, synthesis, and evaluation are considered higher-order thinking skills. Analysis indicates that the learner can deconstruct or break apart the concept. Synthesis indicates that the

Learning Assessment Techniques	Bloom	Anderson & Krathwohl
Virtual labs, computer simulation models, case studies, multiple choice questions Higher order thinking skills	Evaluation Synthesis Analysis	Creating Evaluating Analyzing
Interactive tutorials, simulations, instructional games, case studies	Application	Applying
Simulations, animations, tutorials	Comprehension	Understanding
Flash cards, games, quizzes	Knowledge	Remembering

Figure 22-3 Learning assessment techniques in relation to learning taxonomies.

learner can connect the concept with other concepts and apply it in new ways. Finally, evaluation indicates that the learner can make judgments about how well they understand the concept. Virtual laboratories, computer-simulation models, and case studies assist in the development of higher-order thinking skills in learners. Multiple-choice test questions can also be designed to teach higher-order thinking skills (Lord & Baviskar, 2007).

Drill and Practice

Drill and practice software was among the first educational software introduced. It was relatively simple to produce, and it freed teachers from the mundane chores and repetitive teaching. Flash cards and questions with answers are examples of drill and practice learning methods. Flashcard Friends at http://www.flashcardfriends.com/ is a free website that allows users to create and share flashcards. The users could be teachers and students. Users can also create questions with fill-in-the blanks, multiple-choice, matching, and true and false. Students can collaborate and share the learning resources with others.

Proprietary software such as StudyMate Author® allows faculty to create flash cards for online use in an LMS or downloaded to an iPod, Sony® Playstation Portable, or other small-screen mobile device (Respondus®, 2010). Learners can purchase electronic flash cards online from Skyscape at http://www.skyscape.com and Amazon at http://www.amazon.com. Printed textbooks often include

CD-ROM or a textbook website with flash cards and other interactive learning activities.

Drill and practice can assist the learner to develop the cognitive structure necessary for the kind of reflective thinking that produces critical thinking. The best use of the drill and practice method is as an aid for memorization. Pure memorization provides learning at Bloom's Taxonomy knowledge level, which is essential in many areas to provide a foundation for higher-level learning. For example, it is essential to memorize information such as medical terminology along with rules for combining the terms to create other words to understand the nursing information in texts and articles.

Tutorials

Tutorials are step-by-step programs designed to guide learners to understand information. Well-designed tutorials are interactive when the learner is presented with learning content and then provided with self-assessment multiple-choice questions to assess the learning. Most are patterned on a programmed learning model. The quality of a tutorial is evident with the use of branching techniques. At the low end of the continuum are programs that just inform the learner whether the answer is correct. Those at the high end offer more than one explanation for the same phenomenon and provide feedback on incorrect answers.

Tutorials do not have to "tell" the learners what they need to know. Learners can instead be presented with a situation, given the tools necessary to discover the answer, and then allowed to proceed at their own pace. Examples of interactive tutorials are online at Medline Plus (http://www.nlm.nih.gov/medlineplus/tutorials/). The interactive tutorials provide an opportunity for the learners to review the different modules and test their learning.

Simulations

Simulations imitate actual experiences. Simulations have many uses, such as part of an orientation or in-service, a face-to-face classroom or clinical laboratory setting, or as part of a homework assignment. Effective simulations match the learner's knowledge background, or are, at least, only slightly above it, and the point of view addresses the learning needs. Simulations are available on CD-ROM and the Internet.

The Internet provides simultaneous use by a large number of learners. An online flash simulation, Care of a Client with Schizophrenia (http://www.wisc-online.com/objects/ViewObject.aspx?ID=NUR3704), allows the learner to apply knowledge about schizophrenia. Assessing blood pressure is also a complex skill for the novice healthcare provider student. The simulation Assessing Blood Pressure at http://132.241.10.14/bp/bp.html provides essential knowledge about how to take blood pressure and interpret the sounds. The student uses a mouse to "pump" the virtual blood pressure bulb and then releases the valve to hear the sounds. An interactive quiz provides feedback on the learning.

Animations

Animations provide visual representations of difficult concepts, processes, and models. Animations can be created in a number of file formats. One common format used is called Flash. A Flash player, a free download from http://www.macromedia.com/software/flash/about/, may be used to view the files. Animations are best used as a supplement to written information. The KidneyPatientGuide (http://www.kidneypatientguide.org.uk/site/treatment.php) uses several animations to demonstrate concepts related to dialysis, transplants, and diet. The animation is designed for patients but can also be used with nursing students.

Instructional Games

Online instructional games can add a competitive contest aspect to learning. The purpose for the use of games is to motivate students to learn the needed information. Games can foster collaboration, problem solving, and analytical thinking. Learners must be clear about the purpose when using games. They should also be sure that they have the technology hardware and software necessary to play the game. Games that are successful must meet instructional requirements and be enjoyable for players. Games should be appropriate and not trivialize learning content or encourage guessing (Benner, Sutphen, Leonard, & Day, 2010).

Many different types of games and software are used to create them. Hot Potatoes™ software provides a variety of game formats; it is freeware. Some examples of games include those that select letters to identify words or phrases – similar to a popular television show – crossword puzzles, and fill in the blanks (Half-Baked Software Inc., 2010). Quandary allows users to create action mazes, which are interactive online case studies (Half-Baked Software Inc., 2009). StudyMate Author®, a commercial product, allows users to create games such as crossword puzzles, fill in the blanks, and pick a letter that can be uploaded into LMSs (Respondus®, 2010). SoftChalk™, another commercial product, also allows users to create interactive learning resources with a variety of games (SoftChalk LLC, 2010).

Games are also available on the web. The online game Outbreak at Water's Edge: A Public Health Discovery Game at http://www.mclph.umn.edu/watersedge/ uses a Java applet, a program written in Java programming language, to play a game to discover the source of contamination making residents in the local community sick. The game is available in both English and Spanish. The Nobelprize.org website (http://nobelprize.org/educational_games/medicine/) offers fun interactive games on topics that are difficult for learners to understand, such as blood typing, malaria, and the immune system.

Computerized Quizzes and Surveys

Computers allow for many testing functions. Quizzes and surveys provide a means for assessing learning, and are therefore termed **learning assessment**. LMSs and numerous companies include tools to create quizzes and anonymous surveys. Quizzes can be generated using the forms function of word processing software or more sophisticated proprietary software. Quizzes found on the web are often self-tests associated with tutorials. Self-tests are categorized as formative assessments because they provide information about ongoing learning. Quizzes associated with course grades are summative assessments because they sum up learning. Summative tests are given in a secure testing environment.

Quiz Software. Quiz software is specially designed database software with a variety of uses. It allows faculty to create online quizzes either administered on the Web or integrated for use as a testing function within an LMS. Quiz software can also be useful in creating paper tests. Sophisticated testing software allows for feedback for right and wrong answers, the ability to categorize questions, test item analysis, and scoring student performance. Quiz software may allow the teacher to create a test bank of questions for reuse in various classes. Most test scoring software is capable of providing a file for the instruction that can be imported into a spreadsheet or database as part of an electronic grading book.

Question Writer from http://www.question-writer.com/free-quiz-software.html is a free (for noncommercial use) program that allows the creation of multiple-choice quizzes that can be posted to the Internet. Users are able to print out a results report and view question feedback for correct/incorrect responses.

Surveys. Surveys provide a way to aggregate information anonymously from learners. They are often used in LMSs for learning assessment, such as "the muddiest point" technique and course evaluations. The "muddiest point" assessment is one where the student describes a topic that is least clearly understood. Surveys are a tool that provides evaluation information. Several survey services are available on the web. For example, SurveyMonkey (http://www.surveymonkey.com/) and Zoomerang (http://www.zoomerang.com/) provide free and for-purchase survey tools.

SCORM Tools. **Sharable Content Object Reference Model (SCORM®)** refers to a learning module that can be imported into any SCORM-compliant LMS; think of it as one design fits all (Advanced Distributed Learning, 2010). Typically, the SCORM module is designed to include a self-test associated with one or more learning tools such as flash cards, games, and tutorials. The learner has an opportunity to interact with the learning tools and then take the associated self-test. The self-test resides within the SCORM module, as opposed to the assessment/quiz section of the LMS, but the self-test grade is recorded in the LMS grade book.

The concept was developed by the Department of Defense in 2002 to save design costs associated with multiple systems. Course designer tools that are compliant with SCORM standards and specifications can be exported to all the popular LMSs. Examples of software that can be used to create SCORM tools are Hot Potatoes™, Adobe Captivate®, TechSmith® Camtasia®, Articulate®, SoftChalk, and Studymate Author®.

Computer-Adaptive Testing. Computer-adaptive testing is a type of online testing that is familiar to most licensed registered nurses because since 1994 it has been the type of testing done to assess knowledge for licensure. Computer-adaptive testing is designed to make the testing process more efficient because it adapts the questions to the candidate's responses. The nursing licensure exam – the NCLEX exam – is based on the licensure test plan. The difficulty of the question presented on the computer screen is based on the candidate's previous right or wrong response. Candidates who pass can answer 50% or more of the more difficult questions. Those who fail answer 50% or more of the easier questions correctly (NCSBN, n.d.). A simulation of the exam is available at http://www.pearsonvue.com/nclex/#tutorial.

MERLOT: Web-Based Learning Resources

Many e-learning resources are available on the web, but finding excellent resources can be like finding a needle in a haystack. Multimedia Education Resource for Online Learning and Teaching (MERLOT) at http://www.merlot.org is the first place that faculty and students should search (see **Figure 22-4**). MERLOT is an online repository of peer-reviewed learning resources.

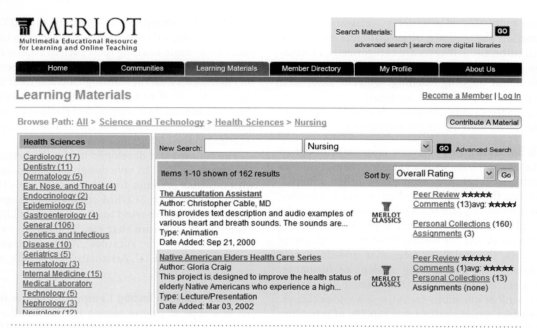

Figure 22-4 MERLOT.

Faculty members or students who wanted to share what they perceived as valuable teaching–learning resources contributed the learning resources you find in MERLOT. The learning resources actually reside in the computer of the author or sponsor. MERLOT simply provides a hyperlink to the resource along with a peer-review rating and comments, user comments, and user-suggested learning assignments. In addition to searching MERLOT, users have the option of searching other digital libraries (federated search). The MERLOT vision is to become the "premiere online community where faculty, staff, and students from around the world share their learning materials and pedagogy" (MERLOT, n.d.).

To take advantage of the community aspects of MERLOT, register for free membership. MERLOT membership has many benefits. Members can

- contribute new learning resources;
- provide users with comments about learning resources;
- publish a user profile to facilitate networking with others who have similar interests;
- save personal collections of their favorite teaching and learning resources;

- build interactive learning web pages by using MERLOT Content Builder; and
- use MERLOT Voices to participate in a collaborative community with others interested in teaching and learning with technology.

MERLOT membership offers faculty members the opportunity to become a peer reviewer in their discipline. MERLOT offers free "Grape (Getting Reviewers Accustomed to the Process of Evaluation) Camp" peer-review how-to courses for faculty who have an interest in learning the peer-review process.

Technologies

The various formats that e-learning takes are discussed as separate entities. Nevertheless, as the power of computers increases, the lines between categories become increasingly blurred. The technologies provide some of the essential mechanisms for e-learning.

Multimedia

Multimedia is used to describe any combination of hardware and software that displays images or plays sound. Today's computers include multimedia software and are equipped with CD-ROM and DVD players. Examples of media players include Windows® Media Player, iTunes®, and Real Player™. Modern media players allow faculty and students to view or create video and audio podcasts, audio files, and **streaming video** related to learning content. Streaming video refers to a technique where a sequence of compressed moving images is sent over the Internet and played by a media viewer as they arrive. Streaming media is a combination of streaming video and audio.

Many nursing textbooks are accompanied by CD-ROMs with videos so that students can hear and see essential concepts related to patient care. Broadband Internet access provides a way to use online multimedia learning resources. The Dalhousie University Common Currency Project (http://currency.medicine.dal.ca/video.htm) has links to videos on nursing procedures and gross anatomy. Martindale's Reference Desk (http://www.martindalecenter.com/) has links to many online multimedia resources for nurses. YouTube (http://www.youtube.com/) includes links to a variety of videos related to nursing and patient education. iTunes U is available using iTunes and has free audio and video educational resources, including entire courses, that can be downloaded to the iPhone, iPad, or iPod Touch.

Virtual Reality

VR is based on illusions. The use of technology is to allow the participant to exist in another reality, experiencing an event that appears real but does not physically exist. The objective is to create a scene in which the participant is free to concentrate on the tasks, problems, and ideas that he or she would face in the real situation. The primary criterion is that the participant be surrounded by an environment and be "inside" the information.

There are two main components of VR. One is the model or visualization that resembles reality and allows manipulation of the environment. Manipulation can be by virtual keyboard enabled with Bluetooth technology that can be displayed on any surface for computer data entry (ThinkGeek, 2010). The second VR component

is an interface that resembles the three-dimensional world. During the VR experience, the "environment" reacts just as it would in the real world.

VR is being used as a training mechanism for nurses learning how to use surgical endoscopic equipment. Nyswaner (2007), a surgery research coordinator, describes the learning challenges associated with video endoscope simulation use: "You need to realize that looking to the right translates into steering to the left. Don't be surprised if it takes a while to get the hang of "driving" [the endoscope] – or that the OR is a high-stress place to learn this skill."

Students can use VR to enhance learning by using online sites such as Open Simulator, Croquet™ or Second Life. Open Simulator, Croquet, and Second Life are online three-dimensional VR environments. Open Simulator (http://opensimulator.org/wiki/Main_Page) and Croquet (http://www.opencroquet.org) are open-source software applications. Second Life (http://www.secondlife.com/) is proprietary. All virtual world participants must first register on the site to obtain a login ID and password and then download virtual world software applications. Participants interact by using **avatars**. An avatar is a fictionalized computer representation of oneself (see **Figure 22-5**). Avatars can be custom designed with different looks. Because avatars can fly, they can "teleport" to different locations.

Many universities have created learning experiences in virtual world environments. Some disease symptoms, such as hallucinations associated with schizophrenia, are difficult to imagine. Virtual Hallucinations is an educational Second Life environment that allows users to experience hallucinations. There are other Second Life educational sites as well, such as Gerontology Education Island.

There are strengths and limitations for using virtual worlds as a part of instruction. Because avatars fictionalize representations of the users, any user disabilities are invisible. Everyone can walk and fly. The sites provide many opportunities for experimentation and research (Skiba, 2007). A potential limitation is that virtual world learning has technical requirements and computer skills that all learners may not have. Navigating

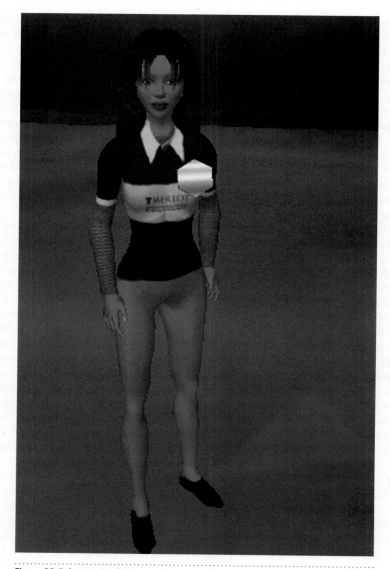

Figure 22-5 Avatar in Second Life.

in a virtual world is a learned skill; fortunately, tutorials and videos are available for use. Learners should have specific learning goals prior to engaging with the learning content. Learners must also be very self-directed; otherwise they could become lost in VR and end up very frustrated. The process to create a virtual world can be time intensive and challenging.

The popularity of Second Life peaked in 2007 (Young, 2010). While there is still a university presence, other universities are exploring some of the open-source virtual world applications.

VR may soon become a standard alternative for learning in higher education. The Kentucky Community and College System (KCTCS) is blazing trails in the use of **simulation-based learning**

(SBL) (KCTCS, 2009). The global Interactive Digital Center (IDC) Consortium has begun showcasing SBL technology for use in higher education and workforce development. SBL uses interactive realistic visualizations. The learner can view or "enter" the visualization (e.g., the cardiovascular system). According to the IDC Consortium, SBL interactions engage the learner and result in "40% greater retention of the subject content with the learner" (Eon Reality, 2008).

A number of resources are available on the use of VR. Ambient Intelligence.org at http://www.ambientintelligence.org/ provides a good starting point. The site links to other websites, journal articles, and books about the use of VR in healthcare. Although the use of VR in healthcare and nursing education is still in its infancy, we can anticipate that it will become commonplace in the future.

Patient Simulators

Patient simulators allow the learner to practice a patient encounter by providing care to a computerized mannequin. This problem-based learning approach provides opportunities for the learner to develop higher-order thinking skills. The primary objective for the use of patient simulators is to allow the learner to be an actual participant in a patient care situation that would be either too difficult, dangerous, or time-consuming to provide in a real clinical setting (Childs & Sepples, 2006). Mannequins can be low or high fidelity. Low fidelity refers simulations that are not true to life. High fidelity refers to realistic simulated patients or situations. For example, high-fidelity mannequins can be programmed to have heart and breath sounds, breathe, and perform physical acts associated with illness, such as coughing or bleeding (see **Figure 22-6**). High-fidelity patient simulators, such as those noted in **Table 22-1**, are used in many nursing programs.

Bearnson and Wiker (2005) reported the use of patient simulators with nursing students using three different postoperative pain scenarios in three simulated patients. One patient was a healthy adult, and the other two patients had significant comorbidities, such as obesity, coronary artery disease, and hypertension. The students were expected to assess and provide postoperative care based on the different patient responses. As a result of the learning simulation experience, students reported increased knowledge about side effects of medications and different patient responses. They also reported that their self-confidence in medication administration skills had improved.

Research reports on the use of patient simulators indicate that students consistently value the learning experiences (Hoffmann, O'Donnell, & Kim, 2007; Howard, Ross, Mitchell, & Nelson,

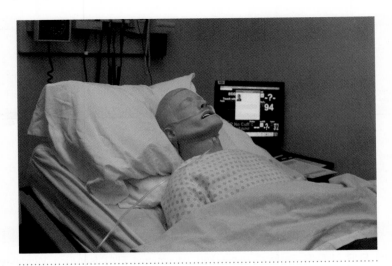

Figure 22-6 Patient simulator.

Table 22-1 Patient Simulation Resources

Examples of High-Fidelity Patient Simulators	Website Address
METIman, PediaSIM, BabySIM, HPS, iStan	http://www.meti.com/which_sim.htm
SimMan®, SimJunior™, SimMom™, SimBaby™	http://www.laerdal.com/nav/207/Patient-Simulators
Virtual I.V.	http://www.laerdal.com/doc/245/Virtual-I-V-Simulator

2010; Kaplan & Ura, 2010). There are, however, downfalls to the use of more complex simulators. Purchase costs for mannequins, hardware, and software and training costs can be prohibitive. Moreover, time is an issue; time is required for faculty training and learning content development (Harlow & Sportsman, 2007; Nehring & Lashley, 2004).

Electronic Health Record Simulation

Due to the complexity of the healthcare setting, simulations are becoming increasingly important. Nursing students are expected to have basic proficiencies prior to providing care to patients/clients in the healthcare setting. The trend to adopt an electronic health record (EHR) has impacted nursing programs. It was easy to simulate paper and pencil documentation, but its use is waning quickly. Nursing programs are adopting the use of a simulated EHR in nursing practice laboratories.

Figure 22-7 is an example of a simulated EHR. The simulated EHR allows the nursing student to practice entering patient documentation, accessing the laboratory, and other testing data, similar to the hospital or clinic work setting. Examples of EHR simulations are NurseSquared (http://www.nursesquared.com/), iCare (http://www.icareacademic.com/), and Neehr Perfect® (http://www.neehrperfect.com/).

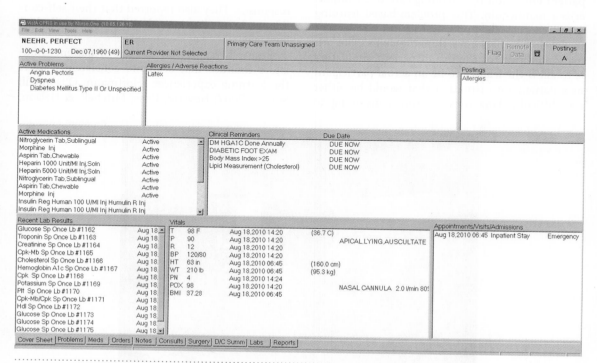

Figure 22-7 Simulated EHR NEEHR Perfect® networked educational EHR featuring WorldVistA. (Courtesy of Archetype Innovations, LLC, 2010.)

Clicker Technology

Clicker technology refers to the personal response systems used in the traditional classroom to provide assessment-centered instruction. Clickers look similar to remote control devices used to control television sets and other media devices (see **Figure 22-8**). Clickers are useful in both small and large classrooms. The two basic requirements for clicker technology are that faculty must have response software loaded on the instructor's computer used in the classroom and the students must each have a clicker or response device. The Clicker Resource Guide at http://www.cwsei.ubc.ca/resources/files/Clicker_guide_CWSEI_CU-SEI.pdf (Adams, CU Science Education Initiative, & UBC Carl Weiman Science Education Initiative, 2009) is an online tutorial designed to assist instructors on the use of clickers. There are numerous types and manufacturers for clickers. Examples of companies that produce clicker software and hardware are iRespond™ (http://

www.irespond.com), TurningPoint (http://www.turningtechnologies.com/), eInstruction (http://www.einstruction.com/), and Senteo™ (http://www2.smarttech.com).

Faculty can assess students' understanding of key concepts by asking students to answer multiple-choice questions projected on a screen in front of the classroom. In this sense, clickers provide assessment feedback on "muddiest points" of learning. The assessment feedback creates the "teachable/learning moment" in the classroom. Because clicker responses can be anonymous, the technology can be utilized to respond to sensitive issues such as ethics and personal beliefs. Reports in the literature support the use of clickers to create an interactive and meaningful learning environment (Berry, 2009; Meedzan & Fisher, 2009; Vana, Silva, Muzyka, & Hirani, 2010). When clickers are assigned to individual students, students can use them to verify class attendance.

Students can obtain clickers in a number of ways. Schools may purchase clickers and distribute them for use in particular classes. A growing number of textbooks support the use of clicker technology. Students may purchase clickers that are associated with a specific textbook, or they may purchase clickers independently through the campus bookstore. Clicker software is also available for use with smartphones, laptops, and tablet computers. An example is eClicker (http://eclicker.com/). The eClicker app is free for students and available for a nominal fee (under $10) for the instructor (Hillegass, 2010).

Web-Based Polling Technology

Web-based polling technology is available for use with online courses to provide assessment-centered instruction. Web-based polling simulates the use of clicker technology. Many of the polling resources are free (see **Table 22-2**). To use a web-based poll in an LMS, the faculty would first create the poll on the polling website. After

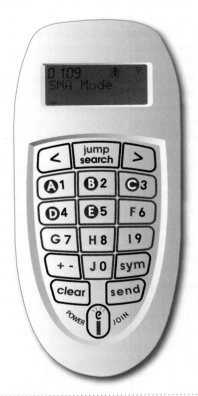

Figure 22-8 Personal response system.

Table 22-2 Free Web-Based Polling Solutions

Polling Solution	Website Address
PollDaddy	http://polldaddy.com/
MicroPoll	http://www.micropoll.com/
Bravenet Web Poll	http://www.bravenet.com/webtools/minipoll/

the poll is created, the user is prompted to copy and paste the code to their course web page and invite participants to vote. The poll provides a link so that participants can view the polling results. Anonymous polling can provide valuable feedback to faculty and students with regard to issues such as personal values, ethics, and beliefs.

Disability-Compliant E-Learning

As more education moves online, the need to make websites available to those with physical disabilities becomes more pronounced. There are special considerations for the design of e-learning for persons with disabilities. The American Disabilities Act (ADA), Section 508, W3C, requires federal agencies to make information technology accessible to qualified persons with disabilities (U.S. Office of Technical and Institutional Services, n.d.). Section 508 refers to the Rehabilitation Act of 1973. The act was amended in 1998 to include electronic and information technology.

As an example of the problem, persons with vision problems use Braille readers to access online information. Websites have to be designed to be compliant with Braille readers. When graphics are used, websites should have alternative text descriptors of the graphic. Additional information on ADA standards for e-learning is available at http://www.access-board.gov/508.htm and http://www.gatech.edu/accessibility.php.

Integrating E-Learning into Educational Programs

Like web-based instruction, other forms of e-learning can be used in a multitude of ways, such as an adjunct to a class, a substitute for a class, or an entire course. Web-based instruction has found uses in all educational venues, including degree programs and CE. E-learning can be of help to healthcare agencies that find it difficult to release employees at given times for classroom sessions. Although there are upfront costs for the technology and software, there are also savings. The costs of faculty and materials, the difficulty

in releasing employees at set times, and the clerical costs of keeping necessary records can all be greatly reduced with appropriate learning management software.

Many vendors now offer e-learning tools that meet the criteria for the mandatory educational programs required by the Joint Commission. For example, Adult CPR Anytime™ Personal Learning Program produced for the American Heart Association includes a DVD to assist with teaching cardiovascular life support (cardiopulmonary resuscitation [CPR]) skills. The minimum competency, basic life support CPR skills, is a standard required competency for nurses and other healthcare providers. Advanced cardiac life support and pediatric advanced life support training is available as e-learning. Users complete the online module and then attend a 2-hour class to demonstrate practice skills.

E-learning is useful for patient education. Office and clinic waiting rooms are excellent locations for the use of e-learning. Patient education can be provided by using CAI in a waiting room as part of a one-on-one session or group teaching. One example is a program designed to teach asthmatic children. Using a combination of simulation with a tutorial and a motivational game, the program was found to significantly increase children's knowledge of self-regulation, prevention, and treatment strategies, as well as increase their beliefs that they had control of their disease (Shegog et al., 2001).

Using Internet access in a waiting room is another approach for providing patient education (Schatell, Klicko, & Becker, 2006). A research study was conducted with 1,804 patients with chronic renal disease to determine their health information literacy with regard to disease management knowledge. The study results indicated that computer access in dialysis center waiting rooms was beneficial because it assisted patients to gain computer technology and information literacy skills necessary with their disease management. Patients and families learned to access Kidney School (http://www.kidneyschool.org), a website with 16 learning modules to assist patients to manage chronic renal disease. Patient survey results on the use of the Kidney School identified many benefits including increased knowledge, better preparation for dialysis, and less fear of dialysis or the future (Medical Education Institute, 2006).

Role of Instructor in E-Learning

The role of an instructor who uses e-learning varies. Although the instructor is an important part of the process, the learners play a key role too. The instructor designs the learning content and facilitates the learning process. Although instructors take more of a "guide on the side" role in the electronic classroom, their focus is still on teaching. The traditional classroom lecture where the voice can convey emphasis might be replaced in the electronic world with narrated PowerPoint slides, podcasts, audio clips, and/or streaming video. The challenge for faculty is in not being able to see the faces of students. As a result, the learners must take on the responsibility of providing feedback on the instruction electronically. Effective faculty–student collaboration often makes the difference between whether learners find success or experience frustration.

Evaluating E-Learning

Evaluating e-learning and determining what computer technology to use depends on the learning module objectives and expected learning outcomes. Bloom's Taxonomy should be used to determine appropriate learning methods. Identifying learning outcomes helps to determine the selection of learning resources that develop psychomotor skills, critical thinking, memorization, or just

knowledge assimilation. The learner's prerequisite knowledge should also be considered.

The one characteristic that sets e-learning above all other teaching mediums, with the exception of a human teacher or live experience, is interactivity. The effectiveness of interaction depends on the mental processing required and the nature of the learner's interaction with the content (Thede, 1995). Several tools are available to assess the quality of e-learning resources. Examples of assessment tools include MERLOT Health Sciences Editorial Board peer-review criteria at http://hercules.gcsu.edu/jsewell/MERLOT/HSPeerReviewGuide.htm, Learning Object Review Instrument at http://www.elera.net/eLera/Home/About%20%20LORI/, and Sharable Content Object Repositories for Education at http://www.sreb.org/programs/edtech/SCORE/index.asp.

Pros and Cons of E-Learning

E-learning and CAI are neither a panacea nor something that will replace teachers. Like all innovations, there are advantages and disadvantages (see **Box 22-1**). One advantage is accessibility. Online learning allows students to access course content anywhere in the world from a computer with Internet access. Online learning accommodates shift work, family obligations, and military duty deployment. Before signing up for a course that

---

BOX 22-1 Advantages and Disadvantages of Distance Learning

Advantages of distance learning
1. Depending on the structure, students can participate in their schedule.
2. Students without easy access to a college can participate.
3. Some agencies have found that offering distance learning as a perk increases retention.
4. Classes in a limited specialty can be offered because of an expanded audience.
5. Access to class is available 24 hours a day, 7 days a week.

6. Learners must think before they express their ideas, thus they cannot speak impulsively. Organizing one's ideas increases learning.
7. All learners must participate.

Disadvantages of distance learning
1. Additional resources are needed to assist instructors and students.
2. Lack of face-to-face contact.
3. May not be suitable to all contents.
4. The technology may contribute to frustration.

BOX 22-2 Successful Online Learners

Learning technology and environment.
The learner:

- Must be very committed and focused on learning. Work and home obligations can be very distracting and can interrupt the learning environment.
- Must give online learning a priority in daily activities.
- Must have access to a working computer with antivirus and antispam protection, an Internet connection, required e-learning software, and a printer. The computer becomes an essential tool for online learning. A computer is as important to an online learner as a motorized vehicle is to a nurse commuting to work in a healthcare agency. To maintain a functioning computer, the learner should:
  - Restrict the use of the personal computer from any other user who may inadvertently download a virus or corrupt the operating system.

- Have a "backup strategy" in case of computer problems. For example, using the college, community library, college, or hospital computer laboratory, or renting a laptop.

Learner qualities. The learner should:

- Be self-motivated and exercise self-discipline; own responsibility for learning.
- Be able to communicate effectively in writing.
- Be open-minded about sharing experiences and willing to learn from others.
- Be willing to ask for help.
- Be respectful of others in the learning environment.
- Participate in the virtual classroom 4–7 days/week.
- Be willing to apply learning to everyday life.
- Have the ability to commit the required number of hours per week for completing assignments and class participation.

uses e-learning, students should make sure that they have the qualities leading to success (see **Box 22-2**).

Students can access the learning resources when they are best able to learn. Online learning allows learners to participate in learning experiences that otherwise are not available outside of real life. It also permits the learners to set their own pace. Another advantage is that, unlike a traditional lecture, learners never have to miss a class; the learning content and class discussion are online. ADA-compliant courses make learning accessible to students who are physically unable to attend class. Courses can be designed to accommodate vision- and hearing-impaired students.

Online learning also has disadvantages. Learners need the required software and hardware. They also need to have a backup plan in case of a computer problem. They need to have sufficient technology skills to allow them to access online courses and to troubleshoot technology glitches. Online learning is a disadvantage to the learner who is not motivated to learn and who does not exercise self-discipline.

Distance Learning and Hybrid Courses

Distance learning is a phenomenon that has been with us since Roman times whenever and wherever a reliable postal service was available. In the United States, correspondence courses have been available since the 18th century. Although correspondence courses are used in many parts of the world, online courses continue to grow in popularity. Face-to-face courses that have a virtual presence in LMSs are known as hybrid courses.

Distance learning means education in which the learners and students are in different locations. Distance education formats differ in the timeframes that they use; some are asynchronous, and others are synchronous (see **Table 22-3**). In the asynchronous format, learners use the learning resources at a time and place that is convenient for them. The asynchronous format is the most common use of LMSs. In synchronous learning, class is held at set times and all participants are "present," either online or in the classroom. Web

TABLE 22-3 Time Criteria Continuum in Distance Learning

Functions	Synchronous	Asynchronous
Meeting times	Set meeting times	No set meeting times
Assignments (includes quizzes and tests)	Set due dates	Students complete assignments when they have time; there is no due date beyond that of the end of the course
Time period of course (most have a given time length from beginning to end of the course)	Starts and ends on a given date	Starts and ends at the convenience of the students
Type of learning	Instructor-led/class discussions	Independent, only feedback is on assignments

conferencing and webinars, often used to provide an educational session, are examples of synchronous learning.

There are many uses for distance learning in healthcare. One of the most widespread uses is for CE. This type of learning is available in different formats; some CE modules are free, and others are available for a small fee. The American Nursing Association provides a comprehensive listing of online CE learning resources at http://nursingworld.org/ce/cehome.cfm. Some of the CE resources are free for members. Most nursing journals that have an online presence provide access to journal articles and an associated quiz for CE credit. Staff educators may find that many of these offerings could be made a part of a staff education program for career ladder programs or other necessary learning.

Full degree programs are also offered online. Accreditation of distance learning is offered by the major college-accrediting bodies just as if the programs were all in a regular classroom. Several certificate programs are also offered online. The various programs vary in their requirements for a presence on campus during the program; some require none, and others may require a weekend presence during each course or a given on-campus presence sometime during the program.

 Future Trends

Ward once said, "If you can imagine it, you can achieve it; if you can dream it, you can become it" (ThinkExist.com, 2010). In 1993, futurist Marc Smith described cyberspace and virtual communities (Smith, 1993). In 1996, Chris Dede portrayed the social aspect of e-learning based on Smith's work: "Social network capital (an instant Web of contacts with useful skills), knowledge capital (a personal, distributed 'brain trust' with just-in-time answers to immediate questions), and communion (psychological/spiritual support from people who share common joys and trials) are three types of 'collective goods' that bind together virtual communities enabled by computer-mediated communication" (Dede, 1996). The imaginations of Smith and Dede helped to set the stage for the Web 2.0 e-learning environment.

Technological advances will continue to impact e-learning and the design of the learning environment. Futurists are now depicting the future of learning/course management systems for "next-generation" learners (Jafari, McGee, & Carmean, 2006). Some predictions are as follows:

- The free Web 2.0 tools will continue to direct future trends in e-learning. LMSs will integrate with other systems.
- The learning environment will have educational equivalents of free Web 2.0 tools such as Facebook, wikis, RSS feeds, and blogs.
- Educational Web 2.0 tools will allow learners to collaborate with others across the world, not simply within a given course.
- The design of instruction and technology used to deliver the instruction will center on the learner's needs (see **Figure 22-9**).
- LMSs will take on some of the smart features of Amazon.com.

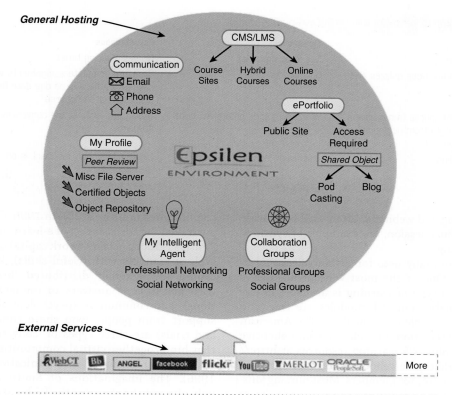

Figure 22-9 Next generation e-learning environment. (From Jafari, A., McGee, P., & Carmean, C. (2006, July/August). Managing courses, defining learning: What faculty, students, and administrators want [Electronic version]. *EDUCAUSE Review, 41,* 50–71. Retrieved November 5, 2010, from http://www.educause.edu/ir/library/pdf/ERM0643.pdf.)

- LMSs will "remember" the students' profile, what they like, and how they learn.
- LMSs will incorporate decision support tools to "remember" where a student was when he or she last exited the course and make recommendations for pertinent learning resources.

The 2011 EDUCAUSE Horizon Report described six technologies likely to impact teaching and learning. The technologies were (1) electronic books, (2) mobile devices, (3) augmented reality, (4) game-based learning, (5) gesture-based computing, and (6) learning analytics (Johnson, Smith, Willis, Levine, & Haywood, 2011). Technological advances and free web-enabled creative resources are empowering the learners to custom design their personal learning environment.

Electronic books are not just a digitized version of the print textbook. The future electronic book allows for note taking and interactive learning. Mobile devices provide for affordable solutions to access the web, use electronic textbooks, use social networking sites, and more. Augmented reality provides a representation of real life with digital images. The concept has fascinating implications for the teaching/learning process. Imagine holding a piece of paper with a blocklike stamp (similar in function to a bar code) on it in front of a computer camera and watching images come to life, allowing you to interact with the images. You probably have encountered the concept, perhaps without realizing it. If you watch television, you probably have viewed some commercial ads with augmented reality. You can learn more about augmented reality at http://www.howstuffworks.com/augmented-reality.htm. Game-based learning, discussed earlier in this chapter, allows for collaboration with others, problem solving, and analytical thinking. Gesture-based computing allows users to provide computer input with body motions. Gesturing can range from swiping a computer screen with fingers to playing virtual golf with a Wii. Learning analytics allows users to analyze data gathered with data-mining tools to improve the teaching and learning experience.

 ## Summary

In the information age, it is imperative that higher education prepare learners to be active, independent learners, and problem solvers. E-learning, when used appropriately, facilitates this process and provides a venue for lifelong learning. E-learning can be classified by the learning method or the technology. There are numerous learning methods including drill and practice, tutorials, simulations, gaming, and testing. Effective learning methods, whether used online or face-to-face, must provide interactivity and prompt feedback to learners. The technology includes multimedia, VR, patient simulators, and clicker technology; each meets different needs.

Using e-learning successfully depends on how it is integrated into the total learning program. The level of interactivity also needs to be considered and matched with program goals. Like all teaching methods, e-learning has advantages and disadvantages. Advantages include interactivity and the flexibility of the medium. Disadvantages can include lack of familiarity with the technology, technology glitches, lack of access, and cost.

With the advent of the Internet, distance learning has become a much more popular method for educational offerings. Programs offered via distance learning vary from correspondence courses and magazine articles to full degree programs. Distance learning requires the development of skills that are not always needed in traditional education including the ability to discipline oneself to set aside time for the program and the ability to communicate effectively in writing.

APPLICATIONS AND COMPETENCIES

1. Discuss uses for multimedia and VR in nursing education.

2. Differentiate between the characteristics of the learning methods drill and practice, tutorial, and game, providing an example that is related to nursing for each one.

3. Identify and analyze an online nursing simulation.

4. Compare the different modes of computerized testing and give examples for appropriate use.

5. Search for an online learning resource of value to nursing and then add it to the MERLOT collection.

6. Discuss the current status of distance education for nursing. Make a list of essential competencies and qualities for successful learners and then compare your list with those listed in this chapter.

7. Evaluate one of your learning experiences by using the seven principles for good practice in undergraduate education. If you are a graduate student, discuss if and how the principles apply to graduate education.

8. One of your functions in a 100-bed hospital is to provide staff education. You wish to integrate e-learning into your organization. Write a proposal that

   a. Interprets the various choices for e-learning.

   b. Discusses the advantages and disadvantages of each.

   c. Provides reasons for using two of these methods.

REFERENCES

Adams, W., CU Science Education Initiative, & UBC Carl Weiman Science Education Initiative. (2009, July 1). *Clicker resource guide.* Retrieved October 31, 2010, from http://cnx.org/content/col10724/latest/

Advanced Distributed Learning. (2010, October 29). *Frequently asked facts about SCORM.* Retrieved October 31, 2010, from http://www.adlnet.gov/Documents/SCORM%20FAQ.aspx

Anderson, L. W., Krathwohl, D. R., & Bloom, B. S. (2001). *A taxonomy for learning, teaching, and assessing: A revision of Bloom's taxonomy of educational objectives* (complete edition). New York, NY: Longman.

Bearnson, C. S., & Wiker, K. M. (2005). Human patient simulators: A new face in baccalaureate nursing education at Brigham Young University. *Journal of Nursing Education, 44*(9), 421–425.

Benner, P. E., Sutphen, M., Leonard, V., & Day, L. (2010). *Educating nurses: A call for radical transformation* (1st ed.). San Francisco, CA: Jossey-Bass.

Berry, J. (2009). Technology support in nursing education: Clickers in the classroom. *Nursing Education Perspectives, 30*(5), 295–298.

Bloom, B. S. (1956). *Taxonomy of educational objectives, handbook 1: Cognitive domain*. New York, NY: Addison-Wesley.

Chickering, A. W., & Ehrmann, S. C. (1996). *Implementing the seven principles: Technology as lever*. Retrieved January 29, 2008, from http://www.tltgroup.org/programs/seven.html

Childs, J. C., & Sepples, S. (2006). Clinical teaching by simulation: Lessons learned from a complex patient care scenario. *Nursing Education Perspectives, 27*(3), 154–158.

Clark, R. C., & Mayer, R. E. (2003). *E-learning and the science of instruction*. Hoboken, NJ: John Wiley & Sons.

Dede, C. (1996). The evolution of distance education: Emerging technologies and distributed learning. *American Journal of Distance Education, 10*(2), 4.

Eon Reality. (2008). *i3D Symposium*. Retrieved October 31, 2010, from http://www.eonreality.com/i3DSymposium/SiMT/FlorenceSC/

Greenberg, L. (2002, December 9). *LMS and LCMS: What's the difference?* Retrieved September 12, 2007, from http://www.learningcircuits.org/NR/exeres/72E3F68C-4047-4379-8454-2B88C9D38FC5.htm

Half-Baked Software Inc. (2009). *What is Quandary?* Retrieved August 31, 2011, from http://www.halfbakedsoftware.com/quandary.php

Half-Baked Software Inc. (2010, June 6). *Hot Potatoes™*. Retrieved October 31, 2010, from http://hotpot.uvic.ca/

Harlow, K. C., & Sportsman, S. (2007). An economic analysis of patient simulators clinical training in nursing education. *Nursing Economics, 25*(1), 23–29.

Hillegass, A. (2010). *eClicker overview*. Retrieved October 31, 2010, from http://bnreclicker.appspot.com/eClicker_Host_Overview.pdf

Hoffmann, R. L., O'Donnell, J. M., & Kim, Y. (2007). The effects of human patient simulators on basic knowledge in critical care nursing with undergraduate senior baccalaureate nursing students. *Simulation in Healthcare, 2*(2), 110–114.

Howard, V. M., Ross, C., Mitchell, A. M., & Nelson, G. M. (2010). Human patient simulators and interactive case studies: A comparative analysis of learning outcomes and student perceptions. *CIN: Computers Informatics Nursing, 28*(1), 42–48.

Jafari, A., McGee, P., & Carmean, C. (2006). Managing courses, defining learning: What faculty, students, and administrators want. *EDUCAUSE Review, 41*(4), 50–71. Retrieved from http://www.educause.edu/ir/library/pdf/ERM0643.pdf

Johnson, L., Smith, R., Willis, H., Levine, A., and Haywood, K., (2011). *The 2011 Horizon Report*. Austin, Texas: The New Media Consortium. Retrieved August 31, 2011 from http://net.educause.edu/ir/library/pdf/HR2011.pdf

Kaplan, B., & Ura, D. (2010). Use of multiple patient simulators to enhance prioritizing and delegating skills for senior nursing students. *Journal of Nursing Education, 49*(7), 371–377.

KCTCS. (2009). *Interactive Digital Center*. Retrieved October 31, 2010, from http://www.kctcs.edu/system_initiatives/interactive-digital-center.aspx

Lord, T., & Baviskar, S. (2007). Moving students from information recitation to information understanding:

Exploiting Bloom's taxonomy in creating science questions. *Journal of College Science Teaching, 36*(5), 40–44.

Medical Education Institute. (2006). Kidney School™: Unique CKD education tool. *In Control, 3*(2), 4. Retrieved from http://www.lifeoptions.org/catalog/pdfs/news/icv3n2.pdf

Meedzan, N., & Fisher, K. L. (2009). Clickers in nursing education: An active learning tool in the classroom. *Online Journal of Nursing Informatics, 13*(2), 19.

MERLOT. (n.d.). *MERLOT: About us*. Retrieved October 31, 2010, from http://taste.merlot.org/

NCSBN. (n.d.). *Computerized adaptive testing (CAT) overview*. Retrieved October 31, 2010, from https://www.ncsbn.org/CAT_Overview.pdf

Nehring, W. M., & Lashley, F. R. (2004). Current use and opinions regarding human patient simulators in nursing education: An international survey. *Nursing Education Perspectives, 25*(5), 244–248.

Nyswaner, A. (2007). "Driver's ed" for the OR nurse. *RN, 70*(3), 45–48.

Respondus®. (2010). *Studymate Author 2.0*. Retrieved October 29, 2010, from http://www.respondus.com/products/studymate.shtml

Schatell, D., Klicko, K., & Becker, B. N. (2006). In-center hemodialysis patients' use of the Internet in the United States: A national survey. *American Journal of Kidney Diseases, 48*(2), 285–291.

Shegog, R., Bartholomew, L. K., Parcel, G. S., Sockrider, M. M., Masse, L., & Abramson, S. L. (2001). Impact of a computer-assisted education program on factors related to asthma self-management behavior. *Journal of the American Medical Informatics Association, 8*(1), 49–61.

Skiba, D. J. (2007). Nursing education 2.0: Second Life. *Nursing Education Perspectives, 28*(3), 156–157.

Smith, M. (1993). *Voices from the WELL: The logic of the virtual commons*. Los Angeles, CA: University of California, Los Angeles.

SoftChalk LLC. (2010). *SoftChalk™*. Retrieved October 31, 2010, from http://www.softchalk.com/

Thalheimer, W. (2006). *People remember 10%, 20%... Oh really?* Retrieved October 31, 2010, from http://www.willatworklearning.com/2006/05/people_remember.html

Thede, L. Q. (1995). *Comparison of a constructivist and objectivist framework for designing computer-aided instruction*. Unpublished dissertation, Kent State University, Kent, OH.

ThinkExist.com, Q. (2010). *William Authur Ward quotes*. Retrieved October 31, 2010, from http://thinkexist.com/quotation/if_you_can_imagine_it-you_can_achieve_it-if_you/15190.html

ThinkGeek. (2010). *Bluetooth laser virtual keyboard*. Retrieved October 31, 2010, from http://www.thinkgeek.com/computing/ keyboards-mice/8193/

U.S. Office of Technical and Institutional Services. (n.d.). *E-learning: Conforming to section 508*. Retrieved October 31, 2010, from http://www.access-board.gov/sec508/e-learning.htm

Vana, K. D., Silva, G. E., Muzyka, D., & Hirani, L. M. (2010). Effectiveness of an audience response system in teaching pharmacology to baccalaureate nursing students. *CIN: Computers, Informatics, Nursing, 29*(6), TC105-TC113.

Young, J. R. (2010, February 14). After frustrations in Second Life, colleges look to new virtual worlds. *The Chronicle*. Retrieved from http://chronicle.com/article/After-Frustrations-in-Second/64137/

CHAPTER 23

Administration Tools for Efficiency

Objectives

After studying this chapter you will be able to:

▶ *Identify the tools necessary to manage business processes in nursing services.*

▶ *Demonstrate basic competencies in spreadsheets and flowcharting in nursing administration.*

▶ *Discuss data management to improve outcomes using quality improvement, benchmarking, and patient care.*

▶ *Explore the use of specialized applications in nursing administration, including scheduling systems and patient classification systems.*

Key Terms

Benchmarking	Gantt Chart
Business Intelligence	Human Resource
Clinical Information Systems	Management System
Consumer Assessment of	(HRMS)
Health Providers and	National Database of
Systems	Nursing Quality Indicators®
Core Measures	(NDNQI®)
Dashboards	Patient Classification
Employee Scheduling System	Systems
Financial Management	Patient Throughput
Flowcharting	Process Improvement
Forecasting	Quality Improvement

There is little doubt that nurse administrators and managers must have competency in a wide range of technology skills to be effective in their roles. According to the American Organization of Nurse Executives (AONE, 2005), one of the five leadership domains is business skills, which includes information management and technology. The use of e-mail, word processing, spreadsheets, and the Internet are basic skills. Beyond these, nurse administrators use management information systems for the purposes of **financial management**, **process improvement**, human resource management, **quality improvement**, **benchmarking**, and **business intelligence**. Because of the nurse administrator's unique role as a leader of nursing services, knowledge of **clinical information systems** is important as well. **Box 23-1** specifies the competencies needed by nurse managers and nurse executives (AONE).

BOX 23-1 AONE Information Management and Technology Competencies

AONE believes that managers at all levels must be competent to
- demonstrate use of e-mail, word processing, spreadsheets, and Internet programs;
- recognize the relevance of nursing data for improving practice;
- use telecommunication devices;
- utilize hospital database management, decision support, and expert system programs to access information and analyze data from disparate sources for use in planning for patient care processes and systems;
- participate in system change processes and utility analysis;
- participate in the evaluation of information systems in practice settings;
- evaluate and revise patient care processes and systems;
- use computerized management systems to record administrative data (billing data, quality assurance data, workload data, etc.);
- use applications for structure data entry (classification systems, acuity level, etc.);
- recognize the utility of nursing involvement in the planning design and choice and implementation of information systems in the practice environment;
- demonstrate awareness of societal and technological trend issues and new developments as they apply to nursing;
- demonstrate proficient awareness of legal and ethical issues related to client data, information, and confidentiality; and
- read and interpret benchmarking, financial, and occupancy data.

Reprinted from American Organization of Nurse Executives, with permission.

Tools

Nurse administrators use various desktop computer applications to increase their efficiency. Basic skills are described in earlier chapters of this textbook. This chapter focuses on unique uses for applications in the work of an administrator.

Financial Management: Spreadsheets

Chapter 8 provides an overview of how to create spreadsheets, insert formulas to perform calculations, and display data in charts. These skills are useful to any nurse manager for following monthly budgets or creating a variance report if the accounting department does not provide one. However, a nurse manager might want to take data available from different sources and create a new spreadsheet to determine if relationships exist between two groups of information.

For example, **Table 23-1** shows sample nursing hours per patient day for registered nurses (RNs) and nursing assistants. Taken alone, the manager can see that nursing hours go up and down depending on the quarter. **Table 23-2** shows the patients' average length of stay (LOS) on the unit for the same time periods. There are variations in LOS between quarters. The manager should consider hours per patient day and LOS simultaneously to see if a relationship exists.

Once staffing and LOS data are entered into the cells of the same spreadsheet, a chart can be created. Examination of a column and line chart reveals that as the number of RN hours goes up (nursing hours are plotted on the left-hand axis), the patient LOS goes down (LOS is plotted on the

Table 23-1 Staffing Report: Hours per Patient Day

	Quarter 1	Quarter 2	Quarter 3	Quarter 4
Registered nurses	9	15	10	12
Nursing assistants	2	3	1	3

Table 23-2 Patient Length of Stay

	Quarter 1	Quarter 2	Quarter 3	Quarter 4
Length of stay	5	3.75	5.25	4.5

right-hand axis). This is an important trend that could be missed when data are viewed independently (see **Figure 23-1**).

The nurse manager must use data to show a need for staffing. Certainly, when staffing is shown to reduce the number of patient days in the hospital, a positive financial impact is produced, and this is a substantial argument for appropriate staffing levels. Other similar comparisons could be made with nurse-sensitive outcomes including falls, pressure ulcers, and infections.

Another way to use a spreadsheet is to trend historical data to forecast for future needs. Unfortunately, in nursing and healthcare, there is no perfect way to predict the demand for services or the supply of nurses to meet the demand. However, nurse administrators can use knowledge of their facilities, historical data, graphing techniques, assessment of trends or seasonal patterns,

and formulas to make reasonable estimates (Finkler, Kovner, & Jones, 2007). Data collection is the first step in **forecasting** future events. The nurse administrator needs to determine what data are most helpful and what length of time would be most appropriate. Finkler et al. suggest using 1–5 years of data for forecasting. If too short a time period is used, false conclusions can be drawn. For example, in **Figure 23-2**, the administrator sees 4 months of data and may think that outpatient surgeries are increasing while inpatient surgeries stay approximately the same.

When viewed within the 5-year period, the administrator can clearly see a seasonal pattern: outpatient surgeries increase during the months of November and December and return to a level of approximately 120 surgeries per month during the rest of the year (see **Figure 23-3**). However, inpatient surgeries begin to increase around July 2007. The administrator knows that a new orthopedic surgeon and a new urologist were recruited to the hospital during that time, which accounts for the increase in inpatient surgeries. This increase can be expected to persist in future years.

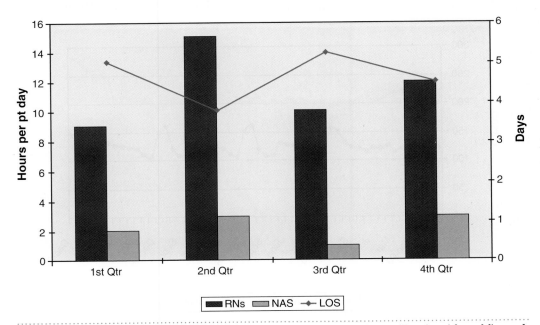

Figure 23-1 Nursing hours per patient day and average patient length of stay. (Reprinted from Microsoft Corporation, with permission.)

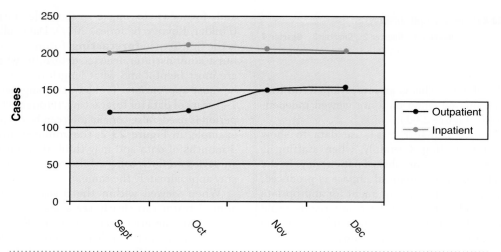

Figure 23-2 Line chart showing number of surgical cases in 4 months. (Reprinted from Microsoft Corporation, with permission.)

Process Improvement

Process improvement is the application of actions taken to identify, analyze, and improve existing processes within an organization to meet requirements for quality, customer satisfaction, and financial goals. Administrators can use a particular strategy such as total quality management, six sigma, or a general process improvement framework called plan-do-check act (Yoder-Wise, 2006). Whatever the strategy used for improvement, an organized approach is necessary to understand the current state of the process and plan for changes to

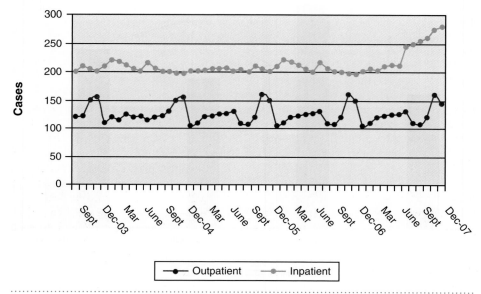

Figure 23-3 Line chart showing number of surgical cases in 5 years. (Reprinted from Microsoft Corporation, with permission.)

Flow before Process Improvement   **Flow after Process Improvement**

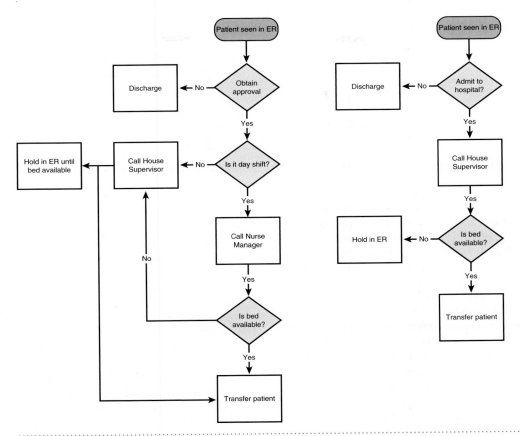

Figure 23-4 Flowchart of admission from emergency room. (Reprinted from Microsoft Corporation, with permission.)

improve outcomes. Process improvement should be an analytical process where tools such as flowcharts, cause-and-effect charts, and other control methods are used to make changes to targeted processes.

Analysis of Processes with Flowcharting

Flowcharting software applications can be useful because nurse administrators can map processes in nursing services. There are many instances in healthcare where care processes need to be examined to make them more efficient or to reduce unwanted variation in care. For example, the movement of patients from the emergency department into a hospital inpatient room for admission is a complicated process. Delays in starting care are unnecessary and costly; analysis through flowcharting may reveal opportunities for improvement in the admission process. In **Figure 23-4**, unnecessary delays can be avoided if the path from decision to admit and the transfer of the patient is a straight line. When multiple decisions need to be made or multiple people are involved, the process becomes more complicated and delays occur. The use of flowcharting is a powerful way to identify steps in a process that can be reorganized for better flow.

A cause-and-effect chart is another useful diagram for nurse administrators to make so that relationships among complex processes are examined.

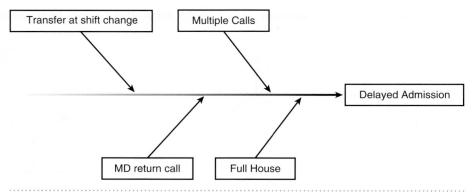

Figure 23-5 Cause-and-effect chart. (Reprinted from Microsoft Corporation, with permission.)

The cause-and-effect chart places the effect at one end of the chart with the many suspected causes branching out from it. The resulting chart resembles a fishbone, thus it is commonly referred to as a fishbone chart. **Figure 23-5** depicts a simple cause-and-effect chart; more complex charts show multiple related causes under each branch.

There are many software options for developing flowcharts. The most readily available are drawing tools included in word-processing packages or presentation software. These tools are usually sufficient unless complicated processes need to be depicted. When a software program is needed with more sophisticated flowcharting abilities, the nurse administrator should analyze the products on cost and capabilities. The Microsoft® product is called Visio®, and other similar products are WizFlow (from Pacestar software©), FlowBreeze Software, SmartDraw®, EDrawSoft©, and ConceptDraw (from Computer Systems Odessa Corp©) to name a few. Most of the products are $50–$200 for a single-user license.

Project Management

Nurse administrators often oversee planning and implementation of complex projects with numerous stakeholders, resources, and financial implications. In many cases, the use of project management software can provide needed organization to keep projects on time and within budget. This type of software is not one that is typically used in nursing administration offices and may need to be purchased.

The benefit of using project management software is the ability to track the project's progress using tools such as a **Gantt chart**, which can show start to end dates and associated costs with tasks (see **Figure 23-6**). Milestones can be marked on the chart so that important parts of a task are highlighted. Links can be made between tasks to depict when tasks need to be completed before others start. Linking tasks is a good practice to use because when a date changes in one task, all other dates are updated to linked tasks. Some project management software can be set to send e-mail reminders to individuals responsible for milestones or tasks within the project. This

Task Name	Duration	Start	Finish		Jan 20, '08	Jan 27, '08	Feb 3, '08	Feb 10,
					S S M T W T F S	S M T W T F S	S M T W T F S	S M T
Analysis of ER admission process	8 days	Wed 1/23/08	Fri 2/1/08					
Setup ER process committee	2 days	Mon 1/21/08	Tue 1/22/08		ER Manager			
Review results of first analysis	2 days	Mon 2/4/08	Tue 2/5/08					
Draft recommendations	1 day	Wed 2/6/08	Wed 2/6/08					
Circulate recommendations	3 days	Thu 2/7/08	Mon 2/11/08					

Figure 23-6 Gantt chart. (Reprinted from Microsoft Corporation, with permission.)

automation frees the administrator to focus on the big picture and leaves the details to the software.

Reports of tasks and costs can be generated. These reports provide a snapshot of the progress, resources, and finances for the project. Depending on the level of integration, these reports can be exported to a spreadsheet application for sharing with others in the organization.

There are many vendors who make project management software for personal computers including Microsoft Project®; Standard Register, which produces SmartWorks®; Inuit QuickBase®; and Experience In Software, Inc., which develops Project Kickstart™. Other options include purchasing a web-based service if the nurse administrator needs to collaborate with others in a multihospital network. Several factors should be considered when making a decision about purchasing project management software. The first is the degree of integration with other administrative tools such as spreadsheets, e-mail, and calendars. The second is the number of users who would access the information contained in the project management software. The third is the security of web-based systems compared with other deployment methods. Finally, the cost of the software should be considered: single-user licenses are relatively inexpensive but do not encourage collaboration. If a nurse administrator needs collaboration and has a secure web solution, the cost of a multiuser license may be well worth the investment.

Human Resource Management

Personnel management is one of the most important parts of the job of a nurse manager. The use of a **human resource management system (HRMS)** is essential for planning and staffing nursing services appropriately. Nursing personnel, staffing, and employment data can be managed with an HRMS, which generally includes four categories: personnel profiles including demographic data, daily work schedules and time-off requests, payroll data, and education and skill qualifications as well as licensure information.

Not only can an HRMS serve as a scheduling system and repository of personnel data, but a productivity module can also be purchased, which can pull nursing data (hours of care-and-skill mix) together with patient data (patient days, average LOS, and patient acuity). This productivity information is critical for nurse managers and nurse administrators to track, trend, and analyze productivity for meaning within their organizations and benchmark against similar organizations across the United States. This is likely the most powerful information that is produced for managers and administrators in healthcare today.

Because regulators and accreditation agencies require information about employees such as competencies, certifications, and evaluations, HRMS may provide a solution to managing these data too. Many HRMSs will contain employee appraisals; orientation checklists; employee competency checklists; development plans; compensation adjustments based on the achievement of personal, unit, or organization goals; and possibly succession plans. The HRMS may also generate reports for the Joint Commission.

Nurse administrators who might be involved in the decision to purchase an HRMS should be certain to view demonstrations from vendors whose products are specialized to healthcare. Because the work of nursing services is so different from manufacturing or other service-related industries, it is important to have systems that meet many specifications. The HRMS needs to meet the following minimum requirements: (1) handle scheduling for 24 hours per day, 7 days per week; (2) accommodate different scheduling rules for units across an entire organization or network; (3) allow for staff self-scheduling; (4) determine the right number and mix of nursing staff for patient needs; (5) provide an analysis of nursing staff usage to manage productivity and support quality patient outcomes; (6) track time and attendance; (7) connect to the payroll system; (8) retain certification and licensure information; and (9) serve as a repository for competency assessments and annual employee appraisals.

Using Data to Improve Outcomes

Quality Improvement and Benchmarking

In the past, nurses have been viewed as an overhead to hospital organizations because revenue was generated by admissions to the hospital, not by the quality of patient care that was provided. This view is changing with pay-for-performance initiative. Nurses are in pivotal positions to improve quality, prevent errors, and improve patient satisfaction in hospitals. For example, if nurses prevent nosocomial infections in postoperative patients, the hospital will receive full reimbursement allowed under the Centers for Medicare & Medicaid (CMS, 2006) regulations for those patients. However, if a patient develops a nosocomial infection, CMS will not reimburse for additional treatment or days of hospitalization associated with the nosocomial infection. In order for excellence in patient care to be the norm for hospitals, nurse administrators must follow the progress of improvements in care and keep nursing staff informed about how their performance affects the hospital's reimbursement.

Not only do nurse administrators engage in quality improvement projects specific to their hospitals, but they must also provide leadership for the hospital's required participation in improvement initiatives mandated by the CMS. These mandated programs include **Core Measures** and **Consumer Assessment of Health Providers and Systems**, Hospital Survey (HCAHPS) (CMS, 2010a; HCAHPS, 2010). In addition, nurse administrators may choose to join the **National Database of Nursing Quality Indicators®** **(NDNQI®)**. These quality improvement initiatives require the nurse administrator to designate staff and resources to the collection of data, aggregation of data for submission to databases, and response to reports.

Core Measures

In 1998, the Joint Commission (2010) in cooperation with the CMS and the Hospital Quality Alliance (HQA) established standardized core measurements required for all accredited healthcare organizations. A few standardized core measurements were required in the first year. In subsequent years, more core measures were added in areas including myocardial infarction, congestive heart failure, pneumonia, pregnancy, treatment of asthma in children, and a surgical care improvement project. Each of these core measures required extensive data collection, aggregation, and reporting to stay in compliance. Once reported, the core

measures are available for the public at http://www.hospitalcompare.hhs.gov.

Consumer Assessment of Health Providers and Systems: Hospital Survey

Beginning in 2007, the CMS in collaboration with the HQA required hospitals to survey patients and families to gather information about their experiences with healthcare (CMS, 2010a). The tool, known as HCAHPS, was developed by the Agency for Healthcare Research and Quality and is a standardized survey tool designed to be administered to a sample of discharged patients. Hospitals are required to submit data to the CMS website so that patients' experiences can be trended over time within one hospital and benchmarked to other hospitals. These data are available to the public to provide accountability in healthcare at http://www.hospitalcompare.hhs.gov.

Hospitals may use a vendor to survey patients or elect to conduct surveys with its employees. Regardless of this choice, surveyors must use a standardized method of collecting data, use a core set of questions (hospitals can add other questions to customize the survey), and submit data within specified timeframes so that comparisons can be made. To date, 10 of the 18 questions are publicly reported. These include six composite topics, one topic on cleanliness, one topic on quietness, and two overall ratings (CMS, 2010b).

National Database of Nursing Quality Indicators®

The quality of nursing care has an influence on a hospital's performance in some of the areas of core measures and patients' experiences in healthcare as measured by HCAHPS. A more direct measurement of the quality of nursing care is possible when nurse administrators choose to participate in the NDNQI®. The American Nurses Association (ANA) in partnership with the University of Kansas, School of Nursing began the development of its safety and quality initiative, which resulted in NDNQI®. After a development period of approximately 4 years, the NDNQI® began accepting data for comparison from hospitals in 1998. The service was free until 2001 when a fee was established for joining the database. In 2010, over 1,500 hospitals participated in the service (ANA, 2010).

The NDNQI® is a national database to which hospitals submit nursing-sensitive data about structure, process, and outcomes of nursing care. The NDNQI® aggregates the data quarterly and returns reports to participating hospitals. Nurse administrators and managers receive unit-level information that is compared across time periods and benchmarked to similar units from other hospitals. The NDNQI® data include nursing hours per patient day, staff mix, falls, nursing turnover, pressure ulcers, infections, restraint use, intravenous infiltration, and nosocomial infection, to name a few (ANA, 2010). More information can be found at http://www.nursingquality.org.

Business Intelligence

Nursing services collect thousands of data elements every day in the delivery of patient care and in management processes such as utilization review, case management, and infection control. More measurements are not needed. In fact, nurse administrators need to focus on a few measurements that are the key drivers of effective, quality care (Frith, Anderson, & Sewell, 2010). Decisions about quality measurements need to be aligned throughout the hospital organization so that they provide information about the outcomes of patient care, patient satisfaction, costs, and revenue. This alignment and linking of data to transform them into information for the purpose of decision making is called business intelligence (Elliot, 2004).

Developing a plan for business intelligence is a strategic process that requires the input of administrators, including the nurse administrator. Information management specialists and nurse informatics specialists have domain knowledge required to develop or select data warehousing software,[1] data integration software, querying software, and dashboard software to present performance indicators. Nurse administrators have domain knowledge of the questions that need to be answered by the data contained in the warehouse. Without an integrated approach with the involvement of administrators from all departments, a healthcare organization can be "data rich and information poor" (Thomas, 2006).

The need for **dashboards** to deliver real-time information on key performance indicators to drive decision making in healthcare has never been greater than today (see **Table 23-3**). Malik (2005) makes an analogy between a pilot's uses of a dashboard of instruments to fly a jet and an administrator's need for a dashboard of key performance indicators to make operational decisions in healthcare. This analogy makes sense if we believe that administrators of complex healthcare organizations need information to make critical decisions just as pilots need information when making decisions while flying. Malik further states that for dashboards to be effective and useful for decision making, they must be SMART.

The use of dashboards in healthcare is playing an important role at senior administrative levels. Dashboards are not just for executives; anyone who has decision-making responsibility should have access to information in the most timely manner possible. Nurse managers need access to real-time data about staffing, productivity, costs, and quality through the use of dashboards to guide operations effectively (Anderson, Frith, & Caspers, 2011).

Patient Care Management

One of the challenges in complex, acute-care hospitals is the workflow, also known as throughput. Delays in patient care as a result of miscommunication, unavailable transport services, overdue room cleaning, and poor patient scheduling decrease patient satisfaction and decrease the profitability of a hospital. Systems are emerging on the market, which have the potential to innovate hospital operations. One such system available from McKesson Corporation is called Horizon Enterprise Visibility™. The system provides a visual presentation of all patients on whiteboards with updates on patients' locations, the status of test results, and updates on discharges, and it communicates this information through existing enterprise software. Another software package developed by CareLogistics™

---

1 See Chapter 9 for more information on data warehousing.

Table 23-3 Effective Dashboards

Synergetic	Dashboard components must work together to relay information on a single screen.
Monitor	Dashboards must display key performance indicators for the user's decision-making needs.
Accurate	Data on the dashboard must be valid and reliable.
Responsive	When key performance indicators are below established targets, a flag or alarm must alert the user.
Timely	Dashboards must display data in real time.

for hospital management delivers innovation in **patient throughput** as well. Workflow is improved by the use of service queues with alerts for priority; synchronization of patient rooms, tasks, equipment, and services; and hospital performance dashboards to keep managers informed in real time.

Employee Scheduling

Even though hospitals continue to function by scheduling nursing staff using a paper system, there are many reasons to change to a computerized **employee scheduling system**. Scheduling nurses' work is a repetitive task, and hours of a nurse manager's time are spent developing biweekly or monthly schedules. Computerized scheduling systems can handle scheduling rules such as master schedules and shift rotations, repeating patterns to make the first draft of a schedule quick. Modifications are more easily made when the availability of nurses shows in the system. Scheduling systems can often prevent errors such as scheduling nurses for a double shift, for overtime, during overlapping shifts, or during requested time off. Often, scheduling systems are capable of generating reports to show the number of productive hours, education, vacation, and family medical leave hours in a period. Some scheduling systems allow the manager to share the schedule with nurses by Intranets, Internet, e-mail, or printing schedules. With an Intranet or Internet interface, nurses can interact with scheduling systems to make requests, view schedules, or fill open shifts.

Some hospitals are successful with centralized, self-scheduling software to fill open shifts (Association of Perioperative Registered Nurses [AORN], 2007). Most of these programs provide a Web-based system for hospitals to use to fill their open shifts. The software matches the qualifications of the RN with the job requirements of the shift and offers an incentive for the RN to bid for the open shift. Hospitals are reporting a reduction of $1–4 million per year in costs for contract labor using this system of competitive bidding for open shifts. Nurses report satisfaction because they see open shifts across the entire hospital, bid for the ones that most interest them, and receive fewer calls at home requesting them to work on their off days (AORN).

Patient Classification Systems (Acuity Applications)

Staffing is one of the most difficult decision-making roles a nurse manager fulfills. **Patient classification systems** were developed to estimate the care needs of inpatients so that prudent staffing decisions can be made. Most patient acuity systems generate data to calculate the number of full-time equivalents needed for a nursing unit (Finkler et al., 2007). Some look at self-care deficits such as those related to activities of daily living, treatments, medications, and patient teaching. Another approach, known as time-based activities, is to assign each task a time based on hospital-specific, predetermined measures. Another method is the use of specific nursing diagnoses based on patient dependency. This approach uses decisions made by the primary nursing care provider.

All patient classification systems depend on accurate and timely data input. Some patient classification systems use computer-based data entry and require the nurse to enter characteristics or tasks that will be used in the scoring of the patient's acuity. Other systems draw data from nurses' documentation in the computerized patient record, which relieves nurses of the additional step of data entry for patient classification. If nurses delay documentation (regardless of the reason), the patient's acuity is downgraded because the documentation of vital signs, education, dressing changes, and other nursing activities are not present in the record to reflect the patient's true acuity.

Clinical Information Systems

Chapter 18 describes clinical information systems in detail. However, a nurse administrator needs to understand the capability and limitations of a clinical information system. Most hospitals have not implemented a fully integrated information system. Fifty percent of hospitals in the United States have clinical documentation systems, but less than 1% of hospitals have a complete electronic medical record (HIMSS Analytics, 2010).

Nurse administrators, in hospitals both large and small, will be faced with the purchase of some type of module for the current information system, bar coding for medication administration, scheduling system, or any number of business applications. Although the nurse administrator may not have knowledge of the technical aspects, the administrator must be the voice of nursing when purchases are considered. Products need to be selected that enhance the work of nursing, not impede it. The nurse administrator is in the best position to advocate for all nursing services and place nurses on purchase committees to make product selections that streamline work processes and put information in the hands of nurses.

The AONE released the guiding principles for the role of the nurse administrator in the selection and implementation of information systems (AONE, 2007). This document clearly states that although the nurse administrator may delegate operational aspects of the acquisition and implementation of an information system, the administrator retains accountability for the process. Some key points include the following: (1) describe the strategic nursing plan so that the chief information officer and members of the task force understand the information needs of nurses now and in the future; (2) know about the planned technology purchases that will occur during the information system acquisition and consider the implications on nursing services; (3) develop an understanding of contracts and legal issues surrounding data ownership; (4) make site visits to hospitals where proposed information systems have been implemented and talk to the chief nurse executives at those facilities; (5) get a clear understanding of the responsibility for training (when, where, how long, who provides, and who pays); (6) develop metrics for implementation and monitor the implementation process using them; (7) include deans from schools of nursing, pharmacy, and others to lessen the impact on their programs; and (8) be prepared for system downtimes.

Starting in 2011, Medicare-eligible hospitals were provided incentives to adopt "certified" electronic health records (EHRs) showing "meaningful use" of information and exchange of health information to improve the quality of healthcare (CMS, 2010b). A phased-in approach to the implementation of EHR was outlined by CMS and the Office of the National Coordinator of Health Information Technology in regulations associated with the American Recovery and Reinvestment Act (Recovery.gov, 2010). Failure to meet meaningful use requirements of EHRs by 2014 will result in reductions in Medicare reimbursement.

The AONE (2010) released a toolkit for the acquisition and implementation of information systems, which provides nurse administrators with three broad suggestions to deal with the new meaningful use legislation: (1) strategize about the implementation of information systems with careful attention to workflow implications, (2) understand the phased-in regulations and use project management to optimize incentives and avoid reductions in reimbursement, and (3) work closely with vendors to ensure that information systems meet certification requirements.

Summary

Nurse administrators, like all other healthcare professionals, use computer applications in their daily work to communicate by e-mail, find resources on the Internet, and develop documents with word processors and spreadsheets. Use of these tools, in addition to applications that can assist in the analysis of processes and in the planning for change, is an essential competency for today's nurse administrator. Moreover, nurse administrators are routinely involved in monitoring data from quality improvement studies (core measures, HCAHPS, NDNQI°, and other measures) to implement change in nursing practice and patient care.

The nurse administrator's need for tools and information to support decisions on financial matters, to develop strategies for improvement in patient care, and to meet regulatory requirements has never been greater. Systems that support administrative work include human resource management systems, scheduling systems, patient management systems, and acuity systems. Information from these systems assists the nurse administrator to use nursing services wisely and to assess the effectiveness of decisions over time.

The nurse administrator should always have a strong voice in the decision to purchase an information system, whether it is a management system or clinical system. This involvement begins well before an information system is selected and continues after implementation to evaluate the performance metrics, costs, and vendor responsibility. The nurse administrator must ensure that decisions regarding clinical information systems, expert systems to support clinical decision making, medical technology, databases, and data warehousing systems that affect nursing services remain within the authority of the nurse administrator because it is this role that retains responsibility and accountability for providing the resources to accomplish patient care in a safe and efficient manner.

APPLICATIONS AND COMPETENCIES

1. Copy the data from the table below into a spreadsheet. Develop a chart (custom type) with a line column on two axes. Place the patient outcomes (falls and pressure ulcers) in the columns and the percentage of RNs on the line.

	Quarter 1	Quarter 2	Quarter 3	Quarter 4
Number of falls	5	8	9	4
Number of pressure ulcers	4	6	7	5
Percentage of registered nurses	0.80	0.75	0.76	0.81

2. Using drawing tools in a word processing software or presentation software, diagram the process for hiring an RN in your organization.
   a. Analyze the process.
      i. Are there ways that the hiring process can stagnate?
      ii. Are there steps that can be streamlined?
   b. Draw the ideal process.
   c. Consider ways to implement change in your organization.

3. Search the Internet and find five software vendors for project management.
   a. List the strengths and weaknesses of each.
   b. Download a trial version of at least two project management software packages.
   c. Develop a Gantt chart for a simple project in your organization to learn to use the software.

4. Go to http://www.hospitalcompare.hhs.gov and compare your hospital's outcome on core measures with three others in your area and two from different areas that have services similar to your own.
   a. Review the following outcomes:
      i. Surgical care improvement/surgical infection prevention
      ii. HCAHPS
      iii. Pneumonia
   b. Develop a plan for improvement in areas where the hospital is below the state and national average.

5. Investigate the use of dashboards in your organization. If dashboards are in use, clarify your understanding of the metrics included on the dashboard. If dashboards are not currently used, develop necessary knowledge of dashboards.
   a. Read more about dashboards from publications in nursing and business.

b. Look for vendors offering healthcare dashboard services on the Internet.

c. Discuss options with the chief information officer.

REFERENCES

American Nurses Association. (2010). *NDNQI® and CMS Reporting*. Retrieved November 2, 2010, from https://www.nursingquality.org/CMS.aspx

American Organization of Nurse Executives. (2005). AONE nurse executive competencies. *Nurse Leader, 3*(1), 15–22. Retrieved November 3, 2010, from http://www.aone.org/aone/certification/docs%20and%20pdfs/NurseExecCompetencies.pdf

American Organization of Nurse Executives. (2007). *AONE guiding principles for defining the role of the nurse executive in technology acquisition, implementation, and evaluation of information technology*. Retrieved November 3, 2010, from http://www.aone.org/aone/resource/PDF/AONE_GP_Technology_and_Acquisition_and_Implementation.pdf

American Organization of Nurse Executives. (2010). *AONE Toolkit for the nurse executive in the acquisition and implementation of information systems*. Retrieved November 2, 2010, from http://www.aone.org/aone/member/ResourceCenter/Toolkits/AONE_Toolkit_Nurse_Executive_Acquisition.pdf

Anderson, E.F., Frith, K.H., & Caspers, B.A. (2011). Linking economics and quality: Developing an evidence-based nurse staffing tool. *Nursing Administration Quarterly, 35*(1), 53–60. Doi: 10.1097/NAQ.0b013e3182047dff

Association of Perioperative Registered Nurses. (2007). Hospitals adopting technology allowing bidding for open shifts. *AORN Management Connections, 3*(11), 1–3.

Centers for Medicare & Medicaid Services. (2006). *Report to Congress: Improving the medicare quality improvement organization program – Response to the Institute of Medicine study*. Retrieved November 3, 2010, https://www.cms.gov/QualityImprovementOrgs/downloads/QIO_Improvement_RTC_fnl.pdf

Centers for Medicare & Medicaid Services (2010a, October 6). *HCAPHS: Patients perspectives of care survey*. Retrieved November 3, 2010, from https://www.cms.gov/HospitalQualityInits/30_HospitalHCAHPS.asp

Centers for Medicare & Medicaid Services (2010b). *Meaningful use*. Retrieved November 2, 2010, from https://www.cms.gov/EHRIncentivePrograms/35_Meaningful_Use.asp

Elliot, T. (2004). *Choosing a business intelligence standard*. Retrieved November 3, 2010, from http://www.businessobjects.com/pdf/solutions/evaluate/evaluating_bi.pdf

Finkler, S., Kovner, C., & Jones, C. (2007). *Financial management for nurse managers and executives* (3rd ed.). St. Louis, MO: Saunders Elsevier.

Frith, K., Anderson, F., & Sewell, J. (2010). Assessing and selecting data for a nursing services dashboard. *Journal of Nursing Administration, 40*(1), 10–15.

Healthcare Quality Information from the Consumer Perspective. (2010). *Hospital survey*. Retrieved November 3, 2010, from http://www.hcahpsonline.org/

HIMSS Analytics. (2010). *Electronic medical record (EMR) adoption model*. Retrieved November 2, 2010, from http://www.himssanalytics.org/

Joint Commission (2010). *Core Measurement Sets*. Retrieved August 21, 2011 from http://www.jointcommission.org/core_measure_set/

Malik, S. (2005). *Enterprise dashboards, design and best practices for IT*. New York, NY: John Wiley & Sons.

Recovery.gov. (2010). *The Recovery Act*. Retrieved September 20, 2010, from http://www.recovery.gov/

Thomas, R. (2006). Information-based transformation: The need for integrated, enterprisewide informatics. *Healthcare Financial Management, 60*(9), 140–142. Retrieved November 3, 2010, from http://www.hfma.org/Publications/hfm-Magazine/Archives/2006/September/Information-Based-Transformation–The-Need-for-Integrated,-Enterprisewide-Informatics/

Yoder-Wise, P., & Kowalski, K. (2006). *Beyond leading and managing: Nursing administration for the future*. St. Louis, MO: Mosby.

CHAPTER 24

Informatics and Research

Objectives

After studying this chapter you will be able to:

▶ Demonstrate basic competencies in statistical analysis software.

▶ Identify sources of data for research.

▶ Discuss the use of data to conduct research in nursing service, education, and administration.

▶ Synthesize research findings in healthcare informatics as evidence for decision making in nursing.

Key Terms

Agency for Healthcare Research and Quality (AHRQ)
Argument
Business Intelligence
Centers for Medicare & Medicaid Services (CMS)
Codebook
Computerized Decision Support Systems (CDSSs)
Data Ferrett
Descriptive Data Analysis

Electronic Medical Records (EMRs)
Statistical Analysis
Evidence-Based Practice
Formula
Healthcare Analytics
Meta-analysis
Microdata
National Institute of Nursing Research (NINR)
Output
Research Utilization

In this data-rich healthcare environment, the need to turn data into useable information is imperative. There is a movement to develop **business intelligence** (also known as **healthcare analytics**), which can integrate financial data, patient data, and quality data to produce predictive analytics for decision makers in healthcare (Anderson, Frith, & Caspers, 2011). Nurse informatics specialists need to understand this next wave of innovation. Moreover, nurses in all roles need skills and tools to summarize sets of numbers into understandable pieces of information and to interpret the meaning of evidence produced through research. The purpose of this chapter is to develop basic competencies in data analysis and research to form a foundation for decision making in nursing and healthcare.

The History of Data Analysis and Research in Medicine and Nursing

The use of data analysis and research in medicine has an interesting history, which began in France and England (Chen, 2003). One of the first instances wherein statistical procedures were used to influence medical decision making was in the early 19th century to demonstrate the harm of performing bloodletting to treat infection. Physicians debated the appropriateness of using mathematics to understand the individual responses of humans to treatments. They argued that medicine was an art that could not be subjected to methods used in science such as astronomy. Even in 1870, when Joseph Lister published his findings on the effect of antiseptic methods in surgery on the mortality rate of patients, physicians rejected the use of statistical methods in medicine. As a professor at the University College in London, Dr. Karl Pearson developed the first inferential statistical methods in the 1880s. The first statistics department was established as the Lister Institute for Preventive Medicine at the turn of the century where Major Greenwood furthered the work of Lister and Pearson (Chen, 2003).

Unfortunately, the use of **statistical analysis** in medicine was not accepted until the 1920s, nearly 100 years after the first use of statistics in medicine (Chen, 2003). By that time, others believed that statistics should be taught to premedical students. Later in the 1940s, the first clinical trial was conducted by the British Medical Research Council to test the effectiveness of streptomycin compared with the usual treatment of bed rest for tuberculosis. Patients' clinical conditions and radiological findings improved when treated with an antibiotic. Following this study, the acceptance of statistics in medicine was secured (Chen, 2003).

The use of statistics and research in nursing has a similar history. The pioneer of statistical thinking was Florence Nightingale, whose work in the 1850s–1860s showed that clean conditions in field hospitals in the Crimean War reduced the mortality rate for soldiers (Brown, 1993). Despite Miss Nightingale's groundbreaking work, the use of statistical analysis and research did not develop until the 1920s when case studies were used to describe the effectiveness of nursing interventions (Gortner, 2000). Afterward, between 1930 and 1960, nursing research in the United States was generally concentrated on nurses, nursing education, and the practice of professional nursing. In 1952, *Nursing Research* was first published; however, the emergence of nursing as a clinical science did not develop until nearly a quarter century later. The **National Institute of Nursing Research (NINR)**, which provided federal funding to nursing studies aimed at prevention of illness, promotion of healthy lifestyles, and support of quality of life, was established in the mid-1980s (Gortner, 2000). Since that time, nurse scientists have been providing research evidence to change traditional ways of caring for patients. This emphasis on **evidence-based practice** is an important step in the development of nursing science and the improvement in patient care.

Use of Technology

Today, statistical analysis and research in nursing are increasing in complexity in large part as a result of the availability of personal computers and statistical analysis programs. Nurse researchers can collect data, manage them in databases, and analyze them with specialized programs. With attention to the principles of data analysis, other nurses (e.g., nurse informatics specialists, managers, educators, clinical nurses, and advanced practice nurses) can benefit from the use of statistical analysis to improve decision making and outcomes.

Personal computers are capable of performing any complex statistical analyses. Commercial statistical analysis programs can be purchased, spreadsheet programs can be used, or free programs can be downloaded from the Internet. Most commercial programs are comparable. Cost and user preference are likely to be the deciding factors. The most popular commercial programs are Statistical Package for Social Sciences (SPSS® provided by SPSS Inc.), Statistical Analysis Software (SAS® provided by SAS Institute Inc.), and Minitab®

Statistical Software (provided by Minitab Inc.). Microsoft Excel® (included with Microsoft Office) and Quattro Pro® (included in Corel® WordPerfect® Office product) are useful because many nurses have software readily available. Free statistical analysis programs are available on the Internet. A comparison of analysis capabilities of free programs is available at http://freestatistics.altervista. org/en/comp.php. Most of these programs are not as user-friendly as commercial software because they do not have a graphical user interface. Instead, they require the use of command lines to input data and run analyses. BrightStat© overcomes this problem, does not require the download of a program because it is an Internet-based program, and provides commonly used statistical procedures.

Statistics Basics

Because data are readily available in healthcare settings today, nurses have an obligation to use them responsibly. Data must be collected, aggregated, analyzed, and interpreted correctly. Nurses who wish to analyze data should refresh their knowledge of statistics either through an academic course or by using reliable sources such as printed textbooks or online textbooks. Several online sites (listed below) are excellent sources of information about the basics of statistics and correct application of statistical procedures to data. Readers are encouraged to review one of the following online sources to understand statistical concepts before undertaking an analysis.

- Statsoft at http://www.statsoft.com/text-book/stathome.html?esc.html&1
- Online statistics: An interactive multimedia course of study at http://onlinestatbook.com/
- Rice virtual lab in statistics at http:// onlinestatbook.com/rvls.html
- Research methods knowledgebase at http://www.socialresarchmethods.net/kb/index.php
- National Library of Medicine: National Information Center on Health Services Research and Health Care Technology at http://www.nlm.nih.gov/nichsr/outreach.html

Using Statistical Software

Simple **descriptive data analysis** can be completed using a spreadsheet. The first step in any data analysis is to put data in the correct format. Enter data on the row with variable labels in the columns. Data that are categorical should be coded with numbers. For example, gender is male or female, but statistical programs typically understand numbers. Change the word "female" into the number "0" and "male" into "1." Make a **codebook** to remember what the numbers mean. The next step is to create or insert **formulas** into the spreadsheet. Fortunately, spreadsheets have built-in formulas for many statistical procedures such as mean, median, standard deviation, variance, and correlation. Users can select a cell on the spreadsheet and insert a formula using the "Insert" menu and clicking "Function." A formula is added by typing the name of the statistical procedure or selecting a category of formula using the drop-down menu. If the category "Statistical" is chosen, a list of statistical formulas is displayed. Users can scroll down until the desired formula is shown. Finally, the numbers that are to be used in the statistical formula are defined by adding them to the "**argument**." This is accomplished by clicking the icon inside the number field. The window minimizes, and the user can select the numbers that are needed. Once the formula is inserted and the arguments are defined, the result of the statistical procedure is displayed.

Spreadsheets also provide graphical presentation of data. As described in Chapter 8, charts can be easily created using the chart wizard. Besides pie, bar, and line charts, scatter charts are used to show relationships between two pieces of data.

Even though spreadsheets can be used to calculate many descriptive statistics, data analysis can be more efficient if a program designed for that purpose is used. A demonstration of analysis is shown using BrightStat©, a free statistical analysis program. Its graphical user interface operates in a manner similar to those in SPSS®, making the demonstration practical. BrightStat© is located at www.brightstat.com, and users can simply register with the site to use it. Users should set their browser options to allow pop-up windows and make sure they have Adobe Flash Player PlugIn. Although there is no users' manual, there are context-specific help screens inside the program.

To use BrightStat©, data from a spreadsheet are uploaded into the program. The spreadsheet should be formatted in the manner described earlier in the chapter. Once the data are available, there are several steps to uploading, browsing, and importing data files (see **Figures 24-1 and 24-2**).

Summarizing data with descriptive statistics using BrightStat© is quite easy. Variables are selected for analysis, and the statistical procedures are chosen (see **Figure 24-3**). More sophisticated statistical analyses such as *t*-test, variance, correlations, and linear regression can be run in BrightStat© too. Graphs can be created including line, bar, scatterplot, histograms, and boxplots. The capability of this free software makes running statistical analyses available to any nurse who needs to find specific answers to questions about patient outcomes, nursing practice, or processes in a healthcare facility. Graphs and statistical analyses are shown in an **output** window, which can be saved inside BrightStat©, exported, or printed.

Research Using the Web

Occasionally nurses need data from sources other than their own facilities to make comparisons. For example, a nurse manager of an emergency department might like to compare wait times for certain diagnoses across all hospitals in the United States. Data are made publicly available using the **DataFerrett**, a browser designed by the federal government (http://dataferrett.census.gov/). A video and tutorial are provided on the website to guide users. DataFerrett is an application that must be downloaded and installed in a local computer. Once installed, users can access public **microdata** (individual responses – not aggregated) from various federal agencies.

Another useful site for health information on the Internet is the **Agency for Healthcare**

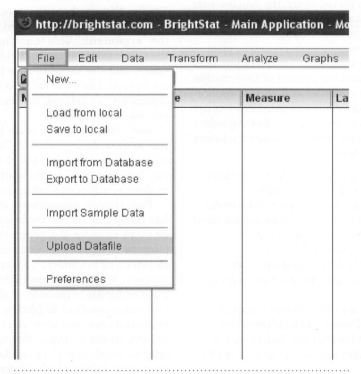

Figure 24-1 Upload data file.

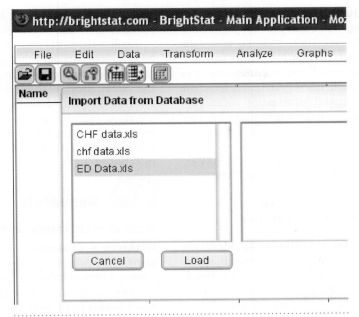

Figure 24-2 Select data file.

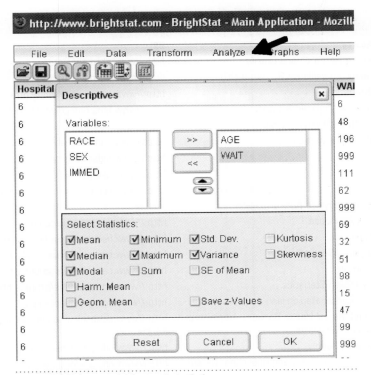

Figure 24-3 Select variables and statistics.

Research and Quality (AHRQ) at http://www.ahrq.gov/data. The AHRQ also provides tools (software downloads), evaluation toolkits, and databases for conducting research. Nurses can use tools to mine for data in several national initiatives (see list below). In addition, nurses can find research on quality, access, cost, and information technology at the AHRQ website. Research findings are synthesized or provided in fact sheets for easy reading.

- Medical Expenditure Panel Survey (MEPS)
- Healthcare Cost and Utilization Project (HCUP)
- HIV and AIDS Costs and Use
- Safety Net Monitoring Initiative

The **Centers for Medicare & Medicaid Services (CMS)** provide access to research, statistics, data, and systems at its website http://www.cms.hhs.gov/home/rsds.asp. Nurses can locate information on patient satisfaction, outcomes of care, and cost. Findings from the required Hospitals

Consumer Assessment of Health Providers and Systems are available for review and comparison.

No discussion of research on the Internet would be complete without looking at the NINR located at http://www.ninr.nih.gov/. Publications from the NINR provide the latest scientific evidence on clinical topics. Monthly summaries of research are made available at http://www.medscape.com/index/section_1221_0. Other Internet sites where useful health statistics can be found are provided in **Table 24-1**.

 Research

Research Utilization in Nursing

Research utilization is critical to the advancement of nursing care and patient outcomes. The consequences of failing to apply research in clinical practice can be harmful to patients. For example, when deaths from sudden infant death syndrome (SIDS) were noticed in the 1970s, it took over

Table 24-1 Helpful Internet Sites to Find Health Statistics

Name of Internet Source	URL
Agency for Healthcare Research and Quality	http://www.ahrq.gov/data/
Behavioral Risk Factor Surveillance System (CDC)	http://apps.nccd.cdc.gov/brfss/
Bureau of Labor Statistics	http://www.bls.gov/bls/safety.htm
Centers for Medicare & Medicaid Services	http://www.cms.hhs.gov/home/rsds.asp
Department of Health and Human Services	
Gateway to Data and Statistics	http://www.hhs-stat.net/
FedStats	http://www.fedstats.gov/
FirstGov	http://www.usa.gov/
Health Insurance Information from the Census Bureau	http://www.census.gov/hhes/www/hlthins/hlthins.html
Health Resources and Services Administration	
Geospatial Data Warehouse	http://datawarehouse.hrsa.gov/
Healthy People 2010	http://www.healthypeople.gov/Data/
Morbidity and Mortality Weekly Report	http://www.cdc.gov/mmwr/weekcvol.html
National Cancer Institute	http://www.cancer.gov/statistics/finding
National Center for Health Statistics	http://www.cdc.gov/nchs/express.htm
National Program of Cancer Registries	http://www.cdc.gov/cancer/npcr/
Substance Abuse and Mental Health Services Administration: National Outcome Measures	http://www.nationaloutcomemeasures.samhsa.gov/outcome/sa_pre.asp
National Vital Statistics Survey	http://www.cdc.gov/nchs/nvss.htm
Web-Based Injury Statistics Query and Reporting System	http://www.cdc.gov/ncipc/wisqars/

20 years to change the practice of positioning babies during sleep to prevent SIDS (Fredriksen, 2006). Even after the American Academy of Pediatrics made the recommendation in 1992 for babies to sleep supine, half of the maternal–child nurses did not change the practice of positioning babies (Moos, 2006). It is the responsibility of every nurse to keep current in practice by using research evidence. There are several ways to stay current: read research literature in the specialty area, subscribe to clinical practice journals, attend professional meetings, and read source documents for new guidelines.

There are other reasons for the failure of clinicians to use research findings to change clinical practice. The first is that research is published in journals to which clinicians might not subscribe. Second, studies with important findings may not be replicated. Single studies are not usually the basis for changing practice. Third, when multiple studies are conducted on a topic, the methods may be so disparate that combining findings into an integrative review or **meta-analysis** may not be possible. Stronger evidence is built through the replication and synthesis of findings to change practice. A good example of the strength of a meta-analysis to change practice is the study

of low-dose warfarin as a prophylaxis for the central venous catheter in patients with cancer (Rawson & Newburn-Cook, 2007). The researchers located randomized control trials by searching for Medline, Embase, Cancerlit, CINAHL, and the Cochran Library. After conducting a meta-analysis procedure, the researchers reported that low-dose warfarin failed to prevent thrombus formation in central venous catheters and was associated with adverse patient outcomes. This study provides clear evidence used to change clinical practice.

The skills needed to find research reports and read and critique them for use in practice begin in a nurse's basic educational program. Faculty in nursing education programs face challenges when introducing evidence-based practice to nursing students. Morgan, Fogel, Hicks, Wright, and Tyler (2007) reported their experiences of teaching students how to search databases for quantitative research associated with health disparity. They reported that undergraduate students need practice and positive reinforcement to improve their health information literacy skills to prepare for the workplace. Students who practice should be able to overcome the challenges of finding and using research in clinical practice. **Table 24-2** provides some learning strategies.

Table 24-2 Learning Strategies to Overcome Challenges Associated With Nursing Research

Challenge	Learning Strategy
Research is intimidating	Attend class and listen to explanations about the research.
	Synthesize literature reviews and discuss the results with faculty.
	Ask faculty for feedback to validate knowledge.
	Practice reviewing research studies, looking for similarities and differences.
Difficulty in identifying research articles	Ask a librarian for assistance in locating journals specializing in nursing research.
	Search digital library databases that index nursing journals.
	Specify research in digital library database queries.
	Ask faculty for feedback on search techniques and quality of search results.
	Practice search skills.
Difficulty in analyzing research results	Learn to identify the sections of a research article in which the results, limitations, and conclusions are summarized.
	Consult research and statistics textbooks to review qualitative or quantitative analysis information.
	Ask faculty for feedback to validate knowledge.
	Practice data analysis skills.

Even though research utilization is clearly important to keep clinical practice safe, there is evidence that nurses in all practice specialties fail to use research. McCloskey (2008) found that nurses report having little access to research findings in their work settings, state that little research is conducted in their clinical areas, and believe that colleagues do not discuss research findings. McCloskey analyzed responses by education (associates, bachelors, masters), years of experience, and roles in the healthcare setting (management, advanced practice, and staff nurse). Nurses with a higher educational preparation and those in management or advanced practice roles reported using research findings more than that by staff nurses and those with an associate degree in nursing. Years of clinical experience were not related to utilization of research findings in changing clinical practice. This research report shows the need for leaders in the healthcare to support, recognize, and reward nurses who use research in clinical practice. Moreover, leaders must develop processes whereby patient outcomes are always viewed through the lens of research literature to ensure that opportunities to implement best practices are not missed. Not only does this benefit patient safety, but it can also have a positive financial influence on the organization to avoid reductions in reimbursement from the CMS for poor quality performance.

Research Findings in Informatics

In a white paper by McCormick et al. (2007), the new focus for research in nursing informatics is outlined. The authors cite the need for a change in the research agenda on the basis of shifting demographics in the United States, escalating costs of healthcare, increasing need for high-quality care, and mounting threats to public health in the 21st century. The agenda calls for the following:

1. Secondary use of clinical data
2. Security, including the use of biometrics, signatures, encryption, and Public Key Infrastructure
3. Aggregation of patient data without the use of identifiers
4. Promoting the use and development of standards

5. Population health
6. Privacy and confidentiality
7. A focus on a National Health Information Network (McCormick et al., 2007, p. 22).

The agenda further calls for nursing informatics research to focus on the improvement of healthcare outcomes by "building the data infrastructure to support quality assessments and improvement and balancing patients interests in privacy protection and protection of their health and safety" (p. 22). This focus on healthcare outcomes demands a shift in the study of perceptions of technology effectiveness to the study of the influence of healthcare technology on financial, quality, and access outcomes.

The following sections describe the current state of research in three major areas: health information technology (HIT), **computerized decision support systems (CDSSs)**, and **electronic medical records (EMRs)**. Although the presentation of research findings is not exhaustive, it does provide readers with a snapshot of topics and methods under investigation in informatics.

Health Information Technology

Adoption of technology and HIT-assisted healthcare is on the rise. The Pew Research Center (2006) reported that in 2000, only 46% of American households used the Internet and 25% of Americans reported using it to obtain health information. Ten years later, the Pew Research Center reported that 74% of households have Internet access and 61% of Americans use the Internet and social networking to access information about health and healthcare (Fox & Jones, 2009). Although seeking health information online is more prevalent now, the impact of that information on Americans' lives is not completely understood. Fox and Jones (2009) reported that only 13% of patients said their health inquiry had a major impact and 44% reported a minor impact. Sixty percent of those patients reported that health information online affected decisions about treatment, 53% said that they asked additional questions in office visits or sought second opinions, and 38% said that their approach to healthy living changed as a result of health information found online. Lacking still are measurements of long-term effects of using online health information sites or changes in health-related quality of life based on information-seeking behaviors.

Computerized Decision Support Systems and Patient Outcomes

CDSSs are information systems deployed for the purpose of improving clinical decision making and patient outcomes. Differential diagnosis, preventive care, disease management, and drug prescribing are the primary support functions provided in CDSS. Studies of the effect of CDSS on healthcare provider performance predominates research literature (see **Table 24-3** for a listing of research studies and outcomes). Development and implementation of CDSSs are varied, leading to problems in integrating findings from research studies

Table 24-3 Research Studies on CDSS

Authors	Function of CDSS	Outcome	Improvement
Cho, Staggers, and Park (2010)	Diagnostic computer-based decision support	Amounts of information preferred by expert and novice nurses	Experts prefer a moderate amount of information and novices prefer high amounts of information
Lee and Bakken (2007)	Diagnosis and management of adult obesity	Adherence to clinical practice guideline	No
Farion et al. (2008)	Diagnosis of acute abdomen	Comparison of accuracy of CDSS and physician to recommend correct triage plan	No
Sintchenko, Iredell, Gilbert, and Coiera (2005)	Antibiotic prescribing in critical care	Patient LOS	Yes
		Defined daily doses	Yes
		Mortality	Same
Kroth et al. (2006)	Documentation of erroneous patient temperature	Improvement in accurate patient temperature	Yes
Cimino (2007)	Information management at the point of care	Provider satisfaction with context-specific information.	Yes
		Provider perception of improvement in patient care	Yes
Garg et al. (2005), review of 100 studies from 1977 to 2003	Systems for diagnosis	Improvement in provider performance	40% of studies
	Clinical reminders for preventative care		76% of studies
			18% of studies
			62% of studies
	Disease management		
	Drug prescribing		
Smith, DePue, and Rini (2007), review of 9 studies from 1986 to 2006	Diagnosis of pain	Information for provider use	Feasibility studies – no comparisons made
	Management of pain		
Lyerla, LeRouge, Cooke, Turpin, & Wilson (2010)	Reminder to nurses to measure Head of Bed (HOB) for ventilator patients	Degree of elevation of HOB and percentage of patients with HOB >30 degrees	Yes

(Garg et al., 2005; Smith, DePue, & Rini, 2007). Other problems exist in this body of literature that call for improvements in future research. Research methodology is usually descriptive or preexperimental; more rigorous designs are needed to test for changes in patient outcomes when CDSS is employed. The CDSSs tend to be stand-alone systems that are not integrated into the EMR. Redundancy in data entry is problematic because of the time requirement and the potential for error. Research in CDSSs needs to focus not only on provider performance but also on the effect of better decision making on patient outcomes.

Research on the Use of Electronic Medical Record Systems

Not only is education and support necessary, but attention to the way EMRs are implemented is important. Gruber, Cummings, Leblanc, and Smith (2009) conducted a systematic review of research literature to examine reported successes and failures. Gruber et al. found 47 success factors and 38 failure factors. The time period most prone to failures was the "go-live" period.

Once the initial go-live period is over, providers can often experience major changes in workflow. Investigating this phenomenon, Lee and McElmurry (2010) conducted an extensive review of literature on workflow postimplementation of EMRs. The authors found that the implementation of an EMR created new work including time-consuming data entry because of structure issues in the EMR, awkward navigation that was not intuitive to healthcare providers, and decreased clinical reasoning ability of healthcare providers because of massive amounts of data. Errors in entering physician orders were reported due to confusing order options and inappropriate order templates. Physicians reported a variety of workflow issues created by EMRs – all stemming from system inflexibility and inappropriate customization. For nurses, documentation completeness was not improved with EMRs, particularly when documentation occurred at the end of shifts rather than in real time. Lee and McElmurry found mixed results regarding nurse attitudes and acceptance of EMRs.

User perceptions of EMRs' usability and of effects on provider behaviors can be found in the EMR literature. Rantz et al. (2010) reported that the evaluation of patients' clinical trends and communication with other healthcare providers was easier after the implementation of the EMR than previous paper systems had been. Nurses and certified nursing assistants expressed concerns about EMRs including inconsistent use of EMRs, such as the use of paper documentation even 6–12 months after the EMR implementation, difficulty for some nursing staff in finding documentation once entered into the system, and late documentation. While implementation at 24 months was perceived by nursing staff as successful, most reported the need for additional staffing during the first 12 months due to increased time for documentation, pulling them away from patient care.

Studies have been conducted to determine the reliability of documentation in EMRs and physician order entry systems. Hakes and Whittington (2008) found no significant difference in documentation time between pre- and post-EMR implementation except when discharging patients to long-term care facilities. This period had a statistically significantly increased documentation time than before EMR implementation. The researchers suggested that patient transition from hospital to long-term care is complex, and EMRs should be designed to better handle the transfer of information to other provider locations. Palchuk et al. (2010) reviewed nearly 3,000 electronic prescriptions, which contained a free-text field. The researchers found 16.1% discrepancies between the e-script and the free-text. The majority (83.3%) of these errors could have led to adverse events or deaths. Pakhomov, Jacobsen, Chute, and Roger (2008) studied the agreement of patient-reported signs and symptoms and the documentation in the EMR. While there were many congruencies between the 1,119 patient self-reports and documentation, there were also many discrepancies. The discrepancies found by Palchuk et al. and

Pakhomov et al. are concerning, and the authors suggested that close attention must be paid to the quality of data entry to assist in the quality of patient care and to provide safe patient care.

Adoption of EMRs does not automatically improve patient outcomes, but some recent studies show promising results. Kazley and Ozcan (2008) investigated the effect of an EMR on 10 process indicators for three clinical conditions: acute myocardial infarction, congestive heart failure, and pneumonia. They found that 4 of the 10 process measures improved after the implementation of EMR. Mortality rates post-implementation of EMRs was studied by Longhurst et al. (2010). They found a 20% decrease in adjusted mortality. In the 18-month study, the researchers found that 36 fewer deaths occurred. Hunt et al. (2009) studied over 6,000 patients during a 24-month period, comparing baseline and post-implementation outcomes for patients with diabetes. Low-density lipoproteins targets and blood pressure control improved over the study period, but mean glycated hemoglobin (HbA1c) did not improve. Patients remained satisfied with their care during EMR implementation.

Researchers who plan to study the impact of using an EMR need to build upon the research base already in place. Assessments of user satisfaction, clinical outcomes, and financial impact are the most widely studied aspects, but there is little consistency in methods or measures. This severely limits the ability to synthesize findings to determine the best practices in EMR planning, implementation, and evaluation. Nahm, Vaydia, Ho, Scharf, and Seagull (2007) suggested tools and methods to study outcomes following EMR rollout. Otieno, Toyama, Asonuma, Kanai-Pak, and Naitoh published results of a new instrument to measure nurses' perceptions on use, quality, and satisfaction with EMRs in 2007. Nurse informatics specialists should use published instruments (if validity and reliability are acceptable) and employ standardized evaluation techniques whenever possible to address the identified shortcomings in the informatics literature.

Summary

Research in medicine and nursing has a short history. Most scholars point to the beginning of clinical trials in the 1940s as a significant marker. Since that time, healthcare professionals have engaged in research to find the best way to produce good patient outcomes. Personal computers are now capable of performing complex statistical analyses that were not possible before the 1990s. Data are available in healthcare settings through EMRs, administrative databases, and the Internet. These advances in technology make the need to produce evidence more urgent. Decision makers at the bedside, in board rooms, and in educational settings need to understand the effects of current practice on outcomes to assess the need for change. The ability to provide meaningful information from discrete data is here and must be used.

Evidence to guide the practice of nursing informatics is beginning to emerge, and informatics specialists need to keep their knowledge current. Yet, the research methodology used in existing studies is mostly descriptive. More rigorous designs are needed to test the effectiveness of technology to improve patient care and outcomes. Nurse informatics researchers are in a good position to lead change through the use of evidence produced in research.

APPLICATIONS AND COMPETENCIES

1. Copy the data from the table below into a spreadsheet. Perform a statistical analysis to obtain descriptive statistics that summarize the data (complete using spreadsheet or BrightStat©). Remember to split the data by hospital first.

   a. Obtain the mean, median, minimum, maximum, and standard deviation for length of stay (LOS) and age.

   b. Find the frequency count of male and female patients and for type of hospital.

   c. Write a paragraph to summarize the LOS of patients at the rural and city hospitals.

   d. Write a paragraph to describe the age of the patients at both hospitals.

LOS	Age	Gender	Hospital	LOS	Age	Gender	Hospital
3	50	Male	City	4	65	Male	Rural
7	72	Female	City	5	72	Male	Rural
2	45	Male	City	2	68	Male	Rural
8	82	Female	City	7	70	Male	Rural
5	72	Female	City	4	50	Male	Rural
7	85	Male	City	6	62	Male	Rural
3	67	Male	City	5	65	Male	Rural
7	66	Male	City	8	80	Female	Rural
5	62	Female	City	8	71	Female	Rural
10	78	Female	City	5	55	Male	Rural
7	77	Male	City	5	47	Male	Rural
8	81	Male	City	10	77	Female	Rural
6	70	Male	City	10	82	Female	Rural
4	63	Female	City	9	85	Female	Rural
8	90	Male	City	8	76	Female	Rural
8	77	Male	City	7	77	Female	Rural
6	79	Female	City	10	81	Female	Rural
7	82	Female	City	8	67	Female	Rural
3	55	Male	City	7	73	Male	Rural
9	57	Male	City	6	66	Male	Rural
4	60	Male	City	10	63	Female	Rural
5	62	Male	City	9	74	Female	Rural
6	78	Male	City	10	80	Female	Rural
6	73	Female	City	6	72	Female	Rural
7	69	Male	City	6	72	Female	Rural
7	70	Female	City	7	67	Female	Rural
9	77	Female	City	3	73	Male	Rural
2	57	Male	City	4	76	Male	Rural
6	59	Male	City	7	72	Male	Rural
7	52	Male	City	10	88	Female	Rural
6	83	Female	City	3	67	Male	Rural

2. Using the same data set, determine the relationship of age and LOS in each hospital.

   a. Make a scatter chart for both hospitals.

   b. Calculate the correlation of age and LOS at both hospitals.

   c. Write a paragraph to describe the findings.

3. Compare the LOS for males and females at both hospitals.

   a. Run a *t*-test to determine if there is a significant difference in mean LOS.

   b. Write a paragraph to describe the findings.

4. Search for research findings at the AHRQ located at http://www.ahrq.gov/research/.

   a. Find a fact sheet regarding the health of minority women in the United States and summarize the findings.

   b. Look for research synthesis on hospital nurse staffing and quality of care. Summarize the main findings.

5. Search for current nursing informatics research in databases at your local hospital, college, or university. Find at least three research reports in your area of interest. Think about how the research could be used in your work setting.

REFERENCES

Anderson, E. F., Frith, K. H., & Caspers, B. A. (2011). Linking economics and quality: Developing an evidence-based nurse staffing tool. *Nursing Administrative Quarterly, 35*(1), 53–60.

Brown, P. (1993). *Florence Nightingale: The tough British campaigner who was the founder of modern nursing.* Watford, England: Exley Publications.

Chen, T. (2003). The history of statistical thinking in medicine. In Y. Lu & J.-Q. Fang (Eds.), *Advanced Medical Statistics.* World Scientific. Singapore: Publishing Company. Retrieved March 13, 2007, from http://www.worldsci-books.com/lifesci/etextbook/4854/4854_chap1.pdf

Cho, I., Staffers, N., & Park, I. (2010). Nurses reponses to differing amounts and information content in a diagnostic computer-based decision support application. *CIN: Computers, Informatics, Nursing, 28*(2), 95–102.

Cimino, J. (2007). An integrated approach to computer-based decision support at the point of care. *Transactions of the American Clinical and Climatological Association, 188*, 273–288.

Farion, K., Michalowki, W., Rubin, S., Wilk, S., Correll, R., & Gaboury, I. (2008). Prospective evaluation of the MET-AP system providing triage plans for acute pediatric abdominal pain. *International Journal of Medical Informatics, 77*, 208–218.

Fox, S., & Jones, S. (2009). *The social life of health information.* Retrieved December 16, 2010, from http://pewinternet.org/Reports/2009/8-The-Social-life-of-Health-Information.aspx

Fredriksen, S. (2006). Tragedy, utopia and medical progress. *Journal of Medical Ethics, 32*, 450–453.

Garg, A., Adhikari, N., McDonald, H., Rosas-Arellano, M., Devereaux, P., Beyene, J., et al. (2005). Effects of computerized clinical decision support systems on practitioner performance and patient outcomes: A systematic review. *Journal of the American Medical Association, 293*(10), 1223–1238.

Gortner, S. (2000). Knowledge development in nursing: Our historical roots and future opportunities. *Nursing Outlook, 48*(2), 60–67.

Gruber, D., Cummings, G., Leblanc, L., & Smith, D. (2009). Factors influencing outcomes of clinical information systems implementation: A systematic review. *CIN: Computers, Informatics, Nursing, 27*(3), 151–163.

Hakes, B., & Whittington, J. (2008). Assessing the impact of an electronic medical record on nurse documentation time. *CIN: Computers, Informatics, Nursing, 26*(4), 234–241.

Hunt, J., Siemienczuk, J., Gillanders, W., LeBlance, B., Rozenfeld, Y., Bonin, K., et al. (2009). The impact of a physician-directed health information technology system on diabetes outcomes in primary care: A pre- and post-implementation study. *Informatics in Primary Care, 17*(3), 165–174.

Kazley, A., & Ozcan, Y. (2008). Do hospitals with EMRs provide higher quality care? An examination of three clinical conditions. *Medical Care Research & Review, 65*(4), 496–513.

Kroth, P., Dexter, P., Overhage, M., Knipe, C., Hui, S., Belsito, A., et al. (2006). A computerized decision support system improves the accuracy of temperature capture from nursing personnel at the bedside. *AMIA Annual Symposium Proceedings, 2006*, 444–448. PMCID: PMC1839332.

Lee, N., & Bakken, S. (2007). Development of a prototype personal digital assistant-decision support system for the management of adult obesity. *International Journal of Medical Informatics, 765*, 281–292.

Lee, S., & McElmurry, B. (2010). Capturing nursing workflow disruptions. *CIN: Computers, Informatics, Nursing, 28*(3), 151–159.

Longhurst, C., Parst, L., Sandborg, C., Widen, E., Sullivan, J., Hahn, J., et al. (2010). Decrease in hospital-wide mortality rate after implementation of a commercially sold physician order entry system. *Pediatrics, 126*(1), 14–21.

Lyerla, F., LeRouge, C., Cooke, D. A., Turpin, D., & Wilson, L. (2010). A nursing clinical decision support system and potential predictors of head-of-bed position for patients receiving mechanical ventilation. *American Journal of Critical Care, 19*(1), 39–47.

McCloskey, D. (2008). Nurses' perceptions of research utilization in a corporate health care system. *Journal of Nursing Scholarship, 40*(1), 39–45.

McCormick, K., Delaney, C., Brennan, P., Effken, J., Kendrick, K., Murphy, J., et al. (2007). Guideposts to the future – an agenda for nursing informatics. *Journal of the American Medical Informatics Association, 14*(1), 19–24.

Moos, M. (2006). Responding to the newest evidence about SIDS. *AWHONN Lifelines, 10*(2), 163–166.

Morgan, P., Fogel, J., Hicks, P., Wright, L., & Tyler, I. (2007). Strategic enhancement of nursing students information literacy skills: Interdisciplinary perspectives. *The ABNF Journal, 18*(2), 40–45.

Nahm, E., Vaydia, V., Ho, D., Scharf, B., & Seagull, J. (2007). Outcomes assessment of clinical information system implementation: A practical guide. *Nursing Outlook, 55*(6), 282–288.

Otieno, O. G., Toyama, H., Asonuma, M., Kanai-Pak, M., & Naitoh, K. (2007). Nurses' views on the use, quality, and user satisfaction with electronic medical records: Questionnaire development. *Journal of Advanced Nursing, 60*(2), 209–219.

Pakhomov, S., Jacobsen, S., Chute, C., & Roger, V. (2008). Agreement between patient-reported symptoms and their documentation in the medical record. *American Journal of Managed Care, 14*(8), 530–539.

Palchuk, M., Fang, E., Cygielnik, J., Labreche, M., Shubina, M., Ramelson, H., et al. (2010). An unintended consequence of electronic prescriptions: Prevalence and impact of internal discrepancies. *Journal of the American Medical Informatics Association, 17*(4), 472–476.

Pew Research Center. (2006). *Maturing Internet news audience – Broader than deep.* Retrieved March 13, 2008, from http://people-press.org/reports/pdf/282.pdf

Rantz, M., Alexander, G., Galambos, C., Vogelsmeier, A., Hicks, L., Scott-Cawiezell, J., et al. (2010). The use of bedside electronic medical record to improve quality of care in nursing facilities: A qualitative analysis. *CIN: Computers, Informatics, Nursing, 28*(2), 1–8.

Rawson, K., & Newburn-Cook, C. (2007). The use of low-dose warfarin as prophylaxis for central venous catheter thrombosis in patients with cancer: A meta-analysis. *Oncology Nursing Forum, 34*(5), 1037–1043.

Sintchenko, V., Iredell, J., Gilbert, G., & Coiera, E. (2005). Handheld computer-based decision support reduces patient length of stay and antibiotic prescribing in critical care. *Journal of the American Informatics Association, 12*(4), 398–402.

Smith, M., DePue, J., & Rini, C. (2007). Computerized decision-support systems for chronic pain management in primary care. *Pain Medicine, 8*(53), 155–166.

Thakkar, M., & Davis, D. (2006). Risks, barriers, and benefits of EHR systems: A comparative study based on size of hospital. *Perspectives in Health Information, 3*(5), 1–19.

CHAPTER 25
Legal and Ethical Issues

Objectives

After studying this chapter, you will be able to:

▶ Discuss the similarities and differences between professional nursing codes of ethics and professional informatics associations' codes.

▶ Identify at least three ways that privacy of information can be breached.

▶ Identify the strengths and weaknesses of the Health Insurance Portability and Accountability Act.

▶ Discuss current telehealth issues associated with practicing nursing across state lines.

▶ Discuss the pros and cons of the implantable patient identifier using radio frequency identification microchip technology.

▶ Give examples of appropriate and inappropriate professional nurse use of Web 2.0 applications.

▶ Apply the use of copyright law to activities associated with the scholarship of professional publications by nurses.

Key Terms

Center for Nursing Advocacy
Code of Ethics
Code of Ethics for Nurses
Coordinated Licensure Information System
Copyright
Fair Use
Fixed Tangible Medium

Health Insurance Portability and Accountability Act (HIPAA)
Nurse Licensure Compact (NLC)
Privacy Rights Clearinghouse
Restricted License
TEACH Act

Informatics applications and competencies are essential skills for all nurses. The rapid change in technology development behooves us to stay abreast of new knowledge. We need to have factual knowledge of technology changes and the potential implications for making our patients safe. Healthcare personnel and those involved with informatics that have access to confidential information have a special obligation to abide by the professional ethical standards and legal statutes in the handling of information. This chapter addresses the ethical and legal responsibilities of the nurse as they relate to informatics. Topics that are discussed include the pertinent professional codes of ethics, **Health Insurance Portability and Accountability Act (HIPAA)** Web 2.0, telehealth, the implantable patient identifier, and **copyright** issues.

Ethics

Professionals are bound by their pertinent **code of ethics**. A code of ethics is made up of statements of the professionals' values and beliefs, which are based on ethical principles (see **Table 25-1**). According to Curtin (2005), there are three characteristics of ethical choices. First, choices always involve conflict of values that are extremely important. Second, scientific inquiry can only influence the choice made in a value conflict, but it cannot provide an answer. Finally, the process involves deciding which value is most important. Curtin suggests that any decision made about conflicts of

Table 25-1 Ethical Principles

Autonomy	Self Rule/Determination
Beneficence	Doing what is best for the individual
Nonmalfeasance	Doing no harm
Veracity	Truth telling
Fidelity	Honesty
Paternalism	Making decisions on behalf of others
Justice	Being fair
Respect for others	Appreciation for human dignity

fundamental values will have lasting and unexpected consequences on human concern areas. For the public good and protection, professionals who are involved with the use of healthcare informatics "must be bound by ethical, moral, and legal responsibilities" (Curtin, 2005).

The concept of conflicting values is central to informatics. As an example, the ethical principles of autonomy and beneficence are often in conflict when discussing the use of radio frequency identification (RFID) to track the whereabouts of nursing staff or patients and for telehomecare monitoring to assess symptoms changes of patients. Relationships between two or more people are subject to conflict of ethical principles, depending on the situation. Nurses must be knowledgeable about ethical principles, the professional **code of ethics for nurses**, pertinent laws, and conflict resolution skills. Even without a universal structured curriculum in ethics, nurses abide by ethical principles while caring for patients and families. In fact, according to the Gallup Poll, nurses have been named the number 1 ethical professionals since 1999, with the exception of 2001 – the year of the World Trade Center terrorist attacks (firefighters were number 1 that year) (Gallup Inc., 2009).

Code of Ethics for Nurses

Professional nursing associations worldwide have established codes of ethics. Not surprisingly, there are marked similarities between all of them. They all address principles and values of ethical practice, although the exact wording may vary slightly. Professional nurses must adhere to their code of ethics in their personal lives, not just in the workplaces. Informatics competencies and applications pertain to the personal use of the computer as well as the use of health information technology (HIT) in the workplace.

The American Nurses Association (ANA) Code of Ethics for Nurses (2001), available online at http://nursingworld.org/MainMenuCategories/EthicsStandards/CodeofEthicsforNurses.aspx, specifies nine provisions. The code addresses issues that concern acting on behalf of the patient's interests, privacy, and confidentiality. It provides general statements that could be useful when addressing conflicts or dilemmas in interactions with others (within and outside the agency) resulting from the creation of, access to, and/or disposition of electronic health information data.

Simpson (2006) asserts that the ANA Code of Ethics Provisions 3, 5, 7, and 8 are particularly applicable for electronic health information. Provision 3, confidentiality and patient safety, addresses the nurse's ethical responsibility to safeguard the patient's right to privacy. Provision 5, competence and continuing education, addresses the nurse's ethical responsibility to maintain competence and ongoing learning. Provision 7, contribution to practice, addresses the nurse's ethical responsibility to contribute to the scholarship of nursing. Lastly, Provision 8, informing the public, addresses the nurse's ethical responsibility to protect the public from misinformation and misinterpretation.

The **Center for Nursing Advocacy** website at http://www.nursingadvocacy.org/research/codes_of_ethics.html includes a link to the International Council of Nurses Code of Ethics for nurses. The Nursing Advocacy website also has links to Nursing Codes of Ethics for Australia, Belgium, Hong Kong, England, and Canada.

Code of Ethics for Informatics Professional Organization Members

Informatics specialists may belong to one or more informatics professional organizations. Each organization has formulated a Code of Ethics for its members (see **Table 25-1**). Although the principles identified for the various health informatics organizations are implied in the nursing codes of ethics, in this time of worldwide adoption of HIT, it may be pertinent to update the nursing codes so that the ethics associated with information technology become more explicit.

Laws, Rules, and Regulations

Laws state exactly what is expected, unlike codes of ethics, which are open to interpretation. A person or an organization caught breaking a law can expect to be penalized. If the offender breaks a criminal law, the penalty could involve a jail or prison sentence; if it is a civil law, the offender can be fined. Regulatory agencies, such as the State Board of Nursing, Centers for Medicare & Medicaid (CMS), and the Joint Commission provide rules for persons or organizations to follow. A person or an agency not following a rule and caught doing so may be penalized as when breaking a law. The penalty for breaking a rule might be temporary or permanent loss of privileges.

The Reality of Security Breaches

A data security breach is unlawful and can result in fines, imprisonment, or both. When discussing informatics, it is easy to think that security breaches are always done using a computer, but that is not true. These can happen when a truck carrying paper records is involved in an auto accident and overturns, spilling out records; postal mail is tampered with; patient paper files are stolen; when computers or computer drives are stolen or lost; as well as theftwith computers using electronic transmission. The criminal hacker has received lots of media attention because it is possible to steal thousands of records with private information relatively invisibly and quickly. The **Privacy Rights Clearinghouse** (2010) maintains an online record of all types of security breaches at http://www.privacyrights.org/.

According to the website, there are a staggering number of security breaches in recent years. A few examples of the enormous problem are as follows:

- On October 21, 2010, a flash drive with 280,000 patient names, addresses, and personal health information for a health plan corporation was lost or stolen.
- On September 21, 2010, a backup tape drive with patient names, addresses, social security numbers, and diagnoses associated with an allergy clinic was reported as lost.

In reviewing the problem, a recurring theme involves the loss or theft of laptops and portable storage devices (flash drives, backup drives, etc.) Breaches were also a result of hacks, viruses, unauthorized access to digital records, and loss of paper records, although those types of breaches were much less common. In some cases, data on the devices were not encrypted.

The Health Information Technology for Economic and Clinical Health (HITECH) Act that went into effect in 2009 includes rules to ensure the privacy and security of health information. The HITECH Act defined "unsecured protected health information" as well as security "breach" (Department of Health and Human Services, 2009). Unsecured protected health information was defined as "protected health information that is not secured by a technology standard that renders protected health information unusable, unreadable, or indecipherable to unauthorized individuals and is developed or endorsed by a standards developing organization that is accredited by the American National Standards Institute (ANSI)" (p. 5). Breach was defined as "the unauthorized acquisition, access, use, or disclosure of protected health information which compromises the security or privacy of such information, except where an unauthorized person to whom such information is disclosed would not reasonably have been able to retain such information" (p. 6). As a result of the law, many healthcare agencies are taking additional steps to ensure health information privacy and security.

According to the Identify Theft Resource Center (2010), medical/healthcare ranked third (13.1%) behind business (41.8%) and education (15.7%) for the percentage of breaches in 2009 (see **Figure 25-1**). However, medical/healthcare ranked second (10,461,818) for the *number* of breaches (see **Figure 25-2**). The ramifications for those who were affected are potentially devastating if the persons in possession of that private information use it maliciously for personal gain. These examples give credence to concerns that we must do more to protect the private and confidential information of healthcare consumers.

To complicate the issue, the HITECH Act covers hospitals and their associated business associates (HIMSS Analytics, 2009). Large hospitals are at the greatest risk for data breaches. The business

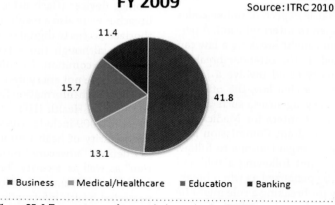

Figure 25-1 Percentage of records breached – 2009.

associates have been less aware of the privacy rulings of the HITECH Act but that must change. All individuals who are responsible for health information must adhere to procedures that keep the information secure and safe.

Prevention of Data Breaches

The prevention of data security breaches is paramount. The actions must be proactive and must involve all employees who have access to protected health information, not just the information technology staff. Healthcare organizations are using risk

assessment to mitigate data breaches. Components of risk assessment are as follows (HIMSS Analytics, 2009):

- Reviewing policies and procedures
- Analyzing system vulnerabilities
- Taking inventory of personally identifiable information (PII) and personal health information (PHI)
- Reviewing pertinent regulations
- Monitoring employee compliance
- Tracking external threats

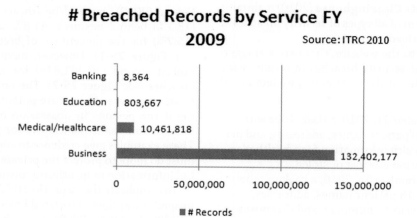

Figure 25-2 Number of records breached – 2009.

In addition to the risk assessment, healthcare agencies are taking measures to prevent data breaches. Data breaches are expensive. In 2009, the average cost of a lost laptop used in healthcare is $43,547 (Ponemon Institute, 2009). The replacement costs of the laptop are just one component of the other costs associated with the loss: cost of employee's time while attempting to recover the loss and reporting the incident, data breach cost, forensics and investigation cost, lost productivity cost, and legal and regulatory cost. According to one study, the average cost for *each* breached record was $204 in 2009 (Ponemon Institute, 2010). The average per-incident cost in 2009 was $6.75 million. Since the public is made aware of data breaches as well as each individual who is affected, reputation is yet another stimulus to prevent breaches. There are several methods that are currently in use. They include (HIMSS Analytics, 2009) the following:

- Performing employee privacy and security training
- Using data encryption software
- Performing an inventory of PII and PHI
- Using data loss prevention software
- Purchasing cyber liability insurance

Privacy and security training must include more than understanding the HIPAA. Employees must understand the differences between a system login, secure access, and data encryption. They must also have the ability and know-how to encrypt files and drives. They must also have plans to prevent the loss of portable computers and drives.

The differences between operating system login, secure access, and data encryption may not be taught in a nursing program or in orientation to a healthcare organization. A system login provides basic protection of personal data and files. To access e-mail accounts and other secure websites, additional logins may be required. A common misconception is that data sent from a secure e-mail server is protected. It is true that the recipient of an e-mail sent from a secure e-mail server does not "see" the message without an additional step to view the message on the encrypted e-mail server. However, if the e-mail recipient is not required to enter a user name and password to view the e-mail, the information is not fully protected.

Encryption software is available without a fee. Users can encrypt the entire computer hard drive or individual folders and files. Encryption software should be a requirement for all portable healthcare agency computers and associated portable devices. To locate encryption software for personal use, consider using an Internet search engine for software reviews on websites such as CNET or on online computer magazines.

Data loss prevention software can be used to track and locate lost/stolen portable computers. The loss-prevention software is proprietary and requires a subscription fee for use. The software is very sophisticated. After the computer is determined as lost or stolen, the owner would contact the software company and the police. When the lost/stolen computer connects to the Internet, the locator software sends a message to the recovery team. The recovery team works with the local police to find the missing computer. If the computer locator software includes data security features, all computer data can be deleted remotely from the missing computer. If the located software package includes geotechnology-locating software, the physical location of the computer can be identified using WiFi or global positioning system technology.

Data loss prevention can also be built into the hardware of a laptop. As an example, Intel manufactures a laptop with hardware that is integrated with data loss prevention software (Absolute Software, 2010). The software uses timers and "poison pills" to block the operating system boot and to secure data. The hardware component prevents computer use even if it is not connected to the Internet or the hard drive is replaced.

The healthcare agency's HIPAA officer and information technology personnel should be able to provide information on data encryption and data loss prevention software. All users of mobile devices must take a proactive stance to protect electronic health information. Inattention to data security can cause devastating results for healthcare consumers whose personal information has been confiscated maliciously by a cyber criminal.

The Limitations of HIPAA Protection

The general public and healthcare professionals have heard so much about the HIPAA that some have come to believe mistakenly that all health records are private and confidential. As an example, in the case of *Beard v. City of Chicago*, a paramedic was terminated from the city's fire department (*Beard v. City of Chicago*, 2004; Terry & Francis, 2007). The plaintiff pleaded that she was discriminated against and cited that others too had taken medical leaves of absence. The fire department happened to keep copies of medical records for all their employees. The fire department staff physician provided the medical records. These were patient records from physicians outside the fire department, with the patient's consent. The fire department resisted providing the records of other employees, citing HIPAA regulations. Of course, the court ruled that HIPAA was not applicable because the fire department did not fall into any one of the three categories that HIPAA covered; it was not a fee-for-service healthcare provider, a health plan, or a healthcare clearinghouse that electronically billed the CMS.

The HIPAA ruling has been criticized for not protecting all private health information. The HITECH Act serves to bridge the limitations of HIPAA. However, if the health information does not fall under HIPAA or the HITECH Act, the information is not protected. Examples include the patients' health record that they have on paper or on their personal computers or the health record on file at their health club.

Legal and Ethical Issues Associated with Telehealth

The Tenth Amendment to the U.S. Constitution guarantees states those powers neither delegated nor prohibited by the Constitution. Under this amendment, individual states have assumed the power to regulate healthcare practitioners for the protection of their citizens. No state, however, has authority over practice in another state. Transport nursing and telehealth both create problems with these assumptions. If a nurse practicing and licensed in state A provides nursing care to a client in state B in which she or he is not licensed, which state has the responsibility and authority to regulate the practice? Malpractice issues associated with telehealth are slowly being addressed. Perhaps the lack of urgency to address this issue relates to the quality of care rendered and lack of need.

The various state boards involved in regulating healthcare practitioners have all been wrestling with the various questions in this issue. Is the care provided at the location of the provider or the patient? Should the healthcare provider be licensed in the state, where the patient resides and the state where the provider is located? Both the American Telemedicine Association (ATA) and the American Medical Association support licensure regulation at the state level (ATA, 2007). The Federation of State Medical Boards developed a framework for regulating interstate practice in 1996. The framework created a "**restricted license**" for practicing telemedicine across state lines; however, the decision to adopt the license was left to the individual state boards. In 2007, the ATA issued a position statement that supported the collaborative agreements between states for licensure of health professionals practicing telemedicine within the United States.

The National Council of State Boards of Nursing (NCSBN) in 1998 endorsed the **Nurse Licensure Compact (NLC)** as a framework for regulating the interstate practice of nursing for RNs and LPNs/VNs (NCSBN, 2010a). Under this concept, nurses holding a valid license in one state could practice (both physical and electronic) in other states, according to the rules and regulations of the states. This is similar to a driving license in which one is licensed in one's state of residence but may drive in another state as long as, while driving in that state, they follow its laws. As of November 2010, 24 states were participating in the NLC (NCSBN, 2010b). The NLC stipulates that certain data about personal licensure be stored in a **Coordinated Licensure Information System** (see Box 25-1). In 2002, the NCSBN adopted a framework similar to the NLC for advance practice registered nurses (APRNs); however, it stipulated that the APRN compact could only be implemented in states that had endorsed the RN and LPN/VN compact.

Implications of Implantable Identification Devices

Use of the VeriMed™ implantable RFID microchip, originally produced by the VeriChip™ Corporation, discussed in Chapter 20, serves to polarize

BOX 25-1 Data Required by the Nurse Licensure Compact Coordinated Licensure Information System

- Name of the nurse
- Licensure jurisdiction(s)
- License expiration date(s)
- Licensure classification(s) and status(es)
- Public emergency and final disciplinary actions (defined by contributing state authority)
- Multistate licensure privileges status

individuals' beliefs. Supporters have praised it as a means of patient identification to expedite safe emergency care, especially for those who may not be able to speak for themselves. Opponents are concerned about issues of privacy and law. The implantable VeriMed™ microchip is about the size of a grain of rice and can be implanted under the skin using a disposable insertion device equipped with a hollow needle (see **Figure 25-3**) (VeriMed™, 2006). To identify the patient, the scanner is held about 3.5 inch from the chip insertion site, which is usually midway on the posterior upper right arm. After the chip is scanned using a handheld device (see **Figure 25-4**), the information is transmitted to a computer application, which displays the patient's medical record number, name, picture, address information, and allergies.

The implantable device was originally marketed for use with patients who have chronic diseases that may require emergency treatment, such as diabetes mellitus and stroke, cognitive impairment such as Alzheimer's disease, and those who have some type of implantable devices such as pacemakers and joint replacements. Proponents envisioned a chip containing a unique patient identifier that would allow healthcare providers access to the electronic health record stored in the NHIN. Supporters stated that the use of the implantable chip is voluntary. The implantable device for humans is no longer marketed since the VeriChip merger to form a company, PositiveID, in 2009. However, PositiveID continues to support patients and healthcare organizations where the chip is in use (PositiveID, n.d.).

The implantable RFID VeriChip was an issue for the American Civil Liberties Union and certain religious conservatives (Bonsor & Keener, 2007). Concerns have been voiced about the loss of individual civil liberties and the possibility of mandatory chipping of humans. Opponents saw chipping as just another way the government is stripping the privacy rights of citizens. In fact, Wisconsin's governor Jim Doyle signed a law against mandatory chipping in 2006 (Spychips.com, 2006). One can only surmise that ethical concerns about

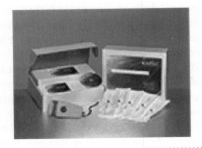

Figure 25-3 VeriMed physician starter kit.

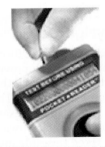

Figure 25-4 VeriMed microchip reader.

human chipping are the reason that the chip is no longer marketed.

Legal and Ethical Issues for the Use of Web 2.0 Applications

Although Web 2.0 applications such as Facebook, blogs, podcasts, video, and picture sharing open up a world of opportunities for sharing thoughts, opinions, and experiences, the use should be approached with measured caution. All shared media are open to the world, including attorneys, nursing colleagues, patients and families, charities, and advocacy associations. Nurse authors who share information on any type of social media must adhere to a set of ethical and legal guidelines. As an example, the owner of the blog is responsible for blog content (Zinn, 2007). Nurses should be familiar with their employer's policies and procedures for social media use by staff members and must avoid all negative references to healthcare agencies or other employers. Shared social media must never contain names or identifiers of patients, families, or other staff members. Moreover, it should not contain any type of information that might *indirectly* identify persons in the clinical setting. All postings should be respectful of others. Dark humor used by some nurses as a coping mechanism in stressful situations is not appropriate within the privacy of the break room and never appropriate in the public blog arena, although the disrespectful behavior has been reported in the literature (The dark world of blogs, 2005). The ethical principle, respect for others, must always be used by healthcare professionals that use Web 2.0 applications.

Copyright Law

The United States Copyright Office defines copyright as a law, Title 17, which provides protection to authorships that are original, thereby protecting intellectual property rights. The keyword in that definition is "original"; examples include books, music, movies, and software. Just about every imaginable **fixed tangible medium** is copyrighted whether or not the individual has applied

for copyright protection. Users should assume that all written or recorded mediums are copyrighted even if there is no © symbol. The copyright protection allows registered copyright owners the right to sue over infringements. The law is available online.

Fair Use

The law does allow for limited use of copyrighted material under the doctrine of **fair use** (U.S. Copyright Office, 2010). Unfortunately, the law provides little direction in determining what amount is fair to use; however, the consideration of the following four factors of fair use should be used as a guide:

1. The purpose and character of the use, for example, nonprofit, educational, news reporting, or commercial
2. The nature of the work, for example, fact, published, unpublished, imaginative
3. The amount of the work used, for example, small amount or a more substantial amount
4. The effect on the author or for permissions with widespread use, for example, little effect or competes with the owner's sales or royalties

Many colleges and universities have learning resources for copyright online. As an example, the University of Minnesota Libraries has a comprehensive, easy-to-use website about copyright at http://www.lib.umn.edu/copyright/. The website includes tools to assess fair use and information on how copyright applies to education.

Not Protected by Copyright

According to the U.S. Copyright Office, there are four exceptions to the copyright law.

- Work that is intangible, meaning that it is not well defined. Examples include unrecorded music or speeches put together without preparation that have never been recorded or written.
- Composites of information with no original author(s). Examples include calendars, height and weight charts, tape measures, and information in a telephone book.
- "Titles, names, short phrases, and slogans; familiar symbols or designs; mere variations of typographic ornamentation,

Table 25-2 Timeline for the Development of the Copyright Law

1440	1710	1790	1895	1978	1980	1998	2002
Gutenberg invented the printing press	Statute of Anne established copyright for owners	U.S. Congress passed 11th copyright law	Printing Act prohibited copyrighting government documents	Copyright protection extended to life of the author plus 50 yr	Copyright amended for computer programs	Copyright protection extended to life of the author plus 70 yr Digital Millennium Copyright Act of 1998	TEACH Act allowed for use of copyrighted works for distance learning[a]

[a]Applies only to nonprofit educational institutions.

From Taking the Mystery out of Copyright (2011) (http://www.loc.gov/teachers/copyrightmystery/text/files/).

lettering, or coloring; mere listings of ingredients or contents" (U.S. Copyright Office, 2010).

- "Ideas, procedure, methods, systems, processes, concepts, principles, discoveries, or devices, as distinguished from a description, explanation, or illustration" (U.S. Copyright Office, 2010).

How long is a copyright in effect? It just depends on when the copyright went into effect and what the status of the law was at that particular time.

History of Copyright

The history of copyright development continues to unfold (see **Table 25-2**). In early history, there really was no need for copyright law, as books were handwritten and very expensive to produce. The invention of the printing press by Johann Gutenberg in 1440 changed things. Authors lost ownership of their creations when the number of printing presses proliferated. In 1710, the Statute of Anne was passed in England to stop bookstores from reprinting books and reaping the associated profits. The Statute of Anne restored rightful ownership back to the authors when it made it illegal to reprint without the consent of the "author or proprietors" of the writings (Library of Congress, n.d.). Eighty years later, in 1790, the U.S. Congress passed the first copyright law protecting the ownership of charts, maps, and books for citizens of the United States for 14 years. If the authors were still living after that time, they could reapply for an extension of their copyright for another 14 years. In 1895, the law was amended to prohibit the copyright of government documents.

Copyright law continued to evolve, protecting poetry, drama, motion pictures, architecture, and music. In 1978, copyright protection was extended to the life of the author plus 50 years. In the meantime, computer technology was developing. The copyright law was amended in 1980 to address computer programs and again in 1998, extending copyright protection to the life of the author plus 70 years. A final significant milestone in the timeline was when the Technology, Education, and Copyright Harmonization (TEACH) Act was passed in 2002. The act allowed for the use of copyrighted material in distance education courses that are provided by accredited nonprofit educational institutions (Library of Congress, n.d.). There are some specific stipulations by this amendment, including that the copyrighted material be used under instructor supervision and that the content should be an integral component of the course.

TEACH Act

Although the **TEACH Act**, passed in 2002, relaxed the copyright law as it applies to distance learning and nonprofit educational institutions, what constitutes fair use is still blurred. In general, the proposed guidelines developed by the Conference on Fair Use (CONFU),[1] held from 1994 to 1996, are taken into consideration when applied to web-based courses (Dobbins, Souder, & Smith, 2005). According to the CONFU, guideline suggestions for

---

1 CONFU was an initiative of the U.S. National Information Infrastructure, which invited representatives from libraries, academic institutions, and industry to define fair use; however, a consensus was never reached.

fair use were as follows: text was 1,000 words or 10% of the work; images were 15 graphics or 10% of the total collection; music was 30 seconds or 10% of the total composition; and video was 3 minutes or 10% of the total video. Faculty and students should follow their institutional guidelines for the interpretation of copyright fair use. There may be differences of opinion about requirements for the use of copyrighted media in password-protected course management systems and general use on the web.

Plagiarism

Quoting a sentence, a few words, or paraphrasing an idea of another's work and giving credit to the author is considered fair use under copyright law; however, not giving the author credit is considered plagiarism (USG Online Library Learning Center, n.d.). Plagiarism is the same as stealing another's intellectual property and is unethical. The origin for the word "plagiarism" is Latin, and it means kidnapper (The University of Melbourne, 2010). If there is a question about the need to obtain permission for the use of a more substantial amount of the material, the author should be contacted for permission.

Use of word processors and the Internet makes it easy to avail the copy and paste functions when writing. Some writers may be tempted to steal the written words and use them as their own. What they may not realize is the Internet also provides a means for others to detect the plagiarism using tools like search engines or plagiarism detection software. Writers should take care when paraphrasing and quoting and use appropriate citation.

A periodic review of good tutorials on the topic is one way of becoming more conscientious about appropriate citation and referencing. The San Jose' public library at http://www.sjlibrary.org/services/literacy/info_comp/plagiarism.htm has good information on the topic and includes an animated tutorial. Most public, school, and college libraries have pertinent online resources on avoiding plagiarism.

Copyright Issues Associated with Google Book Search

In 2005, Google made the news when it launched the "Google Print" Library Project to scan books and make them searchable on the web (Google, 2010a). Google renamed the project "Google Book Search" later that year. The inception of the project began in 1996 with a research project at Stanford University by two computer science students, Sergey Brin and Larry Page. The Google search engine was the consequence of their research. The research entailed creating a search engine for book information.

Google Book Search at http://books.google.com/ provides a way to search, browse, purchase, or borrow a book from an online library (Google, 2010b). Google has collaborated with a number of large libraries internationally, including Columbia University Library, Harvard University, and Oxford University, for the liberty to scan their book collections and make that information available online. Proponents of Google Book Search state that Google is actually helping publishers and authors by making the books available to the public and that the project is assisting in the sale of books. It allows access to rare books that are otherwise unavailable and too fragile to be viewed by the public. The Google book project moves the access to books residing in a digital library to the user.

Those opposed to the project state that the Google Book Project is a copyright infringement and violates fair use practice. The problem is that Google has not asked for the permission of authors of copyrighted books. As a result, several lawsuits, including those by the Authors Guild, were filed against Google (*District Court Rules in Perfect 10 v. Google*, 2006). On November 19, 2009, the court ruled on an amended agreement to settle the lawsuit. As of November 2010, the agreement had not been finalized by the court (Google, 2010c).

The Google Book Search Help Center notes that Google does respect the copyright law by the way the books are displayed. If Google does not have permission from authors or publishers' participants, the only book information displayed is that similar to a card catalog citation. Google suggests that the use of Google books is analogous to visiting a bookstore and thumbing through the books. The Google Book project has challenged copyright law while at the same time changed to cohabitate with the intention of copyright law.

Summary

Informatics is associated with multiple legal and ethical issues. This chapter has focused on a few issues in detail that were not addressed in previous chapters. Ethical issues in informatics have been addressed by professional organizations' codes of ethics. As technology matures and evolves, professional codes of ethics must be updated to ensure that patient information issues are clearly addressed. Professionals are constantly being asked to balance the risks associated with patient autonomy and the greater good. The use of RFID technology using the implantable MediChip with patient and medical record number identification is an example that was explored. Telehomecare monitoring is another example that was provided. Does telehomecare monitoring invade the patient's privacy and/or does it provide unnecessary opportunities for security breaches?

There are strengths and weaknesses in the HIPAA law. The law was crafted with the introduction of the electronic transmission of patient record information for CMS billing. Because nurses and the general public have heard so much about the law, we have begun to develop misconceptions that HIPAA protects all patient information. There are concerns about the lack of adequate protection for electronic health records and personal health records. The HITECH Act was passed to provide additional security for health information.

Because boards for professional nursing practice rules vary from state to state, there is no uniform way to license practice that crosses state lines. The NCSBN did develop the compact licensure agreement, but the decision to have a licensure agreement is still at the state level. The implication for nursing is that the telehealth nurse may have to obtain a license to practice in each state practice area, if those states do not have an agreement. Nurses who practice across state lines must also be aware of the differences in state board rules and regulations for all states in which they are licensed.

Finally, there are legal and ethical issues associated with copyright. Copyright law has evolved so that it now covers all fixed tangible media whether or not the owner has paid a fee and registered their copyright with the government office. Copyright registration provides a mechanism for the owner to sue for infringements on unauthorized use. There is still no agreement on what constitutes fair use; the answers lie in "it depends" on when, where, why, and how the information is used. We are cautioned to notify the copyright owner to clarify any question about fair use. Even if the medium is not copyrighted, as is the case with government documents, we must always provide credit to the source to avoid plagiarism. Plagiarism is ethically wrong because it entails stealing the creation of others.

The legal and ethical aspects associated with informatics are very complex and constantly changing. Ignorance of the law has never provided any protection. What it means is that in addition to changes in practice, nurses must also stay abreast of the associated legal and ethical issues. It also means that to protect patient information, we must advocate for the necessary technology and policy changes.

APPLICATIONS AND COMPETENCIES

1. After reviewing the different codes of ethics discussed, select one for nursing and one other. Discuss the similarities and differences. Is nursing management of patient health information explicit enough? If not, make at least one recommendation for a change in the code.

2. Explore the Privacy Rights Clearinghouse website http://www.privacyrights.org/ on the subject of data breaches. Discuss at least three recent health information breaches and identify strategies to prevent those breaches.

3. Discuss the strengths and weaknesses of the HIPAA and the HITECH Act.

4. Identify one strategy that could be used to protect the privacy of the electronic health record and the personal health record. Explain how the strategy could be applied.

5. Discuss the pros and cons of the implantable patient identifier that uses RFID microchip technology.

6. Conduct a search for nurse-authored features that use Web 2.0 applications. Were you able to identify any legal or ethical issues for the content that was displayed? Discuss your findings.

7. Compare and contrast the use of copyright law when writing a journal article versus the design of a personal blog space or Facebook posting.

REFERENCES

Absolute Software. (2010). *Built-in protection in laptop PCs improves compliance with new healthcare rules.* Retrieved November 3, 2010, from http://www.intel.com/Assets/PDF/whitepaper/health-323461.pdf

ATA. (2007, March). *Licensure portability.* Retrieved November 4, 2010, from http://www.americantelemed.org/files/public/policy/Licensure_Portability.pdf

Beard v. City of Chicago, 299 F. Supp. 2d 872 C.F.R. (N.D. Ill, 2004).

Bonsor, K., & Keener, C. (2007, November 5). *How RFID works.* Retrieved November 4, 2010, from http://electronics.howstuffworks.com/gadgets/high-tech-gadgets/rfid.htm#

Curtin, L. L. (2005). Ethics in informatics: The intersection of nursing, ethics, and information technology. *Nursing Administration Quarterly, 29*(4), 349–352.

The dark world of blogs. (2005). *Nursing Standard, 19*(50), 12.

Department of Health and Human Services. (2009). *Guidance specifying the technologies and methodologies that render protected health information unusable, unreadable, or indecipherable to unauthorized individuals for purposes of the breach notification requirements under Section 13405 of Title XIII (Health Information Technology for Economic and Clinical Health Act of 2009).* Retrieved November 3, 2010, from http://www.hhs.gov/ocr/privacy/hipaa/understanding/coveredentities/hitechrfi.pdf

District Court Rules in Perfect 10 v. Google. (2006, February 17). *Tech Law Journal.* Retrieved from http://www.techlawjournal.com/topstories/2006/20060217b.asp

Dobbins, W. N., Souder, E., & Smith, R. M. (2005). Living with fair use and TEACH: A quest for compliance. *CIN: Computers, Informatics, Nursing, 23*(3), 120–124.

Gallup Inc. (2009, November 22). *Honest/ethics in professions.* Retrieved November 1, 2010, from http://www.gallup.com/poll/1654/honesty-ethics-professions.aspx

Google. (2010a). *About Google books.* Retrieved November 4, 2010, from http://books.google.com/googlebooks/about.html

Google. (2010b). *Library partners.* Retrieved November 4, 2010, from http://books.google.com/googlebooks/partners.html

Google. (2010c). *Google books settlement agreement.* Retrieved November 4, 2010, from http://books.google.com/googlebooks/agreement/

HIMSS Analytics. (2009, November). *2009 HIMSS Analytics report: Evaluating HITECH's impact on healthcare privacy and security.* Retrieved November 3, 2010, from http://www.himssanalytics.org/docs/ID_Experts_111509.pdf

Identify Theft Resource Center. (2010, March 24). *2009 data breach stats.* Retrieved November 3, 2010, from http://www.idtheftcenter.org/ITRC%20Breach%20Stats%20Report%202009.pdf

Library of Congress. (n.d.). *Timeline of copyright milestones.* Retrieved November 4, 2010, from http://www.loc.gov/teachers/copyrightmystery/text/files/

NCSBN. (2010a). *About.* Retrieved November 5, 2010, from https://www.ncsbn.org/156.htm

NCSBN. (2010b). *Map of NLC states.* Retrieved November 6, 2010, from https://www.ncsbn.org/158.htm

Ponemon Institute. (2009, April 22). *The cost of a lost laptop.* Retrieved November 3, 2010, from http://www.ponemon.org/local/upload/fckjail/generalcontent/18/file/Cost%20of%20a%20Lost%20Laptop%20White%20Paper%20Final%202.pdf

Ponemon Institute. (2010, January 25). *Ponemon study shows the cost of a data breach continues to increase.* Retrieved November 3, 2010, from http://www.ponemon.org/news-2/23

PositiveID. (n.d.). *HealthID.* Retrieved November 4, 2010, from http://www.positiveidcorp.com/health-id.html

Privacy Rights Clearinghouse. (2010, October 29). *Chronology of data breaches.* Retrieved November 3, 2010, from http://www.privacyrights.org/data-breach/new

Simpson, R. L. (2006). Ethics and information technology: How nurses balance when integrity and trust are at stake. *Nursing Administration Quarterly, 30*(1), 82–87.

Spychips.com. (2006, May 31). *Wisconsin bans forced human RFID chipping.* Retrieved November 4, 2010, from http://www.spychips.com/press-releases/verichip-wisconsin-ban.html

Terry, N., & Francis, L. P. (2007). Ensuring the privacy and confidentiality of electronic health records. *University of Illinois Law Review.* Retrieved from http://www.law.uiuc.edu/lrev/publications/2000s/2007/2007_2/Terry.pdf

The University of Melbourne. (2010, October 25). *Academic honesty & plagiarism.* Retrieved November 4, 2010, from http://academichonesty.unimelb.edu.au/plagiarism.html

U.S. Copyright Office. (2010, August). *Copyright basics.* Retrieved November 4, 2010, from http://www.copyright.gov/circs/circ01.pdf

USG Online Library Learning Center. (n.d.). *Plagiarism.* Retrieved November 4, 2010, from http://www.usg.edu/galileo/skills/unit08/credit08_03.phtml

VeriMed™. (2006). *VeriMed™ patient identification.* Retrieved August 30, 2011, from http://www.verimedinfo.com/

Zinn, J. (2007). The benefits and problems of using health care blogs. *Nurse Author and Editor Newsletter, 17*(3). Retrieved from http://www.nurseauthoreditor.com/article.asp?id=87

APPENDIX A

Computer Hardware Overview

Key Terms

Black hat hacker	Permanent memory
Bug	Physical
Bus	Random access memory
Cold boot	(RAM)
Compatibility	Read-only memory (ROM)
Driver	Reboot
Hacker	Surge protector
Lithium-ion batteries	Temporary memory
Logical	Universal serial bus (USB)
Nickel–cadmium batteries	Warm boot
Nickel–metal hydride battery	White hat hacker
Object	

In healthcare education, the purpose and parts of a stethoscope are explained before how to use the stethoscope to listen to heart and lung sounds. To be effective in using the stethoscope, a clinician needs to know when to use the bell and when to use the diaphragm. In the same way, it is imperative to have some understanding of how and when to use the tool of informatics, the computer.

 ## The Computer

A complete computer system is the integration of human input and information resources using hardware and software. In computer terms, hardware refers to objects such as disks, disk drives, monitors, keyboards, speakers, printers, mice, boards, chips, and the computer itself. Software includes programs that give instructions to the computer that make the machine useful. Information resources are data that the computer manipulates. Human input refers to the entire spectrum of human involvement, including deciding what is to be input and how it is to be processed as well as evaluating output and deciding how it should be used. This appendix focuses on the computer and the associated hardware components.

Computer Misconceptions

When computers were new, there were many fears and misconceptions about using them. Some of these were computers can think, computers require mathematical genius to be used, and computers make mistakes (Perry, 1982). Today there are other misconceptions, perhaps born of familiarity, which can be dangerous to users. It is important to understand that computers cannot think, and they are not smart. Incidents like the one in which Deep Blue (the nickname given to an IBM computer specially designed to play chess) won a chess game against world champion Garry Kasparov led to such misperceptions (Computer History Museum, 2011). Consider the game of chess. Although there are many possible combinations, there are a given set of moves, rules, and goals that make it a perfect stage to display the potential of computers. Deep Blue is a very powerful computer, capable of quickly analyzing hundreds of millions of possible moves and responding according to rules (known as algorithms) that were part of the software that beat Kasparov. It made use of these qualities to beat Kasparov. It did not use thinking in the human sense. To read more about the history of computer chess, go to http://www.computerhistory.org/chess/index.php.

The thought that only mathematical geniuses can use computers, although just as false, continues to flourish. This belief is linked to the development of the first computers as a means to "crunch numbers," or process mathematical equations. Hence, in colleges and universities, many computer departments are still housed in, or closely related to, the departments of mathematics. It did not take experts long to translate the mathematical concepts into everyday language, an accomplishment that made the computer available to everyone, regardless of level of proficiency in math.

The last myth, that computers make mistakes, makes it a wonderful excuse for human error. This was well illustrated by a cartoon in the early 1990s that showed a man saying, "It's wonderful to be able to blame my mistakes at the office on the computer, I think I'll get a personal computer." Computers act on the information they are given. As one humorist said, "Computers are designed to DWIS, or Do What I Say." As many a user will tell you, they resist with great determination any inclination to DWIM, or "Do What I Mean!" Unlike a colleague to whom you only need to give partial instructions because the person is able to fill in the rest, a computer requires complete, definitive, black-and-white directions. Unlike humans, computers cannot perceive that a colon and semicolon are closely related, and in many cases, a computer believes that an uppercase letter and a lower case letter are as different as the letter A from the letter X. This is known as case sensitivity. There are no "almosts" with a computer.

Computer Characteristics

A computer accomplishes many things that are otherwise impossible. When programmed properly, it is superb in remembering and processing details, calculating accurately, printing reports, facilitating editing documents, and sparing users many repetitive, tedious tasks, which frees time for more productive endeavors. Remember, however, that computers are not infallible. Being electronic, they are subject to electrical problems. Humans build computers, program them, and enter data into them. For these reasons, many situations can cause error and frustration. Two of the most common challenges with computers are "glitches" and the "garbage in, garbage out" (GIGO) principle. That is, if data input has errors, then the output will be erroneous.

Anyone who had been using a computer when it crashed or "went down" may have experienced a guilty feeling that she or he did something wrong. Unless she or he were purposely engaged in something destructive, that person did not cause the crash; she or he just found a flaw in the system that was inadvertently created by the programmer(s). There are times, however, when crashes occur for seemingly no reason. Computers, regardless of their manufacturer, will sometimes, for unknown reasons, perform in a totally unexpected manner (Perry, 1982). This is as true today as when computers were new. The good news is that this is much less apt to happen despite the complexity of today's computers.

Given the complexity of programming, it is not unusual to find "bugs" or glitches in a new system. You may have experienced a problem when a new information system was installed at your place of work. If you should be the unfortunate one who discovers a bug, you can help the programmers to correct it by carefully communicating the actions you took that preceded the problem (as far as you can remember), and the exact result. If an error number was presented on the screen, be sure to include this in your communication. Finding the problem is usually harder than fixing it. The hardest mistakes to fix are those that cannot be recreated.

Digital Native or Digital Immigrant?

Are you a digital native or digital immigrant? Marc Prenky (Prensky, 2001) states that digital natives grew up with computers. They are comfortable with computers, surfing the Internet, emailing, gaming, and social networking. Prensky asserts that digital natives are "native speakers" of the digital computer language. Digital natives are very comfortable with using the Internet as a primary source of information.

On the other hand, digital immigrants were born before computers were popular. Prensky says that digital immigrants have a "digital language accent," for example, printing out email or turning to the Internet as a secondary source of information. If you have not grown up using computers, your attitude about their use may range from curiosity and excitement to complete dislike, frustration, and fear.

Addressing fears takes time for both a trainer and the individual experiencing the fears. One-on-one sessions for the person affected may be necessary and save time in the long run by preventing frantic calls to the help center. Studies show that the learning patterns of those afraid of computers can be improved by treating the bodily symptoms of anxiety and providing distracting thought patterns (Bloom, 1985). Techniques such as teaching relaxation methods before starting any hands-on training often helps, as does giving the anxious trainee something to repeat internally, such as, "You're in control, not the computer." If you can reframe your negative feelings to positive feelings of excitement about discovery and new opportunities, it will be possible for you to overcome your anxieties.

Other helpful techniques include recognizing and accepting fear. One method is to have trainees check off from a list of possible feelings (e.g., panicky, lost, curious) those that they are feeling, a practice that can help them face their fears. Inherent in all these terrors is the fear of failure and of looking incompetent in front of their peers. This may be especially evident in people who see themselves as having a high degree of competence in their profession and to whom people look for answers. Therefore, placing themselves in a learning situation can be very threatening to their self-image.

If you are calling your information services (IS) department for help, it is sometimes difficult to understand what you are being told. One remedy for this is to say, "I just don't get it. Could you please explain it like you were talking to your non-computer-using mother?" We all tend to downgrade the knowledge that we possess, believing that others also possess this knowledge, which causes us to provide explanations that are unclear. IS department personnel are just as susceptible to this condition as nurses are when we talk with our patients.

Types of Computers

The progress in computers is measured by generations, each of which grew out of a new innovation (**Table A-1**). Computer sizes vary from supercomputers intended to process large amounts of data for one user at a time to small palmtop computers. Each type has its niche in healthcare. However, it is becoming increasingly difficult to classify the different types of computers, because smaller ones are taking on the characteristics of their bigger brothers as the amount of space needed for processing lessens.

Supercomputers

Technically, supercomputers are the most powerful type of computers, if power is judged by the ability to do numerical calculations. Supercomputers can process hundreds of millions of instructions per second. They are used in applications that require extensive mathematical calculations, such as weather forecasts, fluid dynamic calculations, and nuclear energy research. Supercomputers are designed to execute only one task at a time; hence, they devote all their resources to this one situation. This gives them the speed they need for their tasks.

Mainframes

The first computers were large, often taking up an entire room. They were known as mainframes and were designed to serve many users and run many programs at the same time. These computers continue to be the backbone of many hospital information systems.

Servers

A server can be a mainframe or personal computer (PC) that is connected with other computers or terminals for the purpose of sharing databases, programs, and files. Server software allows these computers to perform functions like email exchange or off site storage of files.

Thin Clients

Thin clients are today's version of the videotext terminal. These are computers without a hard drive and with limited, if any, processing power. Besides costing much less, thin clients do not need to be upgraded when new software is made available because they do not contain any applications. Because they do no processing, older PCs can function in this capacity instead of being retired.

TABLE A-1 The Five Generations of Computers

Generations Dates Innovation
1. 1940–1956 vacuum tubes
2. 1956–1963 transistors
3. 1964–1971 integrated circuits
4. 1971–present microprocessors
5. Present and beyond artificial intelligence, which includes voice recognition. Includes devices that respond to natural language.

Webopedia Staff. (2010, October 8). *The five generations of computers.* Retrieved January 27, 2011, from http://www.webopedia.com/DidYouKnow/Hardware_Software/2002/FiveGenerations.asp

Personal or Single-User Computers

PCs are designed for one individual to use at a time. PCs are based on microprocessor technology that enables manufacturers to put an entire processing (controlling) unit on one chip, thus permitting the small size. When PCs were adopted in business, they freed users from the resource limitations of the mainframe computer and allowed data processing staff to concentrate on tasks that needed a large system. Today, although capable of functioning without being connected to a network, in businesses including healthcare, PCs are usually connected or networked to other PCs or servers. They still process information, but when networked, they can also share data.

In information systems, PCs often handle the tasks of entering and retrieving information from the central computer or server, although thin clients may be used for this purpose instead. When a full PC is available on the unit, personnel can use application programs such as word processing. PCs are available in many different formats such as a desktop or tower model and mobile Internet devices (MIDs).

Desktop and Towers. The original PC was a desktop model. You are probably familiar with these. The traditional desktop computer has a computer processor, monitor, and mouse. The computer processor component may be placed vertically on the desktop, inside a desk cabinet, or built into the monitor. Some desktop computers classified as "all-in-ones" have the processor built into the monitor and use a wireless keyboard and mouse for data input. A touchscreen monitor may be used for data input instead of a mouse.

Mobile Internet Devices. The term for the class of mobile computers is MIDs or mobile Internet devices. As computer usage became popular, people found that they needed the files and software on their computer to accomplish tasks away from their desks. The first mobile computer that made this practical was really more transportable than portable. Developed in the 1980s, it was about the size of a desktop and had a built-in monitor. Toward the end of the 1980s, the transportables were replaced by true portables: laptops, or computers small enough to fit on one's lap. As technology continued to place more information on a chip, mobile computers became smaller. Mobile computers are commonly classified as laptops, tablet PCs, tablets (includes e-book readers), netbooks, personal digital assistants (PDAs), and smartphones.

Laptops have some drawbacks. The screen is usually smaller than the one in a desktop, and the resolution may not be as crisp. Keyboards are also smaller. The mouse, or pointing and selecting device, can be a button the size of a pencil eraser in the middle of the keyboard, or a small square on the user end of the keyboard, or a small ball embedded in the keyboard. Some users purchase docking stations for their laptops. The laptop can be placed in the docking station (may be called a port replicator, or notebook extender), which is connected to hardware such as a larger monitor, keyboard, separate mouse, and printer. A port replicator enables the user to have access to these devices when at their desk, but makes it easy to remove the laptop and enjoy its portability, albeit, without the hardware connected to the docking station. Some healthcare organizations use laptops for point-of-care data entry at the bedside or any place where care is delivered.

The tablet PC a is variation of the laptop. The tablet PC has a screen that swivels and folds so that it looks like a book. A tablet PC also has a touchscreen and includes a special stylus for pen writing capabilities. The pen writing capability has handwriting recognition that converts it to text.

A tablet is a computer with only a flat touchscreen. Instead of a keyboard or mouse, data is input using a fingertip or stylus. Many smartphones, e-book readers, and media players are classified as tablets. A tablet often has a much longer battery life than a laptop or tablet PC.

The netbook, a scaled down version of a laptop, was introduced in 2007. The netbook is lighter and less expensive than a laptop. They lack an optical drive (CD/DVD capabilities), have less power, smaller monitors and keyboards than a laptop PC. The screen sizes vary from 5 from 10 inches and the weight ranges from 2 to 3 pounds.

Batteries

One thing that all portable electronic devices share is a need for a rechargeable battery. Keeping

batteries charged in healthcare agencies can be a difficult process. A multitude of devices we use in healthcare are battery powered, for example, intravenous (IV) controllers, pumps, dopplers, otoscopes, cardiac defibrillators, laptop PCs, and medication carts. Selecting equipment with the right battery and caring for it properly will increase the battery life and length of time it will power a device. This time is related not only to the care a battery receives but also to the type, size, and age of the battery. As batteries age, they lose the ability to retain a full charge (Wikipedia Contributors, 2010a). There are several types of batteries: nickel–cadmium, nickel–metal hydride, lead–acid, and lithium-ion. With the exception of the lead–acid battery, any of these can be found in mobile computing devices (Buchmann, 2006b).

Nurses often find themselves having to make decisions about the purchase of equipment that is battery powered. To that end, we need to be knowledgeable about the various types of batteries. Two resources that extend the information included in this textbook are How Stuff Works (http://www.howstuffworks.com/battery.htm) and Wikipedia (http://en.wikipedia.org/wiki/Battery_(electricity)).

Nickel-Based Batteries

The **nickel–cadmium batteries** were the first batteries used in laptops. They are relatively heavy and need to be fully discharged occasionally to avoid decreasing the usage time. This need is a result of crystalline formation on their cells, which decreases the length of time the battery can be used. Their life can be extended if they are fully discharged once every 3 months. They are useful where extended temperature range will be experienced and long life is needed. The **nickel–metal hydride battery**, an outgrowth of the nickel–cadmium battery, may be found in mobile phones and laptop computers. Although at first it was thought that it did not suffer from the same memory problem as the nickel–cadmium battery, it has been found to have this problem too, although to a lesser degree.

Lithium-Ion Batteries

The trend today is toward **lithium-ion batteries**. These batteries have a typical life span of 2 to 3 years whether or not they are used because of loss of capacity through cell oxidation, although they are continually being improved (Brain, 2006; Buchmann, 2006a). These batteries respond better if they are only partially discharged, and frequent full discharges are avoided. To maintain the battery life, charge the battery more often or use a larger battery. A lithium-ion battery must have a protection circuit to shut off the power source when it is fully charged. Overheating may result if this is not present and can cause batteries to explode. Since about 2003, the search for cheap batteries has produced a flood of counterfeit batteries that do not have this protection. This is why manufacturers advise customers to buy only approved batteries.

Battery life is documented with watt hours. MIDs often use lithion-ion with either an unspecified number or three, six, or nine cells; the greater the number of cells, the heavier the battery. The actual battery life will probably be less than noted in the manufacturer's information (Lyons, 2009). Batteries are tested in ideal conditions, with a minimal processor speed, the screen dimmed, and wireless turned off. In reality, users that use devices with lithion-ion batteries prefer features that diminish the battery life.

Battery Self-Discharging

If you have ever used a laptop, you may have noticed that after it has been unplugged for a while, the battery charging light comes on when you plug the computer into an electrical outlet. This is a result of self-discharge, from which all batteries suffer (Buchmann, 2005). Interestingly, it is highest right after charge. The nickel-based batteries lose 10% to 15% of capacity in the first 24 hours after charge, which levels off to 10% to 15% a month. Lithium-ion batteries self-discharge only about 5% in the first 24 hours and then 1% to 2% in a month. Higher temperatures will increase the self-discharge rate which doubles roughly with every 18°F (10°C) rise in temperature. Leaving the battery in a hot car will create a noticeable energy loss.

 PC Systems

Desktop and laptop computers consist of at least three components: a display screen, a keyboard for entering data, and the system components generally housed in a rectangular box often referred to as the CPU (central processing unit). These parts provide the input, processing, and output functions needed by a computer.

Surge Protectors

Computers, whether mobile or stationary, need a continuous nonvariable supply of power. Their operation can be affected by a power surge. Although the power surge may be generated by the electrical company, in some homes this can occur when a large electrical device such as an air conditioner comes on. To protect against this, all computers come with some degree of built-in surge protection. When this protection is inadequate, the motherboard, or heart of the computer, may be damaged. For this reason, it is a good idea to use a separate, high-quality **surge protector**. If you use a DSL (digital subscriber line) or a modem to connect to the Internet, use a surge protector that allows you to connect the telephone line since the phone line can also conduct high voltages. Some surge protectors include a battery backup which will allow you time to power down the computer in the case of a power outage. No surge protector, however, will protect from a lightning strike. Some users elect to unplug their computer and monitor altogether during thunderstorms.

How a Computer Works

Did you ever wonder how a computer works? It requires a combination of components that are connected together with communication and power cables. The processing part of a computer consists of a motherboard, a CPU, bus, and cards. Consider watching a video that provides a tour of the inside of a PC at http://videos.howstuffworks.com/howstuffworks/23-computer-tour-video.htm.

Motherboard

The motherboard is the main circuit board with connecting points that determines the type of computer and power supply that the computer can support. The motherboard typically contains the CPU, the basic input–output system (BIOS), memory, and connections to all ports, expansion slots, disks, and all input-output devices. It contains the chip that is the microprocessor or CPU.

A chip is a small box with prongs that enables it to be attached to the motherboard.

CPU/Microprocessor

The CPU is the heart or brains of the computer; it controls what the computer does. Some computer types such as supercomputers or mainframes may have many CPUs. PCs, however, have a single CPU that consists of a single chip called a microprocessor. The CPU consists of an arithmetic logic unit (ALU), a control unit, and some memory registers. The ALU performs all arithmetic and logical operations such as calculating a formula or comparing two items. The control unit directs the flow of information in the computer. It can be thought of as a combination traffic officer and switchboard. It gets instructions from memory, interprets them, directs them, and makes certain they are properly executed. It performs these operations in nanoseconds (one billionth of a second) so that to a user the results appear instantaneous.

These chips, smaller and thinner than a baby's fingernail, come in different varieties. They may be referred to by manufacturer and number or name (e.g., Pentium Intel Current, Athlon AMD Pentium, and Celeron Intel.). All chips with the same number or name are not the same, however. Differences may include power management modifications for battery-run computers or the speed at which the chip accomplishes its tasks. The processing speed is referred to as the clock speed of the computer. The clock speed determines how often a pulse of electricity "cycles" or circulates through the circuits, and hence, how fast information is processed. The more cycles per given time period, the greater the processing speed will be. Clock speed is measured in hertz, which is one cycle per second. Computers today are capable of speeds in the gigahertz (GHz) range (one billion hertz).

The speed of processing is also affected by what is called "word size." This is not related to a word as we know it in reading, but to the number of bits that a computer processes at one time. If a CPU processes 32 bits of information at a time, it is said to be a 32-bit computer, and its word size is 16 bits. A computer that processes 64 bits of information at one time is a 64-bit computer and has a word size of 64 bits. The 64-bit computer, of course, is faster and handles large amounts of RAM (randam access memory) more effectively than the 32-bit computer.

The Bus

The speed with which the computer returns results is affected not only by the speed of the CPU but also by the speed and width of a device called a **bus**. Like a bus one sees on a highway, a computer bus is a mode of transportation for data. Physically, a bus is a collection of wires that transmits data from one part of a computer to another, such as from the CPU to the main memory. It also transmits information about where the data should go. Like a CPU, the bus is measured by the number of bits it transfers at one time and the speed of this transfer.

Cards

Many of the functions that a computer performs are regulated by cards that are inserted into slots on the motherboard. These cards, which like the motherboard are printed circuit boards, are used for things such as the video display, RAM, sound, telephone modem, network connections, and expansion.

How a Computer Works with Data

A computer does all its work on the basis of whether electronic circuits are on or off. In giving information to the computer, these conditions are represented by a one (1) if the circuit is on and a zero (0) if it is off. Because only 1s and 0s are used, the data are said to be binary system data (Roberts, 2009). The decimal system with which we are familiar is base 10, that is, we start expressing our numbers by reusing the last numbers in multiples of 10, for example, the number 11 reuses the 1 from the 10 and adds the 1, 20 reuses the 2 and adds numbers zero to nine, etc. In a binary system, which is base 2, numbers are reused starting with 3. Besides the binary system, two other numbering systems may be seen in computers: octal or base 8, and hexadecimal, which is base 16. To learn more about the binary system, go to a tutorial at http://www.youtube.com/watch?v=ETsfylK7kzM.

Bits and Bytes

The amount of data that can be represented by one circuit is formally called a binary digit and is usually referred to as a bit. Bits hold only one of two values: 0 or 1. They are the smallest unit of information that a machine can hold. When eight of these bits are combined, there is enough memory, or on-off switches, to represent a letter, number, or other character. This amount of memory is called a byte.

ASCII

To make it possible for data to be exchanged between computers, standards were set very early in the evolution of the computer for how the on-off switches in a byte would be used for each character. The standard for PCs is the American Standard Code for Information Interchange (ASCII). Under this system, each character on the keyboard is represented by a number.

Memory

To work with data, to store it, and report it to users, computers need two types of memory: temporary and permanent. **Temporary memory** is what the computer uses to hold program instructions and data that are being created, edited, or used by a user. Anything temporary that the memory contains is deleted when the computer is turned off, unless it is a permanent resident on the computer such as software, or saved by the user when it is something the user created. **Permanent memory** or non-volatile memory is a form of storage. Permanent memory saves any changes in the software or files created by the user when the power is turned off.

Temporary Memory (Primary Memory)

Temporary memory is available for the software you use and the files you create. A file is anything that you create on a computer, including a word-processed document or a presentation slideshow. There are two types of temporary memory. One is the memory that you, the user, have access to for the software you are using and the files that you create and is called **random access memory (RAM)**. The second type is preprogrammed and unchangeable by the user and is known as **read-only memory (ROM)**.

Random Access Memory. RAM is the working or primary memory of the computer. It is temporary, or what is termed "volatile," and everything in it is lost when the computer is turned off unless it has been stored or saved. RAM is the memory area, where the software that is stored on a drive, often the main internal storage device of the computer known as a hard drive, is put when you ask to use a program such as a word processor, or a Web browser. RAM also stores the files on which you are working. When you close the program, it is erased from memory, but not from its storage place. To preserve the files that you create using a program, you must save the file before closing it or the program, or shutting down the computer.

When you open a program or a file, you are not removing it from its storage place but asking that a copy of the program or file be placed in RAM for your use. The original, however, remains on the storage device unless you give a command to delete it. What is not in storage, however, is any change you make to a file after it has been saved. That is, if you retrieve a file from storage and make changes to it, what is in storage is the file that was there when you retrieved it or last saved it. Thus, you must resave a file for it to reflect what is currently in RAM. What does not need to be resaved is the application program because you have generally not changed it, but just used it. In the rare instance that you have made any changes to the program itself, such as changed what it contained on the top of the screen, you will be asked if you want to save these changes. If you like your changes, click Yes.

The amount of RAM that is needed depends on how the computer will be used. If all a computer will be used for is accessing the Web and perhaps a little word processing, it will need only enough RAM to accommodate the operating system's requirements and the applications. Users who routinely keep several programs open at once will want more than the minimum amount of RAM. When the RAM is inadequate to the tasks it is being called on to do, the computer slows down. This is caused by the computer having to exchange parts of the application that are in RAM with the parts that are on a disk that are now needed. Because this exchange is slower than the immediate access that RAM provides, the program slows down. Graphical programs such as picture-editing programs and many games require a lot of RAM; hence, those who wish to use a computer for this purpose will want as much RAM as possible. Because the amount of RAM that a computer can access is dependent on the processor, one needs to have this information before deciding which computer to buy. A good rule of thumb is to buy as much RAM as the processor in the computer will support.

Read-Only Memory. The second type of memory, ROM, can only be read by the computer; no information can be written to it and no information can be erased or deleted from it. The users' only awareness of ROM may be when they see information flashing on the screen when the computer is turned on. The information in ROM is written to a chip before it is installed at the factory. It has no relationship to programs installed by a user or any data that a user creates on the computer. The set of instructions it contains are part of the processor of the computer. ROM is used to store critical programs that all computers need, such as the program that boots (starts) the computer. The BIOS, built-in software that determines what the computer can do without accessing any additional software, is usually found on a ROM chip. The last instruction that the BIOS (basic input/output system) executes is to look for an operating system and install it.

Cache. Cache, which is pronounced "cash," is a special high-speed storage mechanism that permits rapid access to frequently used data. It may be an independent storage device, or a reserved section of main memory. Cache is often used by hard drives, CPUs, and Web browsers. You may have heard the term "cache" in connection to your Web browser's memory or history of recently viewed pages. Two types of caching are commonly used in PCs: memory caching and disk caching. In memory caching, a special high-speed static RAM known as SRAM contains the data. In disk caching, the hard drive's hardware disk buffer stores the most recently accessed data from the disk. When there is a need to access data from the disk, the computer first checks the disk cache, because retrieving data from there is faster than from the disk.

Measurement of Memory

The measurement of memory of any type is based on the byte, or the amount of memory required to store one character, such as the letter "L." It is expressed by placing prefixes in front of the word byte that denote increments of approximately 1,000. A kilobyte is 1,024 bytes, whereas a megabyte is more than 1 million bytes. Although the prefixes in Table A-2 are from the decimal system, the words they create do not represent numbers divisible by 10 because the amounts are translations from the binary numbering system. The same prefixes are used to describe the number of hertz or the measurement of the computer's clock speed. Thus a GHz would be 1,073,741,824 Hz or cycles per second.

Secondary or "Permanent" Memory

Secondary memory provides a form of permanent storage for a computer. This type of storage is permanent only in that the user determines whether or not this data will be retained. Except for files in ROM, a user can delete any data in secondary memory. For many programs and users, this type of storage is on the computer's hard disk, (a large storage device internal to PCs). For those who might be concerned that they would accidentally delete an application program from the hard disk, be assured that this action requires a great deal of effort and is very unlikely to be done accidentally. Additionally, a copy of any application programs on the computer should either be on another storage mechanism that is not attached to the computer, or available from the Internet. Many devices are used to provide storage. They employ either magnetic or optical methods of storing data.

Table A-2 The Bytes	
Name	**Number of Bytes**
Kilobyte	1024
Megabyte	1024^2
Gigabyte	1024^3
Terabyte	1024^4
Petabyte	1024^5
Exabyte	1024^6
Zettabyte	1024^7
Yottabyte	1024^8

Magnetic Storage. Magnetic storage takes advantage of the on-off capacity for bytes that a computer uses and stores information by making the polarity of a magnetic field positive for the 1 or "on" bytes and negative for the 0 or "off" bits. Audio and videotape, examples of earlier magnetic storage devices have since been replaced. The computer hard drive is a type of magnetic storage device still currently in use (Wikipedia Contributors, 2010b).

Hard Drive

What is called a hard drive is a large capacity storage disk. Hard drive storage capacity in today's PCs is measured in gigabytes (GB) and terabytes (TB) storage. On home PCs and many that are found in agencies, a hard drive, which is internal to the computer, is installed. Usually named "C:" this drive contains the operating system. Users often install the software that they have purchased on this hard drive, although some will use a program from another source. All hard drives must be formatted for use with the operating system. See Box A-1 for information about maintaining a hard drive.

External hard drives or storage devices that can be connected to the computer when desired are also available. The portable drives are often used for backing up information on the computer and storing pictures and video. External hard drives usually come preformatted for use with Windows and/or Mac operating systems. When selecting an external hard drive, look for storage space, backup/synchronization software, and transfer speeds. The latest drives use USB 3.0 technology (discussed later in this appendix). Information stored on internal hard drives uses the same method as on smaller removable disks.

Flash Drive. A flash drive is a flash memory storage device that plugs into a universal serial bus (USB) port. One can think of it as both the drive and the disk in one, although the similarity ends there. Flash memory is memory that can be erased and reprogrammed in units termed "blocks." It differs from the more common type of erasable memory by erasing and rewriting these blocks in a "flash" from which its name is derived (Schulz, 2007; Wikipedia Contributors, 2010c). Disks write and rewrite using individual bytes. Flash drives are popular because they are rewritable, can hold up to several gigabytes of information, and are small, fast, reliable, relatively inexpensive per byte, and portable. They are also easily lost!

One caution with flash drives, including card readers for cameras: unlike other nontemporary memory, a flash drive is the drive and disk in one small piece of hardware. Consequently, the power that they need is derived from the computer itself. Although they can be inserted into a USB port with the computer on, they should be removed with more thought and never in the middle of being written to or reading from them. The safest way to remove them is to right click the Safely Remove Disk icon in the lower right corner of the screen (if it is not visible, click the "<" at the end of the icons. Then follow the steps in **Figure A-1**.

Optical Disks. An optical disk is one that is written to and read by light (Smith, 2009). Data are recorded on optical disks by using a laser to burn microscopic pits onto the surface. Another laser beam is shone on the disk to read them. The pits are detected by changes in the reflection pattern. When a reflection is detected, the bit is on; when there is no reflection, the bit is off. Together with flash drives, they have replaced diskettes for storage.

The three kinds of optical storage used in computers today are the compact disk (CD), the digital versatile disk (DVD) and the Blu-Ray Disc™. CD storage originated on the same disks that we use in audio disks. A CD can store about 650 to 700 megabytes of data. CDs can contain audio, video, or both on the same disk. CDs have been replaced in many cases by DVDs. The amount of data that a DVD can store varies from 4.7 to almost 10 GB depending on the disk. Most software sold today is on a CD or DVD; thus, drives that will access either are standard equipment on newer computers. Blu-Ray discs (BD) are an emerging medium currently used for file storage, high definition video, and PlayStation 3 video games. Blu-Ray gets its name from the violet colored laser used to read the data. BDs hold 25–50 GB of data. The BD players are backward compatible and can play CDs and DVDs (Blue-Ray Disc Association, 2008).

Box A-1 Maintaining a Hard Drive

As you continually use your hard drive, saving, deleting, saving again a file, the access to files on the hard drive slows down. This occurs because the filing system (FAT or NTFS) saves files in those sectors you see in Figure A-1, but often a file size exceeds the size of the sector (technically known as clusters). When that happens, the filing system looks for the next vacant sector on the disk and makes a note of where on the disk the next part of the file is located. This creates files that are fragmented, or files with parts stored randomly around the disk.

When we request that a file be retrieved, the filing index tells the read/write head on the disk drive where on the disk to find the file. When it has to keep moving around the disk to find all the parts of a file, or to save one, these processes slow down. To put the disk back into a condition in which all parts of all files are contiguous, a process known as defragging the disk should be done periodically. How often depends on the type of use as well as the size of the hard drive.

To make this task easy on Microsoft Windows® computers, a program called Disk Defragmenter exists that performs this task. This process can take an hour or several hours depending on both the size of your disk and how long it has been since you last used this accessory. To access this program in Windows® XP:

1. Close all programs that are running, including your screen saver.
2. Delete any unwanted programs or files.
3. Click the Start button.
4. Select All Programs.
5. Then select:
   a. Accessories > System Tools
   b. Disk Defragmenter
6. Select the disk to be defragged > Analyze
7. If the disk is ≥10% fragmented, Select the Defragment button.
8. A user interface will show you the progress. Leave the computer alone until the process is completed.

Some people feel that checking the disk for bad sectors should be performed before trying to defragment the disk. To do this:

1. Close all programs.
2. Click the Start button.
3. Select Computer (or My Computer).
4. Right click the disk you wish to check.
5. Click Properties.
6. Click the Tools tab.
7. Click Check Now under Error-checking.
8. You will be prompted to restart the computer to begin the error-checking function.

The Windows® Vista 7 operating systems automatically defragments the disk on a set schedule as well as looks for and repairs bad sectors. If you wish to do this manually:

1. Click the Windows logo in the lower left corner.
2. Click Computer in the right column.
3. Right click the disk you wish to check.
4. Select Properties.
5. Click the Tools tab and make your choice.

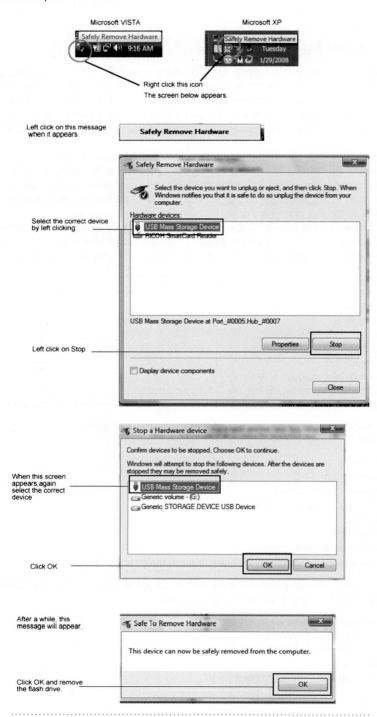

Figure A-1 Safely removing a flash drive.

Today's new computers have drives that are capable of not only reading and writing data from these disks. Whether you can write to an optical disk is dependent not only on the drive but also on several other things, including the type of disk you are using and the available software. Information about the type of disk, whether a CD-ROM (read only), a CD-RW (read/write), a DVD that is read only, or a DVD with read/write capabilities, and whether it supports a double layer will be available on the label of the container in which you purchase the disk. Software affects not only if the computer can write to a disk, but is also a component of the speed with which data is written to the disk. The amount of available space on the disk and the RAM in your computer also affect the speed that the drive writes data. If you will be burning video DVDs or BDs for patient education or other uses, it would be wise to investigate the many options available for making a video, including the aspect ratio and video format that are available in the help feature for the computer operating system.

Optical disks have several advantages, including size, and not being subject to corruption from magnetic fields or to "head" crashes. They are, however, not immune to damage from scratches or high temperatures. See Box A-2 for information on caring for optical disks.

Impermanence of Storage Media

From the preceding text, it is evident that the type of "permanent" storage available is still changing. Optical disks are not immune to obsolescence. A good rule of thumb is to update the storage media used every time you buy a new computer. The most versatile storage method today is probably a flash drive that attaches to what is called a **universal serial bus (USB)** port.

Permanently Destroying Data on Disks

Today many computers in healthcare agencies have data on them that would violate the Health Insurance Portability and Accountability Act (HIPAA) or other privacy acts if it were released. Although your PC is not protected by HIPAA, you probably have files with private information

Box A-2 Caring for Optical Disks

DO
1. Keep the disks clean.
   a. Clean with a clean cotton cloth by wiping from the center to the outer edge, not around the disk, which can cause scratches.
   b. Use isopropyl alcohol or methanol or CD/DVD/BD cleaning detergent for stubborn dirt.
2. Handle the disk by the center hole, or the edges. Some disks are two-sided, so be careful of both sides.
3. Put the disk back in a hard plastic case as soon as you eject it from the computer.
4. Store the disk:
   a. Upright like a library book.
   b. In moderate temperatures.
   c. Away from smoke or other air pollutants.
   d. Out of sunlight.
5. Label the plastic case containing the disk, not the disk.
6. Realize that the length of time before data is corrupted on an optical disk is directly proportional to the conditions under which it is stored and the quality of the disk.
7. Update the storage mechanism with every new computer.

DO NOT:
8. Attach an adhesive label to the disk. The adhesive in the label can corrupt data within a few months.
9. Write on or scratch either side of the disk with any object. Pens or pencils scratch the surface and solvent-based markers may dissolve the protective layer.
10. Expect data on an optical disk to last longer than 5 years.

Smith, J. (2009). *Computer basics: Storage optical disks*. Retrieved January 27, 2011, from http://www.jegsworks.com/Lessons/lesson6/lesson6–9.htm

such as your social security number and/or banking account numbers. All confidential information should be removed prior to discarding an old computer or the associated drives.

Reformatting a hard drive only erases the filing, or address of the files on the disk, but leaves the files intact. In Windows OS prior to NT and 2000, the file system was called File Allocation Table (FAT or FAT32). Windows NT, 2000 and later use New Technology File System (NTFS) to provide an improved method for securing files (VistaHunt.com, n.d.-a, n.d.-b). Unless the disk is wiped clean, old files can be retrieved by any number of products easily obtainable on the Web (Beal, 2009; PC World, 2010).

A more permanent form of disk cleansing is called disk wiping, or sometimes, a data dump (Beal, 2009). Disk-wiping applications use different algorithms (processes), but essentially they rewrite the entire disk with either a number or zero, and then the disk is reformatted. The more times the disk is rewritten and formatted, the more thorough the wiping process is. A government's standard (*DoD 5220.22-M*), which provides medium security, requires three repeats of a two-step process. Each time the process is performed, two passes are made; first the drive is overwritten with ones, and then with zeros. After the third time, a government-designated code of 246 is written on the drive, which is verified by a final pass using a read-verify pass. To find disk wiping software, search the Internet using the terms "disk wipe software."

Peripherals

A peripheral is any external device such as a keyboard, monitor, or mouse, which is connected to the computer. Because they are external in desktops, it is easy to see that these are peripherals. On laptops, however, the connection of keyboards and monitors is internal. In general, peripherals are the devices that allow inputting of data to a computer and outputting of information from a computer. Besides these obvious peripherals, there are many others such as printers (output) and scanners (input) that allow humans to use computers.

Digital Cameras

Digital cameras are finding a place in healthcare for purposes such as recording the healing progress of wounds. Text descriptions cannot compare with a picture in letting clinicians and patients see healing progress.

SCANNERS

Scanners take a picture of a document and then allow users to save this as a file. Unless there is character recognition software available, any text that is scanned will be in a picture format and uneditable. Additionally some healthcare agencies are inputting clinical records to electronic health records by scanning free text. Even when character recognition software is used to translate the words in the "picture" to text, the result needs to be checked for accuracy. Further, unless the form that is scanned is especially designed for scanning, this free text is unstructured and not easily used for reporting information from data.

Clinical Monitors

Clinical monitors can be part of a network and monitored at a central location. They can also be programmed to provide alarms, either at the central station or to individual pagers, when the monitor shows something beyond the norm. Clinical monitors whether attached to a network, or not, can allow patient data such as that produced by cardiology or fetal monitors to be directly input to a computer. The advantage of computerized clinical monitoring is that it allows one person to monitor many patients at once as well as provide notification of problems. It should never be allowed to reduce nurse–patient interaction.

Connecting Peripherals

A peripheral is connected to a computer through a port. Although today the USB port is the de facto standard for PCs, in the past there were other types of ports such as serial and parallel. Computers manufactured in recent years do not have serial or parallel ports.

USB PORT

A USB port or universal serial bus is a standard that was originally created to connect phones to PCs in 1996 (Anton, 2009; Hoy, 2010). It is the standard port for connecting peripherals to PCs, replacing older serial and parallel connectors. These ports are a thin slot, about half inch by one fourth of an inch, which are found on the sides of laptops and on the front of newer desktops or towers. The port is designed with a solid piece in one part so that USB device can only be inserted one way (see Figure A-2).

The original, USB 1.0, port was capable of transmitting data at only 12 megabits (Remember, it takes 8 bits to form a byte, which is required to transfer one letter) per second, which made it useful for only mice and keyboards. This easy connection method, however, created a revolution that resulted in devices such as flash drives, external hard drives, and webcams, which needed faster transmission speeds. Faster connection speeds were met in 2000 with the USB 2.0 technology, which transmits information at 480 megabits per second. USB 3.0 technology was released in 2010. USB 3.0 transmits information at 5 gigabits per second, which is ten times faster than USB 2.0 and faster than the new FireWire 3200.

Firewire

FireWire originated in the mid-1980s as a high-speed data transfer method for Macintosh internal hard drives (Nathanael & Penrod, 2006). Apple presented this technology to the Institute of Electrical and Electronics Engineers (IEEE), who in December 1995, released IEEE 1394, which is an official FireWire standard. It was often referred to as FireWire 400 and had transfer speeds of 100 to 400 megabits per second. In April 2002, the IEEE released a new standard for FireWire 800, which can transfer data at 786 megabits per second.

FireWire 3200, released in 2010, can transfer data at 3.2 gigabits per second (Wikipedia Contributors, 2010d) (see Figure A-3).

Although its speed is faster than USB 2.0 ports, it is impractical for low-bandwidth devices. This fact, together with the knowledge that only Macs include FireWire ports by default, has kept it out of the mainstream. Because of its superior ability to transfer uncompressed video from digital camcorders, it is found on many digital camcorders. Most digital cameras, however, still use USB to transfer images because USB ports are today standard equipment on computers.

Infrared Port

An infrared (IR) port is a connection on a computer that uses IR signals to wirelessly transmit information between devices such as a PDA and a computer. It has a range of about 5 to 10 feet. Most handheld devices have the capability to communicate via IR ports that allow the device to directly interface with another device to exchange data.

Infection Control

Computers, particularly keyboards, have become commonplace in healthcare settings and are easily contaminated with potentially pathogenic microorganisms (Rutala, White, Gergen, & Weber, 2006). Many studies have demonstrated the presence of these organisms, not only in healthcare agencies but also on a nurse's home computer (Anderson & Palombo, 2009; Fukada, Iwakiri, & Ozaki, 2008;

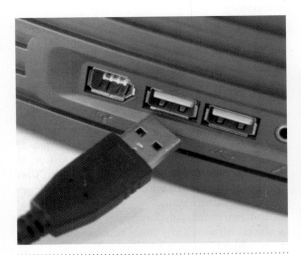

Figure A-2 USB Port.

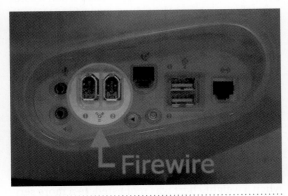

Figure A-3 Firewire.

Hospital computer keyboards and keyboard covers harbor potentially harmful bacteria, 2005; Po, Burke, Sulis, & Carling, 2009). These studies also demonstrated that these organisms can be spread to patients. Although hand washing before touching a keyboard or any other computer part can help, all computer peripherals in a room should be routinely cleaned with a solution recommended by infection control personnel. If possible, engineering the physical environment to prevent contamination should also be done.

Computerese

Many computer-related terms are used in discussion, instruction, and advertising. Although they are not strictly hardware terms, they can often be confusing. If one watches a computer when it has just been turned on, one will see different types of information flashing across the screen. This information is produced by what is called the "booting" process. Booting refers to all the self-tests that a computer performs and the process of retrieving, either from the BIOS or a disk, the instructions necessary to allow the user to start using the computer.

The term "**reboot**" means to restart the computer. A **warm boot** is restarting the computer without turning it off, a selection that is offered when one elects to start turning off the computer. A **cold boot** is starting the computer when the power is completely off. Avoid cold boots if you can, because the jolt of electricity received each time the computer is turned on may shorten its life span. Warm boots are often used when a computer freezes or crashes. It erases information in RAM, which often eliminates memory conflicts that may have caused the problem. These conflicts can be caused by different programs trying to store data in the same location. If a warm boot fails to notify the programs that it is time to stop fighting for the same space and give control back to the user, the machine must be turned off for a cold boot.

A **bug** is a defect in either the program or hardware that causes a malfunction. It may be as simple as presenting the user with a blood pressure chart when a weight chart was requested, to a more serious defect that causes the entire system to crash.

Compatibility refers to whether programs designed for one chip will work with an older or newer chip, or whether files created with one version of a program will work with another version of the same program. Most computer chips and software are backward compatible, that is, they will work with older versions of a program or files created with an older version of a program. Some are not, however, forward compatible, or the situation in which an older program does not recognize files created by a newer version of the same program. This is particularly true of spreadsheets, databases, and presentation programs.

A **driver** is a software program that allows data to be transmitted between the computer and a device that is connected to the computer. Drivers are generally specific to the brand and model of the device. They may come with a new peripheral, or can often be downloaded from the vendor's Website.

Although the term **hacker** originally meant a person who enjoyed learning about computer systems and was often considered an expert on the subject, mass media have turned it into a term to refer to individuals who gain unauthorized access to computer systems for the purpose of stealing and corrupting data. The original term for such a person was cracker. Today, differentiations may be made by using the term **white hat hacker** for a person who uses his or her computer knowledge to benefit others. **Black hat hacker** is the term used for those who use their computer skills maliciously.

When used with a computer, the terms "logical" and "physical" refer to where data are located in the computer. The **physical** structure is the actual location, whereas a logical structure is how users see the data. For example, when a user requests information about laboratory tests, he or she may see the indications for the test, the normal values, the cost of a test, and the patient's test results. Although this information may be presented as one screen, which is a **logical** structure, different pieces will have been retrieved from different files in different locations, which is the physical structure of the information.

Another potentially confusing computer term is object. Although the more common use of the term "**object**" is for a physical entity, or at least a picture on the screen, to a computer, an object is anything the computer can manipulate. That is, an object can be a letter, word, sentence, paragraph, piece of a document, or an entire document. Objects can be nested, that is, a word is an object nested within a sentence object. A paragraph is an object that is contained in a document. When an object is selected, clicking the right mouse button presents a menu of properties of that object that can be changed.

Summary

Understanding how computers function forms the background for a beginning understanding of informatics. Computers are devices, which, although we may anthromorphize them, are still inanimate objects. Computers do not think; they need explicit instructions and are incapable of interpreting gray areas. This is not to say that gifted programmers cannot make one think a computer is behaving in a seemingly human manner.

Like informatics, computers have many different types and parts. When all these parts function together along with human interventions, the results benefit healthcare. Regardless of size, all computers possess some given parts, a CPU, memory, storage devices, and ways to both enter and retrieve data. How many and how much of each of these parts a computer needs depends on the function the computer is intended to serve and often the depth of the owner's pocketbook. Understanding the function of each of these parts allows nurses to creatively and effectively use a computer both professionally and personally.

Computers, however, are not without their hazards in healthcare. Their parts, particularly mice and keyboards, are capable of harboring pathogenic microorganisms, which have been known to create infections in patients. Data that they can contain could create harm if it became known; hence, computers that will need to be discarded must have their internal storage devices thoroughly wiped before being released.

REFERENCES

Anderson, G., & Palombo, E. A. (2009). Microbial contamination of computer keyboards in a university setting. *American Journal of Infection Control, 37*(6), 507–509.

Anton, B. (2009, June 26). *A history of the USB standard.* Retrieved March 23, 2010, from http://ezinearticles.com/?A-History-of-the-USB-Standard&id=2532259

Beal, V. (2009). *How to completely erase a hard disk drive.* Retrieved March 17, 2010, from http://www.webopedia.com/DidYouKnow/Computer_Science/2007/completely_erase_harddrive.asp

Bloom, A. J. (1985). An anxiety management approach to computer phobia. *Training and Development Journal, 19*(1), 90–94.

Blue-Ray Disc Association. (2008). *History of Blu-Ray.* Retrieved February 13, 2010, from http://www.bluraydisc.com/

Brain, M. (2006, November 14). *How lithion-ion batteries work.* Retrieved March 23, 2010, from http://electronics.howstuffworks.com/lithium-ion-battery.htm

Buchmann, I. (2005, November). *The secrets of battery runtime (BU31).* Retrieved March 23, 2010, from http://www.batteryuniversity.com/parttwo-31.htm

Buchmann, I. (2006a, September). *How to prolong lithium-based batteries (BU34).* Retrieved March 23, 2010, from http://batteryuniversity.com/parttwo-34.htm

Buchmann, I. (2006b, November). *What's the best battery?* Retrieved March 23, 2010, from http://www.batteryuniversity.com/partone-3.htm

Computer History Museum. (2011). *Mastering the game: A history of computer chess.* Retrieved January 27, 2011, from http://www.computerhistory.org/chess/index.php

Fukada, T., Iwakiri, H., & Ozaki, M. (2008). Anaesthetists' role in computer keyboard contamination in an operating room. *The Journal Of Hospital Infection, 70*(2), 148–153.

Hospital computer keyboards and keyboard covers harbor potentially harmful bacteria. (2005). *Hospitals & Health Networks, 79*(5), 81–82.

Hoy, M. (2010, February 8). *USB 3.0 vs. USB 2.0 vs. FireWire: What's the big difference?* Retrieved March 23, 2010, from http://www.associatedcontent.com/article/2666601/usb_30_vs_usb_20_vs_firewire_whats.html

Lyons, D. (2009, January 29). Hurry up and type. *Newsweek, 153*(26), 27. Retrieved from http://www.newsweek.com/id/202572

Nathanael, & Penrod, L. (2006). *Firewire vs. USB: A comparison.* Retrieved August 30, 2011, 2011, from http://www.directron.com/firewirevsusb.html

PC World. (2010, January 10). *How to completely erase a hard drive.* Retrieved March 23, 2010, from http://www.pcworld.com/article/157126/how_to_completely_erase_a_hard_drive.html

Perry, W. E. (1982). *Survival guide to computer systems.* Boston: CBI Publishing Company.

Po, J. L., Burke, R., Sulis, C., & Carling, P. C. (2009). Dangerous cows: an analysis of disinfection cleaning of computer keyboards on wheels. *American Journal of Infection Control, 37*(9), 778–780.

Prensky, M. (2001). Digital natives, digital immigrants: Do they really think differently? *On the Horizon, 9*(6), 15–24. Retrieved from http://www.marcprensky.com/writing/Prensky%20-%20Digital%20Natives,%20Digital%20Immigrants%20-%20Part2.pdf

Roberts, B. (2009, February 21). *Computer tutorial how binary code works.* Retrieved January 27, 2011, from http://www.youtube.com/watch?v=ETsfylK7kzM

Rutala, W. A., White, M. S., Gergen, M. F., & Weber, D. J. (2006). Bacterial contamination of keyboards: efficacy and functional impact of disinfectants. *Infection Control and Hospital Epidemiology*, 27(4), 372–377. Retrieved from http://www.unc.edu/depts/spice/dis/ICHE-Apr2006-p372.pdf

Schulz, G. (2007, May 8). *What's the difference between flash memory and conventional RAM*? Retrieved March 23, 2010, from http://searchstorage.techtarget.com/generic/0,295582,sid5_gci1254237,00.html

Smith, J. (2009). *Computer basics: Storage optical disks*. Retrieved January 27, 2011, from http://www.jegsworks.com/Lessons/lesson6/lesson6-9.htm

VistaHunt.com. (n.d.-a). *NTFS*. Retrieved March 23, 2010, from http://www.vistahunt.com/file-systems-in-windows-vista.html

Vistahunt.com. (n.d.-b). *What's special in file systems in Windows Vista*. Retrieved March 23, 2010, from http://www.vistahunt.com/file-systems-in-windows-vista.html

Wikipedia Contributors. (2010a, March 15). *Battery (electricity)*. Retrieved March 21, 2010, from http://en.wikipedia.org/w/index.php?title=Battery_%28electricity%29&oldid=350043603

Wikipedia Contributors. (2010b). *Computer data storage*. Retrieved March 23, 2010, from http://en.wikipedia.org/wiki/Computer_data_storage

Wikipedia Contributors. (2010c, March 23). *Flash memory*. Retrieved March 23, 2010, from http://en.wikipedia.org/wiki/Flash_memory

Wikipedia Contributors. (2010d, March 22). *IEEE 1394 interface – Wikipedia, the free encyclopedia*. Retrieved March 23, 2010, from http://en.wikipedia.org/wiki/Firewire

Index

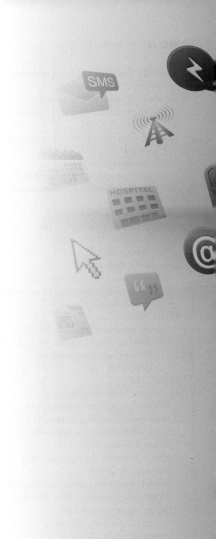